HISTORY TAKING AND PHYSICAL EXAMINATION
Essentials and Clinical Correlates

History Taking and Physical Examination

Essentials and Clinical Correlates

Norton J. Greenberger, MD
Peter T. Bohan Professor, Chairman
Department of Medicine
University of Kansas School of Medicine
Kansas City, Kansas

Daniel R. Hinthorn, MD
Professor of Medicine
Division of Infectious Diseases
University of Kansas School of Medicine
Kansas City, Kansas

With 369 illustrations, 55 in full color

Mosby Year Book

St. Louis   Baltimore   Boston   Chicago   London   Philadelphia   Sydney   Toronto

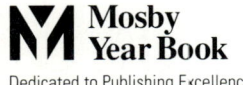
Mosby Year Book
Dedicated to Publishing Excellence

Sponsoring Editor: Robert Farrell
Developmental Editor: Emma Underdown
Production Manager: Gayle May Morris
Production Editor: Donna L. Walls
Design: David Zielinski
Illustrations: Holly R. Fischer and Valorie Loomis

Copyright © 1993 by Mosby–Year Book, Inc.
A Mosby imprint of Mosby–Year Book, Inc.

All rights reserved. No part of this publication may be reproduced, stored in a retrieval system, or transmitted, in any form or by any means, electronic, mechanical, photocopying, recording, or otherwise, without prior written permission from the publisher.

Permission to photocopy or reproduce solely for internal or personal use is permitted for libraries or other users registered with the Copyright Clearance Center, provided that the base fee of $4.00 per chapter plus $.10 per page is paid directly to the Copyright Clearance Center, 27 Congress Street, Salem, MA 01970. This consent does not extend to other kinds of copying, such as copying for general distribution, or advertising or promotional purposes, for creating new collected works, or for resale.

Printed in the United States of America

Mosby–Year Book, Inc. Company
11830 Westline Industrial Drive
St. Louis, Missouri 63146-3318

Library of Congress Cataloging-in-Publication Data
Greenberger, Norton J.
    History taking and physical examination: essentials and clinical correlates / Norton J. Greenberger, Daniel R. Hinthorn.
       p.   cm.
    Includes index.
    ISBN 0-8016-6646-5
    1. Medical history taking. 2. Physical diagnosis. I. Hinthorn, Daniel R. II. Title.
    [DNLM: 1. Diagnosis. 2. Medical History Taking—methods.
    3. Physical Examination—methods. WB 205 G798h]
    RC65.G74 1992
    616.07'5—dc20
DNLM/DLC
for Library of Congress   92-12911
                                                                                       CIP

93 94 95 96 97 GW/UN/VH 9 8 7 6 5 4 3 2 1

Acknowledgements

Several individuals have contributed greatly to this book. First, we thank our secretaries, Shirley Sears, Ruth Stricklen, Margaret McNamara, and Bea Coleton, for their fine efforts in the preparation of the manuscript. Second, we thank all the reviewers who aided in the development of this textbook, as peer review is an essential element in this process. In particular, Sir John Walton reviewed the chapter on the neurologic examination, Dr. Winston Mebust the chapter on the male genitalia, Dr. Charley Norris the sections on the ear, nose, and throat, Dr. Theodore Lawwill the section on the eye, Dr. William Ruth the chapter on the respiratory system, and Dr. Marvin Dunn the chapter on the heart. A special recognition is needed for Dr. Allen Erenberg, who contributed to the pediatric examination chapter.

Third, we thank the physicians who provided photographs, roentgenograms, and imaging studies. This group includes Doctors Theodore Lawwill, Linda Harrison, Solomon Batnitzky, James Kalivas, Loren H. Amundsen, and William S. Royster. Fourth, our artists Holly Fischer and Valorie Loomis provided outstanding drawings, and our photographer Stephan Spector took numerous photos that have clearly complemented the text. Fifth, Emma Underdown of Mosby–Year Book has been particularly helpful in the final preparation of the manuscript.

Finally, we thank our wives, Joan Greenberger and Aletha Hinthorn, who not only provided continuous emotional support, but who also proofread much of the manuscript.

Preface

During the past 2 to 3 decades, widespread and truly impressive advances in diagnostic technology have enabled physicians, residents, and medical students to establish diagnoses with accuracy and safety undreamt of 30 years ago. This technology is available, convenient, efficient, accurate, and frequently reassuring to both patients and doctors. However, it is also being used inappropriately and is costly, contributing in a very real way to the rapidly escalating cost of health care. Most importantly, this reliance on technology has contributed to the relative lack of history-taking and physical-examination skills of medical students and residents as compared with the skills of their counterparts of 20 to 30 years ago.

Another pertinent factor is that the education of medical students with regard to physical diagnosis has changed significantly. Physical diagnosis courses are often disjointed and inserted piecemeal into a curriculum overcrowded with conventional courses. A sense of how to take information from the history and examination and from that construct a working diagnosis often remains underdeveloped. It is this decision-making process that is key to the practice of sound patient care.

A need exists for the physicians of the 1990s and beyond to fully develop their history-taking and physical-diagnosis skills, for several reasons:

- Numerous factors, including technology, have eroded the traditional doctor-patient relationships.
- Too much emphasis on technology leads to incompletely developed basic skills.
- Technology is fallible, and overreliance on such tools is potentially harmful.
- The vast majority of patients are seen in an ambulatory setting in which technology is not available. Such patients often present with undifferentiated problems for which a well-done history and physical examination will point to the current diagnosis or diagnoses.
- A carefully performed history and physical examination will establish the correct diagnosis in the vast majority of patients encountered.
- History taking and physical examination embody both the art and science of medicine, of taking raw information and turning that into a workable plan of medical care.

We have written this textbook to provide students with a rational, effective, practical, and thorough approach to history taking and physical examination. We have emphasized the considerable information that can be gained, the inferences that can be drawn, and the next steps to be considered in differential diagnosis. After the introductory chapter, each chapter provides detailed information about the techniques of history taking and physical examination for each organ system. The final chapter discusses the special consideration of the pediatric examination. Special considerations of the geriatric patient are discussed in each chapter as appropriate.

Our emphasis is on the common entities a medical student can expect to see. The large number of tables, figures, and line diagrams are designed to enhance the student's understanding of these key concepts. Furthermore, case vignettes and tables illustrate how the history and physical examination can be used as a springboard to choosing additional definitive diagnostic tests when these are indicated. Each chapter includes sample questions to ask of patients, along with an explanation of what the question is trying to elicit. A summary checklist at the end of each chapter reminds the student of the key concepts covered.

Our approach underscores the importance of the history and physical examination and correlates information from both with the next logical steps. As such, the book will be useful not only to second-year students beginning their study of physical diagnosis, but also to junior and senior students as well as resident physicians. We intend this book to help physicians of the 1990s and beyond to most effectively use the patient/physician encounter to render safe, appropriate patient care. With this goal in mind, we invite the reader to approach with enthusiasm the building block of clinical medicine: the history and physical examination.

Norton J. Greenberger
Daniel R. Hinthorn

Contents

1. The Medical Interview and Physical Examination, 1
2. The Head and Neck, 38
3. The Respiratory System, 70
4. The Heart, 125
5. The Abdomen, 199
6. Male Genitalia, 262
7. Female Genitalia, 280
8. The Breast, 316
9. The Musculoskeletal System, 333
10. The Neurologic Examination, 382
11. The Psychiatric Evaluation, 426
12. The Skin, 442
13. The Pediatric Patient, 480

A through E. Appendices, 496

HISTORY TAKING AND PHYSICAL EXAMINATION
Essentials and Clinical Correlates

CHAPTER ONE

The Medical Interview and Physical Examination

CHAPTER OUTLINE

Techniques for the Medical Interview
Prepare yourself to meet the patient
Review identifying data
Prepare for the interview
Initiate the interview
Establish rapport and develop a good bedside manner
Techniques of questioning
Ending the interview and the examination

Components of the Medical Interview
Chief complaint
History of present illness
Past medical history
Family history
Social history
Review of systems

The Medical Interview in Special Situations
Pediatrics
Pregnancy
Geriatrics
Patients who do not speak your language
Blind patients and those unable to hear or speak
Psychiatric patients
Addicted patients
Patients with organic brain syndrome
Patients with differences in sexual orientation
Hostile patients

Diagnostic Reasoning

Making the Physical Examination an Active Process

Techniques for Performing the Physical Examination

Summary

Patients seek advice of physicians to help solve problems of illness or to cope with issues of daily living. At the patient's bedside, the clinician brings together the art and the basic sciences of medicine. He* obtains the medical history—the story of the patient's symptoms, past illnesses, and family history—and performs the physical examination. The medical history does more than obtain the scientific data necessary for good medical care; it also begins to build a bond of trust between clinician and patient. Trust is important later when the patient is asked to undergo expensive or painful tests or to take medications faithfully. Finally, the medical history allows observation of the patient's behavior and responses. Together the history and physical examination are useful in deducing probable diagnoses of the patient's disease.

As you read further, you will learn key symptoms patients bring to their clinicians. A few key complaints are commonly associated with dysfunction of each system. By asking about onset of complaints, the tempo of progression of symptoms, and other related health concerns, you will be able to develop a tentative diagnosis or differential diagnosis. This will allow you to thoughtfully perform the physical examination and order appropriate tests.

Techniques for the Medical Interview

Most people's initial contact with the health care system occurs as the patient first meets the clinician and gives the account of the clinical illness. From the physician's standpoint, the medical history is the single most important component in that contact. Diagnoses are made more often from the history during the medical interview than from the physical examination or laboratory studies. From the patient's standpoint, the ability to relate to and trust the physician are most important. To satisfy the objectives of each, the physician must demonstrate his concern for the patient in several ways while seeking the necessary information.

Prepare Yourself to Meet the Patient

Attention to appropriate dress and grooming before the interview will create a favorable first impression. This shows appropriate respect for the patient and for our role as physician. Not only do patients expect a physician to look neat and smell clean, but they expect students to wear clothing appropriate for physicians in their geographic area. In some geographic areas, and in certain clinical areas within a geographic area, the attire the physician selects may be less formal.

Usually physicians are not expected to dress as casually as does the patient. For men, neckties, dress shirts, and white jackets are usual. For women, dress shoes, hose, and business-style clothing are appropriate. Both sexes should avoid wearing jogging shoes except under special circumstances, such as when on-call. Males should keep beards and mustaches groomed so that these do not brush across the patient's face during the eye examination. Females should have controlled hair so that it does not get in the patient's face.

When dealing with children, wearing white coats may frighten them needlessly.

---

* Throughout the text both patients and physicians will usually be referred to as "he" rather than the more cumbersome (s)he or he/she. We have no sexist intent in continuing to use traditional language.

> ### Definition of Terms
>
> *Symptoms* are the experiences that suggest disease or physical dysfunction described in the history by the patient or occasionally by a family member. Pain, itch, or cough are examples of symptoms.
>
> *Signs* are found on examination, when abnormal structure or function suggests the presence of disease. A heart murmur is an example of a sign. Certain symptoms may be signs; an example might be skin rash of which the patient may complain (symptom), or may be found on examination (sign) (see also Appendix B).
>
> *Diagnosis* is the term used to name the cause of the patient's signs and symptoms. For example, the symptom "itch" may be explained by the diagnosis "allergy." By making a specific diagnosis, one distinguishes the patient's illness from illnesses with similar manifestations. The clinician is then able to apply knowledge to this patient that has been learned from other patients with similar conditions.
>
> The terms disease and syndrome have similar meanings, and each is a diagnostic term. *Disease* refers to groups of signs and symptoms indicating abnormal organ structure or function; for example, heart disease or lung disease. *Syndrome* refers to signs and symptoms that occur together involving multiple organs. The signs and symptoms may affect diverse sites. For example, toxic shock syndrome is characterized by diarrhea, reduced blood pressure, skin rash, red conjunctivae and oral mucosa, mental confusion, and abnormal liver and kidney function. Later the skin peels from the fingertips. Toxic shock is called a syndrome, not a disease, even though it is caused by a toxin produced by *Staphylococcus*.
>
> *Differential diagnosis* refers to the different possible diagnoses, the diseases and syndromes that might reasonably explain some or all of the patient's signs, symptoms, abnormal laboratory results and other studies.

Review Identifying Data

The review of identifying information, letters from referring physicians, and data from previous evaluations begins the process for interns, residents, and staff physicians, but this information is not usually available to students beginning physical diagnosis. Patients referred by local physicians to a teaching hospital often have a letter of referral explaining the problem needing evaluation. Patients expect their physician to have reviewed these documents.

Medical students often do not have access to some or all of the patient's previous medical record at the initial contact with a patient. If the patient asks about this or appears reluctant to talk about the history, you may explain to the patient the procedure you are following as a student in physical diagnosis:

- *I am a second-year medical student learning to take medical histories. Your consenting to talk to me will not affect your medical care because I am just learning what questions to ask. But each physician begins like this in training. If it would be alright, I'd like to go ahead and ask you some questions about your illness and health.*

- As a clinical clerk in the third year, the response may be a little different because you will be a member of the patient care team.
- *I would really like to hear about your illness from you directly, if you don't mind. It will allow us to get to know one another, and you can fill me in on the details of how you really felt and how this illness has influenced your life. Some of those sorts of things may not be available in the copies of charts we receive.*
- *If it wouldn't be too hard on you to talk with me before I review these, I'd appreciate it. I like to be able to make my own mind up about the diagnosis before someone else tells me what they think. Sometimes we can find new, important clues that may be helpful.*

Prepare for the Interview

Time constraints are recurring problems for the clinician and patients. Punctuality has been defined as showing value for another person's time. Should you be late in initiating the patient's scheduled interview, give recognition of the delay to reduce the patient's animosity. That word of apology demonstrates your value for the patient and his time.

Before initiating the interview, see that the patient appears comfortable and that the lighting is adequate. Beware of sitting between the patient and the light from a window. This gives a silhouette effect and makes it difficult for the patient

---

Prepare for the Interview

Consider the Patient's Time

Be punctual; apologize if late
Avoid interruptions if possible

Arrange for Privacy

Verbal, visual
Psychologic, actual

Consider Physical Comfort

Temperature, drafts
Hang coats patient carried in

Avoid

Interviewing with desks or furniture between you and patient
Sitting too close or too far from patient (about 3 to 6 feet is best)
Bright lights or a window behind your back, which might blind patient
Eating, drinking, or smoking during interview

Try to

Sit during interview
Choose positions so that your eye level is about that of the patient
Take enough time with patient so you do not appear rushed
Exhibit appropriate bedside manner

to see facial expressions. When possible, before starting the interview take care of matters that might interrupt and interfere with communication by closing doors or turning off the television.

Attention to modifying the environment can help the patient relax and give a complete history. If possible, the patient should be taken to a private room for the medical history and the physical examination. When in a semiprivate hospital room, the other patient and visitors or family members of either patient may embarrass him, causing him to omit sensitive items.

As you take the history in a two-patient room, decide whether the question you ask requires psychologic privacy or actual privacy. Psychologic feelings of privacy can be attained by drawing the curtain between beds. This action provides actual privacy for the physical examination and psychologic privacy for the history. Even though many patients feel freer to talk when the curtain is drawn, you may prevent future unpleasantness between roommates by using care in your questioning.

If the patient's history is overheard, the roommate may worry. For example, if a patient says he has been exposed to tuberculosis and later has a cough, his roommate may worry about contracting tuberculosis. Some patients worry about catching cancer, leukemia, or acquired immunodeficiency syndrome (AIDS). Actual privacy is desirable when asking potentially embarrassing questions (e.g., about human immmunodeficiency virus [HIV] antibody status, sexual history, addiction to drugs or alcohol). Pursue these later when either patient is taken from the room.

The patient's family members may inhibit complete disclosure of illnesses or symptoms. A spouse, parent, or adult child may wish to stay in the patient's room during the history and physical examination. At times it may be best to allow the family member to stay for a portion of the interview. Later during the interview or physical examination, ask the relative to leave for a few moments. This will allow important elements of history to be filled in with the patient alone. Conversely, family members can often add important information. They may feel freer to give additional history outside the room, away from the patient.

Initiate the Interview

The initial contact begins when the patient is greeted. Repeating the patient's name, the physician verifies both the name and pronunciation. If the name is unusual, ask the patient to spell and pronounce his name. Unfortunately, beginning clinicians often fail to recognize the importance of remembering patient's names. Often a medical student may recount the entire medical history,

Initiate the Interview	
Greet the patient by name (first and last)	Put patient at ease
Introduce yourself	State purpose of interview
Shake hands	Obtain consent to proceed

physical examination, and laboratory studies, yet be unable to recall the patient's name. Memory aids may assist in name recall.

Unless the patient is a child or is much younger than the physician, the patient should not be called by the first name. Women are sensitive to male physicians demeaning them in this way. A general rule is that an adult patient may be called by his first name if he expects to call you by your first name.

Along with greeting the patient by name, shake hands with the patient, whether male or female. This initial touch helps to set the patient at ease. Inform the patient of your position as interviewer by using a statement such as:

- *Hello, Mr. Jones, I am Anne Brown, a sophomore medical student learning to take medical histories and perform physical exams. I believe Dr. _____ has spoken to you about my seeing you this afternoon? I would like to ask you some questions regarding your medical history and do a physical examination.*
- Some patients decline to be interviewed or examined. It is not the patient's duty to allow himself to be examined by a student. To be brought into such personal confidence is a privilege our society bestows on few besides clinicians. If the patient declines to be interviewed, politely inquire why.
- *Would you please tell me why you don't want to continue with your medical history?*

Then exit the room and contact your supervisor.

Several things should be avoided in initial contact. First, avoid shifty eyes. With a pleasant facial expression, look directly at the patient without staring. When meeting the patient for the first time, do so while the patient is still dressed. Finally, avoid calling the patient auntie, mother, dearie, dad, or grandma; doing thus quickly arouses irritation.

Establish Rapport and Develop a Good Bedside Manner

After the introduction, make a conscious effort to be certain the patient feels comfortable talking with you. Patients feel at ease when they sense the physician accepts them unconditionally. It is important for each clinician to have his own moral codes, but the medical interviewer does not show disapproval for differing moral codes of patients concerning such areas as drug addiction, promiscuity, homosexuality, or obesity. Showing acceptance of the patient as a person does not indicate approval of the patient's life choices. Only after dealing compassionately with the patient and demonstrating that he is valued as a fellow human being can the examiner expect the patient to consider medical, ethical, or social recommendations that involve sensitive areas of his life.

Clinicians often use the word "rapport" when referring to relationships with patients. This is a harmonious relationship in which patient and clinician are cooperating on a friendly basis, often with a special affinity felt by each. Rapport can often be initiated by taking a bit of time with the patient before starting the medical questioning. During this time questions may be asked about the patient's city or place of residence. Finding a person known to each, or a common topic of interest, adds to rapport. Actually the clinician is showing interest in the patient as a person, not just in his illness. On the other hand, if the patient is in pain or is pressed for time, making small talk implies the patient's problems are not taken seriously. The patient's behavior and symptoms are good clues as to the approach the physician should take.

Patients expect physicians to have a "good bedside manner." From the

> **Cultivating the Style Important in the Good Bedside Manner**
>
> I. Nonverbal style in the good bedside manner
>   A. Use personal grooming usually identified by patients as typical for clinicians.
>   B. Sit (standing implies you are pressed for time) near patient (but not too close; i.e., not within his personal comfort zone, nor so far away that he feels you think he has a communicable illness). Avoid having a desk between you and the patient.
>   C. Look directly into the patient's eyes, but look away (at your note pad) periodically so as not to appear to be staring.
>   D. Maintain a friendly, helpful facial expression. Avoid a show of anger, disgust, or dislike.
>   E. Respect the patient. Avoid showing your disapproval for moral codes different from your own (e.g., homosexuality, alcoholism, obesity, or drug abuse). These can be dealt with objectively (not emotionally) later if needed because of the patient's problems.
> II. Verbal choices in good bedside manner
>   A. Speak directly to patient, tell him your name and what you wish to do.
>   B. Verify the name of the patient. Pronounce and learn his name. Use it in your conversation with the patient.
>   C. Put the patient at ease by being sure he is comfortable.
>   D. Show empathy for the patient, his problems, and how they affect his life. By empathy, we mean consider yourself to be a participant with the patient in trying to solve his problems. Show you care and will help him seek answers.
>   E. Communicate in a tone of voice, speed of words, and choice of words that are similar to those of the patient. You want the patient to sense your warmth towards him, that you are not merely following your own agenda or your list of questions.
>   F. Show concern for the patient's emotions, don't overlook them. If the patient cries, shows anger, or is silent, respond with a statement about it and a question to let the patient explain the reason.

patient's standpoint, this means that the physician shows appropriate concern, demonstrates respect, and listens and responds to the patient. What the patient desires is an empathetic clinician who understands his emotions and concerns. Such a clinician shows respect for the patient, for his thoughts and feelings. He cares about the patient and demonstrates that concern. When a physician appears or even feels impatient, bored, or uncaring, the likely results are an inability to obtain important information and causing the patient to look for another physician.

The clinician who wins the confidence and friendship of his patient will accomplish much more than the clinician who is confrontational, putting the patient on the defensive.

A cheerful attitude with an optimistic outlook gives the patient confidence and security. However, be realistic. Avoid prematurely acting like everything will be all right, or having a cheerful attitude when the patient or a family member is suffering or dying.

> **Lack of Certain Qualities may Jeopardize a Good Bedside Manner**
>
> Lack of knowledge of medical sciences without a willingness to seek help (read about it, consult articles, obtain consultation with peers).
> Bungling incompetence in history, examination, or technical procedures (such as blood drawing).
> Lack of real concern about patient (patients can often see through to true feelings).
> Lack of self-control (verbally lashing out).
> Lack of common courtesy or politeness (mistreating associated health-care workers, nurses).
> Failing to exhibit reasonably good manners personally.

Not everyone has a "good bedside manner" naturally, but these skills improve with effort. Both verbal and nonverbal skills are involved. Physicians show empathy (capacity to participate in another's suffering) nonverbally by a caring attitude and verbally by using language attuned to the patient's feelings. Use genuine warmth in questioning—do not rush through the questions on the database. Three techniques can be learned to show empathy, respect and concern: (1) choice of words, (2) tone of voice, and (3) body language.

The beginning clinical student will wish to avoid the following errors, which fail to show empathy. A patient says a disaster has occurred in his family. The student without an empathetic bedside manner might reply in a conversational tone, "It must have been terrible." The right words, but the wrong tone, have been used, and the student failed to show empathy. Also, beware of reassuring too soon with statements such as, "Don't cry, it'll be alright," unless you are certain you are correct. That response is telling the patient, "I don't want to see you get emotional about it. That makes me uncomfortable."

An example of a response that shows empathy might occur when a patient begins to cry. The physician with the "good bedside manner" stops questioning and gently tries to understand factors involved in this emotional upheaval. He responds, "I can see this really bothers you a lot, doesn't it?" He allows the patient to open up and say more.

The nonverbal empathetic attitude may be shown by sitting near the patient, neither too distant nor too close inside his personal zone of comfort. Look at the patient, make eye contact, but do not stare at him. Take as few notes as is compatible with being able to recall significant details.

On the other hand, sitting across a writing desk from the patient tends to place a barrier both physically and emotionally. When the clinician is not looking at the patient's facial expressions, not listening to his choice of words, and not following up on historical clues, significant components of the history may be lost. Certainly such a physician is not cultivating a good bedside manner.

Techniques of Questioning
BEGIN THE INTERVIEW

Begin the interview by allowing the patient to tell the story in his own way. Open-ended questions are used to facilitate the flow of the history. Specific questions are used later to clarify specific details. This approach allows the patient

Techniques of Questioning
Listen to what patient says and respond appropriately. Ask open-ended questions initially. Clarify potential leads. Target specific responses for probing questions. Be aware of jargon and their meanings. Ask for permission to discuss potentially embarrassing topics.

time to respond and shows interest. Failure to take time to allow the patient to express his problem in his own way can give the feeling of disinterest and may result in a poorly formulated history.

The clinician seeks the answer to the question, "What are the complaints that prompted the patient to seek medical advice?" Examples of short, open-ended questions to begin the history would be the following:

- *What complaints have brought you to the clinic today? What sort of problems have you been experiencing?* These questions elicit problems of concern to the patient and usually elicit the chief complaint(s). Next the appropriate response would be, *Would you tell me more about it?*
- After allowing the patient to tell his story, clarify the time sequence of the illness. The specific problem that caused him to seek medical attention at this particular time may be unclear without asking questions.

KEEP THE INTERVIEW FLOWING

Use questions to clarify potential leads, give clues to unexplored problems, and resolve apparent inconsistencies. The goal is to understand the patient better, to develop a differential diagnosis, and finally to single out a likely diagnosis that would explain the patient's problems. After the patient has finished the spontaneous history, direct questions are often needed to refresh the patient's memory. Examples would be:

- *Have you had shortness of breath with this?. . . . Fever?. . . . Cough?*
- *Has the pain radiated anywhere?. . . . Where?. . . . Any clue as to why?*
- *Have your menstrual periods stopped?. . . . When?*

During the history one tries to understand a patient's use of colloquial terms. An example of the choice of words preventing communication is demonstrated in the following sequence. The clinician asked, "Have you been having diarrhea?" The patient replied, "No, doc." Again the physician tried, "Have you had any loose stools?" The reply, "No." Continuing to question about bowel habits finally prompted the patient to say, "You know doc, I've been having this runnin' off now for several days." The level of education and choice of terms are important in communication.

FOLLOW POTENTIAL LEADS

The importance of following the patient's lead during history taking cannot be overemphasized because clues may otherwise be missed.

1. Think about what the patient is saying and respond appropriately.
2. While the patient talks, consider other information needed such as symptoms, timing, response to symptoms, and self-medication.
3. Encourage the patient to talk by using nonverbal communication such as nodding, looking interested, and leaning forward.
4. Briefly repeat what the patient has said to encourage him to continue, "You had diarrhea. . . ."
5. Ask the patient to clarify what he means by certain words in common usage that have different meanings for different people, such as "flu," "dizziness," and "colic."
6. Show concern for the patient's feelings by matching your tone of voice with his, with facial expressions, and by appropriate pauses to show added concern.
7. Be very careful in confronting the patient with what appears to be an inconsistency in the history lest the patient be put on the defensive. An example of how to do this correctly would be, "I don't understand how you can tell me the pain is so severe when you are smiling all the time."
8. Help the patient analyze how this illness has affected his life. "It must be very difficult for you to be unable to work. Are you able to manage financially? How does your family respond? Does there seem to be any relationship between your abdominal pain and the pressure to pay your bills?"

AVOID REFUSALS TO DISCUSS CERTAIN TOPICS

Certain topics in the history are very embarrassing for some patients: the bowel history, menstrual history, sexual history, or use of alcohol, drugs, and tobacco. If the patient may be embarrassed by a question, try asking for permission to ask the question. An example:

- *It is part of our routine to ask questions relating to the sexual history of our patients. These types of problems can be important in other diagnoses, too. Would it be alright for me to ask you some questions along this line?*

Ending the Interview and the Examination

Finally, after finishing questions, ask the patient:

- *Is there anything you would like to tell me that we have not discussed?* On some occasions the patient will tell the real reason for coming to the physician. Statements such as, "My friend was just diagnosed with breast cancer, and I wanted to be sure that I don't have a malignancy," may surface for the first time.
- Before stopping, stand and make a statement that lets the patient know the interview is over.
- *I appreciate your talking to me today about these things. Now I'd like to begin doing the physical examination.*

Finally, some techniques are useful in terminating the examination. Certain types of interviews (especially the psychiatric examination) need to have a winding down in which the patient is told that he has only a few minutes left to talk. This allows him time to voice any unfinished questions or comments. Similarly, other medical interviews and examinations may require a summary statement of what has been discussed, sometimes with thanks to the patient for his participation. The patient needs to have the feeling that the interview has been effective and that something has been gained.

Components of The Medical Interview

The comprehensive medical interview comprises six major categories. These are ordinarily discussed in the order listed in the box, but variations from this sequence may be useful when the patient volunteers information out of the usual order.

Chief Complaint

The chief complaint (CC) is the problem that prompted seeking medical attention. The CC may not be the first thing the patient says. For example, a patient may say, "I have come to have my gallbladder removed." The CC would actually be the symptoms that have caused the gallbladder to be the object of focus, such as, "I've been bloated and nauseated," or "I have pain here in my side."

It is useful, but not mandatory, to obtain the CC in the patient's own words. By so doing, the clinician avoids ascribing to the patient symptoms that were not actually experienced. By recording the patient's symptoms the clinician keeps from making premature and occasionally misleading judgments about the diagnosis.

More than one problem may be presented as the CC. When CCs are multiple and one problem does not stand out as causing the patient to seek medical care, use the following format to record the information:

CC: 1. Chest discomfort
2. Diabetes not under control
3. Ingrown toenail
4. Skin rash in groin

History of Present Illness

The patient begins by developing the story about each of the CCs in his own words. While listening, be alert to time of onset, sequences of events, changes in complaints, and descriptions of symptoms. Knowledge of disease natural history and the typical association of symptoms in various illnesses allows the clinician to anticipate and later inquire about symptoms the patient may have failed to recall.

At other times, a patient will not discuss his symptoms, but persist in telling the

---

Basic Components of the History

CC — Chief complaint
HPI — History of present illness
PMH — Past medical history
FH — Family history
SH — Social history
ROS — Review of systems

history in terms of diagnostic labels and previous therapy. In such cases, intervene and ask a question such as:

- *Now when you had the diagnosis of pneumonia a few weeks ago, what symptoms did you experience before you started to take the erythromycin? Would you tell me more about the progress of each of these symptoms?* The patient's actual symptoms and *not* the interpretation or diagnosis is important in the history of the present illness.

Medical histories are often too brief because they fail to pursue the patient's symptoms in sufficient detail to allow diagnostic reasoning, which includes formulation of a differential diagnosis and later a specific diagnosis. The complete history leads to the correct diagnosis more often than any other single technique—more often than the physical examination and all the laboratory and x-ray studies combined. But the specific disease actually predetermines which of these, history, physical, lab or x-ray studies, will reveal the diagnosis.

Just as the patient's initial words may not actually be his CC, merely recording the information the patient says about his health is not a medical history. The medical history begins with information the patient volunteers, includes clues from skillful questioning, and requires analysis and reorganization.

When written for the medical record, the history of the present illness (HPI) must nearly always be an edited account of what the patient has said. The HPI should usually begin at the beginning and give a chronologic development of the problem(s). Symptoms need to be recorded regarding location, severity, tempo, quality, and what relieves or aggravates them.

A history given spontaneously is useful, but the history becomes a much more important tool when tentative diagnostic hypotheses are kept in mind during the history. The novice can usually keep one or two possibilities in mind. The experienced clinician may be able to look for five or six diagnoses at once. The object is to listen for information and ask questions to find whether the history supports a tentative diagnosis under consideration. This process is ongoing throughout the entire interview, physical examination, and later analysis of laboratory and radiographic data.

Clues that do not fit the hypotheses being considered may require that the differential diagnosis be modified. Alternatively, new facts bring to mind other questions that support or exclude the diagnosis. Thus the differential diagnosis is a dynamic list of possible diagnoses for a given patient.

Clearly, greater knowledge of diagnoses allows the more experienced clinician to quickly recognize diagnostic possibilities and to ask the appropriate differentiating questions.

Past Medical History

Asking about previous illnesses prompts the patient to recall all types of past events of pediatric, medical, surgical, psychiatric, and obstetric significance. Ask about previous hospitalizations, childhood and adult illnesses, surgical procedures, and psychiatric illnesses. In this category, ask specific, direct questions:

- *Have you had any serious illnesses? In childhood? Adult years? Operations? When and why?*

Pursue immunizations, previous diseases, allergies to medications, other allergies, use of medications, drugs of abuse, environmental hazards, toxic chemical exposures, habits, diet, sleep, and travel. Exposure to known or potentially sick people, pets, or wild animals may give important clues that might not be volunteered. Such information may contribute to the HPI, and these questions often bring up problems the patient has forgotten to mention.

While taking the medical history, the patient may digress from the HPI into past medical history, family history, or social history. At that time it may seem natural to follow up by taking the remainder of the past, family, or social history before returning to additional specific questions about the present history. Items of past history, family history, or social history that are pertinent to the history of present illness may be recorded in the written HPI. Otherwise, those items are placed under the proper topic headings.

Family History

Inquire about family members, illnesses, state of health or cause of death, age, where they live, and who they depend on for support. Include parents, grandparents, spouse, aunts, uncles, siblings, in-laws, children, and grandchildren. Do any disorders occur in family members (e.g., heart disease, diabetes, thyroid disease, high blood pressure, anemia, cancer, epilepsy, headaches, strokes, tuberculosis, kidney disease, mental illness, other)? If these do occur in several relatives, construct a family tree similar to those used in genetics to show disorders. (See Appendix E.)

Social History

The object of the social history is to find how the patient's daily activities may influence his health. A useful starter is:

- *Tell me about your typical day, during the week and on weekends. Begin at 6 AM and take it around the clock until 6 AM the next day. What is your work like? Home life? Religious beliefs? Stressful situations? Important events now and in the past? What does the future hold for you?*
- Obtain information about smoking (i.e., how much and what), use of alcohol (quantitate), and use of illegal and prescription drugs. Ascertain how these affect the patient.

Review of Systems

To discern whether other symptoms may be present but neglected, the system review focuses on each part of the body systematically to give opportunity for recall of potential problems. Questions focus on each organ system or may be modified to cover each body region beginning at the head and working down. The box at the end of the chapter lists specific areas to cover in the systems review.

The Medical Interview in Special Situations

During the medical history, patients may demonstrate behaviors that impede the progress of taking the history: anger, silence, overtalkativeness, and others (Table 1-1). The physician should strive to show a mature response, analyzing the possible reason for these behaviors.

TABLE 1-1: Behavior of Patients That Pose Problems for Physicians

Behavior	Possible Reason	Response of Physician
Anger, hostility, or sarcasm	• Response to illness • Long time response pattern • Clinician late for appointment	• Feels anger in return (avoid showing it) • Feels threatened • *You're angry, want to tell me what is wrong?*
Aggressiveness	• Personality disorder • Used to hide feelings of dependency or inferiority	• Anger in return (avoid) • Difficulty in interview
Crying	• Clue to emotions, anger, fear, depression	• Quiet acceptance • Offer tissue • Ask reasons
Demanding	• Feels neglected or not treated as he deserves	• Tempted to be angry • Power struggle (better to negotiate)
Seductive	• Patient's fantasies • Patient may be hysterical • Physician's dress or demeanor misled the patient	• Maintain professional attitude • Be careful of patient's feelings • Avoid excessive empathy or reassurance, which might be misinterpreted
Silence	• Offended patient • Too many questions too rapidly • Patient thinking of answers • Shy or embarrassed patient • Hostility or depression	• Often feels uncomfortable • Ask about reason: *Are we going too fast?* • *You seem to have trouble talking about this*
Overtalkative	• Patient may just be talkative • May be aggressive • Unable to sort out unimportant versus important details • Nervousness	• Impatience, exasperation • Give patient a few minutes to talk without restrictions • Try not to use open-ended questions • Do not let impatience show
Paranoia	• Underlying personality disorder • Believes there is some devious plan about him • Reassurance is threatening	• Must avoid anger in response • Reassure that he is being treated as any other patient

Modified from Benstein L, Benstein RS: *Interviewing,* ed 4, Norwalk, Conn, 1985, Appleton-Century-Crofts.

Special Concerns in Taking the Medical History

Pediatrics
Pregnancy
Geriatrics
Patients who do not speak your language
Blind patients or those who cannot hear or speak
Psychiatric patients
Addicted patients
Patients with organic brain syndrome
Patients with differences in sexual orientation
Hostile patients

TABLE 1-2: Emotions Patients Show During Medical Interviews

Emotion	Patient's Feelings	Patient's Manifestations
Anger	• Loss of control • Feels powerless	• Outbursts toward student or physician • Criticism of someone, perhaps previous physician
Anxiety	• Loss of control • Guilt • Frustration • Helplessness • Aloneness	• Restlessness • GI symptoms • Headache • Frequent sighs • Trembling
Depression	• Futility • Inadequate and worthless feelings • Defeated • Suicide	• Slowed speech • Sad look • Crying • Insomnia • Loss of energy, fatigue • Mysterious symptoms
Denial	• Believes he will be cured despite fatal illness	• Acts and makes decisions as if he did not have a fatal illness
Projection	• Believes his own emotions are being shown by others	• Hostile patient believes others are hostile to him
Regression	• Returns to an earlier, safer era of life	• Becomes dependent on others • Needs love and attention of significant others

Patients at any age, of any sex, and with varied underlying disorders may manifest emotions as indicated in Table 1-2. As manifestations are exhibited, carefully consider clues as to what the patient is feeling.

Pediatrics

Several special concerns are addressed in the pediatric history and physical examination. For a complete discussion of the pediatric examination, see Chapter 13. For children, focus on birth, prenatal, and neonatal histories. The feeding history is important, along with growth and development. Ask about diseases peculiar to childhood, such as measles, chickenpox, and streptococcal infections of the throat. Also investigate the potential for familial or metabolic disorders and exposure to toxins (e.g., lead paint).

Depending on the child's age, obtain the CC and HPI from the child in the presence of the parent, grandparent, caretaker, or guardian. Within the written introduction to the history, a statement of who the historian was (e.g., parent or child) and the reliability of the historian is appropriate.

The mother's health before and during the pregnancy may be important. Whether the mother received medications or had any illnesses during pregnancy, the amount of weight gained during pregnancy, the approximate duration of the pregnancy and labor, and any unusual vaginal bleeding may signal sequelae in the child. Seek to determine the birth weight and whether any difficulties occurred during labor and delivery. Consider the Apgar score (0 to 10 scale, 10 being best) when ascertaining whether immediate difficulties at delivery occurred.

The neonatal period covers from birth to 4 weeks of age. Potential problems to consider include respiratory difficulties, early recognition of congenital defects, jaundice, convulsions, or infections.

The eating history and feeding problems of the neonate or the child may give a clue to areas for concern. Were supplemental vitamins and iron given? What formula was used? Was honey included in the formula? At what age were specific foods introduced?

The growth of the child, with height and weight at various ages, are ranked on developmental charts, and activity milestones are important in determining whether a child later has normal development.

With a few exceptions, childhood illnesses should now be prevented by immunizations. Impetigo, scarlet fever, and chickenpox remain important diseases for which we do not currently immunize. Record the ages at which immunizations were given, including those for *Hemophilus influenzae* type B, diphtheria, tetanus, pertussis, oral polio, measles, mumps, and rubella.

Pregnancy

Some women are happy to learn of being pregnant, but many are not. Because many conceptions are not planned, it may require time for one or both parents to accept this pregnancy. Questions you may consider asking include:

- *Is this your first pregnancy?*
- *What was the outcome (living child, miscarriage, or abortion) of each previous pregnancy?*
- *How many children do you take care of (may include own children and children from a previous marriage of spouse)?*
- *Did you have any special problems during the previous pregnancies (e.g., blood pressure problems, eclampsia, proteinuria, weight loss or gain, nausea, vomiting)?*
- *Have you had any problems in carrying a previous pregnancy to term (40 weeks), in delivery, or after giving birth (postpartum period)?*
- *Did you breast feed? Do you wish to do so with this child?*
- *Was this pregnancy planned? Does it pose any special problems?*
- *Were you using birth control? What methods?*

Geriatrics

Older patients (over 70) and the very old (over age 85) are as different as people in any other category. Generalizations can be made regarding the health concerns of elderly people, as they acquire more disorders themselves or see their friends get sick and die. In this book, considerations of age-related changes are integrated into the individual chapters rather than discussed separately in a geriatrics chapter.

Common problems include the following:

- Loneliness (as they outlive their friends or are incapable of getting out to visit).
- Fears of becoming incapacitated and being placed in a nursing home (such people are valued very little by society).
- Fear of acquiring cancer.
- Depression (as personal self-image deteriorates from youthful self).
- Fear of leaving the house at night (crimes against the elderly).
- Excessive medications prescribed by physicians (treating each of several diseases, drug interactions, overdosing caused by age-dependent reduction in renal function).
- Poor dietary intake.

Common health problems related to functional decline or disease in the very old include confusion, falls, decubitus ulcers (bedsores), urinary tract problems (hesitancy in starting the stream in men, infections in women), difficulty getting out of bed, and stopping eating or drinking.

Besides asking questions to explore the above situations, consider asking the following:

- *Tell me what it feels like to be 95 (or whatever age the patient is) years old?*
- *How do you spend a typical day?*
- *What is a typical meal like for you? How has your weight been doing?*
- *Who are your friends, and how often do you get together? And with your family?*
- *What do you worry about most?*
- *What are your plans for the future?*
- *Have you fallen recently? How did it hurt you?*
- *Do you have any problem with urination (or voiding)? Would you describe those for me?*

Patients who do not Speak Your Language

As the number of people from foreign countries immigrate to the United States, more language problems arise. Often someone can be found among the hospital employees such as a nurse, janitor, maid, or other person who will be willing, even eager, to translate. Thus in large hospitals, Vietnamese, Chinese, Japanese, Spanish, and other languages are usually spoken by several people. Most hospitals or clinics keep a list of such people who have indicated a willingness to translate.

Otherwise, bilingual pronunciation guides are available. In the absence of either of these options, signaling the patient to pantomime or to write the problem may be the best the clinician can do actively.

Use care not to overinterpret nor underinterpret what a patient says who can speak only a little English. Often the history gets inadvertently altered in this setting.

Blind Patients and Those Unable to Hear or Speak

For some obscure reason, when we talk to patients who are blind, we too often raise the volume of our voices. Blind patients can usually hear, often more acutely than can sighted persons.

The patient who cannot hear can often read lips if you speak slowly and enunciate clearly. However, sometimes clarifying questions will need to be written to them. These patients respond in writing.

Patients who are on a mechanical ventilator are not able to speak because of the endotracheal tube in the larynx. They can hear questions asked but must respond by gestures or by writing.

Psychiatric Patients

Patients who exhibit psychotic or emotional problems may take one of many different appearances (see Chapter 11).

Some patients will exhibit flight of ideas and be unable to follow a thought to a logical conclusion. Others may be paranoid. Delusions, illusions, and hallucinations are typical of psychotic patients. When these events become evident, some additions to the usual medical history will be needed to help establish the patient's psychologic problem and to pursue the nature of any concomitant medical problems.

Addicted Patients

In our society many people are addicted. These people have a need or desire to continue the focus of addiction. Examples include minor addictions such as to caffeine, food, and exercise, and major addictions such as to alcohol, illegal drugs, pornography, and sex. Major addictions became so pervasive as to modify a person's life-style to satisfy the addiction. Each of these addictions, minor and major, may have health consequences.

To obtain information about addictions, questions may be asked directly or indirectly. Often the direct approach is not rewarding because persons addicted do not wish to admit addiction, even to themselves. The reason for seeking medical care may be caused by the addiction or by an entirely different problem, in which case the patient may have no desire to stop addictive habits.

When taking the history from the alcoholic, ask questions such as the following:

- *On an average day, how many drinks do you have before breakfast?*
- *What type of alcoholic beverages do you usually consume and how much of each (wine, beer, whiskey)?*
- *Do you eat food or do you omit food when you drink? How often?*
- *Do you ever lose consciousness or lose control when you drink? ever harmed yourself or someone else?*
- *Have you ever experienced withdrawal symptoms (DTs)?*
- *Do you wish to stop drinking? why?*

The user of illicit drugs is in a precarious position. When he admits his use to you, he is saying that he broke the law. As a physician, you must not try to satisfy your idle curiosity about his drug suppliers lest you learn too much about covert drug and gang activity and thereby be perceived as a threat to those persons.

Examples of appropriate questions follow:

- *I need some information about what types of drugs you use and how you use them. I do not want to know who your drug suppliers are. If I ask you anything you don't want to talk about, just say so and we'll move on to another topic.*
- *Do you ever use intravenous drugs? What, and how often?*
- *Do you ever use a needle that someone else has used?*
- *Do you clean needles? How? Are you able to obtain sterile needles every time?*
- *What kinds of reactions have you had after taking drugs? Any bad reactions?*
- *Have you ever had to do things to obtain drugs that you are not happy about (traded sex, harmed someone)?*
- Use care if the patient tells you about committing illegal activities. Consult with your supervisor or the hospital attorney. Because the chart is a legal document, it is important to be careful about any details entered into the medical record.

Patients with Organic Brain Syndrome

Patients who are demented pose special problems. The patient with Alzheimer's disease may or may not be able to give the history, depending on the stage of disease.

A patient who has had multiple strokes may be equally demented, depending on brain structures involved. The chronic alcoholic with Korsakoff's syndrome (see Chapter 11) may appear to be making perfectly good sense, then you find out later that he has been confabulating, covering for those areas of memory that are faulty.

Patients with Differences in Sexual Orientation

When taking a history, do not assume that a patient is having sexual activity, nor that sexual relations are with one member of the opposite sex in a monogamous relationship. Instead, questions may progress in a manner similar to the following:

- *Tell me about your sexual practices.*
- *Are you currently having sexual activity with anyone?*
- If the reply is "Yes, with my spouse," usually no other question is needed. However, if a sexually transmitted disease is a consideration, you may say, *I don't want to offend you, and you don't need to answer this if you don't wish to, but is there anyone else you have been having a relationship with?*
- *Have you ever had same-sex relationships?*
- *How many (total) sexual partners have you had?*
- *Do you find sex satisfying? Why or why not?*
- *Do you ever have sex for money or drugs? Have you always insisted on or worn a condom? What safe-sex techniques do you practice?*
- *Have you had any sexually transmitted diseases (syphilis, "bad blood," gonorrhea or clap, venereal warts, chlamydia, hepatitis B)? Any possible exposure to AIDS?*
- *Have you ever been abused sexually? What have you done to put this behind you and to learn to cope with it? Do you feel that you need more help with this?*

Hostile Patients

Patients may be hostile because they are upset at the physician for being late, at the medical student for coming in to see them when they expected a staff physician, because they are sick (why me?) or because they are just usually hostile toward others.

- You may defuse this situation by saying (when you walk into the patient's room), *I'm sorry I'm so late. Am I keeping you from something you need to be doing?* If there is, you may quickly ascertain the CC and determine if a later visit would be better. For hostility becoming manifest later in the interview, you may say, *I can see you really are upset about something. Have I done or said something to upset you? I'm awfully sorry if I have. Do you want to tell me about it?*
- For patients who are upset at having a medical student enter the room to do the history and physical, it is a good policy for the student to say *I'm very sorry you're so upset at my being here. Dr. _____ has asked me to see you and to take your medical history and perform an examination. If you really don't want me to continue, I will stop now and let him know.*
- For patients who distrust physicians generally, an intern, resident, or staff physician may say, *I understand your concerns about your health and about whether you can trust me. My policy is always to let you know what I am thinking and why. After the history and exam, I'll explain what we plan, and I'll be sure to tell you about the results and what those results mean to you. We'll just look at these reports together in your chart. I don't want to hide anything from you that you want to know about. And I won't tell anyone besides Dr. _____ (the attending physician) anything without your permission. Is there any other area of concern that bothers you now?*

The inexperienced clinical student and sometimes even physicians are tempted to overstep the bounds of information gathering and prematurely give advice (Table 1-3). Inexperience, discomfort in patient contact, feeling rushed for time,

TABLE 1-3: Responses of Clinicians and the Message Conveyed to the Patient

Response of Clinician	Example	Outcome of Message
Advice giving	• *If I were you, I would....*	• If successful, patient has learned little; becomes dependent if mechanism not understood. • If unsuccessful, blames physician.
Asking irrelevant questions	• Use of a question to avoid period of silence.	• Information gathered may not be something clinician desires to or is qualified to handle. • May be used to avoid expression of deep feelings about a topic under discussion.
Avoidance	• Staying away from patients who are upset, demanding, hostile, dying, or have AIDS or cancer.	• Patient feels isolated, lonely. Patient loses trust in clinician. This makes care more difficult.
Changing subjects	• Not answering the patient's questions, trying to protect him.	• Desire to avoid talking about a subject; this interferes with modification of feelings.
Double questions	• *Have you had fever and vomiting?*	• This is an attempt at time saving but may result in ambiguous responses, wasting time.
False answers	• *Don't worry, it'll be all right.*	• Not effective in quieting patient because this relys on falsification or avoidance. Says to patient either problem does not exist, or he is worrying excessively.
Valid assurance (appropriate)	• Understanding and correct information given.	• Patient feels respected, listened to, and understood instead of overwhelmed with advice or platitudes.
Why questions	• *Why did you do it?*	• Although this may be seeking information, it can imply disapproval.

Modified from Benstein L, Benstein RS: *Interviewing*, ed 4, Norwalk, Conn, 1985, Appleton-Century-Crofts.

or not knowing what to say contrast acutely with appropriate assurance given to the patient in a timely manner.

Diagnostic Reasoning

During early clinical training, students find constructing a differential diagnosis for a patient's problems difficult. The mature clinician ordinarily constructs the differential diagnosis by thinking of clinical patterns of diseases affecting patients. Not only does he consider signs and symptoms, but also factors such as age-related illness, the epidemiologic trends of disease, illnesses common in the community, familial diseases, the time course of the illness, and the statistical likelihood of a given disease. Two terms are often applied to the immediate recognition of a diagnosis, "augenblick" and "gestalt." When the observed clinical features allow an immediate diagnosis, *augenblick* indicates the diagnosis was made with the speed of blinking the eye. Those who use the term *gestalt* indicate that the summation of the units trigger recognition of the composite diagnosis.

Even experienced clinicians are not always able to make rapid diagnoses. Often they need to use a reasoned approach, as does the beginning student, to formulate a differential diagnosis of difficult clinical problems. A technique for formulating a differential diagnosis table for a single problem has been described. Table 1-4 shows a partial construction of such a table for a patient complaining of headache. Across the top of the page are placed anatomic structures dealing with the area of the body to which the complaint refers. On the vertical axis, classic pathologic disease processes are listed. At the boxes made by the intersection of rows and columns, possible diagnoses are placed in each. Diagnoses are refined by reviewing with the patient other questions to identify those diagnoses which seem to be more likely. When a patient has several problems for which differential diagnosis tables can be constructed, diagnoses on more than one of the tables may be more likely to apply. Not only does the clinician use the history and examination to assist in defining the likelihood of diagnoses in the matrix, but laboratory and x-ray studies are used.

To derive a single diagnosis from the differential diagnosis, keep several factors in mind. For most patients, a single diagnosis that explains the patient's illness will usually have a higher probability of being correct than two or more diagnoses to explain signs and symptoms. In contrast, certain patients often have several diagnoses at the same time, such as geriatric patients, patients with AIDS, and patients who have had extended hospital stays. The inexperienced clinician will often try to include uncommon diseases high in the differential diagnosis. Certainly rare diseases occur, but the old adage "common diseases are common" should be remembered for routine diagnosis.

To sort out the most likely diagnosis from the differential diagnosis list, keep in mind a few hypotheses that may explain the patients' symptoms. While the patient is giving the history, formulate questions to help differentiate possible diagnoses. By the time the history is completed, you may have changed the list of possible diagnoses several times based on the patient's responses. Then use the physical examination to explore these possibilities.

Diagnostic errors do occur and have been studied (Table 1-5). Students may make errors in omission, but with experience in taking histories and performing examinations, the errors in diagnosis move toward the bottom of the table (especially the "no-fault" type).

Make the Physical Examination an Active Process

Beginning students of clinical medicine often think the physical examination is a passive process, that the clinician merely goes through the steps in performing an examination looking for whatever abnormality may be present. This is not the case. The clinician has asked himself and the patient many questions during the medical history. During the examination he searches for clues that support, fail to support, or make unlikely specific diagnoses. The examination becomes an active process. Even early in training before diagnostic reasoning is developed, it is appropriate to ask oneself general questions about findings during the examination. Questions to demonstrate some of these possibilities are listed in the box on pp. 26-28.

The experienced clinician is frequently able to determine more from the physical examination than is the beginning student. Occasionally both find this puzzling, but the reason is twofold. First, the experienced clinician thinks of the

Text continued on pg. 28.

TABLE 1-4: Considerations in Differential Diagnosis of Headache*

Process	Skull	Meninges	Vessels	Brain	Sinuses	Eyes	Jaw and Teeth	Neck and Back Muscles	Ears
Congenital	• Sickle cell	• Spina bifida	• Bleed • Aneurysm		• Hypoplasia				
Environmental	• Trauma				• Pollen/pollution	• Eye strain	• Malocclusion	• Stresses	
Endocrine						• Cataract (diabetes)			
Genetic			• Stroke		• Kartagener's syndrome	• Dislocated lens			
Iatrogenic		• After lumbar puncture	• Caffeine withdrawal	• Pseudotumor	• Recent nasogastric tube	• Poor lens (glasses) corrections	• Poor fit of dentures		
Infectious	• Osteomyelitis	• Bacterial/viral/fungal meningitis		• Brain abscess • Encephalitis	• Sinusitis	• Conjunctivitis	• Abscess	• Myopathy	• Otitis
Inflammatory			• Temporal arteritis		• Allergies	• Iritis	• Temporal mandibular arthritis	• Myopathy	
Mechanical	• Old or recent fracture		• Migraine	• Contusion	• Sinuses filled	• Foreign body	• Grinding teeth	• Imbalance	• Chloesteatoma
Neoplastic	• Paget's			• Tumor	• Tumor	• Melanoma			
Psychologic				• Stress					
Unknown etiology		• Sarcoidosis	• Vasospasm • Hydrocephalus						

Format adapted from Fulop M: Teaching differential diagnosis to beginning clinical students, *Am J Med* 79:745-749, 1985.

*This format will assist you in learning how to construct a differential diagnosis. As you mature in medicine, you will follow this technique less and less rigidly, but you will begin to think in clinical patterns (during your junior and senior years).

TABLE 1-5: Errors in Diagnosis

Reason for Error	Examples	Outcome	Back-up Mechanism to Make Diagnosis	Future Consequences
(1) Error from history	• Failure to ask about hunting and rabbit exposure.	• Diagnosis of tularemia not entertained or refers patient	• None unless physician happens to order titer	• Prolonged illness
(2) Error from examination				
(a) Exam was incomplete	• Pelvic exam deferred.	• Pelvic mass missed	• Referral to Ob/Gyn for annual pelvic exam	• If no referral or exam, delay in diagnosis
(b) Skill of examiner incomplete	• Cardiac auscultation performed, mitral rumble not heard (because of skill or training).	• Mitral stenosis not considered as a possible cause of patient's problem	• Chest x-ray study, ECG, or other tests may suggest mitral stenosis	• Patient not warned about the need for antibiotic prophylaxis with dental procedure and may develop SBE
(c) Exam room inappropriate	• Room too noisy to hear soft cardiac sounds.	• Patient suffering prolonged		
(3) Errors from faulty cognition				
(a) Failure to trigger diagnostic hypothesis (physician does not know or does not consider the possible diagnosis)	• Failure to consider *Clostridium difficile* as cause for diarrhea 1 week after discharge from hospital (IV antibiotics had been given for another problem).	• Prolonged, debilitating diarrhea	• Pseudomembranes seen if sigmoidoscopy performed	• Needless other tests done to evaluate diarrhea
(b) Faulty framing of context (wrong emphasis placed on patient's symptoms, signs, or other data)	• Lady with abdominal pain, vomiting, weight loss, wide pulse pressure, brisk reflexes evaluated for GI problem; hyperthyroidism not considered until atrial flutter developed.	• Delay in diagnosis and some tests performed that were not needed	• Diagnosis made as disease progressed	• Patient suffering prolonged because of delay in diagnosis

Adapted from Kassirer JP, Kopelman RI: Cognitive errors in diagnosis: in situation, classification, and consences, *Am J Med* 86:433-441, 1989.

Continued.

TABLE 1-5: Errors in Diagnosis—cont'd

Reason for Error	Examples	Outcome	Back-up Mechanism to Make Diagnosis	Future Consequences
(c) Errors in assessing disease prevalence (believing the findings in a patient warrant looking for a rare disease, when a common disorder is more likely)	• Man with injured spinal cord with urinary tract infection and severe hypertension evaluated for pheochromocytoma (rare disease) with conflicting test results.	• Many needless laboratory studies performed.	• Nephrology consultation gave correct diagnosis of spinal cord disease with urinary tract infection (common complication of Foley catheter).	• Progression of disease and possible consequences (e.g., chronic pyelonephritis)
(d) Error in interpreting clinical data (unless a piece of datum is highly specific, a positive is likely to be a false positive if the disease is rare)	• Patient has plasma gastrin level checked, and it is very high. The patient is believed to have the Zollinger-Ellison syndrome (rare) rather than recognizing need to repeat the test, as it may be a false positive.	• Could lead to inappropriate tests or surgical procedures	• Consultation with surgeon or gastroenterologist	
(e) Errors in beliefs about the mechanism of patient's problems	• Patient presents with shortness of breath and swelling of ankles. Clinician correctly diagnoses congestive heart failure but fails to consider a recent painless myocardial infarction as the cause.	• Patient not managed correctly for underlying problem	• If ECG is performed or cardiac enzymes checked, may reveal diagnostic abnormalities	• Possibilities for early intervention for heart rhythm disturbances and for repeat infarctions not considered

(f) Error in applying clinical axioms (e.g., Sutton's law; after Willy Sutton, who, when asked why he robbed banks, is supposed to have said, "You go where the money is")

- Young woman presented with right upper quadrant abdominal pain and diarrhea. Ultrasound of liver showed multiple hypoechoic masses that raised diagnosis of abscess or tumor. Some clinicians wanted to do needle aspiration invoking Sutton's law. Wrong. CT showed a vascular hemangioma.

- Change in patient management

(g) Errors in verifying previous diagnostic labels

- Man had adrenal tumor removed. Pathologic diagnosis was pheochromocytoma. Recurrent retroperitoneal bleeding prompted one of the physicians to reconsider diagnosis. Further studies confirmed the tumor to be angiosarcoma.

- Correct diagnosis looked for and found only after treatment failure

- The consulting oncologist recognized that retroperitoneal bleeding was unusual following pheochromocytoma

(h) No-fault errors (diagnostic clues point to a common diagnosis when, actually, a rarer cause is present but is masked by the appearance of more common possibility)

- Woman returned from foreign trip with diarrhea; she had eaten food from restaurants not recommended. Stool exam showed two parasites, for which she was treated. Diagnosis was parasite-induced diarrhea. Diarrhea worsened. Later she was found to have a very rare metastatic tumor of the liver secreting vasoactive intestinal peptide, which caused the diarrhea.

- Radiographs, scans, and laboratory studies.

Questions for the Examiner to Ask Himself During the Examination

Blood Pressure

- Is the arm in the standard position when the blood pressure is measured?
- In which arm is the blood pressure higher?
- Is the blood pressure higher in the legs compared with the arms?
- Does the blood pressure increase or decrease when the patient sits up from supine or stands from sitting?
- If the blood pressure was high, does it decrease to normal when measured again after a few minutes?

Temperature

- Was the temperature taken orally, axillary, rectally?
- What kind of a thermometer was used: the dot apparatus, electronic thermometer, or a mercury thermometer?
- Does the temperature change during the day?
- When is the temperature highest: early morning, midafternoon, or evening?

Pulse and Respirations

- What was the pulse rate? Rhythm?
- Does the pulse vary with respirations?
- What was the respiratory rate? Are respirations regular or irregular? Any patterns?

General Appearance

- What is the general attitude and appearance of the patient?
- How does he respond to you?
- Casually look for abnormalities and normal variations in face and hands while you are talking to the patient

Eyes

- Are the conjunctivae pale, erythematous?
- Do the sclera have pingueculae, ptyergia, or other markings?
- Is arcus senilis present at the margin of the cornea?
- When a flashlight is shined in one eye, do both pupils constrict? Do pupils change size when patient looks at objects close, then afar?
- Is the red reflex present or absent?
- When the flashlight is swung to the other pupil, do both remain constricted?
- Are each of the extraocular muscles functioning normally?
- On funduscopic examination, are the lens and vitreous clear?
- Observe vessels as they cross the margin of the optic disc. Draw the general configuration of the arteries and veins. When arteries and veins cross, does nicking occur?
- What are the appearance and sizes of the arteries and veins?
- Are hemorrhages or exudates of the retina present?

Nose

- Is the septum deviated?
- Which turbinates are seen? Are they red, swollen, dripping, bleeding?
- Any tenderness when palpating over the frontal or maxillary sinus?

Questions for the Examiner to Ask Himself During the Examination—*continued*

Teeth and Mouth

- Are the patient's gums and gingiva in good health? Receding from the teeth?
- Are the gums red or inflamed?
- Are the teeth in good repair or do they have cavities? Plaque?
- Does tapping a blunt object against each tooth elicit tenderness?
- Does the patient have halitosis? Why?
- Are the anterior and posterior tonsillar pillars and the tonsils intact? Is exudate, erythema, or swelling of the tonsils evident?
- Does the patient have inclusions in crypts?

Ear

- Are abnormalities of the pinna present?
- Is cerumen present in each external canal?
- What is the general appearance of the light reflex on the tympanic membrane (TM)? Is it bulging, perforated, draining?
- Does the TM move well when the patient blows his nose while occluding the nostrils?
- Can the chorda tympani be seen behind the TM?

Neck

- Are the carotid pulses equal bilaterally?
- Is a bruit present over the carotids?
- Is the thyroid gland enlarged by observation or palpation?
- What about tenderness over the thyroid or a bruit over the thyroid?
- Is the patient's neck stiff?
- Are any nodes palpable in postauricular, postcervical, or anterior cervical positions?

Chest

- Is the patient breathing normally? If not, what type of abnormality?
- Are breath sounds apparent over each bronchopulmonary segment? Delineate each bronchopulmonary segment projected onto the chest wall.
- If abnormal sounds are present, where is each, and describe.
- Is the chest wall tender? Is the patient's back tender to percussion?
- Are the breasts equal in size, symmetric, tender, have lumps or nipple discharge? Are the axillary nodes or epitrocheal nodes palpable?

Heart

- Examine the patient sitting, supine, and in left lateral decubitus position.
- Is the first or the second sound louder? At which area?
- After focusing on the second heart sound in the pulmonic area, are two components present?
- Gradually inch from that location. Can the two components of the second heart sound be heard in the aortic area and the mitral area? How does the second sound split with respirations?
- Is a systolic murmur present? Does it radiate into the neck? Where over the

Continued.

> **Questions for the Examiner to Ask Himself During the Examination — *continued***
>
> precordium is it loudest? What happens to the intensity of the murmur if the patient sits up? Stands? Reclines on left side?
> - Listen with the bell towards the apex for an S_3.
> - Listen from the lower left sternal border towards the apex with the diaphragm for an opening snap.
> - Does clenching the fist tightly enhance the intensity of the murmur or decrease it?
> - Listen for S_4, S_1, clicks, S_2, OS, and S_3 individually.
>
> **Abdomen**
> - Are the liver and spleen palpable?
> - Does the umbilicus feel normal?
> - Is the cecum or the sigmoid colon palpable? Tender? Fecal filled?
> - Are masses present?
> - Are bruits heard over the aorta, femoral arteries, the iliacs?
> - Does the patient have costovertebral angle tenderness to percussion?
>
> **Vascular**
> - Are the femoral pulses full? Popliteal? Dorsalis pedis, posterior tibial? Carotids? Equal bilaterally?
> - Are bruits present?

differential diagnosis and searches for other possible associations while examining the patient. For example, the finding of petechiae on the palate will bring to mind the possibility of endocarditis. When he finds this, the experienced clinician will especially look for splinter hemorrhages and conjunctivae petechiae, examine the palms and soles, auscultate for a heart murmur, and palpate for splenomegaly. Items that might be overlooked by the novice will all be found by the experienced examiner. Knowledge of diseases and their associated physical findings contributes to the examination.

Second, knowledge of the differential diagnosis becomes important when palatal petechiae are found. The beginning student sees palatal petechiae and says, "uh-huh." The experienced clinician notes the palatal petechiae, thinks rubella, looks for a rash, palpates for posterior cervical nodes, and asks about joint discomfort. Still thinking of the palatal petechiae, he considers infectious mononucleosis and looks for adenopathy, hepatic tenderness, an enlarged spleen, or a rash. Still considering palatal petechiae, he entertains the diagnosis of streptococcal infection, checks the temperature, examines the pharynx closely, and looks for anterior cervical adenopathy. Finally, he thinks about endocarditis and makes the observations mentioned above. Thus a single clue may prompt a more careful diagnostic evaluation of selected parts of the physical examination according to the differential diagnosis being contemplated.

> **How Physical Exams are Performed: Regional Considerations**
>
> | | |
> |---|---|
> | Vital signs | Breasts, anterior chest, sitting |
> | Skin and general inspection | Cardiac sitting, supine |
> | Head | Abdomen |
> | Eyes | Rectal |
> | Ears | Genitalia |
> | Nose | Musculoskeletal and vascular |
> | Throat/neck | Neurologic |
> | Hands and arms | Psychiatric |
> | Posterior chest sitting | |

Techniques for Performing the Physical Examination

The patient is prepared for the physical examination by asking him to remove all clothing except the lower undergarments and to wear a short cloth or paper gown that opens in the back. The patient's legs are usually covered with a short (draw) sheet.

The physician enters the room after the patient has changed to the gown and washes his hands at once. The examination is not performed as it is written for the medical record, but is performed by anatomic regions as listed in the accompanying box.

The vital signs will usually be taken first. Check the blood pressure in each arm with the patient sitting and the elbow supported on a desk. On a complete evaluation, check blood pressure with the patient supine, sitting, and standing to look for postural decreases in pressure. If the blood pressure measurement is higher than normal, retake the blood pressure and the pulse after 15 to 30 minutes. Check the temperature and pulse rate. The radial pulse rate is ordinarily counted for 15 seconds, the result multiplied by 4 and recorded as the pulse rate. Respirations are counted for 30 seconds and multiplied by 2. Check the temperature.

Then generally inspect the patient. Observe the hair, color, texture, eyebrows, eyelashes, use of makeup, lips, ears, hands, palms, nails, arms, feet, and legs. Note any skin changes or lesions (see Chapter 12). Check vision with a Snellen eye chart, using either the wall or the pocket version (see Chapter 2). For routine bedside evaluation of vision, ask the patient to read from a magazine with each eye closed or from a book with and without glasses. Observe the conjunctivae, pupils, and irises with a penlight. Then examine the mouth, throat, and teeth. The funduscopic examination follows.

Evaluate the ears beginning with the pinna, the external ear, the ear canal itself, then the tympanic membrane with the otoscope (see Chapter 2). Change the otoscope speculum so that the nose can be inspected. Inspect the nasal septum and the lower and middle turbinates and mucosa. Use a tuning fork to perform the Weber and Rinne tests and a ticking watch (if available) to test hearing.

Move to the backside of the patient at this point, inspecting the back and the posterior portion of the head and neck. Ask the patient to flex the neck, to turn it from side to side, and to bend down (see Chapter 2). Observe the muscle groups along each side of the vertebral column for evidence of scoliosis. Palpate the neck for posterior and anterior cervical nodes, and palpate the thyroid using hands around the neck from both sides.

Ask the patient to breath deeply while you observe chest symmetry (see Chapter 3). Test vocal fremitus and percuss the level of the diaphragm on both sides. With the patient breathing through the mouth, perform auscultation, comparing sequentially one side of the chest with the other.

Next examine the patient from the front. Inspect the breasts (both men and women) at this time. Then ask the patient to lie down and complete the remainder of the breast exam (see Chapter 8). This includes examination for axillary nodes, supraclavicular nodes, and epitrochlear nodes. Again inspect, palpate, percuss, and auscultate. Evaluate breath sounds bilaterally. Auscultate the heart sounds with the patient sitting.

Evaluation of the heart continues with inspection, palpation, percussion, and auscultation, first sitting, then supine (see Chapter 4). Correlate the jugular veins with cardiac findings with the thorax and head of the patient elevated to 30 degrees. Examine the carotid pulses and the carotids.

Next inspect the abdomen (see Chapter 5). Follow inspection by auscultation before percussion or palpation. After listening for bruits and bowel sounds, percuss gently for liver and spleen size and for abdominal masses, including a full bladder. Palpate first gently and superficially, then follow by deeper palpation for liver or spleen enlargement, masses, kidneys, or other organomegaly.

Next inspect the groin and palpate for pulses, enlarged nodes, and hernias (see Chapter 6). Inspect the arms and legs and palpate pulses and joints (see Chapter 9).

The neurologic and psychiatric examinations are performed next as indicated by the patient's complaints and other findings on the examination (see Chapters 10 and 11). Finally, the rectal and genital examinations complete the exam (see Chapters 6 and 7).

Use a standard format for recording in the medical record, the patient's hospital or clinic chart. The material in the box that ends this chapter provides a standardized format.

Suggested readings

Berstein L, Berstein RS: *Interviewing,* New York, 1985, Appleton-Century-Crofts. *An excellent paperback that gives lots of help on conducting the medical interview.*

Fulop M: Teaching differential diagnosis to beginning clinical students, *Am J Med* 79:745-749, 1985. *This article popularizes the table format of how to construct a differential diagnosis for students who have not yet learned about many disease processes.*

Kassirer JP, Kopelman RI: Cognitive errors in diagnosis: instantiation, classification, and consequences, *Am J Med* 86:433-441, 1989. *Clinicians make errors in diagnosis for many reasons. This article analyzes why.*

Oboler SK, LaForce FM: The periodic examination in asymptomatic adults, *Ann Intern Med* 110: 214-226, 1989. *Epidemiologic standards have been used to show what parts of the periodic physical examination are likely to be productive in the patient without symptoms of disease.*

Smith RC, Hoppe RB: The patient's story: integrating the patient- and physician-centered approaches to interviewing, *Ann Intern Med* 115:470-477, 1991. *The patient-centered interview, letting the patient tell his story in his way is contrasted with the physician guiding the interview. The latter leads to patient dissatisfaction and doctor-shopping.*

Format for Recording Information Obtained from the Medical Interview and from the Physical Examination

Patient Identifying Data

Patient's name, age, address, and telephone number.

Date the history. Where was it taken. Name of informant? Reliability? Name and address of referring physician.

Chief Complaint(s)

Use the patient's own words and avoid medical terms in the chief complaint. If the patient has several chief complaints, number them and give the history of the present illness for each one.

History of Present Illness

Give a chronologic narrative of the chief complaint(s). For patients having chronic illnesses, give the reason the patient is seeking medical attention at this time. Include pertinent positives and negatives ordinarily asked in the system review pertaining to the patient's problem. Try to avoid medical diagnostic labels, but discuss the patient's signs and symptoms that may have prompted another physician to use the diagnostic label.

Past Medical History

Major illnesses experienced by the patient including childhood and adult years. Ages at each of these.

Injuries, operations and ages.

Immunizations (DPT, rubella, smallpox, polio [oral versus inactivated], mumps, pneumococcal, measles, influenza, *Haemophilus influenzae,* type B, others).

Allergies, medications, food, contact, asthma. Blood transfusions and dates? Date of last chest x-ray film, last Papanicolaou's test, mammogram. Results? Skin tests for tuberculosis?

Use of medications? Nonprescription medications? Habits including tea, coffee, alcohol, tobacco, laxatives, marijuana, mind altering social drugs, birth control pills, health food store supplements.

Family History

Father, mother, age, if living; age at death; state of health and previous illnesses.

Siblings and children of patient, illnesses previously, ages at death.

Family members who have had the following: Stroke, diabetes, hypertension, heart disease, tuberculosis, alcoholism, jaundice, bleeding tendency, obesity, gout, asthma, mental illness, cancer, or other? If yes, who, relationship, age, and outcome. For familial disorders, draw the diagram of the pedigree.

Personal (Social) History

Place of birth, residence, occupation, marital status, number of children, ages and sexes of children, military experience, foreign travel, religion, brief description of a typical day (include eating, sleeping, and exercise habits).

Review of Systems

General

Weight, weight at age 18

Maximum, minimum, recent change of weight and how much

Appetite, weakness, fatigue, fever, chills, night sweats, anorexia, syncope, insomnia, sleeping habits

Skin

Color change, itching, rash, moles and change, hair and change, nails and change, infections, tumors

Head

Headaches, trauma

Eyes

Vision, glasses, contact lenses, blindness or blind spots, scotomata, pain, tearing, redness, itching, burning dryness, glaucoma

Ears

Hearing, deafness, discharge, pain, vertigo, tinnitus

Nose and sinuses

Decrease of smell, bleeding, dryness, discharge, obstruction, pain, sinusitis, hay fever

Mouth

Dental caries, painful teeth, bleeding gums, sore tongue, postnasal drip, oral ulcers, thrush, lip lesion, fever blisters, canker sores

Throat

Sore throat, hoarseness, painful swallowing, tonsillitis

Neck

Stiffness, decreased motion, pain, lumps in neck, swollen glands, goiter

Continued.

**Format for Recording Information Obtained from the Medical Interview
and from the Physical Examination** — *continued*

Breasts
  Lumps, discharge, pain, bleeding, nipple retraction, change in size, tenderness
Respiratory
  Cough, sputum, color, frequency, pleurisy, hemoptysis, wheezing, dyspnea, chest pain, recurrent respiratory infection, exposure to tuberculosis, positive TB skin test
Cardiac
  Chest pain, dyspnea on exertion, orthopnea, paroxysmal nocturnal dyspnea, murmur, palpitations, edema, cyanosis, syncope, history of rheumatic fever, previous electrocardiogram results
Vascular
  High blood pressure, phlebitis, varicosities, claudication, Raynaud's phenomenon
Gastrointestinal
  Nausea, vomiting, belching, dysphagia, heartburn, antacid use, hematemesis, food intolerance, indigestion, jaundice, clay-colored stools, dark urine, fatty or greasy food intolerance, change in bowel habits, constipation, laxative or enema use, hematochezia, melena, fissures, rectal abscess, diarrhea, bloating, hemorrhoids, hernia
Urinary tract
  Dysuria, hematuria, frequency and volume, polyuria, hesitancy, inability to start stream, incontinence, nocturia, renal stones, history of infections
Female reproductive
  Menarche age, climacteric age, postmenopausal bleeding, menorrhagia, postcoital bleeding, leukorrhea, pruritus, history of venereal disease, obstetric history (gravida, para, live births, abortions, living children, complications of pregnancy), libido, contraceptive methods, dyspareunia, menstrual flow (light, heavy, number of pads used per day, passage of blood clots), regularity, dysmenorrhea, vaginal/pelvic infections
Male reproductive
  Penile discharge, skin lesions, circumcised, history of venereal disease, serology, testicular pain or mass, fertility, impotence, libido
Hematologic
  Anemia, easy bruising, easy bleeding, bleeding gums, lymphadenopathy
Musculoskeletal
  Muscle pain, cramps, weakness, atrophy, trauma, tenderness, joint pain (heat, redness, stiffness, deformity), fracture, kyphosis, scoliosis, lordosis

Endocrine
  Heat or cold intolerance, excessive sweating, change in hair distribution or coarseness, breast change, voice change, polydipsia, polyuria, polyphagia, goiter, change in hat, glove, or shoe size
Central nervous system
  Headache, syncope, seizures, vertigo, blindness, diplopia, paralysis/paresis, tremor, ataxia, dysesthesia, dysarthria, incoordination, tics, fainting, blackouts, numbness, tingling, memory loss
Psychiatric
  Nervousness, depression, hyperventilation, insomnia, thoughts of suicide, emotional instability, illusions, delusions, hallucinations, memory impairment, memory loss, nightmares, tension

Physical Examination
Vital signs
  Temperature, respiration, pulse (regular/irregular), height, weight; blood pressure (supine, sitting, standing) in right arm, left arm, leg
General appearance
  Nutrition, body habitus, apparent age, color (black, white, Indian, Mexican-American, jaundice, pale), distress, obvious mental disease, constant coughing, voice abnormality, or cyanosis—note patient's behavior and movement during interview
Skin
  Normal, dry, moist, coarse, smooth, rash, scars (draw general body diagram indicating position of scars), moisture, temperature, baldness, hair amount, texture and distribution; describe lesions, abnormal pigmentations, tumors, nail changes, needle tracks, bruises, hirsutism, petechiae, purpura, telangiectasia, or nevi
Lymph nodes
  Normal, enlargement, consistency, mobility, tenderness; note anterior and posterior cervical, superclavicular, epitrochlear, axillary, inguinal, and femoral nodes; record size of nodes in centimeters if enlarged
Head
  Size, shape, symmetry, contour, tenderness, bruits; in children, check if fontanelle is closed
Eyes
  External: conjunctivae, sclerae, pupil size and reaction, ptosis, arcus senilis, protrusion, gross visual acuity, visual fields by confrontation, extraocu-

**Format for Recording Information Obtained from the Medical Interview
and from the Physical Examination — *continued***

Eyes — cont'd
 lar movements, reaction to light and accommodation, nystagmus
 Funduscopic: red reflex, lenticular opacity, optic disc, arteries, veins, hemorrhages, exudates, microaneurysms, photophobia

For visual fields by confrontation, draw diagram indicating area of abnormal field; for funduscopic abnormalities also draw diagram indicating site and type of abnormality

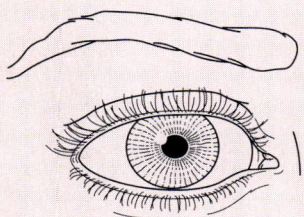
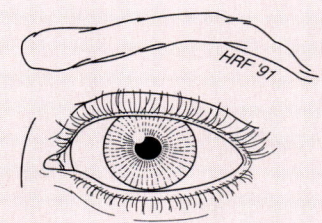

Ears
 Normal, pinna, tophi, external canal, tympanic membrane, discharge, cerumen, hearing, Weber's test, Rinne test

Nose
 Normal, septum (deviation or perforation), mucosa, airway obstruction, discharge, enlarged turbinates, polyps, sinus tenderness; if sinus disease suspected, transilluminate sinuses

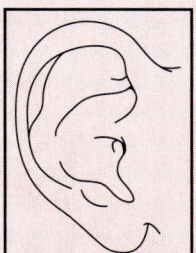
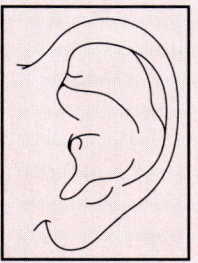

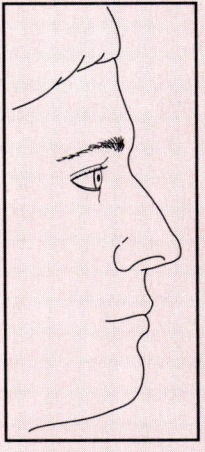

Continued.

Format for Recording Information Obtained from the Medical Interview and from the Physical Examination — continued

Mouth and throat
Normal, odor of breath, color and appearance of lips, tongue, gums; conditions of teeth including caries, dentures (remove to examine palate), tonsils, uvula, soft and hard palate, larynx, epiglottis, gentle percussion of teeth, salivary glands, rigidity or limitation of motion, thyroid, trachea, venous distention, anterior cervical nodes, submaxillary nodes, posterocervical nodes, carotid and jugular pulses, and bruits

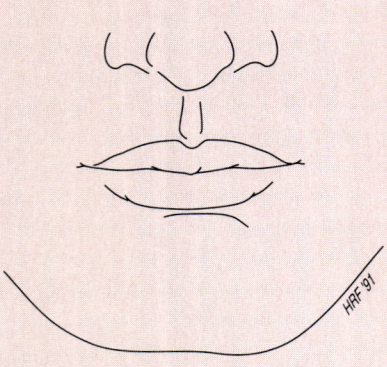
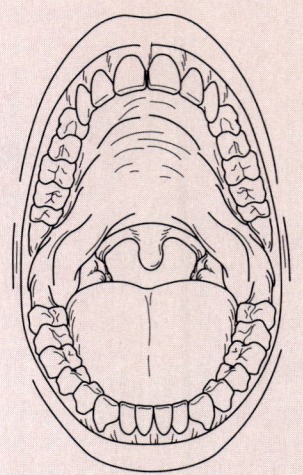

Breasts
Size, consistency, symmetry, tenderness, palpable masses, retraction, ulceration, asymmetry, dimpling, discharge from nipple, gynecomastia

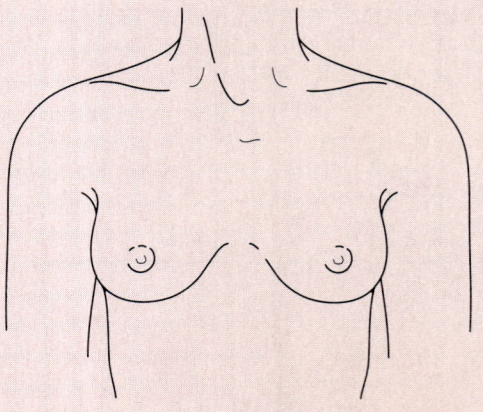

Format for Recording Information Obtained from the Medical Interview and from the Physical Examination—*continued*

Back
Mobility, kyphosis, lordosis, scoliosis, tenderness on palpation or percussion, tenderness to CVA percussion, sacral edema

Thorax
General configuration, symmetry, movement with respiration

Respiratory
Inspection: labored, shallow, Kussmaul, periodic, or other breathing; use of accessory muscles in breathing
Palpation: palpate for areas of tenderness (costochondral junctions), access respiratory excursion
Percussion: diaphragm excursion, symmetry, dullness, hyperresonance
Auscultation: crackles, wheezes, rubs, rales, rhonchi, egobronchophony, whispered, pectoriloquy, fremitus

Heart
Inspection: precordium for abnormal pulsations, heaving, or bulging; point of maximal impulse
Palpation: precordium for shocks, thrills, rubs
Percussion: heart size
Auscultation: ascultate at valve areas, rate, rhythm; quality of heart sounds; extra sounds S_4, M_1, T_1, ES, MSC, A_2, P_2, OS, S_3; draw diagram indicating timing of extra sounds, murmurs and rubs; note areas where each sound is most intense

Abdomen
Inspection: scaphoid, flat, distended, obese, dilated veins, scars, striae gravidarum; describe intrinsic movement, scars, hair distribution
Palpation: tenderness, rigidity, rebound, guarding, mass, fluid wave, hernia, liver span, spleen, kidneys, referred pain
Percussion: tympany, shifting dullness, sizes of organs or masses
Auscultation: bowel sounds (pitch, absent, rushes), rubs, bruits; note abnormalities on appropriate diagram

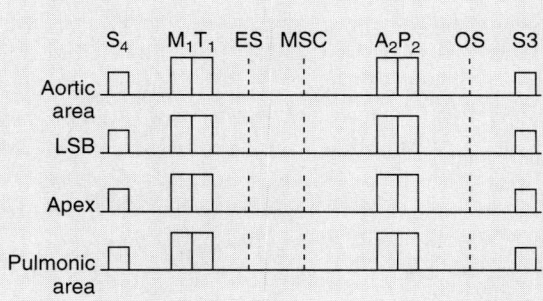
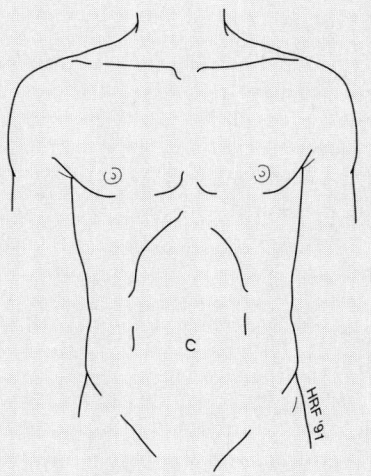

Format for Recording Information Obtained from the Medical Interview and from the Physical Examination—*continued*

Extremities
Joint swelling, tenderness, redness, heat, deformity, and limitation of motion; edema (if pitting is present, grade 1+ through 4+), cyanosis, varicosities, ulceration, clubbing, rash on palms or soles, color and temperature of legs, hair growth on legs, calf tenderness, muscle weakness, condition of nails (e.g., pitting, lines, configuration, tinea)

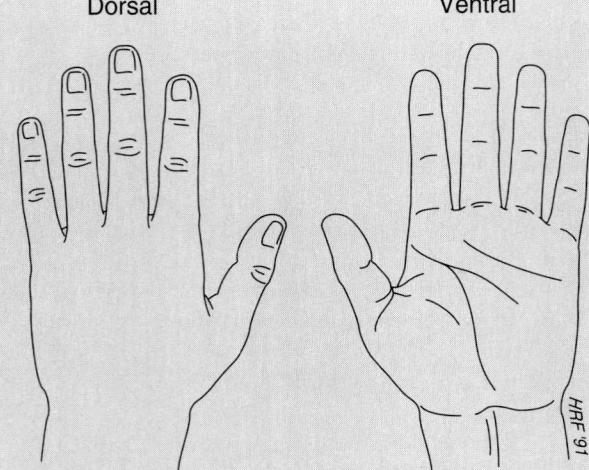

Vascular examination
Peripheral pulses: carotid, brachial, radial, femoral, popliteal, dorsalis pedis, posterior tibial; also record hyperactive, abnormal, or bruit

Male genitalia
Penis, circumcised, scrotum, hair distribution, testes (size, tenderness, masses), epididymis; transilluminate scrotal enlargements; urethral discharge (amount, color, consistency)

Female genitalia
External: hair distribution, labia, clitoris, introitus, urethra, perineum, Bartholin's glands, Skene's glands, urethra
Internal: vaginal walls and discharge, cervix, uterus (size, shape, mobility, consistency), adnexa including ovaries, cul-de-sac, pain with cervix movement, Papanicolaou's test or maturation index taken, rectal, rectovaginal exam

Rectal examination
External skin and skin tags, sphincter tone, hemorrhoidal veins, masses, presence of fecal material in rectal vault, polyps or masses, prostate (size, consistency, shape, tenderness, nodules)

Neurologic
Mental status: appearance (disordered, average, neat, bizarre), psychomotor activity (slow, average, fast), affect (average, exaggerated, labile), mood and attitude (detached, sad, suspicious, hostile, demanding, obstinate, anxious, friendly, seductive, helpless, cooperative), speech and associations (disorganized, loose, circumstantial, logical), thinking style (concrete, functional, abstract), intelligence (retarded, dull, normal, bright), memory impairment (remote, recent), judgement (poor, good), disorientation (time, place, person), insight (little, average, good), suicidal ideation (threat, attempt, no information)
Cranial nerves: (I) smell; (II) visual fields and vision; (III, IV, and VI) pupils, ptosis, EOM, nystagmus; (V) corneal, masseters, temporal, pin and touch; (VII) brow, mouth, nasolabial fold, taste; (VIII) Rinne and Weber's tests, whispered voice; (IX and X) swallow, uvula, gag, phonation; (XI) sternocleidomastoid, trapezius; and (XII) protrusion of tongue, tremor, fasciculation, atrophy

Format for Recording Information Obtained from the Medical Interview and from the Physical Examination—*continued*

Neurologic—cont'd

Reflexes: (a) stretch jaw, brachioradialis, biceps, triceps, knee, ankle; (b) superficial reflexes (abdominal, cremasteric, plantar); (c) frontal lobe reflexes (suck, snout, palmomental, grasp); note relaxation phase of stretch reflexes, normal or prolonged

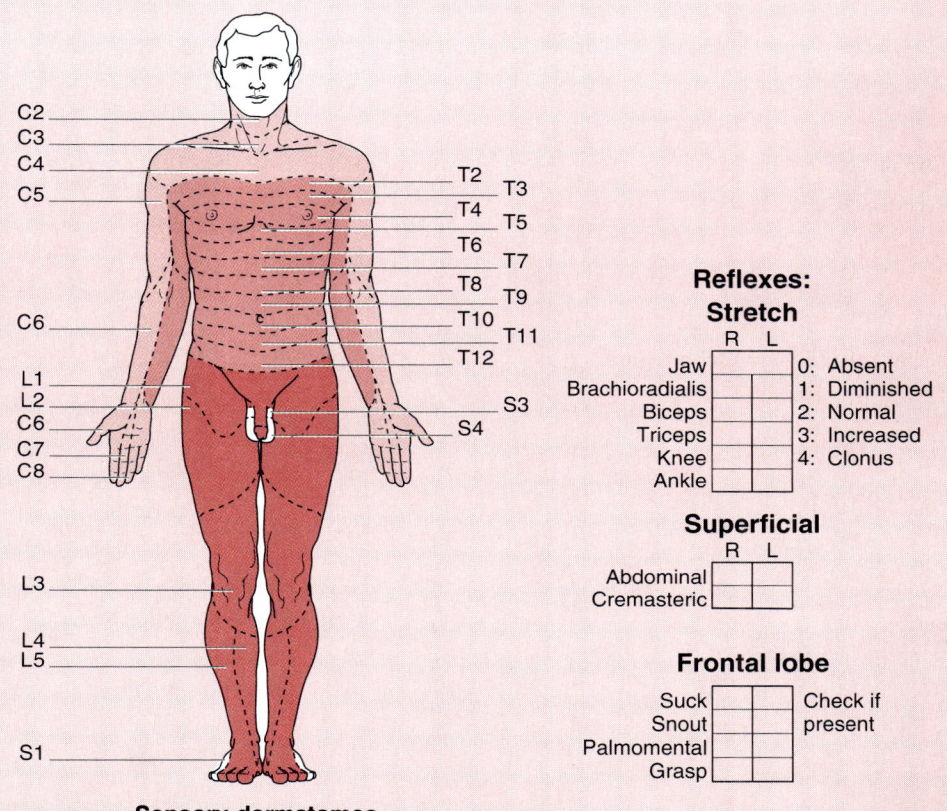

Sensory dermatomes

Motor: muscular strength (hemiparesis, hemiplegia, proximal weakness), muscular tone (flaccid, spastic, rigid, cogwheel), muscular volume (atrophy, hypertrophy), involuntary movements (tremor, dystonia, asterixis, chorea)

Coordination and cerebellar: limb (F-N, F-F, H-K, rapid alternating), gait (walk, heel, toe, tandem), Romberg (normal, abnormal), finger to nose, finger to finger

Sensory: note dermatome distribution; peripheral—pain, touch, temperature, vibration, and position; cortical—two-point discrimination and object identity; meningeal signs—Brudzinski, Kernig, neck rigidity

Synthesis

Problem list
Differential diagnosis for each major problem.
Plan for evaluation (laboratory studies, x-ray films, medication, surgical procedures).
Signature of historian
Date

CHAPTER TWO

The Head and Neck

CHAPTER OUTLINE

Eye, Ear, Nose, Mouth, and Throat

The Eye

History Taking
Loss of vision, changes in vision, complaints concerning sight
Diplopia
Eye pain
Excessive lacrimation and ocular discharge
Scotomata

Physical Examination
General inspection
Eyelids
Conjunctiva
Sclera
Globe
Cornea
Iris and pupils
Ocular motility and extraocular movements
Visual fields' testing
Funduscopic examination
Visual acuity

The Ear

History Taking
Ear pain
Hearing loss and deafness
Tinnitus
Vertigo

Physical Examination of the Ear
Earlobe
External auditory canal
Tympanic membrane
Testing hearing

The Nose

History Taking
Epistaxis
Nasal discharge
Facial pain and chronic sinusitis

Physical Examination of the Nose
Nares, turbinates, and septum
Sinuses
Miscellaneous abnormalities

The Mouth, Throat, and Neck

History Taking
Painful ulcers and sores in the mouth and tongue
Bleeding gums
Abnormal taste
Sore throat
Hoarseness
Difficulty swallowing

Physical Examination of the Mouth and Throat
Lips, mouth, buccal mucosa, gums, teeth, and palate
Tongue
Salivary glands
Pharynx
Larynx
Neck

Summary

Eye, Ear, Nose, Mouth, and Throat

Visual complaints are some of the most common reasons patients seek a physician. Loss of vision, changes in vision, and complaints concerning sight warrant careful evaluation. Specific problems such as cataract and glaucoma merit referral to an ophthalmologist. Eye trauma should alert the examiner to the possibility of corneal ulcers, abrasions, and retinal detachment. Diplopia should raise the question of a lens or corneal abnormality, cranial nerve palsies, ocular muscle problems, and even brainstem problems. The eye may also offer clues to the diagnosis of and severity of systemic diseases such as diabetes mellitus and hypertension. It is important that the examiner gain expertise in recognizing papilledema because this sign of increased intracranial pressure (ICP) mandates a thorough evaluation.

Several simple and often neglected bedside or office tests can be used to evaluate hearing. A common and often neglected cause of impaired hearing in the elderly is excess cerumen in the ear canal. If a question remains about a patient's hearing, and especially if he reports a recent, abrupt change, refer the patient for an audiogram.

Sore throat is a very common complaint and is usually caused by viral or bacterial upper respiratory infections (URIs). Hoarseness is a symptom that may reflect systemic diseases such as hypothyroidism and lung cancer. Thyroid diseases (i.e., hypothyroidism and hyperthyroidism) are quite common and must be considered in a variety of clinical settings.

THE EYE

History Taking
Loss of Vision, Changes in Vision, Complaints Concerning Sight

In evaluating complaints concerning loss of or changes in vision, it is important to ask whether such symptoms are monocular or binocular. Sudden monocular changes in vision should raise the question of disorders such as amaurosis fugax, migraine headaches, retinal detachment, retrobulbar neuritis, vitreous hemorrhage, central retinal artery occlusion, and uveitis. Binocular loss of vision may be caused by cortical blindness or hysteria, although the latter diagnosis should not be a primary initial consideration. Other important considerations in loss of vision are: (1) the time course during which the symptoms developed (i.e., sudden or gradual); and (2) what additional symptoms, if any, accompanied the visual loss.

SUDDEN LOSS OF VISION
Amaurosis Fugax

Amaurosis fugax is defined as a transient painless loss of vision in one eye indicative of retinal ischemia usually caused by ipsilateral carotid artery stenosis or embolization to the retinal artery. It is frequently recurrent. Classically, there is abrupt onset of monocular visual loss that lasts 5 to 15 minutes. The patient often states that, "It seemed as if a shade or curtain fell over my eye." If amaurosis fugax is caused by recurrent embolization from carotid artery plaques, other

Key Symptoms in the Evaluation of the Eye	
Sudden Loss of Vision, Changes in Vision, Complaints Concerning Sight • Amaurosis fugax • Migraine headaches • Retinal detachment • Vitreous hemorrhage • Retrobulbar optic neuritis • Central retinal artery occlusion • Uveitis	**Gradual Loss of Vision** • Cataracts • Glaucoma • Optic nerve compression by mass lesion • Optic neuropathies • Increased intraocular pressure • Macular degeneration • Cortical blindness • Presbyopia • Diplopia • Eye pain • Photophobia • Glaucoma • Excessive lacrimation and ocular discharge • Scotomata

lateralizing symptoms such as transient contralateral numbness, paresthesias, and weakness may be elicited in addition to visual loss.

Migraine Headaches

Migraine headaches can cause transient visual loss in one or both eyes. Accompanying symptoms usually facilitate the diagnosis of migraine. In addition to headaches, patients frequently complain of scintillating or unformed flashes of light, dazzling zigzag lines, scotomata, tinnitus, and dizziness. If evidence of bilateral visual field defects is elicited, it suggests involvement of the visual cortex in the occipital lobes. For a detailed discussion of factors triggering migraine headaches, see Chapter 10.

Retinal Detachment

Flashing lights, floating specks, halos, and blurring of vision *preceding* visual loss should suggest a retinal tear or retinal detachment.

CASE 2-1 Sudden Loss of Vision

A 29-year-old woman noted a sudden decrease in vision in her right eye. For the 2 weeks preceding this event she had also noted numbness and paresthesias in her hands and some difficulty with coordination. Physical examination revealed evidence of nystagmus and retrobulbar optic neuritis involving the right eye. In addition, there were physical findings indicative of cerebellar dysfunction (incoordination, impairment of rapid alternative movements, pastpointing). This constellation of clinical features led to detailed studies that confirmed the diagnosis of multiple sclerosis in which the cardinal symptom was sudden loss of vision in one eye.

Vitreous Hemorrhage

Vitreous hemorrhage is a fairly frequent complication of diabetic proliferative retinopathy (i.e., new vessel formation and scarring). Such vitreous hemorrhage often causes sudden blindness.

Retrobulbar Optic Neuritis

The term *retrobulbar optic neuritis* refers to a syndrome characterized by the rapid development over hours or days of impaired vision in one or both eyes. The most common cause of unilateral retrobulbar neuritis is multiple sclerosis. Other less frequent causes include encephalitis, uveitis, and central nervous system (CNS) fungal infections. Frequently, no obvious cause is evident. Characteristically, patients with retrobulbar neuritis note loss of central vision with some preservation of peripheral vision. Spontaneous recovery of vision frequently occurs within a few weeks.

Central Retinal Artery Occlusion

Central retinal artery occlusion can occur with temporal arteritis and cause sudden blindness; this is but one form of anterior ischemic optic neuropathy, a condition caused by interruption of the blood supply to the optic nerve. The diagnosis of temporal arteritis should be considered when a pentad of findings (i.e., headaches, musculoskeletal complaints [polymyalgia rheumatica], fever, anemia, and a raised erythrocyte sedimentation rate) is present. This diagnosis is frequently confirmed by noting granulomatous arteritis in temporal artery biopsy specimens.

Uveitis

Inflammation of the uveal tract (i.e., iris, ciliary body, and choroid plexus) causing uveitis can also result in abrupt loss of vision. Importantly, ocular pain is almost always present. Uveitis occurs with several disorders, including connective tissue diseases (e.g., rheumatoid arthritis, systemic lupus erythematosus [SLE]), histoplasmosis, sarcoidosis, tuberculosis, ulcerative colitis, and Behçet's syndrome.

GRADUAL LOSS OF VISION

Cataracts

Cataracts are defined as opacities in the lens. Patients with cataracts often note halos around lights, and their vision becomes blurred in bright light. The latter symptom results from increased light causing pupillary constriction, which, in the face of lenticular opacities, causes impaired vision.

Glaucoma

Glaucoma is a disorder in which elevated intraocular pressure (IOP) transmitted through the aqueous humor damages the optic nerve. It is the most common cause of gradual visual loss in individuals over age 50 years.

Optic Nerve Compression by a Mass Lesion

Intracranial neoplasms can directly involve the optic nerve and cause gradual loss of vision. Such neoplasms include meningioma, melanoma, and retinoblastoma.

CASE 2-2 Headaches and Loss of Vision

A 49-year-old man noted the gradual onset of fatigue, weight gain, and enlarging hands and feet, and his family noted that his facial features were coarsening. He also complained of headaches, decreased vision, and increased frequency of urination. Physical examination revealed facial characteristics strongly suggestive of acromegaly. Importantly, visual field testing revealed a bitemporal hemianopsia. The patient was also found to have developed diabetes. A CT scan of the head along with elevated serum growth hormone levels confirmed the diagnosis of a functioning pituitary adenoma that was impinging on the optic chiasm.

Optic Neuropathies

Several diseases can affect the optic nerve, causing an optic neuropathy and visual loss. Some of the more important causes include demyelinating diseases such as multiple sclerosis, drugs such as ethambutol, toxins such as methyl alcohol, and hereditary optic atrophy.

Increased Intraocular Pressure

Any disease process that causes increased IOP, such as intracranial mass lesions (e.g., tumor, abscess, bleeds), can result in gradual visual loss.

Macular Degeneration

Any disease process that results in macular degeneration can be expected to cause visual impairment.

CORTICAL BLINDNESS

Cortical blindness is one of the few causes of binocular irreversible blindness. It usually results from cerebrovascular insults with infarction of the visual cortex in both occipital lobes. Such patients often have other neurologic stigmata of multinfarct dementia (see Chapter 10). The diagnosis of cortical blindness should be suspected in patients with *binocular blindness* (total blindness or at best only perception of light flashes) but with preservation of pupillary responses to light and full excursion of the extraocular muscles (see below).

PRESBYOPIA

During the fifth decade and thereafter, the ability of the lens to accommodate decreases, resulting in progressive difficulty in reading, especially fine print. This change of vision, which is part of the normal aging process, is termed *presbyopia*.

Diplopia

Diplopia (Table 2-1) is defined as double vision and in its most common form the binocular fusion of images is impaired. With a complaint of double vision it is important for the examiner to first check and determine if diplopia is present with only one eye open. *Monocular diplopia* should suggest either a lens or a corneal abnormality. *Binocular diplopia* should suggest one of the following problems:

- Cranial nerve palsy
- Ocular muscle problems

TABLE 2-1: Common Eye Symptoms

Symptoms	Causes
Diplopia	• Lens or cranial abnormality
	• Cranial nerve palsy (see Table 2-2)
	• Ocular muscle problems
	• Orbital mass/inflammation
	• Myasthenia gravis
Eye pain	• Increased ICP (aneurysm, meningitis, cavernous sinus thrombosis)
	• Contiguous strictures (sinusitis)
	• Foreign body
	• Conjunctivitis
	• Iritis
	• Corneal abrasion
Photophobia	• Corneal inflammation
	• Iritis
Burning/itching	• Inflammation or irritation caused by infection, allergies, or irritants
Scotomata	• Retinal lesions
	• Demyelinating diseases
	• Intoxications (methyl alcohol)

- Orbital masses or inflammation
- Brainstem problems such as ischemia caused by vertebral basilar transient ischemic attacks

The sudden onset of diplopia suggests a problem either with an insult to the macula or with neuromuscular control of the eye position. The abrupt onset of diplopia with pain suggests either cranial nerve or orbital involvement. Diplopia without pain but with a decreased variation should raise the question of myasthenia gravis. Finally, if diplopia is binocular, the examiner should determine whether it is horizontal or vertical (see below). Some typical questions to ask are as follows:

- *Have you had changes in vision, in one eye or both eyes?*
- Has the change in your vision been gradual or abrupt?
- Have you had other symptoms with the changes in your vision? Any headaches? Flashes of light? Tinnitus? Dizziness? This constellation of clinical features suggests migraine headaches.
- *Have you experienced numbness, paresthesia, or weakness?*
- Has your transient loss of vision been associated with difficulty swallowing (dysphagia), dizziness, or transient loss of consciousness? This constellation of clinical featuures suggests TIAs.

Eye Pain

It will be recalled that the eye is innervated by the ophthalmic division of the fifth cranial nerve. Further, the dura mater is also innervated by a branch of the fifth cranial nerve; consequently, intracranial processes such as aneurysms, mass lesions, meningitis, cavernous sinus thrombosis, and migraine can give rise to eye pain. Eye pain (see Table 2-1) can also arise from contiguous structures, especially sinusitis involving the ethmoid, frontal, and sphenoid sinuses. Acute increases in IOP frequently cause deep-seated eye pain as well as blurred vision. The cornea is quite pain-sensitive, so injury to normal corneal epithelium often results in rather intense discomfort. *Photophobia,* or eye pain on exposure to light, is experienced with inflammation of the cornea, ciliary body, and iris. Therefore, with complaints of eye pain and photophobia or blurring of vision, the examiner should suspect involvement of deeper structures.

The triad of symptoms including facial pain, headache, and photophobia is common with viral infections. Burning or itching discomfort indicates inflammation or irritation caused by infections, allergies, or irritants (e.g., chemical, foreign body).

Several disorders are associated with eye pain and visible lesions. The list, by no means complete, includes:

- Conjunctivitis
- Foreign body
- Corneal ulcer
- Stye (hordeolum)
- Chalazion
- Scleritis (iritis)
- Iridocyclitis

Finally, acute increases in IOP, as frequently occurs in glaucoma, can result in eye pain.

Excessive Lacrimation and Ocular Discharge

Excessive lacrimation occurs with URIs, allergies such as hay fever and seasonal rhinitis, irritation secondary to a foreign body, and obstructed lacrimal ducts. Purulent discharge from the eye occurs with bacterial infections (staphylococci), conjunctivitis with secondary infection, hordeolum, and chalazion.

Scotomata

The term *scotomata* refers to specific areas or islands of impaired vision. A retinal lesion causes arcuate scotomata, whereas macular disease causes central scotomata and disturbed vision, especially for straight lines *(metamorphopsia)*. Optic nerve disease (demyelinating or infiltrative) causes centrocecal (macular area and blind spot) scotomata, and intoxications (methyl alcohol) causes central or centrocecal scotomata.

Physical Examination of the Eye

General Inspection

Note whether the patient uses glasses or contact lenses. Initial inspection of the eyes will disclose whether the position of both eyes is normal; whether there are any obvious abnormalities in the eyelid, conjunctiva, or cornea; and whether xanthelasma is present. These eye structures and some of the diseases affecting them are discussed in detail below (Fig. 2-1).

Eyelids

PTOSIS

Ptosis is defined as failure of the eyelids to open fully; one or both eyes can be affected. Ptosis can be congenital or occur with several disorders, including myasthenia gravis, Horner's syndrome, and encephalitis.

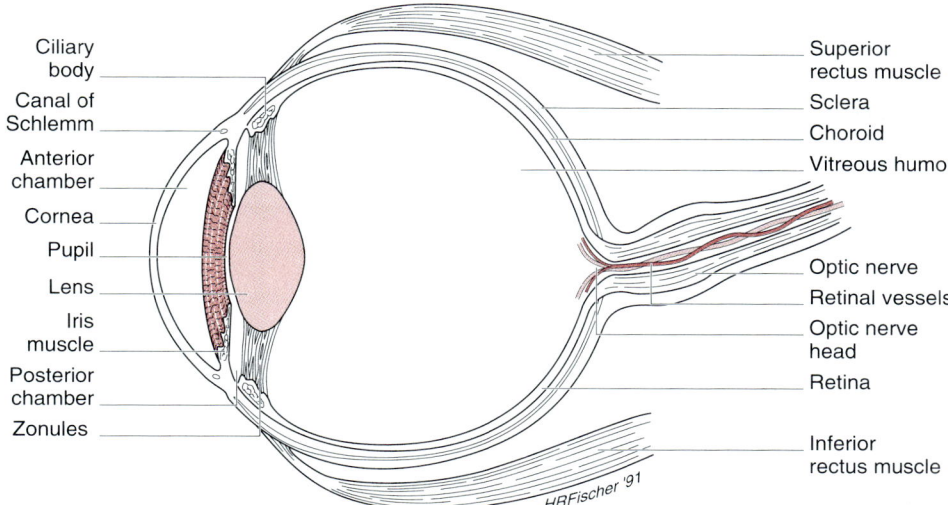

Fig. 2-1 Anatomy of the eye.

FAILURE TO CLOSE

The eyelid(s) fail to close because of partial or complete paralysis of the orbicularis oculi muscles, as occurs in Bell's palsy.

LID LAG

Lid lag is assessed by the examiner holding either his index finger or a light in the midline above the patient's eyes and then moving it downward rapidly and noting whether the globe delays in following the movement. This is also evidenced by white sclera appearing between the iris and upper lid margin.

STYE (HORDEOLUM)

A stye is a small abscess in the eyelid caused by an infection of one of the sebaceous glands of Zeis, which open into the hair follicles (Plate 1). It appears as a small pustule and is painful.

CHALAZION

Chalazion is an acute inflammation of the meibomian gland that results in a cyst and produces, in essence, an internal stye.

Conjunctiva

CONJUNCTIVITIS

Conjunctivitis is usually obvious on inspection and is caused by infections, allergies, and irritants (Plate 2). Secondary infection often results in a purulent exudate.

PETECHIAE

Conjunctival petechiae (minute reddish spots containing blood) are present in several disorders, including blood dyscrasias, clotting disorders, and bacterial endocarditis.

SUBCONJUNCTIVAL HEMORRHAGE

Subconjunctival hemorrhages are caused by extravasation of blood in the conjunctiva and occur under various conditions, including trauma (often occult), coughing, sneezing, and weight lifting. They are transient.

Sclera

The sclera is the fibrous coat of the eyeball.

SCLERITIS

Scleritis (inflammation of the sclera) occurs in several conditions, including collagen diseases such as rheumatoid arthritis and lupus erythematosus (Plate 3). Severe focal necrosis with scleritis in rheumatoid arthritis is termed *scleromalacia perforans.*

OTHER ABNORMALITIES IN DISEASE STATUS

Blue sclerae are pathognomonic of the disorder *osteogenesis imperfecta;* the blue shade results from a very thin sclera in which the choriod plexus shows through. Brown sclerae are observed in the disorder *alkaptonuria* (hereditary metabolic disorder) and are also noted in normal black men. Yellow sclerae, termed *scleral icterus,* usually indicate the presence of jaundice and should raise the question of liver disease or hemolytic anemia.

Globe

EXOPHTHALMOS

Exophthalmos is defined as prominence or protrusion of the eyeball to such an extent that the eyelid will not cover it. Bilateral exophthalmos is classically present in Graves' disease and also occurs in acromegaly and cavernous sinus thrombosis. Unilateral exophthalmos should raise the question of orbital tumor, abscess, cellulitis, or fracture. Proptosis refers to forward replacement of the eyeball (Plate 4).

EYE SIGNS IN HYPERTHYROIDISM

The eye signs of hyperthyroidism include:

- Exophthalmos
- Lid lag
- Stare
- Infrequent blinking
- Difficulty with convergence

Cornea

SCARS, ABRASIONS, AND ULCERS

Scars, abrasions, and ulcers are frequently secondary to trauma and may not be clearly evident (Plate 5). Special techniques may be required for their full assessment.

KERATOCONJUNCTIVITIS SICCA

Keratoconjunctivitis sicca is an inflammatory condition resulting from lack of tears. It is frequently associated with dry mucous membranes resulting from lack of salivary secretion (xerostomia). The triad of keratoconjunctivitis sicca, xerostomia, and rheumatoid arthritis is termed *Sjögren's syndrome.*

INTERSTITIAL KERATITIS

The triad of findings of interstitial keratitis, deafness, and notched teeth is known as *Hutchinson's triad* and is one manifestation of congenital syphilis.

ARCUS SENILIS

Arcus senilis is a gray band of opacity around the cornea and is a fairly frequent accompaniment to the aging process.

KAYSER-FLEISCHER RINGS

Kayser-Fleischer (KF) rings are circular bands of brownish pigment covering the lateral and medial margins of the cornea. They are caused by deposition of excessive amounts of copper in Descemet's membrane. Accordingly, they are found in disorders wherein excessive copper accumulates in the body, classically Wilson's disease but also primary biliary cirrhosis and primary sclerosing cholangitis.

PINGUECULAE

Pingueculae are small yellowish elevations of the conjunctiva near the corneal margin, usually on the nasal side, caused by hyaline degeneration of subconjunctival connective tissue. Brownish discoloration of pingueculae is found in Gaucher's disease.

Iris and Pupils

The pupil is the aperture in the iris through which light enters the eye (see Fig. 2-1). The iris is a thin circular disc, perforated centrally but a little to its nasal side by the pupil. The iris contains (1) the pupillary sphincteric muscle, under parasympathetic control, which constricts the pupil and (2) radiating muscle fibers, under sympathetic control, which dilate the pupil. The pupils reveal information about the integrity of the brainstem and local conditions affecting the eye. The pupils should be round, regular, and equal in size.

ANISOCORIA

The term *anisocoria* refers to unequal pupils, which can be caused by either miosis or mydriasis of one pupil (see below).

PUPILLARY REACTION TO LIGHT

Ask the patient to fixate his eyes straight ahead on a distant object. Then bring a penlight from the side obliquely across the patient's eye and note whether the pupillary response is appropriate (i.e., constriction). The lack of a direct response indicates damage to the afferent pathway—either the retina or optic nerve—and is a sensitive test of early degenerative changes in the optic nerve. Abnormal direct pupillary responses also occur with brainstem injury (see Chapter 10).

CONSENSUAL REACTION TO LIGHT

Stimulation of one eye directly normally evokes an indirect or consensual response (constriction) in the opposite eye. An absent consensual response usually indicates a lesion in the oculomotor nerve, ciliary ganglion, or Edinger-Westphal nucleus.

MARCUS GUNN PUPIL

When the examiner's pen light is switched rapidly from one eye to the other, the other eye initially constricts. The Marcus Gunn response refers to a pupil that dilates as light swings to it. In other words, pupillary constriction to an indirect response is better than that to direct light. The Marcus Gunn pupillary response indicates either severe macular disease or optic nerve disease in the affected eye.

CONVERGENCE

Convergence (inward movement of eyes along with pupillary contraction to a moving object) is tested by having the examiner position either his index finger or the patient's index finger in the midline at eye level 15 to 20 inches away. The index finger is moved to the bridge of the patient's nose, and the examiner notes whether pupillary constriction occurs, as well as the point at which convergence of the eyes stops (normally a few inches from the nose). Impaired convergence is often present in Graves' disease.

ARGYLL ROBERTSON PUPIL

The Argyll Robertson pupil indicates a form of central nervous system (CNS) syphilis (tabes dorsalis). It is characterized by the following abnormalities:
1. Weak or absent pupillary constriction on direct exposure to light
2. Normal response to accommodation
3. Failure of the pupil to dilate with painful stimulation or after administration of atropine

ADIE'S PUPIL

Adie's pupil is a pupil that is larger than its fellow and reacts poorly to light. The reaction to both light and accommodation is delayed or sluggish. It is often confused with Argyll Robertson pupil. One or both eyes may be affected.

MYDRIASIS

The term *mydriasis* refers to abnormal dilation of the pupil. Mydriasis occurs with third cranial nerve palsies (diabetes, aneurysms), increased IOP, midbrain lesions, deep coma, brain death, and often drugs such as atropine and sympathomimetic drugs. Artificial eyes can also give the appearance of mydriasis.

MIOSIS

The term *miosis* refers to abnormal constriction of the pupil. This occurs with iritis, miotic drugs (narcotics), and paralysis of the cervical sympathetic nerves.

HORNER'S SYNDROME

Horner's syndrome is characterized by ptosis, miosis, anhydrosis, and enophthalmos. It is caused by a lesion involving the superior cervical ganglion (bronchogenic carcinoma) or cervical sympathetic nerves.

Ocular Motility and Extraocular Movements

ABNORMAL POSITIONING OF THE EYES

Abnormal positioning of the eye or *nonparalytic strabismus* (squint) is seen most commonly in children. Deviation of the wandering eye inward (nasal) is termed *esotropia* and outward (temporal), *exotropia*. Abnormal positioning upward is termed *hypertropia* and downward, *hypotropia*.

NYSTAGMUS

Nystagmus is a condition in which the eyes move in a more or less rhythmic manner from side to side, up and down, or in a rotary manner from the original

TABLE 2-2: Innervations and Actions of the Extraocular Muscles (see also Fig. 2-2)

Eye Muscle	Innervation	Primary Action	Defect with Nerve Palsy
(1) Medial rectus	Oculomotor (III)	• Adduction (eye moves nasally)	Oculomotor (III) nerve palsy classically results in ptosis and inability to elevate or adduct the eyes. Common causes include diabetes, aneurysms, and midbrain lesions.
(2) Inferior rectus	Oculomotor (III)	• Depression (eye moves downward)	
(3) Superior rectus	Oculomotor (III)	• Elevation (eye moves upward) • Adduction	
(4) Inferior oblique	Oculomotor (III)	• Elevation • Abduction • Extorsion	
(5) Superior oblique	Trochlear (IV)	• Depression • Intorsion • Abduction	
(6) Lateral rectus	Abducens (VI)	• Abduction (eye moves temporally away from nose)	Affected eye cannot cross the midline on lateral gaze.

The mnemonic LR_6SO_4 indicates that the lateral rectus is innervated by the sixth cranial nerve and the superior oblique is innervated by the fourth cranial nerve. The other four ocular muscles are innervated by the third cranial nerve.

point of fixation. The to-and-fro movements are of two types, jerk and pendular. *Jerk* refers to alternating slow drift and quick corrective movements, whereas *pendular* refers to smooth oscillations. The pattern of nystagmus may be horizontal, vertical, rotary, or mixed. A few nystagmoid jerks can be normal at the extreme position of lateral gaze. Sustained nystagmus, however, is always abnormal. The new development of nystagmus should raise the question of several disorders, such as:

- Demyelinating disease (multiple sclerosis)
- Labyrinthitis (viral/bacterial)
- Drugs (phenytoin)
- Wernicke-Korsakoff syndrome
- Ménière's disease
- Brain tumors

EXTRAOCULAR MOVEMENTS AND CRANIAL NERVE PALSIES

It will be recalled that (1) the medial and lateral rectus muscles are responsible for movement of the eye in a horizontal mode, (2) the superior and inferior rectus muscles are the effectors for movement in a vertical plane, and (3) the superior and inferior oblique muscles are responsible for rotational movements of the eye (Table 2-2).

The term *conjugate* gaze means that both eyes move in the same direction, whereas *disconjugate* gaze indicates a divergence in eye movement. A *gaze palsy* is defined as an inability to look in a given direction. The extraocular movements are tested by asking the patient to follow either the examiner's index finger or a test object as it is moved through the six cardinal positions of gaze (Fig. 2-2): (1) upward, (2) downward, (3) to the upper right, (4) to the lower right, (5) to the

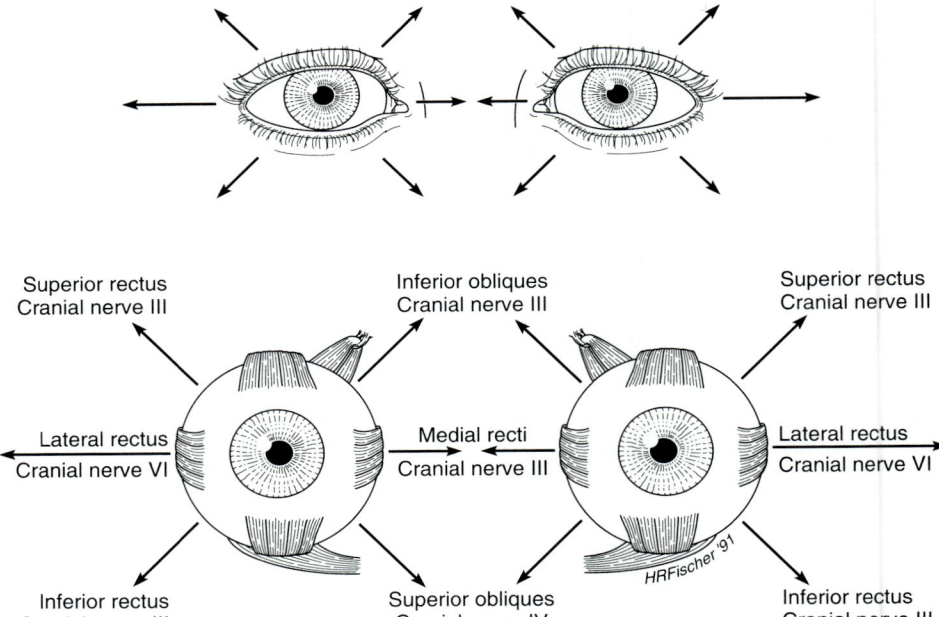

Fig. 2-2 The six cardinal positions of gaze.

upper left, and (6) to the lower left. A weakness in specific extraocular muscles usually indicates a problem in the cranial nerves that innervate them. For example, the levator palpebrae, superior, medial, and inferior rectus, and inferior oblique muscle are innervated by CN III. Thus, a third nerve palsy classically results in ptosis and inability to elevate or adduct the eyes. Common causes of third nerve palsies include diabetes mellitus, aneurysms, and midbrain lesions at the level of the superior colliculus. The superior oblique muscle is innervated by CN IV, and the lateral rectus by CN VI; a lesion affecting the latter cranial nerve results in paralysis of lateral gaze.

Finally, convergence is tested by having the patient focus on the examiner's finger as a test object as it is moved in the midline to a point close (2 to 3 inches) to the patient's nose.

DIPLOPIA

Please review the background material on diplopia, above. When testing extraocular movements and for cranial nerve palsies, the patient should be asked whether he sees one finger or two as the examiner's finger is moved through the six cardinal positions of gaze.

Visual Fields' Testing

The visual fields are initially assessed by confrontation testing (Fig. 2-3). You should stand about 2 to 3 feet in front of the patient and ask him to fix his gaze on your nose with one eye while he covers the other eye with the palm of his hand. The visual fields are divided into four quadrants by imaginary horizontal and vertical lines passing through the reference point, the nose. Begin by positioning one finger to the extreme temporal side of the field being tested. Ask the patient when he can just see your finger. Next ask him to indicate when your finger is moving and when it stops. Finally, test whether the patient can identify one, two, or three fingers that you may display. This sequence is repeated with the opposite

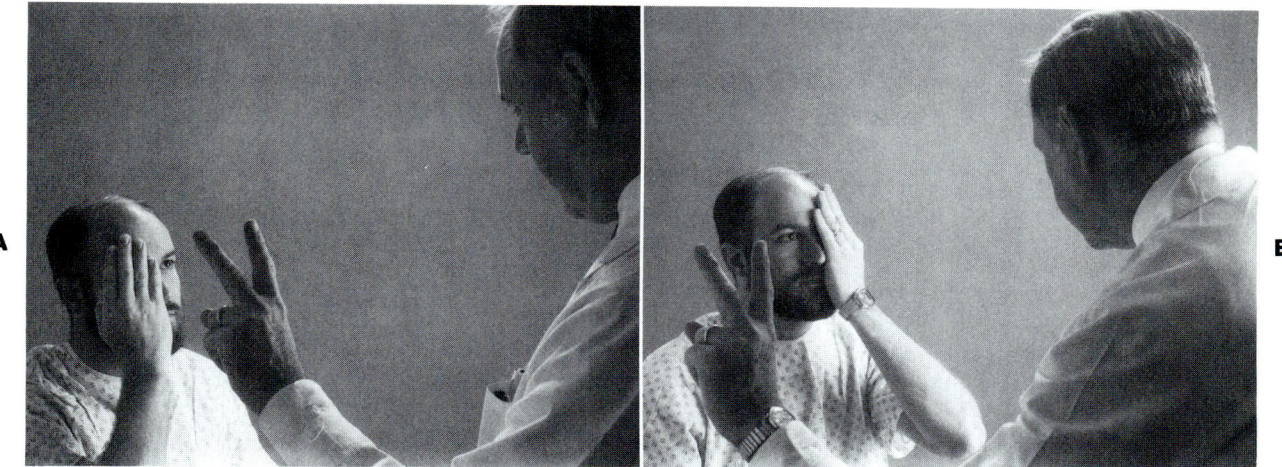

index finger assessing the nasal visual field of the same eye. After the horizontal fields for one eye have been tested, assess the vertical fields in the same manner. This entire sequence is then repeated for the opposite eye.

Fig. 2-3 Visual field testing by confrontation. Note in **A** that the examiner's two fingers are just coming into view in the nasal field of the left eye. In **B**, the two fingers are coming into view in the temporal field of the right eye.

VISUAL FIELD DEFECTS

A schematic representation of the common visual field defects is shown in Fig. 2-4.

Complete Monocular Blindness

Complete monocular blindness can be caused by a lesion in the optic nerve or retina.

Bitemporal Hemianopsia

Bitemporal hemianopsia is caused by a lesion, such as a pituitary tumor, at the optic chiasm.

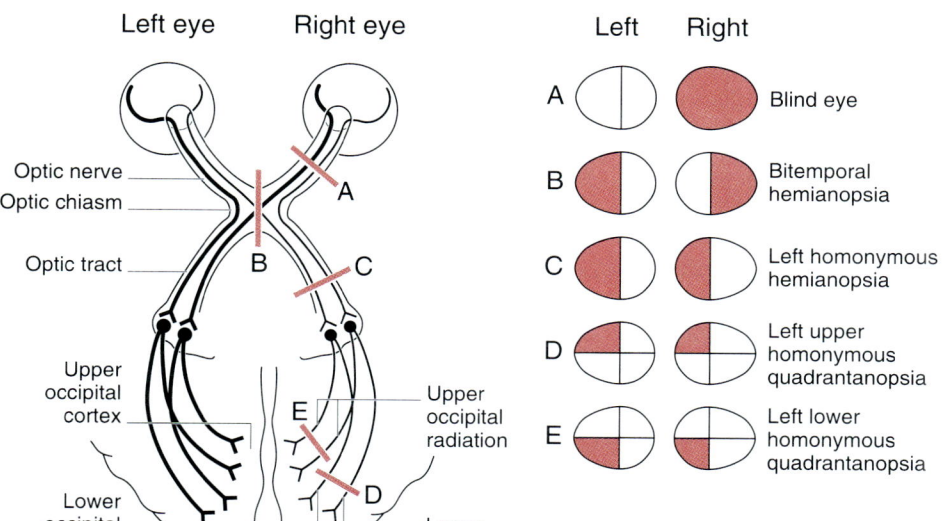

Fig. 2-4 Visual pathways from the retina to the occipital cortex. The effect of the fields of vision produced by lesions at various points along the optic pathway is shown on the right.

Homonymous Hemianopsia

Homonymous hemianopsia, which consists of a temporal field cut in one eye and a nasal field cut in the opposite eye, is commonly caused by a lesion in the optic tract, as may occur after a middle cerebral artery thrombosis or embolism.

Nasal Hemianopsia

Nasal hemianopsia is usually caused by an ipsilateral lesion in the optic nerve.

Quadrant Hemianopsia (Quadrantanopsia)

The loss of a quarter of a visual field is termed a *quadrant hemianopsia* or a *quadrantanopsia* and may reflect a lesion in the optic radiations past the geniculate body. Such a defect may be caused by a brain neoplasm.

Homonymous Hemianopsia with Central Vision Preserved

Homonymous hemianopsia can occur, but with central vision preserved.

Funduscopic Examination

TECHNIQUE

The funduscopic examination should be carried out with the room darkened. Alternatively, a 10% phenylephrine solution can be used to achieve pupillary dilation. The patient should be sitting facing you. Ask him to look straight ahead with both eyes fixating on a distant object. Hold the ophthalmoscope in your right hand when examining the patient's right eye. Place your left hand on the patient's forehead and use the thumb to retract the eyelid, expose the pupil, and prevent blinking. Use the right eye to examine the patient's right eye. Initially set the lens at +8 or +10 diopters and hold the instrument about 10 to 12 inches from the patient's eye. Shine it into the pupil to detect the normal red reflex. Move the ophthalmoscope nearer the eye while observing the cornea and lens and gradually reducing the lens power. The optimal magnification will vary, but in the absence of refractive error in you and patient, the retina will usually be in clear focus when the lens power is zero. This entire process is repeated for examination of the left eye. The technique of the ophthalmoscope examination is illustrated in Fig. 2-5.

THE RED REFLEX

The normal red reflex will not be visible if lens cataracts are present. Rather, black spots or shadows will be observed. Drusen are small hyaline bodies appearing behind the retina.

OPTIC NERVE HEAD

The optic nerve fibers arise from cells in the ganglionic layer of the retina and pass in a compact bundle, approximately 25 mm long, from the back of the eye to the optic chiasma (Fig. 2-6). The optic disc is round or oval vertically and appears as a yellowish white plate with clearly defined margins. The center of the optic disc is white in comparison with the periphery and constitutes the physiologic cup. It is white because it lacks nerve fibers. Retinal vessels (arteries and veins) enter and emerge from the optic disc. Because this area is also devoid of nerve fibers it appears pale yellow (Plate 6-A).

In optic atrophy, the optic disc appears white (Plate 6-B); this can occur with demyelinating diseases such as multiple sclerosis, chorioretinitis, and tabes dorsalis.

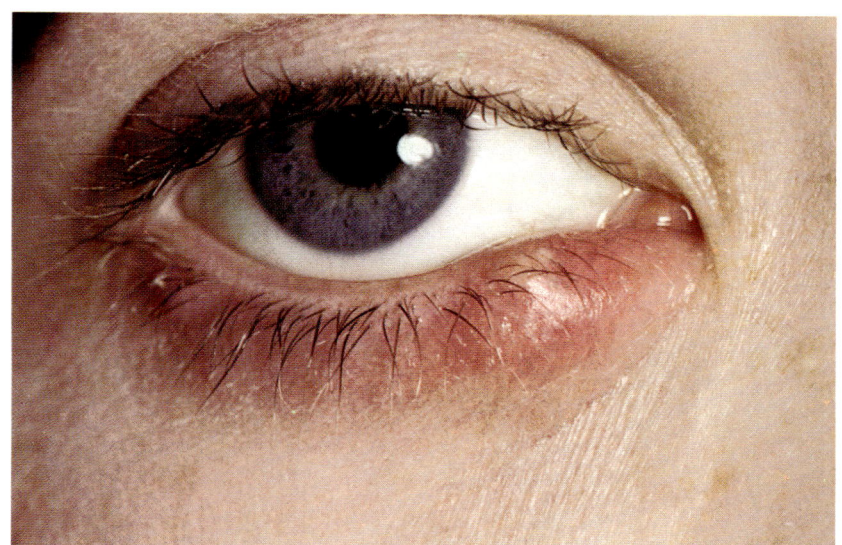

Plate 1 Sty. (From Bedford MA: *Color atlas of ophthalmological diagnosis,* ed 2, St Louis/London, 1986, Mosby-Year Book/Wolfe).

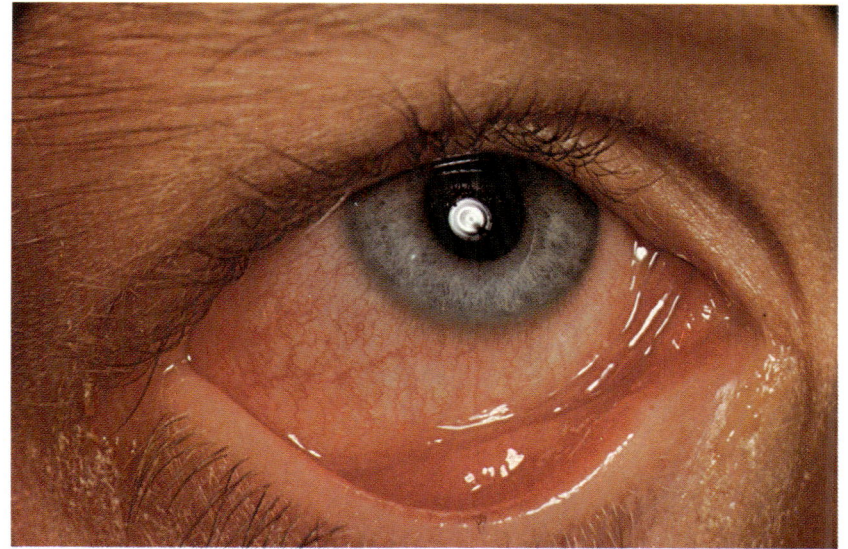

Plate 2 Conjunctivitis. (From Bedford MA: *Color atlas of ophthalmological diagnosis,* ed 2, St Louis/London, 1986, Mosby-Year Book/Wolfe).

Plate 3 Scleritis.
(From Bedford MA: *Color atlas of ophthalmological diagnosis,* ed 2, St Louis/London, 1986, Mosby-Year Book/Wolfe).

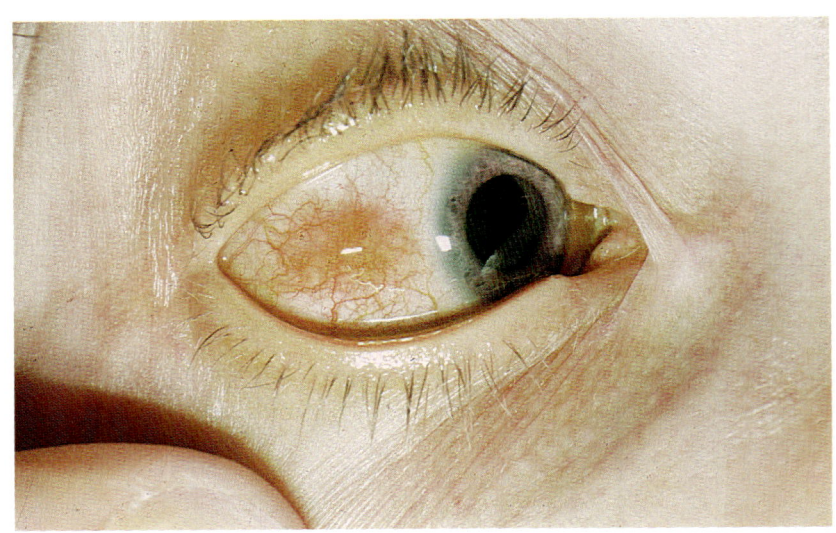

Plate 4 Proptosis in hyperthyroidism.
(From Bedford MA: *Color atlas of ophthalmological diagnosis,* ed 2, St Louis/London, 1986, Mosby-Year Book/Wolfe).

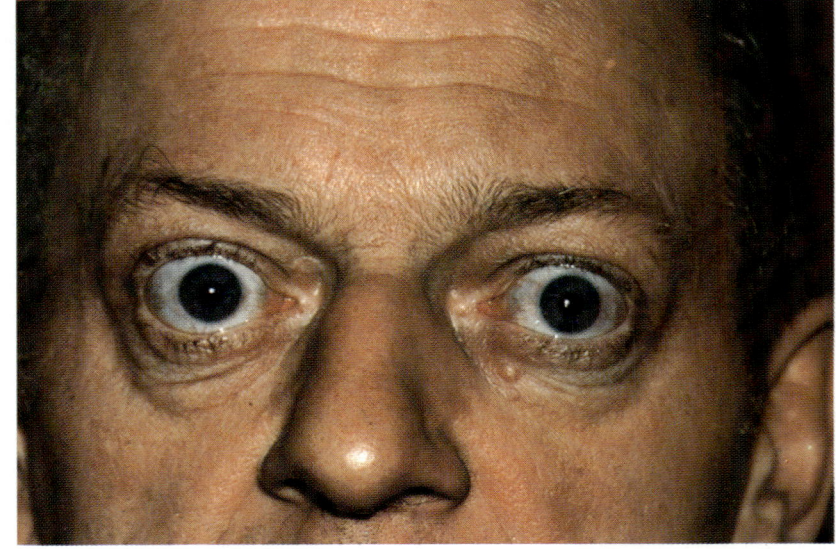

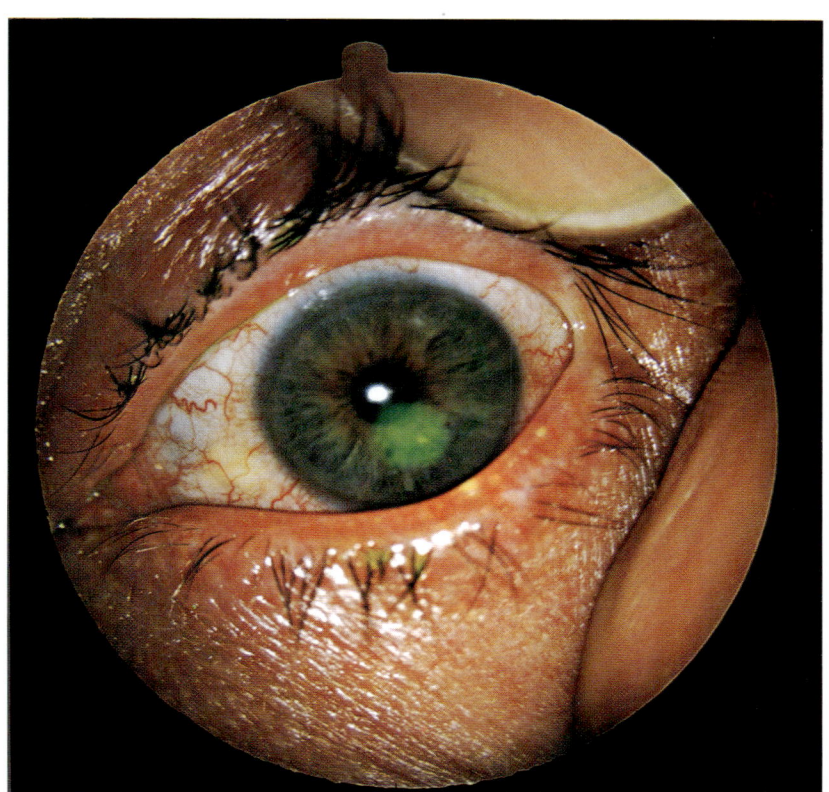

Plate 5 Traumatic corneal ulcer.
(From Bedford MA: *Color atlas of ophthalmological diagnosis,* ed 2, St Louis/London, 1986, Mosby-Year Book/Wolfe).

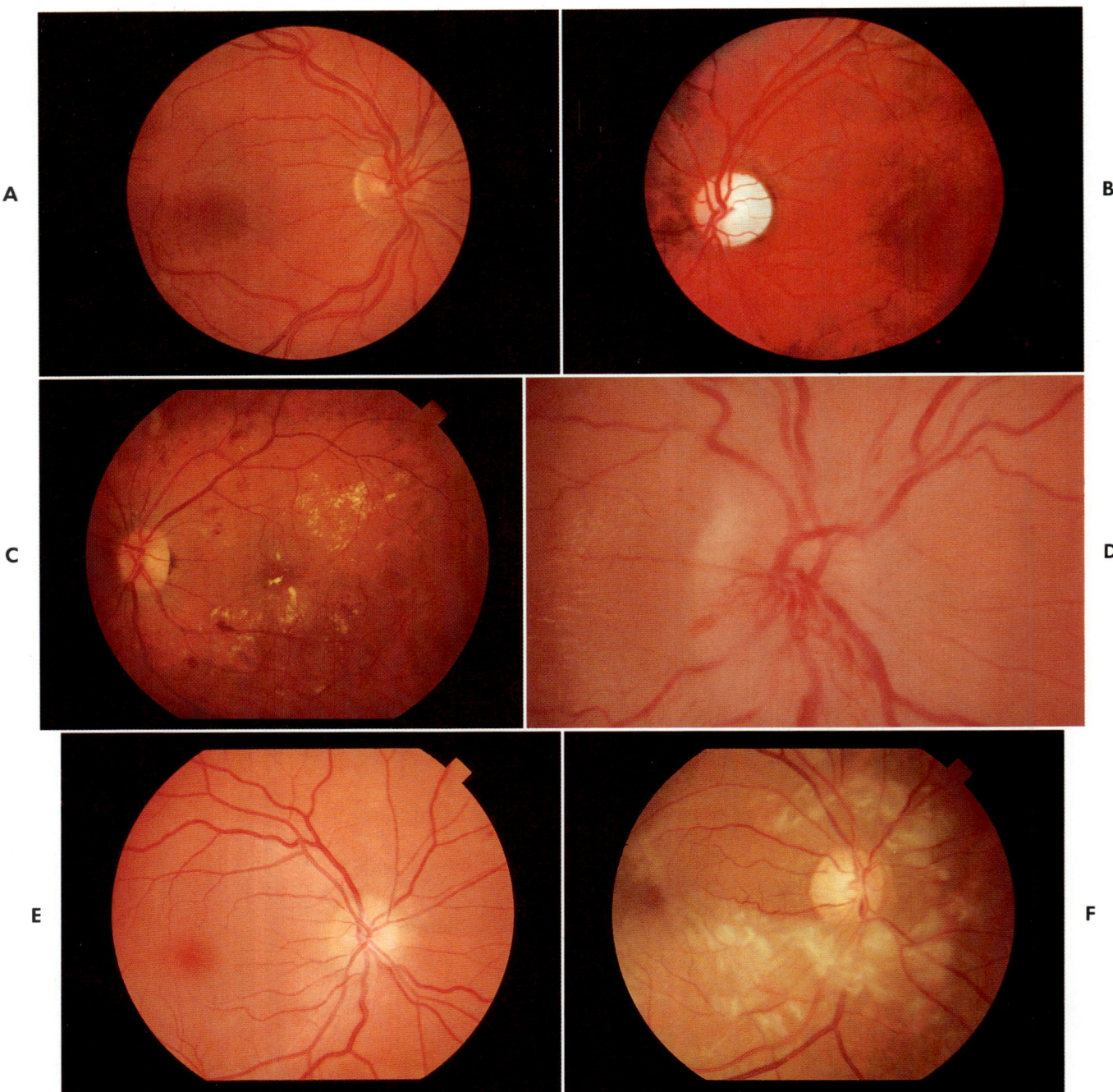

Plate 6 Fundus views. **A,** Normal fundus. **B,** Optic atrophy. Note extreme pallor of optic nerve head. **C,** Diabetic retinopathy. Note microaneurysms, dot hemorrhages, and yellow exudates. **D,** Papilledema. Note indistinct or blurred margins of the optic disc as well as vessel engagment. **E,** Pseudotumor cerebri. Note blurring of disc margins. **F,** Hypertensive retinopathy with grade 3 changes. Note arteriolar narrowing and cotton wool exudates.

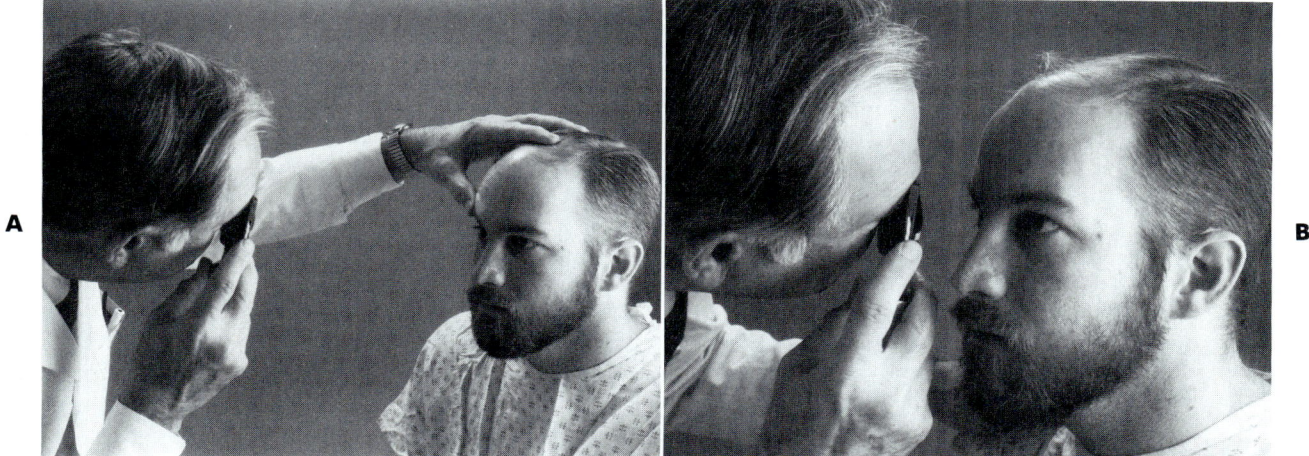

Fig. 2-5 Technique of funduscopic examination.

VESSELS

The retinal arteries and veins are branches of the superior and inferior nasal and temporal arteries and veins. The retinal arteries are bright red, pulseless, and contain a thin bright line running along the middle, which is light reflected from the vessel wall. The retinal veins are darker red and may pulsate; these lack the central stripe (see Plate 6-A). The veins are a bit wider than the arteries, with a ratio of 4:3. This ratio is altered by narrowing of the arteries (as in hypertension), dilation of the veins (as in congestive heart failure), dysproteinemias, and in hypoxemic COPD. The areas where veins and arteries cross should be observed carefully for venous nicking or tapering (see Plate 6-A).

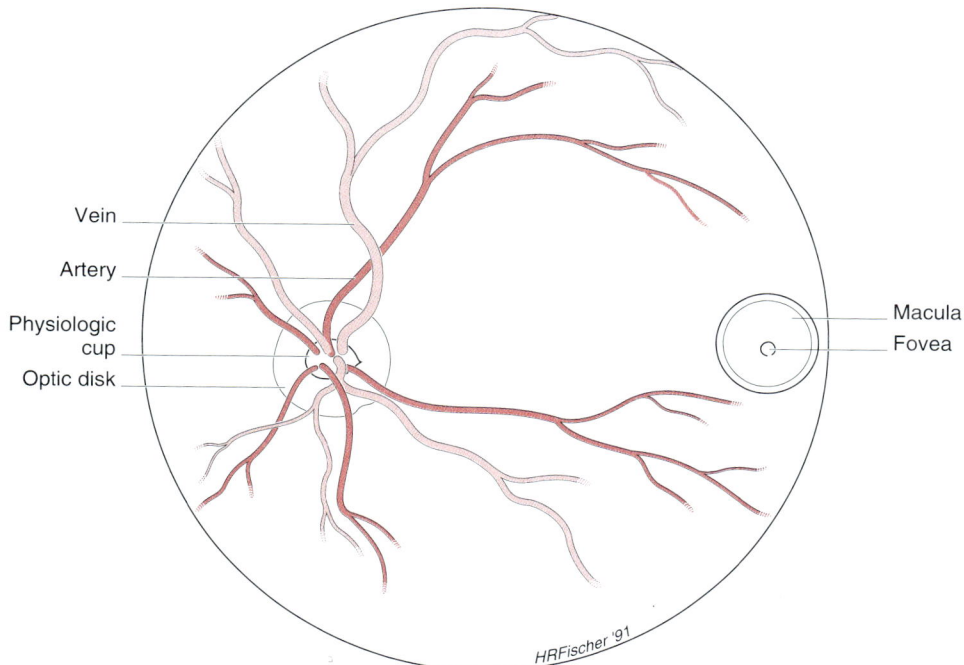

Fig. 2-6 Optic nerve head: retinal landmarks.

MACULA

The macula is that area of the retina containing yellow luteal pigment. It is approximately 2 to 5 mm in diameter, lies 3 mm (2 to 3 disc diameters) lateral to the optic disc, and appears as a smaller, darker red area in the retina. The fovea centralis lies in the center of the macula and is responsible for accurate central vision (see Plate 6-A). Examination of the macula is often difficult because illumination of this area causes discomfort. Macular degeneration is an important cause of progressive visual loss.

HEMORRHAGES

Retinal hemorrhages are observed most commonly in the accelerated phase of hypertension and diabetes mellitus. Less common causes of retinal hemorrhages include bacterial endocarditis, leukemias, hemostatic disorders, SLE, and retinal vein thrombosis. Flame-shaped hemorrhages are more characteristic of hypertension, whereas the "dot-and-blot" hemorrhages are more commonly found in diabetes. The dot-and-blot hemorrhages may be difficult to distinguish from microaneurysms, which are distinct round red spots (often present in clusters) characteristic of diabetic retinopathy. In proliferative diabetic retinopathy new vessels (neovascularization) may be seen both near the optic disc and in the periphery. It bears emphasizing that the retina must be examined carefully in all diabetic persons for stigmata of diabetic retinopathy (Plate 6-C).

Small hemorrhagic spots with central white areas *(Roth's spots)* were originally described in bacterial endocarditis but may also occur in collagen diseases, dysproteinemias, leukemias, and pernicious anemia.

EXUDATES

Two types of exudates may be seen. The first, "soft" or *cotton wool* exudates, are gray to white areas with ill-defined fluffy borders resembling small clouds. They result from infarcts of the retina caused by occlusion of the arterioles and occur in the accelerated phase of hypertension as well as in other disorders of the microcirculation. *Hard exudates* are dense, well-defined, creamy white spots with sharp edges. They are formed by lipid-laden macrophages deep in the retina in the site of old hemorrhages. Hard exudates are observed in chronic renal failure and diabetes mellitus.

PAPILLEDEMA AND PAPILLITIS

Papilledema is defined as swelling or edema of the optic disc caused by increased ICP. The increased ICP effects compression of the central vein of the retina, so return of blood from the eye is impaired. In its early stage, papilledema may be difficult to recognize with certainty. The earliest sign of papilledema is usually engorgement of the retinal veins. Subsequently, the upper and lower nasal disc margins become blurred, the physiologic cup is observed, the temporal margins of the disc become blurred, and pulsations in the veins disappear (Plate 6-D). The major causes of papilledema include brain tumors, malignant hypertension (see below), hydrocephalus, benign intracranial hypertension (pseudotumor cerebri) (Plate 6-E), meningitis, and subarachnoid hemorrhage.

Swelling of the optic disc also occurs in *papillitis,* which is an inflammation of the optic disc or nerve head. Papillitis causes edema of the disc that is indistinguishable from papilledema. However, in contrast to papilledema, visual loss occurs, with scotomas or additional blind spots in the central part of the visual field. Whereas papilledema is nearly always bilateral, papillitis is frequently unilateral. The more frequent causes of papillitis are listed above under the discussions of retrobulbar neuritis, uveitis, and optic neuropathies.

HYPERTENSIVE CHANGES

Systemic hypertension often produces characteristic changes in the retinal vessels (Plate 6-F). Accordingly, the fundi must be carefully examined in all hypertensive patients and especially in patients with accelerated hypertension. Listed below is a system for classifying retinal changes in hypertension:

Grade 1: Focal narrowing of arteries and arterioles.

Grade 2: Generalized narrowing of arteries and arterioles is present, resulting in abnormal vein:artery ratios grade of 3:2. This is often associated with AV nicking and crossing defects. Recall that the arteries and veins share a common sheath, and in arteriosclerosis and/or hypertension, the artery crossing the vein causes the blood flow in the vein to be impaired so that it appears to be capped.

Grade 3: In addition to the above changes, hemorrhages and soft exudates are also present.

Grade 4: In addition to the preceding changes, papilledema is present.

The above findings are illustrated in Plate 6-F.

Retinal signs of arteriolar sclerosis are often present along with the above noted hypertension changes. In addition to the AV nicking and crossing defects, sheathing, or "copper wiring," of the arterioles may be evident.

RETINAL ARTERY AND RETINAL VEIN OCCLUSION

The funduscopic appearances of retinal artery and venous occlusions are shown in Plate 6. Occlusion of the retinal artery classically results in retinal pallor, narrowed retinal arteries, retinal veins that are nonpulsatile, and later on, a cherry-red spot at the macula. The more common causes of retinal artery occlusion include vasculitis (as occurs in temporal arteritis and LE), embolization from a plaque in the carotid artery, dysproteinemias, and cryoglobulinemia. Central retinal vein occlusion results in engorged and tortuous veins that are often disrupted, giving the appearance of railroad "box cars." Edema of the optic disc is often present. The major causes of central retinal vein occlusion include dysproteinemias, polycythemia rubra vera, and sickle cell disease.

MISCELLANEOUS

Angioid streaks appear as pigmented lines radiating outward from the optic disc; they superficially resemble blood vessels. They are classically observed in pseudoxanthoma elasticum.

Visual Acuity

Visual acuity can be checked in several ways. The simplest test is to have the patient read from a newspaper or magazine. In an office setting, ask the patient to read from a standard Snellen eye chart (Fig. 2-7). The results are usually expressed as a fraction, with the numerator being the last line read correctly and the denominator the distance at which the line should be read by a normal person.

If a patient cannot read newsprint or from an eye chart, hold up fingers to see if they can be accurately identified. If the patient cannot identify them, then flash a light beam across the patient's eyes. If the latter is not perceived and the extraocular movements are preserved, suspect cortical blindness. In this setting, the extraocular muscles can be assessed by tapping the side of the patient's head and asking him to look in that direction.

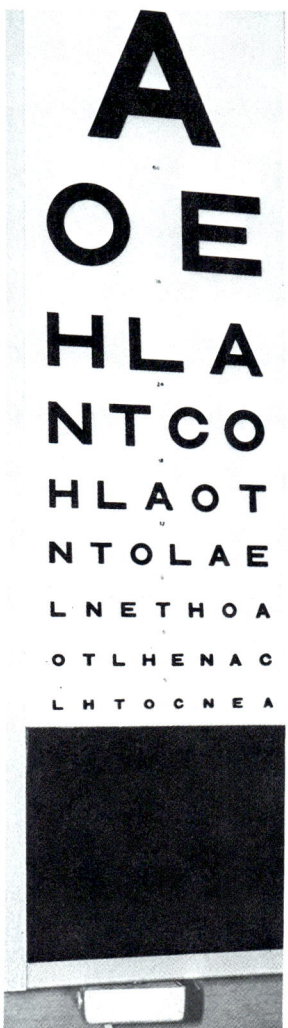

Fig. 2-7 Snellen eye chart. (From Bedford MA: *Color atlas of ophthalmological diagnosis,* ed 2, St Louis/London, 1986, Mosby-Year Book/Wolfe).

THE EAR

History Taking

Ear Pain

Ear pain may be caused by disease processes involving the external auditory canal, tympanic membrane, middle ear, or contiguous structures such as the mastoid part of the temporal bone. Ear pain may also be *referred* from infected teeth, pharyngeal lesions, and temporomandibular joint (TMJ) problems such as occur in rheumatoid arthritis. However, the most common causes of ear pain are inflammation or injury to the external auditory canal and infections of the middle ear. In this connection, external otitis can be caused by:

- Bacterial infections
- Fungal infections
- Swimmer's ear
- Foreign body
- Trauma
- Contact dermatitis
- Herpes zoster
- Trigeminal neuralgia

Otitis media can be either suppurative or serous. *Suppurative* otitis media is nearly always associated with a severe earache. *Serous* otitis media, in which serous fluid accumulates behind the tympanic membrane, is frequently present with URIs, viral exanthems, tonsillitis, and sinusitis. *Mycoplasma pneumoniae* infections may cause a bullous myringitis resulting in ear pain. Finally, a blocked eustachian tube, which can occur with many of the above disease processes, frequently results in ear pain or a very discomforting full feeling in the ear.

Hearing Loss and Deafness

Hearing loss is usually classified as either *conductive* or *perceptive;* the latter is also termed *sensorineural*. Virtually any disease process involving the external auditory canal, tympanic membrane, and osseous bones in the middle ear can interfere with sound transmission and cause a conductive hearing loss. By contrast, sensorineural deafness usually results from abnormalities in the cochlear end organ or auditory nerve. Lesions in the auditory cortex may result in an inability to interpret what is heard; this is termed a *central* hearing loss.

Patients of all ages should be asked about their hearing, and simple tests to

Key Symptoms in the Evaluation of the Ear	
Ear pain	Tinnitus
Hearing loss and deafness	Vertigo

assess their hearing then carried out (see below). The common causes of hearing loss in adults include:

- Presbycusis caused by degenerative changes in the middle ear
- Otosclerosis
- Ménière's disease
- Excess cerumen in the auditory canal
- Ototoxic drugs (aminoglycosides)
- Cerebellopontine angle tumors

The most common causes of hearing loss in infants and children include:

- Maternal infection during pregnancy (rubella)
- Chronic suppurative otitis media
- Ototoxic drugs
- Bacterial meningitis

Cholesteatoma (epidermoid cyst or tumor usually arising in the middle ear or mastoid) is a treatable cause of hearing loss in children and adolescents. Excess cerumen in the auditory canal is a common cause of decreased hearing in the elderly.

Tinnitus

Tinnitus is a continuous sound, usually described as ringing, in one or both ears and is perceived as originating inside the head. Buzzing, hissing, humming, whistling, roaring, or clicking sounds are also frequently reported. Tinnitus occurs as a result of disease processes involving CN VIII and the inner ear and its neural pathways and connections. Tinnitus occurs with acute labyrinthitis, Ménière's disease, and hearing loss from a variety of causes, but especially chronic exposure to loud noises. The complaint of a chronic, pulsating feeling in the ears (i.e., pulsatile tinnitus) should raise the question of a glomus tumor; the latter is characterized as a fibrovascular tumor arising from glomus bodies in the bulb of the internal jugular vein.

Vertigo

Vertigo is the sensation that the outer world is revolving about oneself (*objective* vertigo) or that one is moving in space (*subjective* vertigo). Vertigo, often perceived as a sense of rotation or motion, is variably described as spinning, turning, moving, veering, or following in a circular direction. Patients often complain that their surroundings seem to be whirling about them or that they are in motion when they obviously are not. Vertigo is associated with middle ear disease, disorders of the labyrinthine system, eye disorders, and cerebellar disease. Vertigo occurs commonly with acute toxic labyrinthitis, which in turn often follows viral URI. Ménière's disease, characterized by the triad of hearing loss, tinnitus, and vertigo, is frequently accompanied by nausea, vomiting, and nystagmus. The vertigo present in Ménière's disease is often intermittent and intense.

Benign positional vertigo is a disorder in which transient attacks of vertigo are induced by movements of the head and trunk. For example, looking upward with marked dorsiflexion of the head, turning over in bed, lying down, and sitting in certain positions may cause symptoms. Importantly, attacks can often be induced by asking the patient to carry out the maneuver thought to produce the symptoms.

Finally, in all patients with complaints that sound vertiginous, the examiner must determine whether such complaints actually reflect unsteadiness of gait, postural dizziness or light-headedness, or syncopal episodes.

Physical Examination of the Ear

Earlobe

The earlobe or auricle cartilage may fail to develop; this is termed *microtia*. The auricle should be palpated for the presence of *tophi* (nodular deposits), which, if present, would suggest the diagnosis of gout. In relapsing polychondritis the auricular cartilage undergoes repeated inflammation; consequently, the auricle may be intermittently swollen and red.

External Auditory Canal (Fig. 2-8 and 2-9)

To examine the external auditory canal with the otoscope, first gently pull the auricle up and backward to straighten the canal. Check the canal for excess cerumen, furuncles, and evidence of otitis externa; the latter should be excluded in swimmers and all patients complaining of earaches. Foreign bodies will be obvious.

Tympanic Membrane (see Fig. 2-8 and 2-9)

Check the tympanic membrane for color, integrity, perforation, and evidence of previous infections and/or perforations, which may have resulted in a scarred eardrum. A tympanic membrane that is bulging usually has fluid behind it. A serous effusion gives rise to clear fluid, a suppurative effusion to cloudy yellow fluid, and blood to reddish-brown fluid. As noted above, a bullous inflammation of the tympanic membrane *(bullous myringitis)* is occasionally seen in patients with a *Mycoplasma pneumonia* infection.

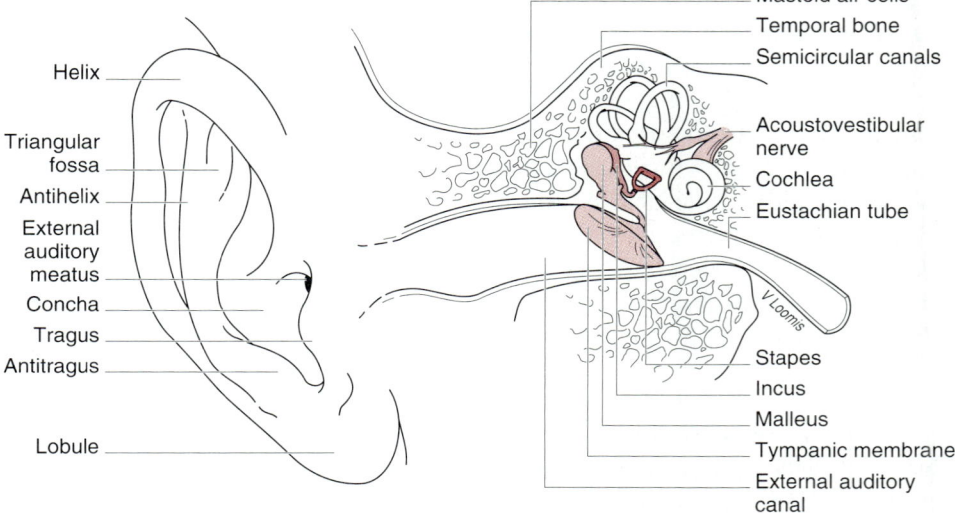

Fig. 2-8 Anatomy of the external, middle, and inner ear.

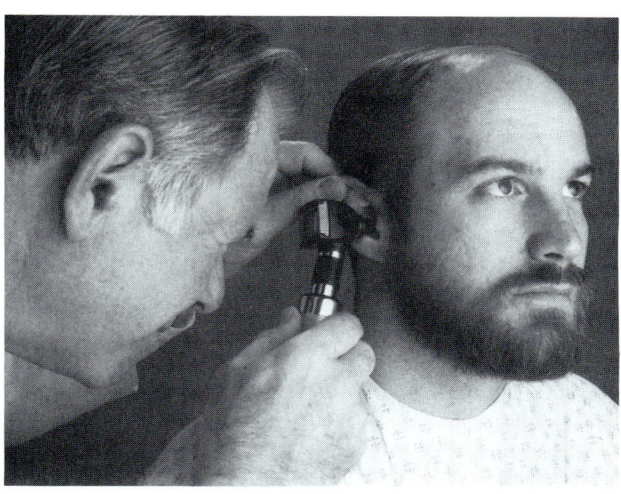

Fig. 2-9 Technique for examining the external auditory canal and tympanic membrane.

Testing Hearing

Some simple bedside or office tests of hearing include the following:

- Rubbing the index finger and thumb together 1 to 2 inches from the patient's ear
- Determining whether the patient can hear a ticking watch or tuning fork
- Determining whether the patient can hear your whispered voice

If a question remains about a patient's hearing and especially if there has been a recent, abrupt change, refer the patient for an audiogram.

The Rinne and Weber's tests can be used to further define hearing loss (Fig. 2-10). For the *Rinne test,* assess the patient's ability to hear a tuning fork by holding the tuning fork near the auricle (AC, or air conduction) and then placing it over the mastoid process (BC, or bone conduction). Normally, sound conducted through air is perceived longer and more clearly than is sound conducted through bone (AC > BC). If BC is > AC, this reversal indicates either middle ear disease or a conductive hearing loss. For *Weber's test,* place a vibrating tuning fork in the middle of the forehead. If the tuning fork is perceived better in one ear (i.e., lateralizes), this suggests either a conductive hearing loss in that ear or a sensorineural loss in the opposite ear.

Fig. 2-10 Rinne and Weber's tests. In **A**, note the tuning fork placed on the midforehead. In **B**, the tuning fork is placed over the mastoid process. For details, see text.

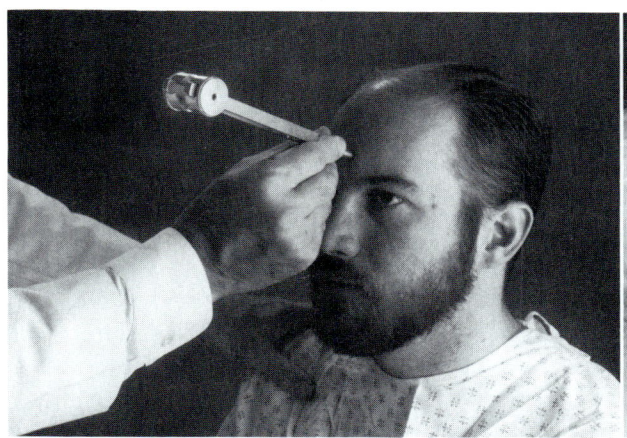
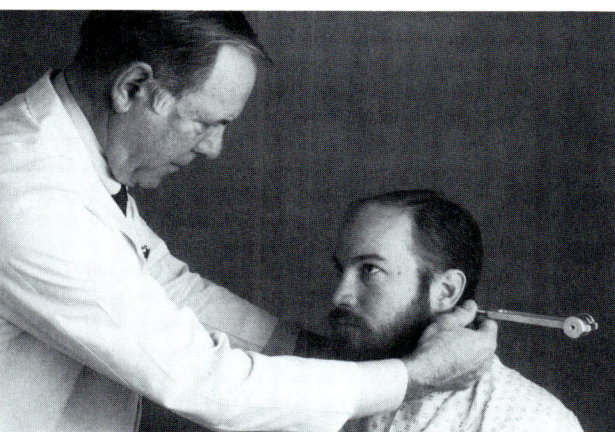

A   B

THE NOSE

History Taking

Epistaxis

Transient epistaxis is a frequent complaint and is most commonly caused by forceful nose-blowing and sneezing, nose picking, and facial trauma with a direct blow to the nose. *Recurrent epistaxis* may be the harbinger of several disorders, including coagulopathies, hypertension, renal failure, cirrhosis, and hereditary hemorrhagic telangiectasia.

Nasal Discharge

Transient nasal discharge is most often caused by the common cold and allergic rhinitis. A purulent discharge, especially if accompanied by fever and facial pain, should suggest acute sinusitis. The development of a persistent, clear nasal discharge after head trauma, especially if unilateral, should suggest an occult skull fracture with leakage of CSF (CSF rhinorrhea). Chronic nasal discharge may be caused by protracted use of nose drops (which are topical vasoconstrictors), cocaine snorting, and chronic sinusitis.

Facial Pain and Chronic Sinusitis

Facial pain, especially if recurrent and accompanied by nasal discharge, should suggest chronic sinusitis. Detailed questions should be asked about:

- The location and pattern of the pain
- Previous workup, if any, for sinusitis (sinus x-ray studies)
- Previous antibiotic therapy
- Whether the patient is known to have nasal or sinus polyps, which, by their location, may predispose to obstruction and the development of recurrent infection

The pain location pattern will vary depending on the sinuses involved. For example, pain above the eyes that is worse after waking up and improves during the day suggests a frontal sinusitis. Pain over the cheeks suggests a maxillary sinusitis.

Physical Examination of the Nose

Nares, Turbinates, and Septum

The nose is examined by tilting the patient's head backwards and introducing a nasal speculum, attached to an otoscope, into the nares (Fig. 2-11). Note the presence of mucus, crusts, foreign material, polyps, and sites of any recent bleeding. Also review the size, color, and mucosa overlying the turbinates; edema and hyperemia of the turbinate is usually quite obvious. Rhinorrhea (excessive mucus secretion from the nose) is associated with URIs, allergic rhinitis, and nonallergic vasomotor rhinitis. The nasal septum is examined for deviation, masses, or perforation. A perforated septum is usually caused by trauma and less commonly by disorders such as Takayasu's arteritis, Wegener's granulomatosis, sarcoidosis, syphilis, and tuberculosis. Nasal polyps can be either sessile or

Key Symptoms in the Evaluation of the Nose
Epistaxis Nasal discharge Facial pain and chronic sinusitis

pedunculated and are found with long-standing allergic rhinitis and triad asthma (asthma, nasal polyps, and aspirin sensitivity).

In patients with a history of recent epistaxis, the primary anterior site is Kiesselbach's area, which is a vascular network in the anterior nasal septum. Some patients have posterior bleeding sites, and, not infrequently, multiple oozing points may be seen.

The technique for examining the nose is depicted in Fig. 2-12.

Sinuses

Palpation over the maxillary or frontal sinuses may cause pain. Transillumination of the maxillary sinuses with a penlight should reveal a clear red-orange image. Failure of the light to be clearly seen suggests chronic sinusitis.

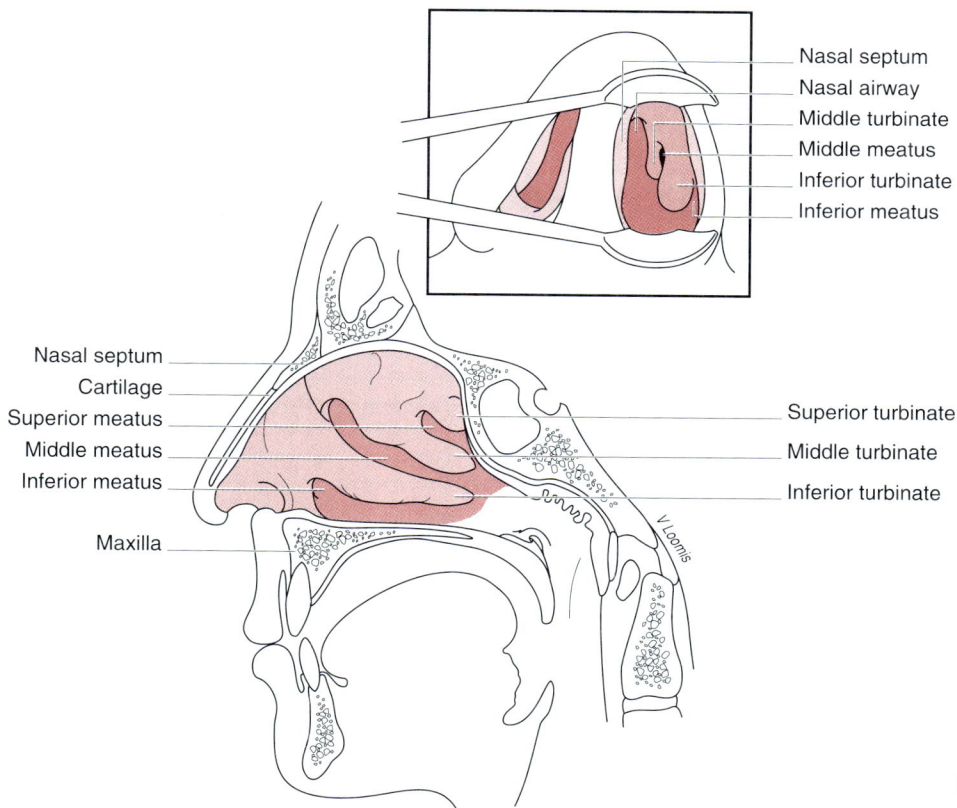

Fig. 2-11 Anatomy of the nares, turbinates, and septum.

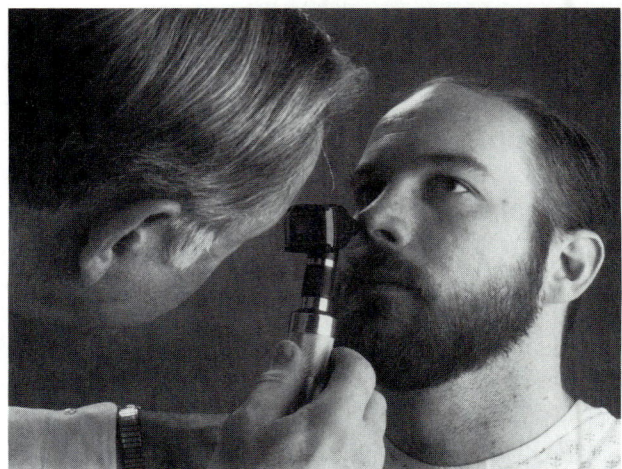

Fig. 2-12 Technique for examining the nares and turbinates.

Miscellaneous Abnormalities

RHINOPHYMA

Rhinophyma is a severe type of acne rosacea found in association with hypertrophy of the skin and congestion of the subcutaneous tissue. The distal two-thirds of the nose undergoes bulbous enlargement and has the appearance of a lobulated tumor.

SADDLE NOSE

The nose appears to be shaped like a saddle with a depressed proximal and prominent lower half. In the preantibiotic era this deformity was commonly associated with congenital syphilis. It is now more likely to result from trauma.

THE MOUTH AND THROAT

History Taking

Painful Ulcers and Sores in the Mouth and Tongue

Oral ulcers are usually painful. The major causes of such ulcers include:

- Recurrent aphthous ulcers
- Recurrent herpes simplex infection
- Other infections such as herpes zoster, tuberculosis, histoplasmosis, and syphilis
- Hematologic disorders such as leukemia, agranulocytosis
- Trauma caused by dentures, foreign bodies, and chemicals
- Cytotoxic drugs or radiotherapy
- Disorders such as erythema multiforme, Wegener's granulomatosis, Stevens-Johnson syndrome, and Reiter's syndrome

Oral carcinomas initially are frequently painless, but as they fail to heal and increase in size, discomfort usually supervenes and occasionally bleeding occurs as well. Behçet's syndrome and histiocytosis X are rare causes of recurrent oral ulcers.

Key Symptoms in the Evaluation of the Mouth and Throat	
Painful ulcers and sores in the mouth and tongue	Sore throat
Bleeding gums	Hoarseness
Abnormal taste	Difficulty swallowing

The most common lesions affecting the oral mucosa are recurrent aphthous and herpetiform lesions. Aphthous ulcers may recur several times a year, usually last 4 to 10 days, and are often preceded by prodromal symptoms such as soreness or burning in the mouth. They are frequently associated with inflammatory bowel disease (ulcerative colitis, regional enteritis) involving the colon.

Primary infections caused by type 1 herpes simplex virus may cause stomatitis or gingivostomatitis. Recurrent infections may result in sores or blisters on the lips and in the mouth. A variety of stimuli may provoke a recurrence, including mechanical trauma, strong sunlight exposure, intercurrent infections, and stress.

Bleeding Gums

The most common cause of bleeding gums is periodontal disease. Blood dyscrasias such as leukemia, other disorders causing thrombocytopenia, and drugs (phenytoin, salicylates) can also cause bleeding gums.

Abnormal Taste

Abnormalities in taste are generally of two types, hypogeusia and dysgeusia. *Hypogeusia* is defined as an impaired ability to taste normally, or a decreased sensitivity to taste. *Dysgeusia* refers to unpleasant tastes. Hypogeusia commonly accompanies URIs, glossitis, and stomatitis. Dysgeusia has been well documented with medications (metronidazole), vitamin and mineral deficiency (zinc depletion), chronic hypercalcemia (hyperparathyroidism), and viral infections (viral hepatitis). Indeed, in patients with viral hepatitis, hypogeusia and dysgeusia are quite common and are the basis for patients frequently complaining that, "cigarettes do not taste right to me."

Salt craving should raise the question of Addison's disease.

Sore Throat

Sore throat is most commonly caused by viral URIs, bacterial pharyngitis (streptococcal), recurrent tonsillitis, and infectious mononucleosis. Monilial and herpetic infections are frequently encountered in immunocompromised hosts. Diptheria, Vincent's angina (fusiform bacillus and *Borrelia vincentii*), and peritonsillar abscess are much less frequent causes of pharyngitis. In patients with the recent onset of sore throat, ask about systemic symptoms (fever, chills), neck discomfort (adenopathy), previous history of streptococcal infections or infectious mononucleosis, and upper respiratory symptoms (coryza, cough, myalgias, headache). The latter constellation of URI symptoms would point toward a viral rather than a bacterial pharyngitis, but this would have to be correlated with the physical examination (see below).

Hoarseness

Hoarseness, or a harsh, rough, grating quality of the voice, may be caused by disease processes affecting the pharynx, vocal cords, or recurrent laryngeal nerve. The new onset of hoarseness that persists always warrants a detailed inquiry. Some of the more common causes of hoarseness include the following:

- Laryngitis caused by viral and bacterial infections
- Vocal cord lesions such as polyps, carcinoma, and tuberculosis
- Excessive use of vocal cords as with politicians on the stump
- Hypothyroidism
- Certain medications such as anticholinergics
- Interruption of the recurrent laryngeal nerve as may occur after thyroid or parathyroid surgery, mediastinal tumors, aortic aneurysm, and bronchogenic carcinoma

With any heavy smoker who inexplicably develops hoarseness, the rule-out diagnosis must be bronchogenic carcinoma.

Difficulty Swallowing

Please see the section on dysphagia in Chapter 5.

Physical Examination of the Mouth and Throat

The technique for examining the buccal mucosa, gums, teeth, palate and pharynx is depicted in Fig. 2-13.

Lips, Mouth, Buccal Mucosa, Gums, Teeth, and Palate

Examine the patient's lips for swelling, melanin spots (Peutz-Jeghers syndrome), telangiectasia (Osler-Weber-Rendu disease), ulcerations, and herpetiform lesions. The latter may occur as raised, erythematous, crusted, or ulcerated lesions in different stages of evaluation.

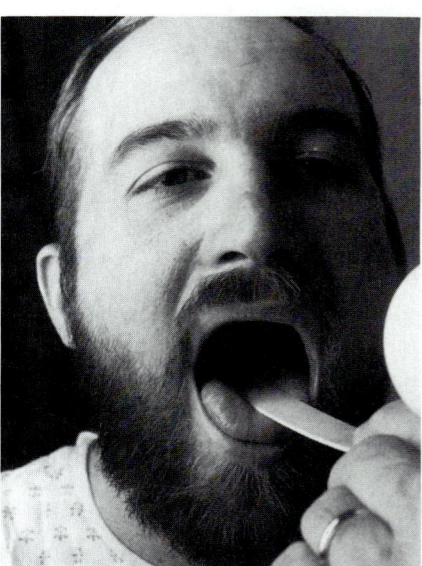

Fig. 2-13 Technique for examining the bucca, mucosa, gums, teeth, palate, and pharynx.

Check the buccal mucosa for ulcerations, inflammation, melanin spots, telangiectasia, and pigmentation (abnormal brown pigmentation of the buccal mucosa is seen in Addison's disease). *Koplik's spots* are white spots on the buccal mucosa opposite molar teeth that precede the typical morbilliform rash of measles.

The gingiva may appear hypertrophied in patients on phenytoin; a dark line above the gingival margin is seen with lead and bismuth poisoning. *Vincent's infection* or *trench mouth* is an acute necrotizing ulcerative gingivitis and stomatitis characterized by painful gingiva, bleeding on pressure, and gingival necrosis and ulceration. Examine the teeth for dental caries and periodontal disease; the latter examination is especially important in patients with diabetes mellitus, as periodontal abscesses can trigger a bout of diabetic ketoacidosis.

Leukoplakia on the buccal mucosa and tongue appears as a whitish raised plaquelike lesion that is clearly a precancerous condition. It is frequently associated with irritation from tobacco use.

Tongue

Carefully examine the tongue for ulcers. All tongue ulcers that fail to heal after 2 weeks should be considered potentially malignant and must be biopsied. Carcinomatous ulcers have a predilection for the sides, base, and undersurface of the tongue. Deviation of the tongue to one side occurs with lesions of CN XII. Further, atrophy of the paralyzed side will result in an appearance of unequal size.

Glossitis (inflammation of the tongue) can occur in several conditions, including:

- Vitamin and mineral deficiencies (vitamin C, niacin, riboflavin, zinc)
- Medications (metronidazole, phenytoin)
- Infections (candidiasis)
- Vitamin B_{12} and folic acid deficiency (pernicious anemia)
- After cytotoxic drugs or radiotherapy

A large tongue *(macroglossia)* is well documented in patients with amyloidosis and acromegaly. Color changes in the tongue may mirror systemic diseases. Thus, a "strawberry" or "raspberry" tongue, which occurs because of hypertrophy of the fungiform papillae, is seen with scarlet fever. A "hairy" tongue, appearing as such especially on the distal half, may reflect fungal infections as well as staining by tobacco or food. A smooth, bald-appearing tongue can be seen with iron deficiency anemia, pernicious anemia, and niacin deficiency.

Salivary Glands

The parotid and sublingual glands can be palpated during the routine examination of the jaw and neck. Bilateral parotid enlargement occurs with chronic alcoholism and mumps. Unilateral parotid enlargement can occur because of parotid tumors. When examining the buccal mucosa, Stensen's duct, which drains the parotid gland, should be easily visualized. Palpation of the cheek over the duct may be painful if suppurative parotitis, nonsuppurative parotitis, or parotid duct calculi is present. Suppurative parotitis is more likely to occur in debilitated and dehydrated patients.

Increased salivation occurs with oral infections, inflammatory conditions, and irritants. Decreased salivation is common with anticholinergic drugs and in Sjögren's syndrome. The latter, which is characterized by dry eyes and dry mouth (keratoconjunctivitis sicca and xerostomia) can be either a primary or a secondary disorder (i.e., associated with other autoimmune diseases such as rheumatoid arthritis).

Pharynx

Depress the tongue with a tongue blade to facilitate examination of the palate, uvula, tonsils, and pharynx. Although streptococcal pharyngitis is classically associated with fever, odynophagia, whitish exudate in the pharynx and/or tonsils, and tender lymphadenopathy and viral pharyngitis with just pharyngitis, this distinction often breaks down. Pharyngitis is also common in patients with infectious mononucleosis.

A whitish dirty brown membrane over the tonsils and posterior pharynx should raise the question of diptheria.

A peritonsillar abscess is characterized by fever, sore throat, cervical lymphadenopathy, and tonsillar enlargement. The abscess can be located anteriorly between tonsils and the anterior pillars, or posteriorly, which results in the tonsils being pushed forward. Pain radiating to ear on swallowing is common.

A retropharyngeal abscess usually manifests as a bulging mass that can expand rapidly and occlude the airway. The associated symptoms are fever, pain, and dysphagia, and, if untreated, stridor may result.

Larynx

The causes of hoarseness are listed above. The larynx and vocal cords usually can be visualized by indirect laryngoscopy.

Neck

The neck (Fig. 2-14) is first inspected for evidence of visible masses, pulsations, obvious goiter, or distended neck veins (the latter are discussed in Chapter 5). A systematic examination of lymph node–bearing areas should include palpation for posterior cervical, anterior cervical, supraclavicular, submental, submandibular postauricular, and suboccipital lymph nodes. If lymph nodes are palpated, record

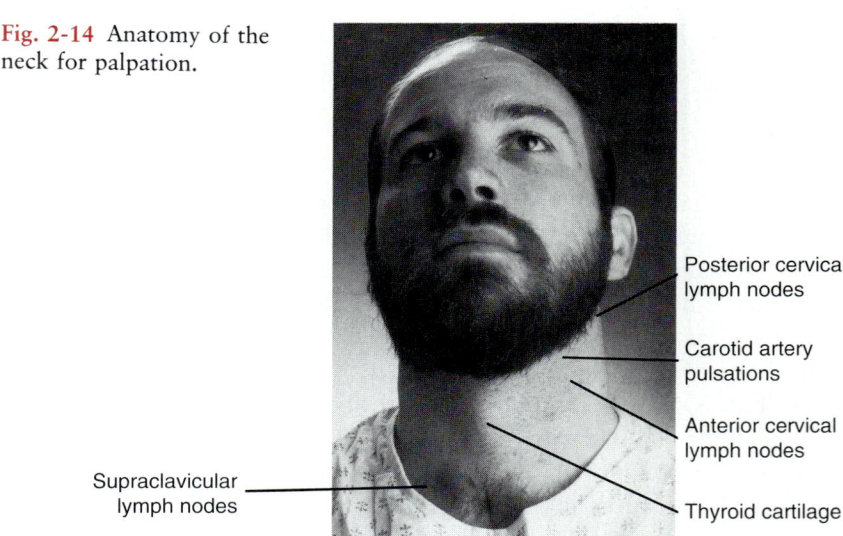

Fig. 2-14 Anatomy of the neck for palpation.

their size, consistency, mobility, and location. The carotid arteries should be palpated and carefully auscultated for evidence of bruits. Asymptomatic carotid bruits are an important physical finding, usually indicating atherosclerotic disease at the carotid bifurcation or the internal carotid artery and an increased likelihood of transient ischemic attacks or strokes in the ensuing 5 to 10 years.

The important steps in the examination of the thyroid gland are shown in Fig. 2-15. First, while facing the patient, have him swallow to see if any masses are evident in the midline just at the level of the thyroid cartilage. Palpation can be carried out from either a posterior or anterior position (see Fig. 2-15). In the posterior position, place your thumb on the back of the patient's neck and curl your index and third finger so they are placed on the trachea at the level of the thyroid cartilage. Palpate gently in the midline and laterally to detect any obvious thyroid enlargement. Next have the patient take some water in his mouth and hold it until your fingers are placed in the position noted above. The patient is then asked to swallow. In this manner, an enlarged thyroid isthmus, enlarged upper and lower lobes, and unilateral thyroid nodules can be better appreciated.

If the physical examination reveals an enlarged thyroid, carefully auscultate the thyroid for bruits. A diffusely enlarged thyroid gland along with a bruit are frequently found in Graves' disease. The thyroid can also be palpated from the anterior position using both thumbs and repeating the above procedures. An enlarged thyroid gland may be caused by:

- Graves' disease
- Nontoxic thyromegaly
- Thyroiditis
- Colloid cyst
- Thyroid carcinoma and, rarely, other neoplasms of the thyroid

Hard-feeling lesions should raise the question of carcinoma or Riedel's struma. An enlarged thyroid gland may also cause tracheal deviation, and patients may also complain of dysphagia.

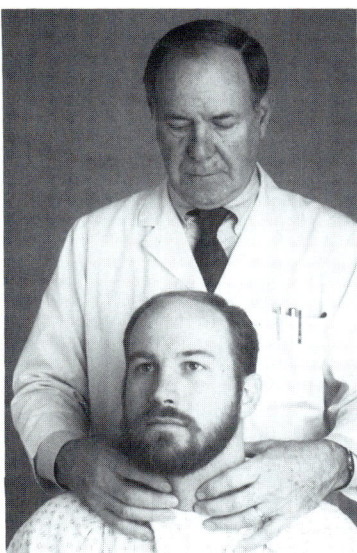

Fig. 2-15 Examination of the neck to assess the thyroid gland.

Summary

The examination of the eye, ear, mouth, throat, and neck is reviewed in the accompanying box.

Checklist for Examination of the Head and Neck

The Eye

General inspection (lids, conjunctiva cornea, xanthelasma)
Lids
- Lid lag
- Ptosis
- Bell's palsy
- Sty (hordeolum)
- Chalazion

Conjunctiva
- Conjunctivitis
- Petechiae
- Subconjunctival hemorrhage

Sclera
- Scleritis

Globe
- Exophthalmos

Cornea
- Scars, abrasions, ulcer
- Cataracts
- Kayser Fleischer rings, pinguecula

Iris and pupils
- Anisocoria
- Papillary reaction to light and accommodation
- Marcus Gunn, Argyll-Robertson, and Adie's pupil
- Mydriasis, miosis
- Horner's syndrome

Ocular motility and extraocular movements
- Nystagmus (horizontal vertical)
- Extraocular movement and cranial nerve pulses
- Tests for diplopia

Visual fields
- Defects by confrontation testing

Fundoscopic examination
- Optic disc
- Vessels
- Macula

Visual acuity
- Eye chart
- Read newsprint

The Ear

Ear lobe
- Microtia, swelling, nodular deposits (tophi)

External auditory canal
- Excess cerumen, otitis externa

Tympanic membrane
- Bulging, scarred, inflamed

Hearing
- Watch, tuning fork
- Rinne and Weber's tests (middle ear disease, conductive hearing loss)

The Nose

Nares, turbinates, septum
- Mucus, crusts, foreign material, polyps, recent bleeding
- Deviation or perforation of septum

Sinuses
- Transillumination

The Mouth, Throat, and Neck

Lips, mouth, buccal, gums, teeth
- Swelling, melanin spots, telangiectasia, ulceration, Koplik spots, periodontal disease

Tongue
- Ulcers, glossitis, atrophy, macroglossia

Salivary glands
- Parotid enlargement

Pharynx
- Pharyngitis, tonsillitis

Larynx
- Can be visualized by indirect laryngoscopy

Neck
- Lymph nodes (Check anterior, posterior, and supraclavicular)
- Trachea (is it midline?)
- Thyroid (is it palpable and enlarged?)
- Carotid arteries (check for bruits)

Suggested readings

Alberti PW, Thurben RJ, editors: *Otologic medicine and surgery,* New York, 1988, Churchill-Livingstone. *A standard textbook.*

Bedford MA: *Color atlas of ophthalmological diagnosis,* ed 2, St Louis, 1986, Mosby-Year Book. *A short, useful color atlas illustrating common ophthalmic conditions. The funduscopic abnormalities associated with a wide variety of conditions are particularly worthwhile.*

Linn JB Jr, Martin JB: Disturbances of smell, taste, and hearing. In Wilson J, et al, editors: *Harrison's principles of internal medicine,* ed 12, New York, 1990, McGraw-Hill, pp 152-156. *A concise summary of symptoms arising from disorders in these organ systems.*

Wray SH, Slanouts TL, Buerde RM: Disturbance of vision and ocular movements. In Wilson J, et al, editors: *Harrison's principles of internal medicine,* ed 12, New York, 1990, McGraw-Hill, pp 143-152. *A concise summary especially useful for the interpretation of ocular symptoms.*

CHAPTER THREE

The Respiratory System

CHAPTER OUTLINE

History Taking
Pulmonary symptoms
Upper respiratory tract symptoms
Past history of pulmonary problems

Physical Examination of the Respiratory System
General examination
Chest anatomy
Inspection
Palpation
Percussion
Auscultation

History and Physical Findings in Selected Pulmonary Problems
Asthma
Atelectasis
Bronchiectasis
Bronchitis
Bronchiolitis
Cancer of the lung
Cor pulmonale
Croup
Cystic fibrosis
Pleural effusion
Emphysema
Epiglottitis
Pneumothorax
Pulmonary hypertension
Pulmonary edema
Historical clues to the etiology of pneumonia

Summary

Disorders of the chest and lungs are increasingly important presenting complaints. Cigarette smoking, noxious inhaled chemicals, and allergies to pollen contribute to symptoms in many of the 20 million Americans with respiratory complaints. Asthma is increasingly important in children, as is cancer and obstructive lung disease in the older population. Massive efforts towards a smoke-free environment should help reduce these numbers in the future, but large numbers of young people are being recruited into the ranks of smokers.

Tuberculosis, once declining in incidence, has undergone a resurgence in immigrants from developing countries, among those with HIV infection, and in homeless people. Because tuberculosis is quite communicable, is both an acute and chronic illness, and reactivates after many years into contagiousness, we may anticipate future problems with it.

In the pulmonary evaluation, the history is generally more important than is the physical examination. Recently, other methods used in diagnosis have undergone changes. Advances in diagnostic techniques, including pulmonary function studies, chest radiographs, CT scans, radionuclide scans, and MRIs, have enhanced the accuracy of diagnosis far beyond the physical examination for certain chest diseases. Nonetheless, other chest diseases require a careful history and examination for diagnosis. These traditional techniques remain important in guiding selection of additional studies.

History Taking

Pulmonary Symptoms

The eight cardinal symptoms of pulmonary disease are listed in the accompanying box.

Wheezing, stridor, and cyanosis may be considered either signs or symptoms, depending on their severity and whether each was recognized by physician or patient. Each of the cardinal symptoms is discussed, considering pulmonary and other causes.

COUGH

The cough reflex can be divided into four distinct components. *Air is inspired into the lungs*, and the *glottis is closed*. *Compression of the lungs* results from contraction of thoracic, diaphragmatic, and abdominal muscles. As the *glottis is opened suddenly,* intrapulmonary pressure expels particles from the trachea or bronchi.

During a vigorous cough, other effects occur. The high positive intrathoracic pressure impedes blood return to the right atrium. During prolonged coughing, blood shunted from the superior vena cava to the facial veins may give the face a cyanotic appearance. Because no venous valves exist between intrathoracic and intracranial veins, the cerebrospinal fluid (CSF) pressure increases in proportion to intrathoracic pressure. Repeated vigorous coughing can cause increased vascular pressure and can even result in petechiae of the face or eyes.

Cardinal Symptoms of Pulmonary Disease	
Cough	Dyspnea
Sputum	Wheezing and stridor
Hemoptysis	Hiccup (singultus)
Chest pain	Cyanosis

CASE 3-1 Cough Caused by Tuberculosis

A 51-year-old man who lived in his car presented with a cough lasting for 2 months, production of yellow sputum several times each day, and a weight loss of 10 pounds. He admitted to having night sweats regularly and needing to change clothes because they were wet with sweat.

Social history revealed that he had been homeless since losing his job 3 years ago. He often shared living space with intravenous drug abusers, but insisted he did not "touch the stuff."

Physical examination showed a thin white man in no distress with crackles heard bilaterally over the bases of both lungs posteriorly. His chest x-ray film showed several calcified granulomas and a small cavity in the right upper lung field. An acid fast stain of sputum smear showed a few acid fast bacilli. Several weeks later, the culture confirmed infection with *Mycobacterium tuberculosis*.

Five types of stimuli produce coughing (see the accompanying box).

Types of questions you ask are based on the causes of the cough. Sample questions would include:

- *Tell me about your cough: how much do you cough, what brings it on, what relieves it?* Try to determine the mechanical cause.
- *Do you smoke or are you exposed to possible respiratory irritants or fumes?*
- *Do you swallow into your windpipe (aspiration)?*

Clues to the Cause of Cough

I. Pulmonary mechanical causes of cough
   A. Inhalation of an irritant as dust, smoke, or foreign body causing intraluminal fluid
   B. Aspiration of pharyngeal contents
   C. Pressure from the serosal surface of bronchus distorting the bronchus
   D. Asthma
II. Inflammatory and infectious causes of cough
   A. Mucous membrane edema
   B. Mucus or pus in trachea or bronchi
   C. Laryngitis
III. Temperature causes of cough
   A. Inhalation of air cooler than ambient temperature
IV. Nonpulmonary causes of cough
   A. Transudate of fluid into alveoli
   B. Pulmonary emboli
   C. Irritation of external ear canal
V. Psychogenic cough
   A. Habitual
   B. Used to get attention, express hostility, or release tension during embarrassment

- *What about wheezing? What brings it on? Exercise? Breathing cold air?* Asthma must be considered as a possibility.
- *Do you cough up phlegm?* This is a clue to bronchitis, pneumonia, or other causes.
- *Do you cough more during the night?* This may be caused by transudation of fluid.
- *Does inserting your finger into your ear cause cough?*
- Could this be habit coughing?

Traction or pressure external to a bronchus, distorting the lumen, may result in cough. Examples include enlarged nodes, tumor, or tension on a bronchus from fibrosis. Aspiration of vomitus or of pharyngeal contents initiates a protective cough reflex. Inhalation of noxious gases, dust, or smoke results in mucosal edema and cough. Interstitial lung disease may cause a nonproductive cough. Pleural effusions that compress the lung produce coughing. Inflammation of mucous membranes and allergies activate cough receptors caused by edema or hyperemia.

Cough may be stimulated by mechanisms not initially of pulmonary origin. Pulmonary emboli may cause cough, along with dyspnea, cyanosis, or hemoptysis. Congestive cardiac failure, especially left ventricular failure, allows transudation of fluid into the alveoli, resulting in cough.

Occasionally cough is of psychogenic origin. Some people develop a habit cough. This may follow a bout of bronchitis. Others use cough to obtain or to divert attention.

Cough is one of a few symptoms potentially more troublesome at night, perhaps because of fewer distractions or the accumulation of bronchial secretions. The smoker's cough characteristically occurs in the morning and produces sputum. When asthmatics cough and wheeze during attacks, the cough is usually dry without sputum *(nonproductive)*.

The patient is not necessarily a good judge of cough frequency—he grows accustomed to it. A family member may give a better history about how often the patient coughs.

The type of cough may be distinctive. In children a most distinctive cough (but less common today) is the whoop heard with pertussis (whooping cough). The child exhibits a burst of 15 to 20 short coughs followed by the whoop. This is a long inspiratory sound caused by air passing between laryngeal muscles in spasm.

Acute laryngitis often results in a painful barking cough. In tracheitis, the cough is harsh and accompanied by substernal chest pain. Initially nonproductive, the cough in tracheitis later becomes painless and productive. Partial obstruction of the trachea or bronchi with a foreign body may produce cough with stridor. In chronic obstructive pulmonary disease (COPD), coughs are characterized by prolonged loose cough expulsion of sputum; wheezing may be associated. In some patients with COPD a wheezing quality is prominent during laughing.

The complications of cough include embarrassment, hoarseness caused by laryngeal irritation, loss of sleep, sore thoracic muscles, and rib fractures. The incessant coughing caused by *Mycoplasma pneumoniae* or uncontrolled asthma may result in rib fractures in young people. Probably chronic bronchitis is most often associated with cough-induced rib fracture, but osteoporosis and metastatic tumor of bone contribute by weakening the bony structure. Cough syncope from cerebral ischemia may follow a prolonged, severe bout of coughing. Petechiae around the eyes are complications of vigorous coughing, especially in patients who have reduced platelet counts, as in leukemia.

SPUTUM

Sputum, or phlegm, is a secretion from the trachea, bronchi, or lungs coughed up through the glottis. A cough with sputum is termed *productive*. Both sputum and cough are abnormal. Even though cigarette smokers accept sputum as normal, production of sputum is always abnormal. Patients often deny or minimize sputum production. Men typically expectorate sputum, and women frequently swallow it. While taking the history and performing the physical examination, ask the patient to expectorate sputum into a cup for examination. Characteristics of sputum are indicated in the box below. Saliva, clear and watery, can be distinguished on gross inspection from sputum, which looks mucoid or purulent and may be clear, yellow, green, brown, or bloody.

Patients estimate sputum quantity poorly unless they save the expectorate. Volume estimates may be stated as a half cupful per day, or a teaspoonful several times daily. During treatment in the hospital or at home, patients should expectorate sputum into measured clear plastic sputum cups for examination and quantitation. Clinical improvement results in reduction in daily volume with changes in color from green or yellow to white or clear.

Many pulmonary disorders are associated with sputum production, including:

- Bronchitis
- Bronchiectasis
- Bronchoalveolar carcinoma
- Pneumonia
- Lung abscess
- Tuberculosis
- Pulmonary edema

Chronic bronchitis is defined by the production of sputum on a daily basis for at least 3 months of a year in 2 consecutive years, or for 6 months continuously without another defined cause of lung disease. Bronchiectasis typically results in

---

Sputum Characteristics

I. Amount (volume): scanty, spoonfuls, or cups
II. Frequency and duration of production
III. Color, taste, odor
    A. Yellow or green suggests infection, (i.e., polymorphonuclear leukocytes), yellow sputum may indicate infection or allergic response (i.e., eosinophils)
    B. Taste—usually metallic (use patient's words)
    C. Odor—foul odor suggests anaerobic bacterial infection, lung abscess, or bronchiectasis
IV. Appearance of sputum in clear sputum cup
    A. After prolonged standing, sputum separates into three layers (bronchiectasis)
V. Viscosity
    A. Mucoid sputum is viscous and difficult to expectorate (early pneumococcal pneumonia or asthma)

large volume sputum production. This sputum characteristically separates into two or three layers while standing in the sputum cup. The characteristics of sputum production are shown in the accompanying box.

HEMOPTYSIS

Hemoptysis is the expectoration (spitting-up) of blood-streaked sputum or of gross blood. Hemoptysis often alarms patients and prompts immediate medical attention. Hemoptysis is defined as expectoration of more than 2 ml of blood. Often blood-streaked sputum is termed hemoptysis without quantitation. The clinician attempts to establish two things regarding hemoptysis: the anatomic bleeding site (Table 3-1) and the underlying cause for the bleeding (Table 3-2).

Bleeding may be caused by one of several pathogenic processes. Bleeding from the nose *(epistaxis)* or bleeding from the GI tract *(hematemesis)* can mimic hemoptysis.

Techniques including ENT examination (see Chapter 2), fiberoptic bronchoscopy, and chest x-ray films may be needed to determine the site of possible hemoptysis.

Historical clues can help differentiate between the causes of hemoptysis listed in Table 3-2. Only a few causes of hemoptysis will be discussed here. The most common causes of hemoptysis in North America are bronchitis and bronchogenic carcinoma. A rust color is characteristic for the bloody sputum of lobar pneumococcal pneumonia.

TABLE 3-1: Symptom: Hemoptysis and Two Potentially Confusing Symptoms

Anatomic Site of Bleeding	Historical Clues	Physical Examination	Other Diagnostic Techniques
Respiratory tract (hemoptysis)	• Blood or blood-streaked sputum coughed up • Sputum present or absent • Tingling in throat • Desire to cough • Blood bright red • May be frothy	• Clues depend on pathologic process • Crackles of pneumonia or pulmonary edema • E-to-A-changes if pneumonic consolidation of lung is present (see pg. 110)	• Chest x-ray film • Fiberoptic bronchoscopy
Nose (epistaxis)	• Recent nosebleed • Bleeding from anterior nares if bleeding site is anterior • Spitting up blood without coughing	• Bleeding site anterior septum; Kiesselbach's area • Indirect exam of larynx and posterior nasopharynx using mirror and headlamp • Gingival bleeding	• Fiberoptic rhinoscopy visualization is replacing indirect (mirror) examination when equipment is available
GI tract (hematemesis)	• Nausea associated • Blood is actually vomited • Blood is dark red color or looks like coffee grounds	• Upper abdominal tenderness • Observation of patient during bleeding episode to differentiate vomiting from hemoptysis	• Upper GI endoscopy • Barium swallow and upper GI roentgenogram

TABLE 3-2: Symptom: Hemoptysis

Pathologic Cause of Hemoptysis	Historical Clues in Addition to Hemoptysis	Physical Examination	Other Diagnostic Techniques
A. Infections			
1. Chronic bronchitis*	• Daily sputum for at least 3 months in 2 consecutive years (no other lung pathology responsible)	• Prolonged exhalation • Expiratory wheeze • No other cause responsible	• Chest x-ray film • Pulmonary function studies
2. Acute bronchitis*	• Recent onset of cough, sputum, fever, sore throat, substernal pain with coughing or breathing	• Exclude other causes • Red mucous membranes • Rhinorrhea common	
3. Bronchiectasis	• Recurrent bacterial infections • Recurrent hemoptysis • Large volume of sputum	• Sputum separates into three layers on standing	• Chest x-ray film • Fiberoptic bronchoscopy • Thin slice CT scan
4. Pneumonia*	• Fever, cough, sputum • Scanty amounts of blood • Rust-colored sputum with pneumococcal pneumonia	• Examination findings of pneumonia	• Chest x-ray film • Gram stain and culture of sputum
5. Lung abscess	• Aspiration during loss of consciousness or seizure • Recent dental procedure or anesthesia • Foul-smelling sputum	• Sputum discolored and fetid odor	• Chest x-ray film • Culture of sputum (for anaerobes if bronchoscopy performed with protected specimen)
6. Tuberculosis	• Age over 60, may be younger • Immigration from third world country • Previous positive skin test • Underlying AIDS	• Crackles; few findings unless advanced disease	• Chest x-ray film • Sputum acid-fast smear and culture • Skin testing
7. Histoplasmosis	• Midwest resident • Exposure to dust from chicken house or starling roost • Flulike syndrome	• Typically nonspecific • Acute illness presents as pneumonia • Chronic may be cavitary or disseminated	• Chest x-ray film • Fungal smear and culture • Bone marrow and sputum cultures • Histoplasma titers
8. Coccidiomycosis	• Desert southwest travel or residence • Oriental race • Valley fever • Skin lesions	• Skin lesions	• Chest x-ray film • Positive serum titer • Culture of sputum

*Common causes.

TABLE 3-2: Symptom: Hemoptysis—cont'd

Pathologic Cause of Hemoptysis	Historical Clues in Addition to Hemoptysis	Physical Examination	Other Diagnostic Techniques
B. Neoplasma			
1. Lung cancer*	• Weight loss • Anorexia • Cigarette smoking	• Unilateral telangiectasia of skin vessels on chest • Localized wheeze over major airway	• Chest x-ray film • CT scan • Fiberoptic bronchoscopy
2. Bronchial adenoma	• Young woman • No other symptoms	• Wheezing over airway	• Chest x-ray film • Bronchoscopy
C. Immune process			
1. Goodpasture's syndrome	• Cough, dyspnea • Men more often affected	• Hypoxia • Renal failure	• Chest x-ray film shows hilar infiltrates • Immune complex deposits shown by immunofluorescence in biopsy of lung and kidney
2. Wegener's granulomatosis	• Sinus pain and drainage • Bloody nasal discharge • Cough, dyspnea, chest discomfort	• Nasal mucosal ulceration • Perforation of septum	• Biopsy shows granulomas and arteritis of upper and lower respiratory tract • Eye, skin, and kidneys often involved
D. Aspiration of foreign body	• Eating peanuts, popcorn, then coughing and inhaling • Patient may or may not be aware of precise timing of aspiration	• Wheezing; stridor acutely • Postobstructive pneumonia if chronically present	• Apparent on chest x-ray film if radioopaque • Bronchoscopy
E. Trauma			
1. Knife or gunshot wound, fractured rib	• Patient relates event • If unconscious rely on exam	• Signs of trauma	• Chest film or rib films show fracture or foreign body
2. Inhalation of smoke or noxious fumes	• Material aspirated or inhaled		
F. Pulmonary			
1. Thromboembolism*	• Surgery • Immobilization caused by other illness • Use of oral contraceptives • Pleuritic chest pain • Recent prolonged car ride allowing venous thrombosis	• Pleural friction rub • Accentuated P2	• Chest x-ray film • Ventilation perfusion lung scan • Pulmonary arteriogram
G. Cardiovascular			
1. Left ventricular failure	• Dyspnea on exertion • Orthopnea • Paroxysmal nocturnal dyspnea	• S3 • Basilar crackles	• ECG • Chest x-ray film

Continued.

TABLE 3-2: Symptom: Hemoptysis—cont'd

Pathologic Cause of Hemoptysis	Historical Clues in Addition to Hemoptysis	Physical Examination	Other Diagnostic Techniques
2. Mitral stenosis	• Same as above • Previous rheumatic fever	• S3 • Opening snap, diastolic murmur with presystolic accentuation	• ECG • Chest x-ray film • Echocardiogram of mitral valve
3. Primary pulmonary hypertension	• Young woman • Chest discomfort • Weakness, fatigue • Effort syncope	• Few physical findings early • P2 is accentuated • Prominent *a* waves on jugular pulse	• Cardiac catheterization
H. Hemorrhagic diathesis			
1. Anticoagulation therapy*	• Takes Coumadin, heparin, or other anticoagulants	• Ecchymoses • Easy bleeding	• Prothrombin time • Partial thromboplastin time • Platelet count
2. Thrombocytopenia (idiopathic or in leukemias)		• Petechiae • Large bruises	• Decreased platelet count
3. Hemophilia	• Family history • Large-joint hemorrhages		• Partial thromboplastin time • Factor assay

Massive hemoptysis is defined as coughing up more than 600 ml in 24 hours. The most common cause of massive hemoptysis is bronchiectasis. Other causes include bronchogenic carcinoma or an aspergillus fungus ball invading a lung cavity. The immediate concern for the patient with massive hemoptysis is hypoxemia rather than the blood loss itself.

Both Goodpasture's syndrome and Wegener's granulomatosis are rare causes

---

CASE 3-2   Hemoptysis versus Epistaxis

A 35-year-old man presented to the emergency department complaining of spitting up blood. He said that he was just sitting around listening to music. He thought he coughed and brought up what looked like a lot of blood—perhaps several teaspoonfuls. He denied having had a nosebleed, cough, fever, pain, or any other illnesses. He said the cough was actually more like clearing his throat.

The physical examination showed no bleeding sites along the nasal septum, a normal appearing throat, and chest clear on auscultation. The chest x-ray film was normal.

Indirect examination using a headlamp and mirrors showed a normal posterior nasopharynx and vocal cords. However, when the otorhinolaryngologist examined the nasopharynx with a fiberoptic laryngoscope, he found a small tumor at the apex that appeared to have bled recently. This was later removed and found to be nasopharyngeal carcinoma.

of hemoptysis. Goodpasture's syndrome results from antibody-induced damage of alveolar and glomerular basement membranes. Hemoptysis is accompanied by cough, dyspnea, pneumonia, and microscopic hematuria. Wegener's hemoptysis is associated with epistaxis, sinusitis, pulmonary infiltrates, and glomerulonephritis, all caused by necrotizing granulomas and arteritis.

CHEST PAIN

Chest pain may originate from intrathoracic or extrathoracic structures. This chapter considers chest pain caused by thoracic structure involvement (see the accompanying box). The differential diagnosis of chest pain is expanded further in Table 4-1 in which cardiac etiologies of chest pain are considered.

Symptoms suggesting that chest pain is not of cardiac origin include the following:

1. Chest pain intensified by breathing is typical of pleural involvement and is termed *pleuritic*. The pain may be described as knifelike or shooting. A pleural friction rub may be heard during auscultation at the site of pleuritic pain. If a pleural effusion develops, the pain may subside. Pleuritic chest pain may be present in pneumonia, pulmonary emboli causing infarction of the lung, tuberculosis, carcinomas, and other diseases involving the pleura. Diaphragmatic irritation by pericarditis or by a subphrenic abscess may also cause pleuritic pain. Involvement of the dome of the diaphragm causes referred pain to the top of the shoulder. When the lateral margin of diaphragm is involved, pain is sensed along the chest wall.
2. Chest pain with local tenderness is characteristically caused by involvement of skin, subcutaneous tissue, fat, breast, or bone. Costochondral joint pain, tender to the touch, is termed *Tietze's syndrome*. The pain of shingles (herpes zoster) begins before the eruption of vesicles and often persists weeks or months after skin lesions are healed. Old healed rib fractures may remain painful, especially during cough.
3. Retrosternal chest pain associated with coughing or breathing is characteristic of tracheitis. Retrosternal chest pain without coughing occurs with pain of cardiac, mediastinal, or esophageal origin.

Chest Pain

Chest Wall Pain

Trauma, recent or old healed rib fractures
Tietze's syndrome
Herpes zoster
Osteoporosis

Breast Tenderness (see Chapter 8)

Mastodynea
Inflammatory or neoplastic disease
Engorgement with milk after parturition

Intrathoracic Structures

Tracheitis
Esophageal pain (see Chapter 5)
Pericarditis (see Chapter 4)
Myocardial (see Chapter 4)
Mediastinal pain
Ruptured esophagus
Large mediastinal nodes
Aortic aneurysm dissection

Chest pain of esophageal origin is discussed in Chapter 5. Painful swallowing is common in herpetic and candida esophagitis and drug-induced ulcerations.

The chest pain of pericarditis is often sharp and intermittent. Pain of cardiac origin may take one of several forms (see Chapter 4).

Pain from esophageal rupture is severe and agonizing. The patient becomes agitated. Similar uneasiness is found after a ruptured aortic aneurysm. By comparison, the pain of myocardial infarction causes the patient to be quiet but apprehensive. Patients with large mediastinal nodes complain of ill-defined retrosternal weight or "oppression."

DYSPNEA

Difficult or labored breathing is termed *dyspnea*. The dyspneic patient requires effort for breathing, which is commonly called shortness of breath. Patients may appear tachypneic (breathing rapidly) to the clinician but not sense shortness of breath and not complain of dyspnea. In contrast, the person who has labored breathing because of physical exercise, or the person hiking above 10,000 feet, may recognize his effort or lack of physical conditioning and may consider his shortness of breath normal. The patient with advanced COPD may not complain of dyspnea, as he reduces activity along with the decreased functional capacity of his impaired lung. Hyperpnea, rapid and deep breathing, may be caused by metabolic acidosis, including diabetic ketoacidosis, renal failure, or lactic acidosis. Such patients usually do not complain of dyspnea because of their altered cerebral function (Table 3-3).

Dyspnea that occurs when the patient is lying flat may be orthopnea or paroxysmal nocturnal dyspnea. *Orthopnea* is dyspnea with onset occurring on lying down. Orthopnea is characteristic of heart failure but is found with obstructive airway disease and bilateral paralysis of diaphragms. Orthopnea is relieved at once by sitting up or by elevating the head and thorax on two or three pillows.

On the other hand, *paroxysmal nocturnal dyspnea* (PND) does not begin at once after lying down, nor is it relieved at once by sitting up. With PND, the patient is dramatically awakened from sleep, gasping for air. The patient senses impending suffocation. Relief usually occurs after a few minutes of sitting or standing. Profuse sweating may follow. During an attack of PND, cough and hemoptysis may be manifestations of pulmonary congestion. PND indicates acute pulmonary edema caused by heart failure. Recurrent episodes cause patients to sleep upright in a chair.

WHEEZING AND STRIDOR

Wheezing is the high-pitched musical breath sound caused by air rushing past secretions, edema, tumor, or an aspirated foreign body. Patients may use the term "wheeze" to describe noisy breathing or even rattling nasal secretions. Wheeze should refer to musical sounds produced lower in the air passages, in bronchi or the trachea. Wheezing becomes louder during exhalation but may also occur during inhalation. Wheezing is a characteristic symptom of asthma (Table 3-4). However, patients with very severe airway obstruction in asthma may have decreasing wheezing as the airway is increasingly obstructed and less air passes by. Many lung diseases are associated with mild wheezing.

A form of asthma termed *silent asthma* is not accompanied by wheezing and is noted by the patient. It is a cause of unexplained cough. In certain people, inhaling cool air may precipitate cough or asthma.

Text continued on pg. 87.

TABLE 3-3: Symptom: Dyspnea

Condition	Historical Clues	Physical Examination	Other Diagnostic Techniques
I. Pulmonary disease A. Asthma	• Triad of dyspnea, wheezing, and cough • Personal or family history of allergies common • Attacks may be provoked by exercise, infection, or stress	• Tachypnea during attack • May be asymptomatic between asthma attacks, during attacks depending on severity, may exhibit air hunger, ashen color, pale or cyanotic mucous membranes • Hyperaeriation of chest with depressed diaphragms • Wheezing on auscultation, prolonged expiratory phase; in severe disease may be unable to move air sufficiently rapidly to produce even a wheeze	• Pulmonary function studies show decreased maximal expiratory flow rate, increased airway resistance, increased static lung volumes, normal or elevated diffusion capacity for carbon monoxide • Blood gas analysis, respiratory alkalosis with hypocapnea, and either normal or reduced arterial oxygen tension
B. Chronic bronchitis	• Cough with expectoration of sputum for at least 3 months in 2 successive years without other diagnostic cause • Wheezing and dyspnea particularly associated with inhaled irritants or with acute respiratory infection • History of cigarette smoking	• During acute exacerbations may appear cyanotic • Tracheal bronchial secretions may be apparent during coughing or laughing • Patient often overweight • Coarse rhonchi and wheezes often present • Cor pulmonale with signs of right ventricular failure occurs late	• Arterial oxygen tension reduced, arterial carbon dioxide tension increased, hematocrit often increased to the polycythemic range, carbon monoxide diffusing capacity normal to slightly decreased
C. Emphysema	• May have a history of either asthma or chronic bronchitis • History of cigarette smoking • Patient may not have history of sputum production • Dyspnea with varying degrees of exertion	• Asthenic body build with weight loss • Tachypnea with pursing of the lips or a grunting sound during exhalation • Neck veins often distended during exhalation but collapse with inhalation • Barrel-shaped chest • Hyperresonant chest by percussion	• Blood gases show arterial oxygen reduced and carbon dioxide tension low to normal • Pulmonary function shows increased total lung capacity and residual volume • Maximal expiratory flow rates are decreased • The carbon monoxide diffusion capacity is reduced

Continued.

TABLE 3-3: Symptom: Dyspnea—cont'd

Condition	Historical Clues	Physical Examination	Other Diagnostic Techniques
C. Emphysema—cont'd		• Decreased breath sounds with end expiration, high-pitched rhonchi • Vertical heart configuration	• Chest roentgenogram shows depressed diaphragms, large retrosternal translucency on the lateral film, and bronchovascular shadows, which do not extend to the periphery
D. Pneumonia	• Cough, chills, and fever • Purulent or bloody sputum • Chest pain	• Fever, tachypnea, tachycardia • With multiple lobes involved in the respiratory distress syndrome, patient may be hypoxic and cyanotic • Decreased respiratory excursion on affected side if pleuritic pain is present • Percussion dullness present if consolidative pneumonia or pleural effusion is present • Auscultation often shows high-pitched inspiratory crackles, bronchial breath sounds, or egophony	• Chest x-ray film localizes pneumonia and shows extent better than does examination • Hypoxia, hypocarbia, and respiratory alkalosis may be present • Blood culture and sputum cultures are needed to delineate microbial etiologies
E. Pulmonary emboli	• A recent auto ride • Prolonged bed rest, especially in hospitals or nursing homes • Use of oral contraceptives • May have no symptoms • Hemotypsis • Pleuritic chest pain	• Tachycardia is the single consistent finding • Pleural friction rub if pulmonary infarction has occurred • Rarely right ventricular gallop, increased intensity of pulmonary valve closure or prominent A-waves in the jugular venous pulse • Examination of legs may show deep venous thrombosis, or abdominal pelvic pain may suggest presence of phlebitis • Loud pulmonary closure sound (P2) • S2 may be widely split with extensive embolic obstruction	• Chest x-ray film may show infiltrate if infarction has occurred • Pleural effusion if infarction has occurred • ECG usually normal but may show shift of the Q-S axis rightward, peaked P waves and S-T changes of right ventricular strain • Ventilation perfusion scan of chest shows normal ventilation with perfusion defects in the area of emboli • Arterial blood gases show hypoxia, hypocapnea, and respiratory alkalosis • Pulmonary angiography may show abrupt vessel "cutoff," filling defects of vessels

TABLE 3-3: Symptom: Dyspnea—cont'd

Condition	Historical Clues	Physical Examination	Other Diagnostic Techniques
F. Cystic fibrosis	• Usually diagnosed in infancy with acute intestinal obstruction (meconium ileus at birth) • History of repeated respiratory infections, especially with *Pseudomonas aeruginosa* isolated from the sputum	• Nasal polyps, sinusitis common • Multisystem involvement • Small stature, clubbing of fingers	• Culture of sputum commonly shows *P. aeruginosa*, often resistant to antibiotics • Male sterility common • Sweat-gland dysfunction shows sweat chloride usually exceeds 70 mEq/L
G. Pneumothorax	• Cyanosis • Chest pain • Pain radiating to neck	• Cyanosis • Shift in trachea away from involved side • Absence of breath sounds on involved side	• Chest x-ray film
II. Heart disease			
A. Congestive heart failure	• Precipitating causes and underlying heart disease both require establishment; seek historical clues for each precipitating cause • Myocardial infarction, secondary to ischemic heart disease with or without chest pain • Systemic hypertension with rapid increase in blood pressure • Excess sodium intake, physical overexertion, or emotional crisis • Arrhythmia, either rapid or slow • Cardiomyopathy caused by rheumatic fever, viral infections, or other causes • Valvular disease caused by infective endocarditis, calcific valvular disease • Symptoms such as dyspnea, orthopnea • Fatigue and weakness • Altered mental state with confusion, headache, insomnia, and impaired memory • Paroxysmal nocturnal dyspnea	• Patient uncomfortable when lying flat longer than a brief time • Cyanosis present with severe heart failure • Tachycardia • Distension of jugular veins • Arterial pulse shows pulsus alternans • Moist inspiratory crackles in posterior lung bases • S_3 and S_4 • Hepatic distension and tenderness • In severe disease, hydrothorax, ascites • Pedal edema • Hepatojugular reflux • Cheyne-Stokes respiration	• Directed toward identifying underlying cause and the immediate precipitating factors • ECG • Chest x-ray film • Kerly's B lines on chest x-ray film • Echocardiography

Continued.

TABLE 3-3: Symptom: Dyspnea—cont'd

Condition	Historical Clues	Physical Examination	Other Diagnostic Techniques
B. Pulmonary edema	• Advanced degree of congestive heart failure • Historical items similar to congestive failure • Patient appears acutely ill with perspiration • Apprehension of impending death • Frothy, bloody sputum	• Patient appears ashen, cyanotic • Rattling sound often apparent during breathing without use of stethoscope • Profuse perspiration • Tachypnea • Tachycardia • Crackles throughout all lung fields	• Medical emergency • Therapy should be instituted concommitant with diagnostic studies • Chest x-ray film shows diffuse increased markings, often cardiomegaly, prominence of upper lobe vasculature, occasional pleural effusions
C. Cardiac asthma (paroxysmal nocturnal dyspnea)	• Severe shortness of breath, commonly at night • Prominent wheezing • Precipitating factors that increase pulmonary vascular congestion (e.g., increased sodium intake, overexertion)	• Tachypnea, tachycardia • Moist crackles in bases of lungs during episodes and often between episodes • Diaphoresis • Cyanosis • Wheezing	• Pulmonary function testing when etiology of dyspnea is not clear • Chest x-ray film • ECG • Radionuclide ventriculography may be helpful to demonstrate reduced ventricular ejection when cardiac and pulmonary asthma are difficult to differentiate
III. Hematologic A. Anemia	• Often asymptomatic when gradual in onset and not severe in degree • Acute anemia may be caused by underproduction of red cells, bleeding, or hemolysis • Rapid uncompensated anemia, patient complains of dyspnea, palpitation, especially with exercise • Symptoms of heart failure if the heart is otherwise compromised • Dizziness, headache, syncope, tinnitus, or vertigo	• Pallor, tachycardia, widened pulse pressure • Active precordium • Lungs are clear • Systolic ejection murmur is common • If caused by hemolysis, and splenomegaly	• Complete blood count • Fecal study for occult blood • Visualization of feces for evidence of blood or black, tarry stools (signifies upper GI bleeding) • Examination of peripheral blood smear • Bone marrow examination • Additional studies if hemolysis appears to be present by decreased haptoglobin, increased serum-free hemoglobin

TABLE 3-3: Symptom: Dyspnea—cont'd

Condition	Historical Clues	Physical Examination	Other Diagnostic Techniques
B. Carbon monoxide poisoning	• Exposure to exhaust leaks from automobiles or other engines • Exposure to improperly ventilated combustion • Exposure to fire in confined space • Symptoms depend on concentration of carbon monoxide to which one is exposed and duration of exposure • Low level mild exposure impairs vigilance and decreases maximal exercise capacity • At increased levels, symptoms may include headache and giddiness • Vomiting, weakness, and lethargy • Obtundation and injury to the myocardium • Unconsciousness • Death	• Sweating, fever • Cherry color of skin and mucous membrane resulting from red carboxyhemoglobin is rare, cyanosis is more common	• 1 ml of patient's blood diluted with 10 ml of water to which 1 ml of 5% NaOH is added will turn oxyhemoglobin brown • Significant levels of carboxyhemoglobin will turn the solution yellow (less than 20%) or pink (greater than 20%)
IV. Metabolic diseases A. Diabetic ketoacidosis	• Diagnosis easier if patient known to have diabetes • Increased urine formation • Altered consciousness or coma • Other causes also need to be considered in the diabetic patient • Anorexia, nausea, vomiting • Many other complications may be present in diabetic ketoacidosis, including gastric dilation, cerebral edema, electrolyte abnormalities, myocardial infarction, various infections, and respiratory distress syndrome	• Kussmaul's respirations, tachypnea, deep breathing • Altered level of consciousness • Body temperature normal or below normal: alternatively, fever may indicate infection • Diabetic retinopathy with microaneurysms, dilated veins, dot-and-blot hemorrhages, cotton wool spots, and hard exudates may be present	• Blood glucose is quite high, 475 ml/dl or more • Serum bicarbonate often less than 10 mmol • Glucosuria

Continued.

TABLE 3-3: Symptom: Dyspnea—cont'd

Condition	Historical Clues	Physical Examination	Other Diagnostic Techniques
B. Other metabolic acidosis			
1. Acute acidosis	• May be no symptoms • Increasing symptoms may include fatigue, stupor, or coma	• Kussmaul's respiration or hyperventilation	• Diagnostic techniques focus on determining the cause for acidosis • Increased acid production • Ketoacidosis (e.g., diabetic, alcoholic, starvation) • Lactic acidosis (e.g., circulatory or respiratory failure, drugs or toxins, enzyme defects) • Poisonings (e.g., salicylates, methanol, ethylene glycol)
2. Chronic acidosis	• Fatigue, anorexia	• Signs often relate to the underlying cause of acidosis (e.g., alcoholism, starvation, uremia, diarrhea)	• Renal failure with uremia • Renal tubular acidosis • Loss of alkali (e.g., diarrhea, carbonic anhydrase inhibitors, ureteral bladder) • Excess intake of aluminum chloride or amino acids
3. Lactic acidosis	• Confusion or obtundation	• Evidence of circulatory insufficiency	• Electrolyte anion gap with decreased bicarbonate, normal glucose, absent ketones
4. Aspirin overdose	• Vertigo, tinnitus, impaired hearing, confusion • Nausea, vomiting • Hyperventilation	• Hyperventilation	• Decreased carbon dioxide • Serum salicylate level usually over 35 mg/dl
5. Ingestion of antifreeze (ethylene glycol)	• May appear intoxicated • Vomiting, stupor, coma	• Tachypnea, bradycardia, hypothermia	• Hypocalcemia, oxalate crystals in urine
V. Neurologic diseases—forebrain disturbance or midbrain lesion	• May occur in congestive heart failure, brain trauma or hemorrhage, or chronic hypoxia or at high altitudes in normal persons • Cheyne-Stokes respiration, alternating apnea and hyperpnea, gradually changing amplitude of breaths		• Chemoreceptors lag behind blood gas changes of lung

TABLE 3-4: Symptom: Wheezing

Condition	Key Elements in Diagnosis
Asthma—triad of cough, wheezing, and dyspnea	• May be episodic or be continuous
Chronic obstructive pulmonary disease	• Production of sputum daily for 3 months or more in 2 consecutive years or for 6 months continuously, without other cause
Cardiac asthma	• Prominent wheezing along with signs of right- or left-sided congestive heart failure
Reactive airway disease	• Wheezing precipitated by breathing cold air, exercise, or noxious environmental exposures
Narrowing of airway by foreign body or tumor	• History of aspiration • Weight loss, cigarette smoking, and other signs suggesting tumor
Epiglottitis	• Fever, dysphagia, hoarseness • Drooling, choking feeling • Adults have swollen neck • Burn injury of epiglottis may also cause acute epiglottitis
Laryngeal edema caused by anaphylactic allergic reaction	• Injection or ingestion of allergen • Swelling of face and pharynx, associated with itching
Foreign body between vocal cords	• Change in voice or complete aphonia • Pain with pricking sensation • May occur during eating • Rapid onset of local swelling, cyanosis, suffocation • May have stridor followed by inability to breathe
Gastroesophageal reflux disease	• Nighttime cough • Frequent throat-clearing

CASE 3-3 Asthma

A 10-year-old boy who had asthma for several years was brought to the clinic by his parents. He had been wheezing all night and was unable to sleep throughout the night following horseback riding. The parents became conserned when they noted an ashen-gray discoloration (cyanosis) around his lips and in his face. He had been using an inhaler and was faithfully taking oral medications.

The physical examination showed an anxious young man with central cyanosis of the tongue and lips. Respiratory excursions of the chest were minimal, and he was using the accessory muscles of the neck to breathe. He had very few wheezes, and breath sounds were poor uniformly.

This patient demonstrated a severe attack of asthma that could have rapidly resulted in decompensation and death. He had few wheezes because he was unable to move air in and out of his lungs. This was a medical emergency requiring immediate and intensive therapy even before other diagnostic tests were begun.

Stridor is a high-pitched crowing sound occurring with inspiration. Stridor indicates severe airway obstruction. Examples include a foreign body or tumor in a bronchus, or spasm or edema of the larynx. Stridor portends total airway obstruction, an impending medical emergency. The patient may need immediate laryngoscopy, endotracheal intubation, or tracheostomy.

Acute epiglottitis in the pediatric patient is characterized by stridor and apprehension. The patient persists in sitting up, drools from the mouth, is unable to swallow, and complains of sore throat. Avoid examining the throat until facilities are available to intubate the patient because the airway may become obstructed by the inflamed epiglottis should the patient begin to cry or gag on the tongue depressor.

Epiglottitis in adults is also an emergency, usually not quite so severe as in children, but manifested by similar signs. Adult epiglottitis is manifested by swelling of the neck, swelling of the epiglottis and uvula, stridor, difficulty swallowing, and the sensation of an object caught in the throat. *Hemophilus influenzae* and viruses are the most common causes of epiglottitis in adults and children. Burns may also cause epiglottitis. Inhaled hot gases may cause bulla on the epiglottis, which can obstruct the airway.

HICCUPS

Hiccups, also termed *singultus,* are not necessarily caused by diseases of the chest. However, mediastinal, pleural, or bronchial problems may result in hiccups. Although many disorders have been associated with hiccups, the etiology often remains undetermined (see the accompanying box).

CYANOSIS

Cyanosis refers to the bluish color of the skin or mucous membranes caused by an excess of reduced (deoxygenated) hemoglobin in the underlying capillaries (Table 3-5). Cyanosis becomes apparent when the amount of reduced hemoglobin (deoxyhemoglobin) exceeds 5 g/dl. In patients who are anemic, cyanosis may not be displayed even in severe hypoxia because of the lower total amount of

---

Symptom: Hiccups

Abdominal Disorders

Hiatal hernia
Space-occupying lesion of liver
Diaphragmatic irritation (e.g., peritonitis, subphrenic abscess, following intraabdominal operations)

Mediastinal Disorders

Phrenic nerve irritation
Bronchial obstruction
Cardiac enlargement
Myocardial infarction
Esophageal obstruction
Pleural irritation

Central Nervous System

Encephalitis
Meningitis
Intracranial tumor or hemorrhage

No Organic Disease

Swallowing air
Excessive tobacco or alcohol use
No cause apparent

TABLE 3-5: Symptom: Cyanosis

Condition	Clues to Diagnosis
I. Central cyanosis	
A. Arterial oxygen has >5 gm/dl desaturated hemoglobin	
1. Respiratory causes	
a. Hypoventilation (asthma, COPD, aspiration of foreign body)*	• Not breathing • Unable to move air in and out because of obstruction
b. Diffusion abnormalities (pulmonary emboli)*	• Ventilation • Ventilation perfusion (VQ) imbalance (VQ lung scan)
2. Cardiac causes	
a. Congenital disease with right-to-left shunt (tetralogy of Fallot)	• Murmurs, ECG, and chest x-ray findings • Cardiac catheterization
b. Pulmonary AV fistula	• Requires angiography for diagnosis
c. Pulmonary edema	• Air hunger, moist rales, frothy pink sputum
B. Shock	• Depends on etiology: myocardial, septic, or other cause
C. Hemoglobin abnormalities	
1. Methemoglobinemia	• Congenital, or acquired following exposure to nitrates, sulfonamides, or primaquine • Brown discoloration of skin
2. Sulfhemoglobinemia	• Binding of hydrogen sulfide to hemoglobin • Oxygen binding site is lost • Oxygen transport reduction is less than expected by patient's color
3. Polycythemia	• Red, dusky appearance not true cyanosis
II. Peripheral cyanosis	
A. Vascular obstruction	• Cyanotic appearance distal to obstruction caused by stasis (e.g., superior vena cava syndrome)
B. Cold exposure	• Females under age 40
1. Raynaud's phenomenon*	• Three-fold color change (i.e., white, blue, then red, especially of fingers)
2. Livido reticularis*	• Persistent lacelike mottled areas on legs
C. Decreased cardiac output	• Heart failure • Cardiogenic or septic shock

*Common causes.

hemoglobin. Central cyanosis is prominent on the lips, tongue, and face. It occurs because of inadequate oxygenation in the lungs or because of diseases that allow blood to bypass the lungs. Peripheral cyanosis involves the hands, cheeks, lips, and ears and may result from cold-induced vasoconstriction with resulting circulatory stasis. Excessive oxygen extraction by the tissues is the cause of peripheral cyanosis.

Two considerations are important in detecting cyanosis: persons with dark complexions may either appear cyanotic when not cyanotic, or their dark skin pigmentation may obscure cyanosis. Alternatively, some physicians find it more difficult to perceive cyanosis than do other physicians.

Besides pulmonary causes for cyanosis, the shock syndrome from nearly any cause, such as cardiogenic shock or septic shock, may result in cyanosis.

An appearance similar to cyanosis may be seen with methemoglobinemia of 1.5 g/dl or sulfhemoglobinemia of 0.5 g/dl. The absolute amount of oxygenated hemoglobin does not prevent the bluish color in any of these three conditions. Indeed, when the required concentration of deoxyhemoglobin, methemoglobin, or sulfhemoglobin is present, the color changes appear.

Argyria is an uncommon slate-blue discoloration distributed throughout the skin that superficially resembles cyanosis, but on closer inspection the two conditions can be distinguished. Argyria is caused by deposition of silver in the dermis, usually derived from medications containing silver.

Upper Respiratory Tract Symptoms

The upper respiratory tract has been discussed in the ear, nose, and throat portion of the history and examination (see Chapter 2). However, because these structures are contiguous with the lower respiratory tract, symptoms commonly coexist. Common symptoms referable to the nose are airway obstruction and nasal discharge. The "runny nose" is properly termed *rhinorrhea* or, if caused by a viral illness, *coryza*. The common cold affects adults 2 to 4 times each year and children 6 to 11 times. Colds are characterized primarily by nasal discharge. Rhinoviruses and coronaviruses most commonly cause cold symptoms, but these viruses may infect the lower airways, causing tracheitis or bronchitis. Allergy to inhaled pollen from dust or grass may result in nasal discharge and sneezing: if the paranasal sinuses become involved, pain or headache may result.

Past History of Pulmonary Problems

After obtaining the history of the present illness, ask about previous respiratory illnesses or symptoms. The questions below are not inclusive but are a guide to encourage patient recall.

- *Have you ever had asthma or an allergy to inhaled allergens, such as pollen?* Determine whether this visit is for a recurrent or a new episode. The problem may be complicated by disease or treatment (e.g., yeast overgrowth with inhaled steroids). Also check for a related problem (e.g., aspirin sensitivity, nasal polyps).
- *Have you ever had pneumonia?* The answer may provide clues to possible associated conditions, such as immune deficiency or tumor. Also check for complications of pneumonia (e.g., bronchiectasis).
- *Have you experienced pleuritic chest pain?* This can be a clue to possible pneumonia, pulmonary embolus, or previous chest wall pain.
- *What about tuberculosis: Ever had a reactive skin test, abnormal chest x-ray, bacillus of Calmette-Guerin (BCG) immunization?* Although common several years ago, tuberculosis is now seen usually in the elderly, Third World immigrants, HIV-positive persons, and the homeless. It is often undiagnosed unless specifically considered, and it is communicable.
- *Have you had chest injuries or operations?* These are usually dramatic, and the patient volunteers this information readily. Consider the potential for late complications (e.g., osteomylitis, pleural thickening).

Patients often fail to recognize relationships between bronchial asthma, allergic rhinitis, and other manifestations of allergy as urticaria, eczema, or angioedema. A detailed history of allergy to trees, grasses, ragweed or other plants, animal dander, foods, and medications may yield clues to the present illness.

In a patient who has pulmonary symptoms, ask about previous pneumonia because chronic pulmonary problems such as bronchiectasis or pulmonary fibrosis may follow pneumonia. For patients who have had pneumonia more than once, consider possible causes of aspiration such as loss of consciousness, drug abuse, or seizures. Recurrent pneumonia also alerts the clinician to possible structural lesions, such as endobronchial carcinoma, a foreign body in a bronchus, bronchiectasis, or cystic fibrosis. Immune defects also may result in recurrent pneumonia. Examples include AIDS, hypogammaglobulinemia, and leukemia.

Because of the recent resurgence in cases, tuberculosis must not be forgotten. Ask patients whether they have had a recent chest x-ray film or a skin test. Adults beyond midlife who initially have a negative PPD test should have a second skin test applied immediately to determine that they actually are not infected. Patients from Third World countries may have been immunized with BCG to reduce personal risk of developing tuberculosis. Initially after BCG immunizations the skin test may be positive, but most patients revert to negative skin tests within 2 years unless they are, in fact, infected with tuberculosis.

Intraabdominal processes that irritate the diaphragm mimic pulmonary disease by causing pleuritic chest pain or shoulder pain. Examples may include subphrenic abscess, splenic injury, intraabdominal bleeding, and pancreatitis with pleural effusion.

After the patient has volunteered information about previous illnesses and injuries, questions may elicit additional clues to pulmonary disease. Items from Tables 3-6 to 3-8 may help the patient's recall.

TABLE 3-6: Clues to Pulmonary Disease from Past Medical History

Clue	Disease Possibility
Infants and Toddlers	
Low birth weight and prematurity	• Respiratory distress syndrome
Sudden onset coughing	• Aspiration
Feeding difficulty	• Aspiration, child may be ill from myriad of causes
Apneic episodes (or sibling died of SIDS)	• Increased risk of SIDS
Recurrent pneumonia	• Cystic fibrosis
	• Immunodeficiency, congenital
	• AIDS
Older adults (age 60 + years)	
Cigarette pack years	• COPD, heart disease
	• Peripheral vascular disease
	• Cancer
Poor dentition	• Anaerobic pneumonia or lung abscess
Night sweats	• Chronic infection
	• Occult fever
	• Neoplasm
Weight loss	• Chronic infection, tumor
	• Malabsorption
	• Diabetes
	• Hyperthyroidism
Previous immunizations for respiratory pathogens	• 23-valent pneumococcal vaccine may reduce risk of pneumococcus infection
	• Influenza virus vaccine

In the child, the history of coughing or difficulty breathing suggests infectious disease, aspiration of a foreign body, or ingestion of a solvent (see Table 3-6). A severely ill baby or the baby with pneumonia may tire quickly, lose appetite, appear cyanotic, or work excessively and perspire while trying to feed. History of sudden infant death syndrome (SIDS) in a sibling suggests increased risk in the patient. Children who choke while they spit up are more likely to aspirate. Recurrent pneumonia in the pediatric age group may be caused by aspiration, cystic fibrosis, or immunodeficiency.

In older adults the history (see Table 3-6) may reveal potential for lung conditions. The number of cigarette packs smoked per day times the number of years smoking gives an estimate of the cigarette pack years. In general, an increasing number of pack years is associated with an increasing risk of chronic bronchitis, emphysema, coronary atherosclerotic heart disease, or lung cancer.

A history of poor dental hygiene is a risk factor for anaerobic aspiration pneumonia or lung abscess. Unrecognized fever may be manifested as sweating during the night. Such night sweats are characterized by soaking of night clothes, often requiring the changing of them. Night sweats may be found in patients with abscesses, cancer, tuberculosis, or AIDS. Unexplained weight loss has diagnostic significance pointing to similar diseases.

A history of immunization against pneumococcus or influenza virus helps in formulating the differential diagnosis.

The social history, including environmental exposures (Table 3-7), contributes to analysis of pulmonary symptoms. Pipe smoking is associated with lip cancer. Cigar smoke, inhaled by some smokers, may be as harmful as cigarette smoke. The lower tar and nicotine cigarettes currently in fashion may reduce the risk of lung and laryngeal cancer, but the added flavoring agents may pose risks yet undefined. Finally, other smoke besides tobacco, such as marijuana or smoke inhalation from a fire, may have deleterious effects.

Nature affords potential exposure to allergens, infective bacteria, or soil contaminated with bird droppings containing fungi. Air conditioning, water cooling towers, and hot water faucets may harbor *Legionella pneumophila*. Central heating with humidifiers has been associated with growth of thermophilic *Actinomycetes*. Water humidifiers or air conditioners support various pathogens. Exposure to other chemicals, dust, irritants, or allergens can occur at the work place.

Exposure to respiratory pathogens may occur from person-to-person contacts. An elderly nursing home patient or the homeless person may transmit *Mycobacterium tuberculosis*. Immigrants from southeast Asia and inner-city drug addicts or homeless people may transmit isoniazid-resistant strains of *M. tuberculosis*. Patients with HIV infection may have and transmit tuberculosis even before AIDS develops.

The family history may be contributory in patients with lung diseases. Several uncommon respiratory diseases have a hereditary component (Table 3-8). Inquiring about respiratory problems in family members may give clues to disease in the patient. Asthma, hay fever, and atopic eczema exhibit familial associations.

Physical Examination of the Respiratory System

General Examination

The physical examination in areas other than the chest may give clues toward the causes or complications of pulmonary diseases (Table 3-9). While taking the

TABLE 3-7: Social and Environmental History in Pulmonary Diseases

Clue	Disease Possibility

I. Tobacco use
  A. Patient smoked
    1. Type (cigarettes, pipe, cigars, chewing tobacco, snuff, smokeless tobacco, nicotine chewing gum)
 	
    2. Duration, number, calculate pack years
  B. Passively inhaled smoke (work or home) as a risk factor
	• Cardiovascular disease
	• Chronic bronchitis and emphysema
	• Cancer of lung, larynx, mouth, esophagus, bladder, kidney, stomach, pancreas
	
	• Small airways' dysfunction
	• Increased respiratory infections in infants

II. Home environment
  A. Allergens
  B. Infective pathogens
	
	• Flowers, trees, housedust, mites, and molds
	• Air conditioning units—*Legionella*
	• Water humidifier—actinomycetes
	• Dust, pathogenic fungi

III. Work environment
  A. Chemical, vapors
 	
  B. Allergens
	
	• Mask, goggles worn?
	• Changes in work procedures? Other workers affected?
	• Type of reaction, protection?

IV. Person exposure	• Tuberculosis • Influenza during epidemics
V. Animal exposure	• Pigeon droppings—*Cryptococcus* • Chicken, bat, or starling guano—*Histoplasma* • Sheep or cattle—Q fever • Parrots, parakeets—psittacosis • Rabbits—tularemia
VI. Travel exposure	• Midwest—*Histoplasma* • Southwest—*Coccidioides* • Southwest Asia—lung fluke (*Paragonimus*), melioidosis, tuberculosis

history, note whether the patient is breathing quietly or appears to be short of breath. Other signs to look for include wheezing, cyanosis, stridor, altered mentation, or restlessness. If the patient shows these signs of distress, the history and exam must be abbreviated to initiate immediate therapy. Later, after the patient is comfortable, the history can be completed.

The odor of the breath may indicate pulmonary disease. Halitosis can be caused by the following:

- Food ingested
- Poor oral hygiene
- Dental caries
- Exudative pharyngitis
- Sinusitis
- Necrotic lesions in mouth or throat
- *Campylobacter pylori* colonization of the stomach
- Lung abscess
- Zenker's diverticulum

TABLE 3-8: Uncommon Pulmonary Diseases with Hereditary Component

Disease	Inheritance	Clinical Manifestations	Other Diagnostic Techniques
Alpha$_1$-antitrypsin deficiency	• Autosomal dominant • 5% to 14% of population is heterozygous	• Develop severe basilar emphysema at early age • Bronchitis is common if patient smokes from age 20 to 40	• Serum protein electrophoresis, alpha$_1$ very low • CXR
Cystic fibrosis	• Autosomal recessive • 1:2,000 to 1:60,000	• Meconium ileus at birth • Bronchiectasis • Pancreatic and hepatobiliary dysfunction • Chronic progressive lung disease with multiple infections • Sterility	• Sweat test chloride above 70 mEq/L • CXR—highly suggestive
Familial interstitial lung disease	• Autosomal dominant	• Lung disease noted by age 30 to 50 years	• CXR
Kartagener's syndrome		• Defect in cilia motility • Situs inversus • Dextrocardia, sinusitis • Bronchiectasis • Nonmotile sperm	• CXR (dextrocardia) • Sinus films

TABLE 3-9: Physical Examination Clues to Pulmonary Diseases

Finding	Significance
I. Respiratory distress	
A. Dyspnea	• Arterial hypoxia, obstruction to airflow through bronchi
B. Cyanosis	• Desaturated hemoglobin exceeds 5 gm/dl
C. Stridor	• Large airway obstruction, potentially life-threatening
II. Aphonia, acute onset	• Laryngeal obstruction
III. Odor of breath	• Foul odor of anaerobic lung abscess, bronchiectasis, dental abscess • Sweet odor of diabetic ketoacidosis • Fishy odor of hepatic failure (fetor hepaticus) • Urinary odor of azotemia • Halitosis in stomatitis, gingivitis, coated tongue, cigarette smoking • Bitter almond odor of cyanide poisoning
IV. Clubbing of fingernails	
A. Lung disease	

1. Lung cancer, primary or metastatic
    2. Bronchiectasis
    3. Lung abscess
    4. Mesothelioma
	• Selective enlargement of distal segment of fingers or toes caused by increased soft tissue at proximal nail bed

B. Heart disease	
1. Cyanotic cardiac disease 2. Infective endocarditis	• As above

TABLE 3-9: Physical Examination Clues to Pulmonary Diseases—cont'd

Finding	Significance

C. GI disease
  1. Regional enteritis
  2. Chronic ulcerative colitis
  3. Cirrhosis of liver
	• As above

D. Idiopathic clubbing	• As above
V. Eyes	
A. Horner's syndrome (anisocoria, ptosis, miosis, anhidrosis)	• Interruption of inferior cervical or superior thoracic sympathetic chain or ganglia • Commonly caused by bronchogenic carcinoma
B. Choroidal lesions	
1. Tuberculosis, granulomas	• Indistinguishable on observation from sarcoid, fungal granuloma • Phylctenular lesions specifically indicate tuberculosis
2. Toxoplasma	• Acute lesions have yellow-white cottonlike patches and indistinct margins and are surrounded by erythema • Chronic lesions are white to gray plaques with black periphery of choroidal tissue
VI. Skin	
A. Malar facial rash with "butterfly" distribution	• Erythematous, flat or raised rash on cheeks • Exacerbated by ultraviolet light • Telangiectasia may develop in lupus
B. Erythema nodosum	• Red, raised tender nodules, especially over extensor surface of lower legs • Primary tuberculosis, coccidioidomycosis, histoplasmosis • Sarcoidosis • Beta-hemolytic streptococcal infections • Leprosy • Lymphogranuloma venerum • Ulcerative colitis, Crohn's syndrome • Medications
VII. Heart	
A. Tachycardia	• Pulmonary embolism • Anxiety states • Fever and infection • Pneumothorax
B. Accentuated P2	• Increased pulmonary arterial pressure occasionally in primary pulmonary hypertension but more often secondary to conditions such as COPD and emboli
C. Distant heart sounds best heard at base and epigastrium	• Barrel chest with increased space between heart and skin • Overinflated lung • Vertical heart • Lower diaphragms

Fecal breath odor is typical of anaerobic lung abscess and bronchiectasis.

Clubbing of the fingernails (see Chapter 12) is characterized by chronic swelling of the proximal nail beds, which distorts the angle between nail and nailbed with a soft puffiness. Viewed from the side, the proximal nail-nailbed angle becomes flat, with the fingernail and nailbed forming an arclike appearance. Viewed from above, the finger (or toe) with advanced clubbing is broadened near the tip. Patients often do not notice the changes of clubbing, partly because the onset may be so insidious. Diseases associated with clubbing include chronic respiratory disease, cyanotic chronic cardiac diseases with arteriovenous shunting, and inflammatory bowel disease.

The eye examination may provide clues to pulmonary abnormalities. Horner's syndrome consists of unilateral ptosis (droopy eyelid), miosis (small pupil), and *anhidrosis* (lack of sweating) on the same side. The cause is commonly lung cancer or another thoracic process that interrupts the superior cervical sympathetic nerve chain, causing the triad of symptoms.

Chemosis, or edema of the conjunctivae, which keeps the lids from closing because of swollen tissues, may be found in hyperthyroidism, allergies, or in obstruction of the superior vena cava. Other associations include COPD, congestive heart failure, and renal failure.

Choroidal tubercles found during ophthalmoscopic examination suggest sarcoidosis or disseminated tuberculosis.

The neck examination may give clues to pulmonary disease. Enlarged right supraclavicular lymph nodes suggest right-sided intrathoracic disease. In contrast, left supraclavicular nodes may be caused by abdominal or thoracic pathologic processes. Supraclavicular nodes on either side may be observed in various diseases such as carcinoma, lymphoma, sarcoidosis, AIDS, syphilis, or tuberculosis. Jugular venous distension in right-sided heart failure may be caused by pulmonary disease (cor pulmonale).

Skin clues to possible thoracic pathologic processes include the malar "butterfly" distribution of rash characteristic of lupus erythematosus. Pulmonary or pleural manifestations of lupus need not accompany the rash. Dilation of small veins over the lower third of the chest is occasionally seen in normal men, but unilateral dilated veins have been described in lung cancer, COPD, and AIDS. Erythema nodosum, small (1 to 3 cm) red nodules on the anterior aspect of the lower legs, sometimes accompanies coccidioidomyocosis, histoplasmosis, tuberculosis, or sarcoidosis. Vesicles of herpes zoster follow a dermatome distribution. Herpes zoster may be associated with severe pain before, during, and after the appearance of vesicles in elderly persons. Zoster pneumonia is an uncommon complication.

Chest Anatomy

The surface anatomy of the chest wall is used to describe the site of a lesion (Fig. 3-1). This is usually done by describing the lesion with reference to such sites as the suprasternal notch, the angle of Louis, the xiphoid process, the midsternal line, the midclavicular lines, or the anterior, medial, and posterior axillary lines, and by giving the number of the rib interspace. To count the ribs or interspaces, locate the sternal angle, which has the second rib attached laterally. By counting down along the sternum, the ribs and interspaces can be identified to the seventh rib.

For women with large breasts, skin and soft-tissue lesions may be described with reference to the nipple instead of the rib interspace. Thus a lesion might be described as being 2 cm from the right nipple at 5 o'clock.

The posterior surface anatomy of the chest is less precise. When a person flexes the head forward, the prominent vertebra is the seventh cervical. The costovertebral angle is formed by the inferior margins of the twelfth ribs and the

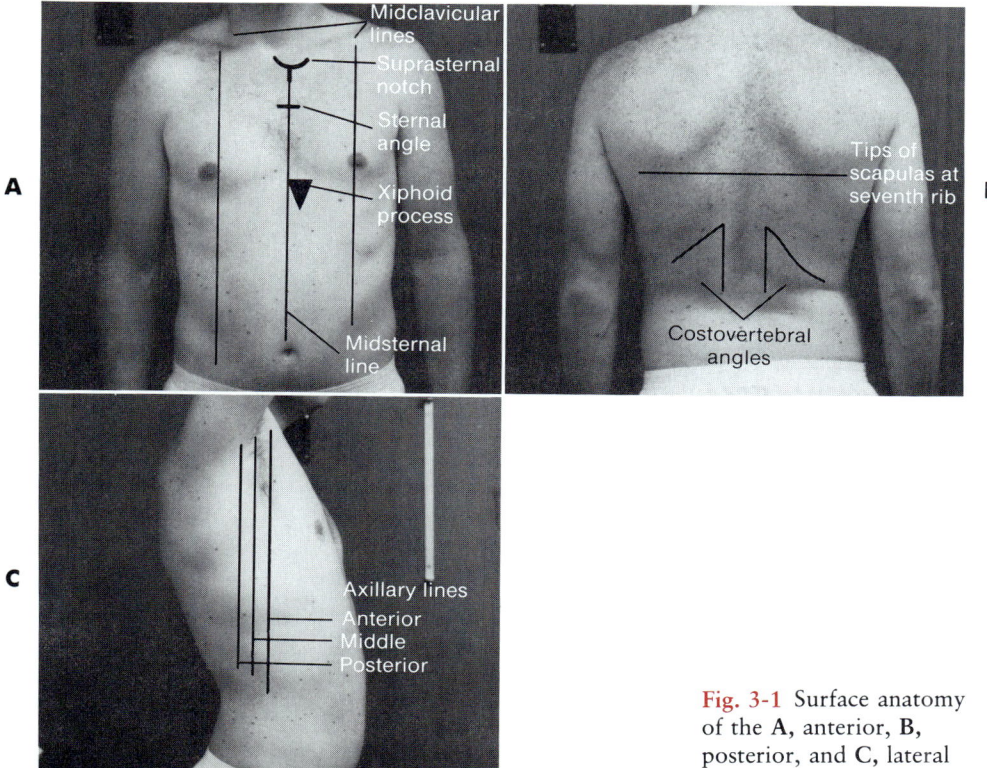

Fig. 3-1 Surface anatomy of the **A,** anterior, **B,** posterior, and **C,** lateral chest.

perpendicular line along the vertebral column. When sitting at rest, the tips of the scapulae extend over the seventh rib.

In examining the lungs, the imaginary projection of lobes and bronchopulmonary segments onto the chest wall becomes important in localizing intrathoracic disease (Fig. 3-2). The right lung has three lobes—the upper, middle, and lower lobes. The left lung has two lobes—the upper and the lower lobes. The left upper lobe lingula corresponds to the right middle lobe. Each lobe is subdivided into bronchopulmonary segments. The lobe or segment involved with pneumonia or tumor determines the site of physical findings.

Inspection

Examination of the chest usually proceeds from the posterior to the anterior chest. Each of the four techniques of examination (inspection, palpation, percussion, and auscultation) is applied, first posteriorly then anteriorly (see the box on pg. 99).

Study of respirations shows that resting adults breathe 12 to 16 times each minute. The respiratory rate in children is somewhat more rapid at 12 to 20 per minute. Most people sigh several times per hour, but repeated deep breathing is abnormal if not done voluntarily. Normal inhalation takes a proportionately longer time in the respiratory cycle than does exhalation. Exhalation is prolonged in asthma or COPD.

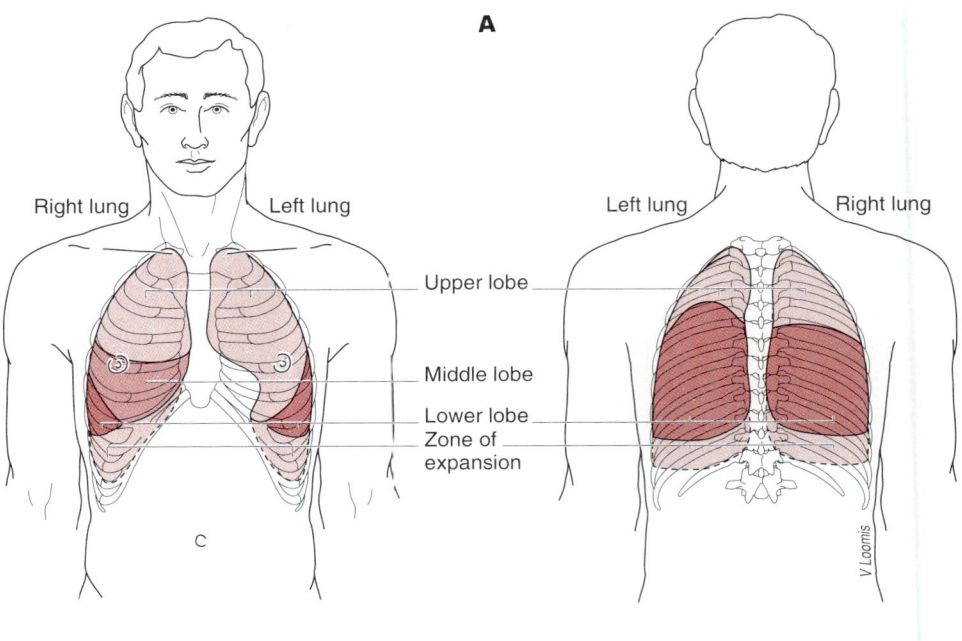

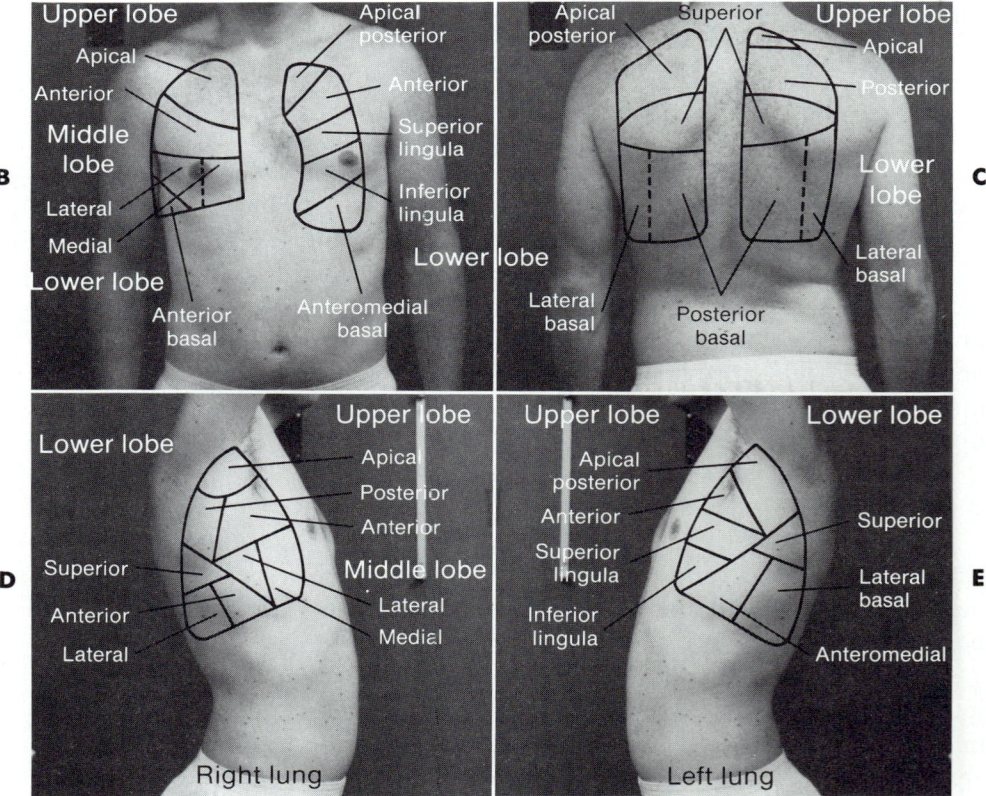

Fig. 3-2 Projections of lobes onto the surface of the chest wall. **A,** Drawing shows orientation. Bronchopulmonary segments. B through E, Views from anterior, posterior, and lateral positions.

> **Examination of the Chest**
>
> I. Inspection of the chest wall
>   A. Respirations
>   1. Rate (breaths per minute)
>   2. Breathing patterns
>   B. General configuration
>   1. Symmetry
>   2. Shape
>   3. Surface deformities (scars, prominences, nodules)
>   4. Trachea (midline, previous tracheostomy)
>   C. Posterior chest wall
>   1. Kyphosis
>   2. Scoliosis
>   3. Lordosis
>   4. Gibbus
>   5. Kyphoscoliosis
>   D. Anterior chest wall
>   1. Pectus carinatum (pigeon-chest deformity)
>   2. Pectus excavatum (funnel-chest deformity)
>   3. Barrel chest
>   4. Flail chest
> II. Palpation of chest
>   A. Palpate abnormalities observed by inspection
>   B. Palpate tender areas
>   1. Costochondral junction tenderness (Tietze's syndrome)
>   2. Broken ribs
>   3. Fracture of clavicle
>   4. Sternoclavicular joints
>   5. Xiphisternal junction
>   6. Pleural friction rub
>   C. Assess respiratory functioning
>   1. Tracheal position
>   2. Chest excursion
>   D. Tactile fremitus
>   1. Decreased or absent (pleural fluid, thickened pleura, emphysema, pneumothorax, atelectasis)
>   2. Increased (more often in males, and in pneumonia)
> III. Percussion of chest
>   A. Techniques
>   B. Percussion sounds
>   1. Tympanitic
>   2. Hyperresonant
>   3. Resonant (normal)
>   4. Dull
>   5. Flat
> IV. Auscultation of chest
>   A. Subtle sources or error
>   B. Normal breath sounds
>   1. Over trachea, bronchi
>   2. Over lung periphery
>   C. Abnormal sounds
>   1. Crackles (rales or crepitations)
>   2. Rhonchi (low pitched)
>   3. Wheezes (high pitched, musical)
>   4. Pleural friction rub
>   5. Vocal resonance (vocal fremitus)
>   a. Bronchophony
>   b. Pectoriloquy
>   c. Whispered pectoriloquy
>   d. Egophony
>   6. Hamman's sign

Bradypnea (Fig. 3-3) indicates a slow breathing rate, found in insulin coma, drug-induced respiratory depression, or increased ICP. *Tachypnea* refers to rapid, shallow breathing. Diseases that restrict the mobility of the lung, cause pleuritic chest pain, or decrease the size of the intrathoracic cavity (e.g., elevated diaphragm) may produce tachypnea. *Hyperpnea* indicates rapid, deep breathing, with increased minute ventilation disproportionate to metabolic needs. *Hyperventilation* is rapid, deep breathing causing overventilation, reducing the carbon dioxide content of the blood. This results in respiratory alkalosis. Causes include anxiety, aspirin overdose, and gram-negative septicemia. *Kussmaul respirations* are characteristically deep, usually rapid breaths (central hyperventilation) typical of metabolic acidosis, particularly diabetic hyperglycemic coma. To compensate

Fig. 3-3 Patterns of respiration that patients commonly exhibit.

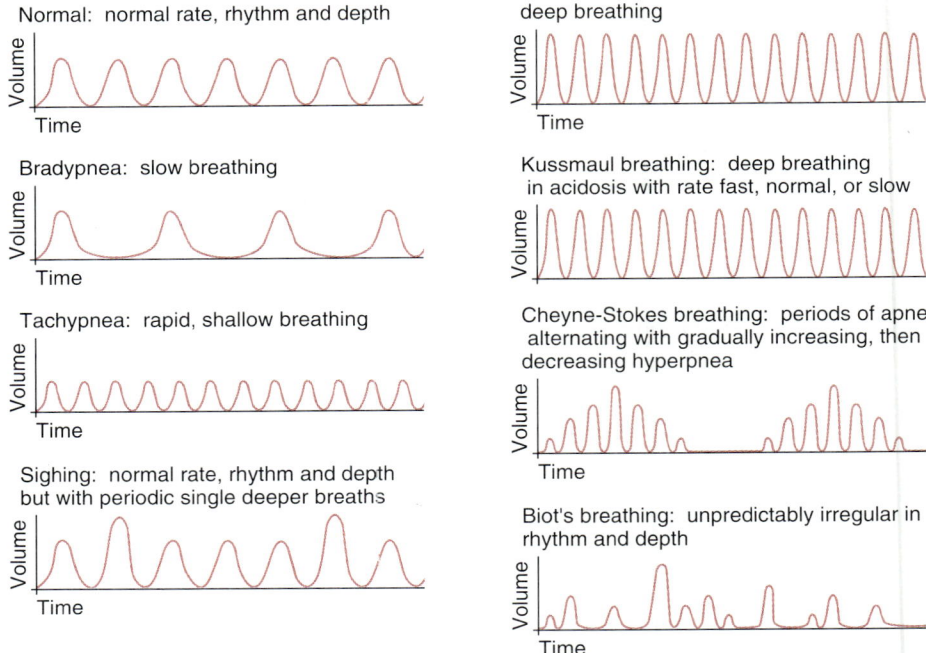

for the increased metabolic acid, there is compensatory breathing-out of carbon dioxide. Other metabolic acidosis, renal failure, and lactic acidosis can cause Kussmaul respirations. Some patients with Kussmaul respirations have a normal rate of breathing but have a larger than normal tidal volume.

Cheyne-Stokes respiration is cyclic (periodic) breathing in which apnea alternates between cycles of gradually increasing, then decreasing hyperpnea. Cheyne-Stokes respiration occurs with cerebral dysfunction. The respiratory centers become less sensitive to minute changes in arterial carbon dioxide tension. As the apnea phase continues, the P_{CO_2} rises. This stimulates breathing, but the patient's carbon dioxide level is lowered so much that apnea results. Causes include congestive heart failure, uremia, meningitis, or pneumonia. Cheyne-Stokes respirations may indicate a grave prognosis, or they may subside without fatal outcome.

Biot's breathing has been termed *ataxic breathing* because of the unpredictable and irregular respirations. Breaths may be shallow or deep and cease for short periods. Biot's breathing may occur with meningitis or other causes of brain dysfunction.

Sleep apnea is a common abnormality of lack of airflow at the mouth and nostrils for at least 10 seconds. Sleep apnea is common in men over age 50, who may have as many as 10 apneic episodes per hour of sleep. The airway is obstructed by relaxed pharyngeal muscles, backward movement of the tongue, upper airway obesity, or enlarged tonsils or adenoids. Arterial oxygen desaturation occurs during apnea. Such persons have chronic sleep deprivation, daytime somnolence, paranoia, hostility, and agitated depression.

For proper inspection of chest and thorax, ask the patient to undress to the waist and be sure the lighting is good. Provide women with suitable gown, open toward the back, so that the portions not being examined may be covered. Begin

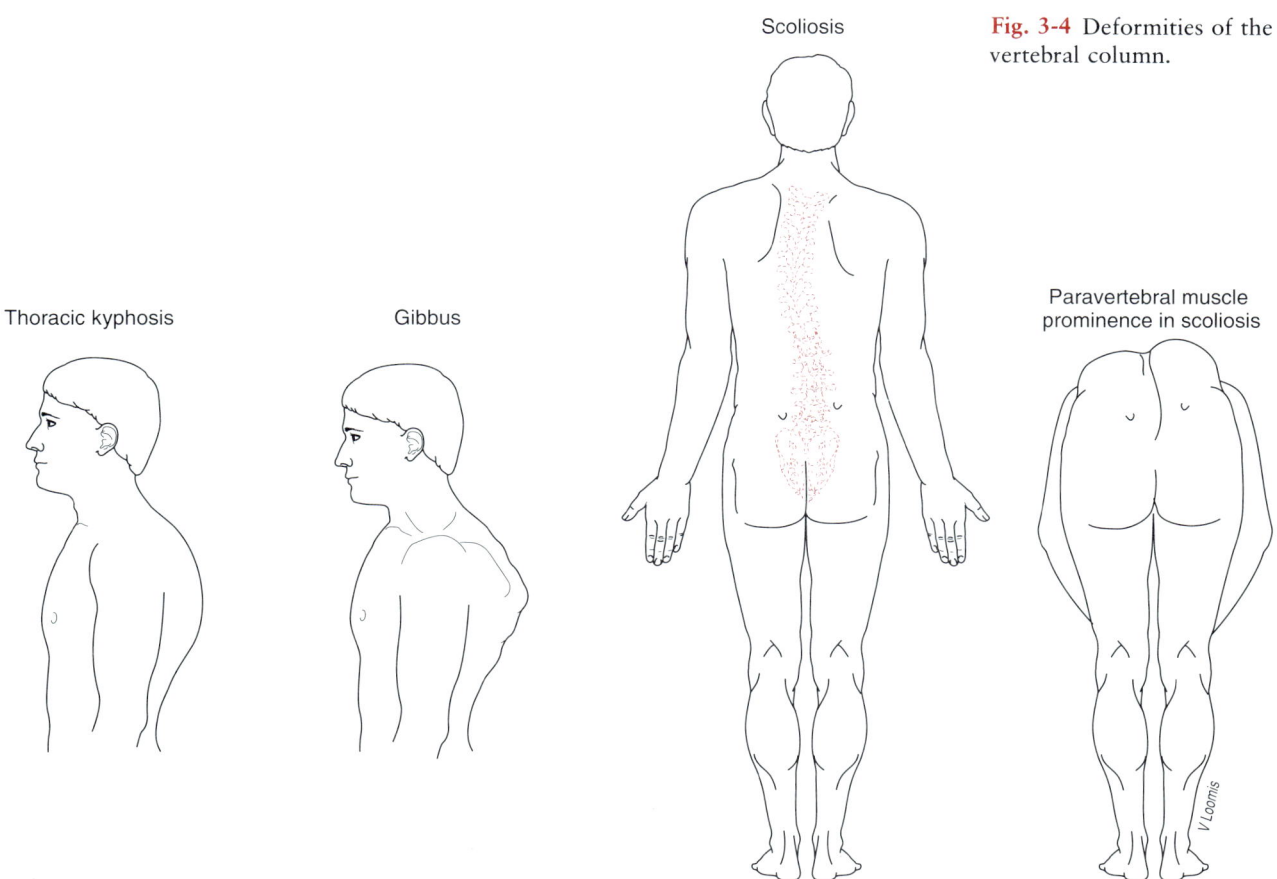

Fig. 3-4 Deformities of the vertebral column.

this part of the examination with the patient sitting, to enable comparison of one side of the chest with the other. Extremely ill and unconscious patients may be examined while supine, rotating them from side to side.

Beginning at the base of the neck, observe the general shape of the neck, arms, and chest. The *buffalo hump*, a fatty deposit overlying C7, is characteristic of Cushing's syndrome (corticosteroid effect). Observe the ratio of anteroposterior chest measurement compared with lateral measurement of the chest; normally this is 5:7. Flat-chested people have an anteroposterior:lateral ratio of 1:2. The configuration of the barrel chest seen in emphysema is more rounded (like a barrel) so that the ratio is approximately 1:1.

Abnormal vertebral column configurations may be found on examination of the posterior chest wall (Fig. 3-4). *Kyphosis* is excessive hunchback curvature of the spine. Mild kyphosis is normally present in the thoracic spine. Excessive kyphosis may be congenital or may develop with aging, causing the "dowager's hump" that results from osteoporosis with compression of vertebrae and narrowing of intervertebral spaces.

Scoliosis is lateral curvature of the spine in an S-shaped formation. Subtle scoliosis may be detected by having the patient bend forward. Instead of the normal symmetric prominence of paravertebral muscles on each side of the vertebral column, excessive prominence of muscles on one side of the spine occurs in scoliosis. *Kyphoscoliosis* is the combination of kyphosis and scoliosis together, abnormal curvature of the spine both in the anteroposterior and lateral dimensions.

Lordosis is the bowing of the spine inwardly, normally found in the lumbar and cervical spines. Lordosis is always abnormal if it is present in the thoracic spine. A few slender people have the straight back syndrome with relative absence of either kyphosis or lordosis along the spine.

Gibbus deformity is a sharp change of the angle of the spine instead of a gradual change. This sharp angulation presents a posterior spine prominence usually caused by destruction of a vertebral body. Gibbus deformity is characteristic of Pott's disease, vertebral tuberculosis.

Checking for maximal expansion of chest circumference may be helpful to the physician. Asthma, emphysema, and pulmonary fibrosis restrict chest excursions. Place a string or tape measure around the chest, then ask the patient to exhale completely and then inhale completely. Note the difference in the measured circumferences. Chest expansion of less than 2 cm is abnormal, whereas expansions of 5 cm or greater are normal. An alternative method of checking expansion of the chest is performed while palpating the back and is described later.

Inspect the anterior chest beginning with the configuration of the neck, arms, breasts, and sternum. Examination of the breasts is discussed in further detail in Chapter 8. Inspect the base of the neck for tracheal deviation and thyroid prominence, and the supraclavicular areas for adenopathy, swelling, and jugular venous pulsations.

Deformities apparent on examination of the anterior chest include barrel chest, pectus carinatum, and pectus excavatum (Fig. 3-5). In *pectus carinatum* (pigeon-chest deformity) the sternum is displaced forward so that the anteroposterior measurement is increased. The sternum has been likened to the keel of a ship (carinate) or the chest of a pigeon. This deformity may be found in those with Marfan's syndrome or rickets or in otherwise normal people.

In *pectus excavatum* (funnel-chest deformity) the lower end of the sternum is depressed inwardly toward the backbone. The configuration is described as resembling a funnel. Pectus excavatum may also be found after rickets or in Marfan's syndrome. Likewise, pectus excavatum may be observed in otherwise normal individuals.

A *flail chest,* caused by multiple fractured ribs, allows one side of the chest to move paradoxically during respirations, opposite to the other side.

Inspection of the normal chest during breathing should show both sides expanding equally and simultaneously. Delayed movement of one side may be caused by pain from pneumonia, pleurisy, or pulmonary infarction. An endobronchial foreign body, a tumor, or neurologic impairment may produce similar findings.

Respiratory distress describes breathing of patients working at breathing, who appear apprehensive, or who are using cervical accessory muscles (sternocleidomastoideus, scaleni, and trapezii) in breathing. These patients may have cyanotic lips, tongue, ears, and fingertips.

Children in respiratory distress may have flared nasal alae or chest wall retractions. Retraction occurs during inhalation, with expansion of the chest and simultaneous inward retraction of the abdominal muscles. Such children are usually breathing rapidly and exhibit a combination of findings. Stridor, wheezing, and grunting noises with respiration may be apparent.

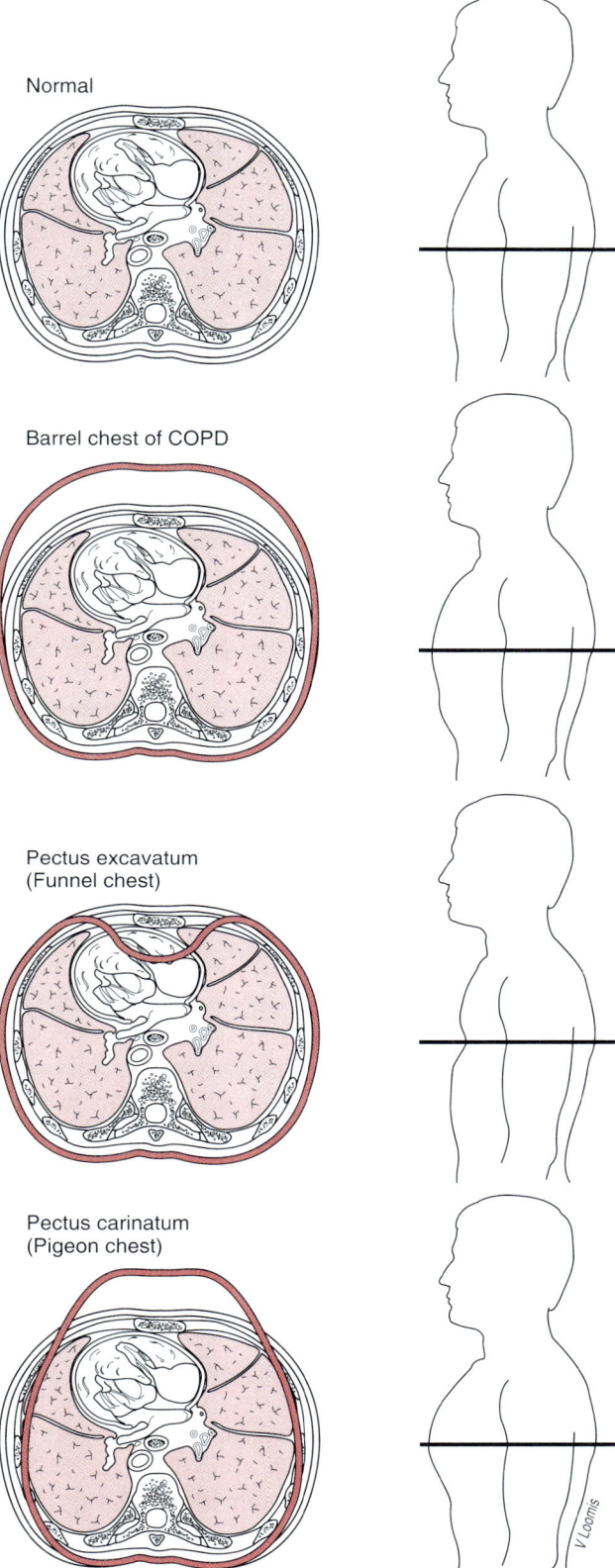

Fig. 3-5 Deformities of the chest wall.

Fig. 3-6 Respiratory expansion. **A,** Position of hands on patient's chest to show respiratory excursion: full expiration. **B,** Hands moved apart when patient takes a deep breath. This shows normal potential for chest expansion with respirations.

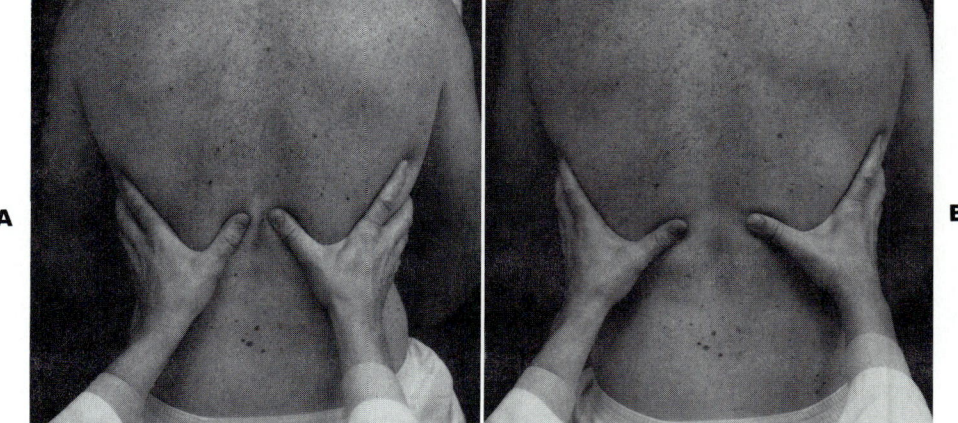

Palpation

Palpate the chest wall using the flat surfaces of the hands and fingers. Palpation of the chest allows the clinician to assess abnormalities observed by inspection, to identify tender areas, to examine other abnormalities, to assess chest excursion as described above, and to observe transmitted vibrations when the patient speaks.

Subcutaneous nodules, lipomas, macules, papules, and petechiae observed by inspection are differentiated using palpation. *Sinus tracts* (tunnels under the skin) allow drainage of serous or purulent material. For example, actinomycosis produces sinus tracts under the skin of the chest in the immunosuppressed patient. Costochondral joint swelling and tenderness *(Tietze's syndrome)* mimics other causes of chest pain. Fractured ribs or clavicle may be suspected because of tenderness on palpation, yet an x-ray study is both more sensitive and specific. The sternoclavicular joint may be warm and swollen in rheumatoid disease, septic arthritis, or disseminated gonococcemia. Normal adults may complain of a tender xiphoid process. Patients with pleurisy may perceive their own friction rub, which can be palpated but is more clearly identified by auscultation.

Subcutaneous emphysema produces a crepitus or crackly sensation when palpated, indicating air moving through the tissues. Subcutaneous emphysema is often caused by disruption of the lower respiratory tract. Examples include the patient with a tracheostomy or the patient with endotracheal intubation who is receiving positive end–expiratory pressure to treat adult respiratory distress syndrome (ARDS).

Palpation is used to assess chest excursion during breathing. The examiner lays the palms of both hands on the back of the chest with the thumbs extended toward the patient's head. The examining fingers are outstretched over the sides of the thorax. As the patient breathes, the thumbs are pulled from the midline, giving an indication of expansion (Fig. 3-6).

The trachea is also palpated during breathing. Normally it descends slightly during inspiration. The suprasternal notch rises slightly as the ribs move towards the head. An uncommon sign is the tracheal tug, felt with the heart beat, called *Oliver's sign*. With the patient sitting, ask him to lift his chin up. Palpate the trachea for a tug or pull. This is caused by an aortic aneurysm or dilated aorta, which pulls the trachea downward by pressure on the left mainstem bronchus.

The trachea may deviate somewhat from the midline toward the right side in older patients. A lateral shift in mediastinal structures can cause deviation toward

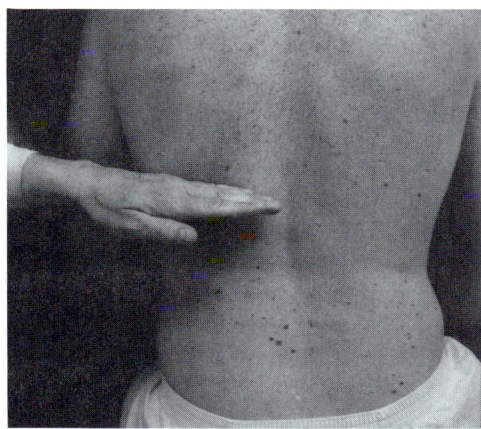

Fig. 3-7 Tactile fremitus using the side of the hand against the chest. Examiner locates level of diaphragm while patient repeats phrase "ninety-nine."

either side. *Pneumothorax* (air between visceral and parietal pleura) shifts the trachea towards the side opposite the pneumothorax. Pneumothorax may occur spontaneously or may follow rupture of a subpleural bleb or a penetrating wound of the chest wall. *Tension pneumothorax* is a medical emergency in which a ball valve mechanism allows air into but not out of the pneumothorax during breathing. Gradually the pressure increases. Other causes of tracheal and mediastinal shift include pleural effusion or empyema. The mediastinum and trachea shift to the opposite side. In contrast, atelectasis of a lobe of the lung shifts the mediastinum and trachea toward the affected side because of loss of volume on that side. Tumor, aspirated foreign body, or mucus plugging of a bronchus are potential causes of atelectasis.

Tactile fremitus (vibration) is assessed by either the palm or the ulnar edge of the hand against the chest wall (Fig. 3-7). Ask the patient to say "ninety-nine" or "1, 2, 3." Vibrations are transmitted to the examining hand from normal lungs. Fremitus is produced by sound vibrations originating in the larynx passing through the lungs to vibrate the chest wall. The lung anatomy allows the transmitted frequency to vibrate the chest wall (Fig. 3-8). Normally, by moving

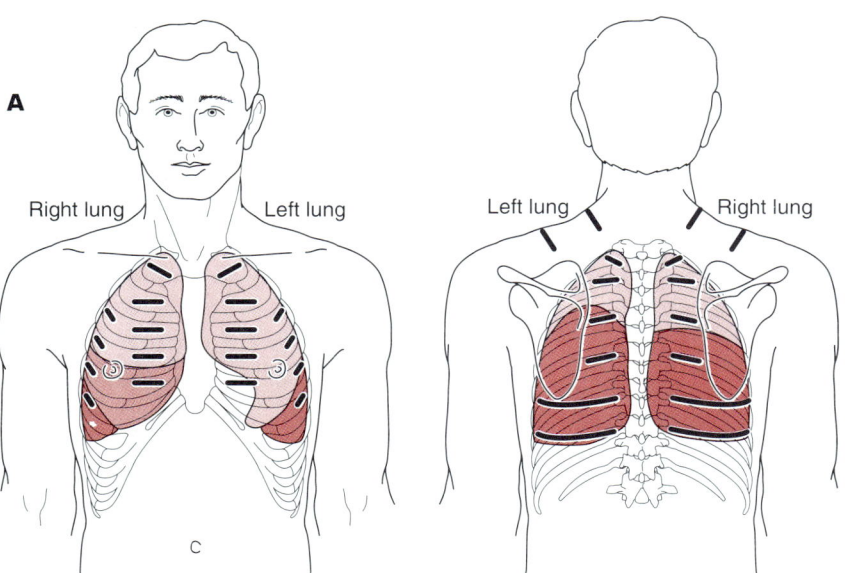

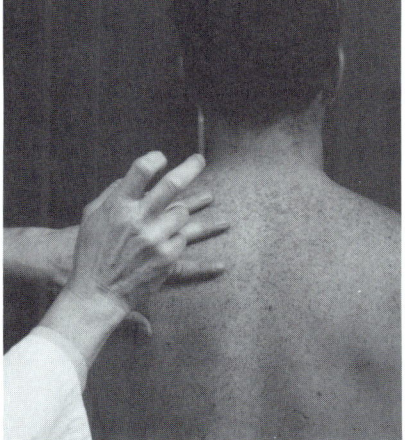

Fig. 3-8 Percussion of the chest. **A,** Drawing shows bars to indicate sites on the anterior and posterior chest to percuss and auscultate. **B,** Posterior view. Tip of third finger of the right hand strikes the distal interphalangeal joint of the left third finger. Entire left third finger is pressed against chest wall. Vibrations are felt and heard. Percuss from above down to and then below the diaphragm.

the examining hand to various levels of the chest, one can compare fremitus and find the levels of the two leaves of the diaphragms. Fremitus is increased in deep, resonant voices and decreased in high-pitched voices. Fremitus is increased in pneumonia with pulmonary consolidation. Fremitus is absent below the level of the fluid in pleural effusion or empyema because the fluid between the lung and the chest wall reduces transmission of vibrations. Other causes of decreased fremitus include pleural thickening, pneumothorax, atelectasis, and emphysema.

Percussion

Percussion (mediate percussion as opposed to direct percussion) is performed by laying the palm and fingers of the examining hand against the chest and striking the distal interphalangeal joint of the left middle finger with the tip of the right middle finger. The striking finger is partially flexed, the right wrist relaxed similar to that of the concert pianist. The objective is to transmit vibrations to the underlying chest wall. The middle finger of the left hand laying flat against the chest will feel a difference in vibrations depending on the deep structures. An audible tone is also present and varies depending on deeper structures. Air-filled normal underlying tissues vibrate responsively and are termed *resonant*.

Percussion of the posterior chest should begin at the apex of one side followed by percussion of the opposite side (see Fig. 3-8). In sequence, percuss down the back, first on one side, then the other from apex to diaphragm. Diaphragmatic excursion can be assessed by percussing both sides first with deep inhalation and then with maximal exhalation (Fig. 3-9). Normal diaphragmatic excursion is 3 to 5 cm. Anterior percussion dullness is higher on the right than on the left. The borders of the mediastinum and heart can be percussed when light percussion is used.

Three to five percussion sounds are described, depending on the clinician (Table 3-10). Percussion over the periphery of the normal chest gives resonance. An increased ringing quality is *hyperresonance*. This may be found in emphysema or pneumothorax. Increased resonance is called *tympany*. Tympanitic sounds are

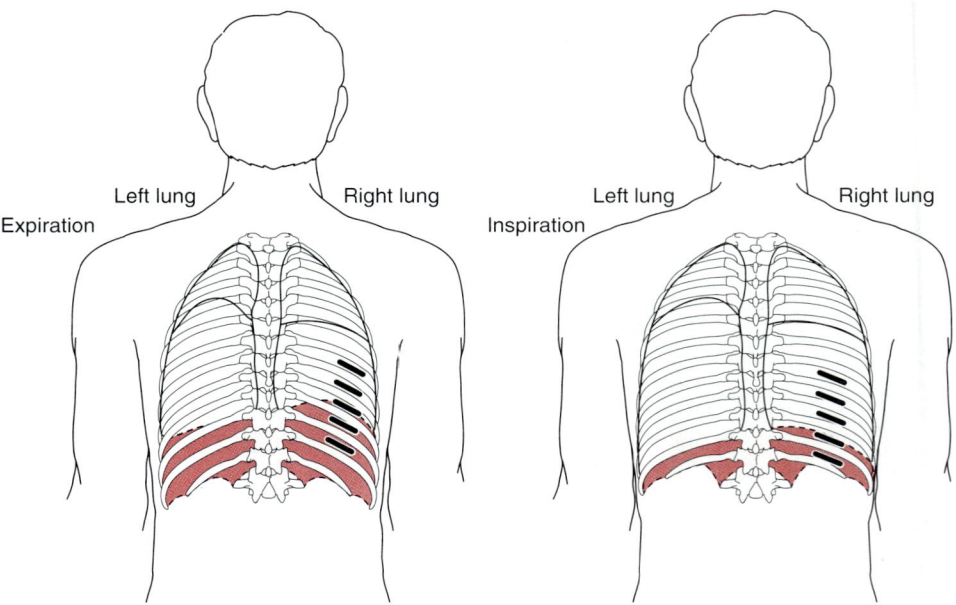

Fig. 3-9 Sites to percuss levels of the diaphragm to assess diaphragmatic expansion.

TABLE 3-10: Percussion Sounds

Sound	Description	Association
Flat	• Very dull without ringing tones	• Heard over large pleural effusions
Dull	• Decreased resonance	• Heard over the liver or over pleural effusions
Resonance	• Normal sound with some ring	• Normal chest, laterally
Hyperresonance	• Increase in ringing tones	• Heard over chest hyperexpanded as in emphysema
Tympanitic	• Even more ringing	• Heard over air-filled stomach or distended intestines

heard from percussion over air-filled structures such as the gastric bubble or gas-filled intestines. Usually hyperresonance, not tympany, is heard in percussion of the chest.

On the other hand, two tones describe reduced resonance: dullness and flatness. *Dullness* is a decrease in resonance, normally found over the liver, spleen, or below the diaphragm. Pleural fluid, empyema, or consolidation of lobar pneumonia results in dullness to percussion. *Flatness* describes extreme dullness with few or no ringing tones. Examples may include pleural effusions, massive pulmonary consolidation with tumor, and pneumonia. Solid masses tend to dampen the vibrations, giving a flat or dull tone. Solid masses more than 5 to 6 cm away from the chest wall usually cannot be detected by percussion. Small lung lesions not adjacent to the chest wall ordinarily do not give a dull percussion note. However, pleural fluid does so, and percussion may readily suggest as little as 200 to 300 ml of fluid.

The patient's illness may require the clinician to percuss when the patient is in the supine position or lying on the side. If the patient's spine is in an **S**-shape, the ribs may be closer or further apart than normal. This relationship changes the percussion note unless pillows are placed under the patient to straighten the vertebral column.

Caveats in percussion include the following:

1. Remember that pleural fluid requires a few minutes to settle completely into dependent positions after the patient moves from the recumbent position to sitting. Thus wait until after the patient has been sitting before beginning to percuss.
2. Patients who have COPD and emphysema may exhibit hyperresonance so that cardiac dullness is nearly undetectable.
3. In emphysema the diaphragms posteriorly are much lower than is normal by percussion.
4. The inexperienced examiner may neglect to move the right breast of a woman to percuss for dullness of right middle lobe pneumonia, typically behind the right breast. This clue to pneumonia would then be missed.

Auscultation

The choice of stethoscope for chest examination is not so critical as the choice for cardiac auscultation. A stethoscope should be used with both the diaphragm

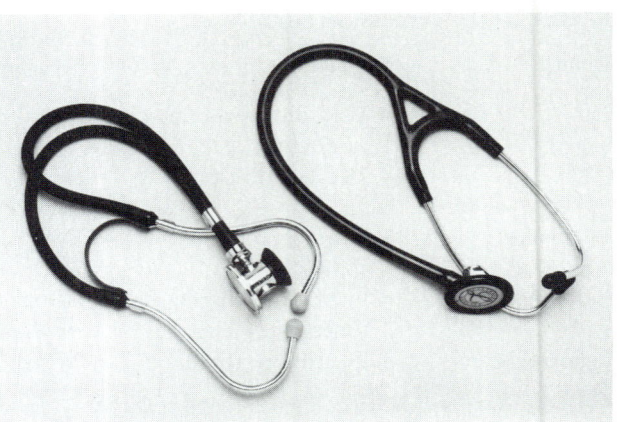

Fig. 3-10 Use of the stethoscope.

and bell functions. These may have two separate heads, one head that can be rotated, or one head that changes from bell to diaphragm function with pressure (Fig. 3-10). When the bell is lightly placed against the skin, low-pitched sounds are heard better. The diaphragm placed firmly against the skin is used for high-pitched sounds. Most of the sounds that reach the chest wall from the bronchi and lungs are of low frequency; thus the bell should be used in preference to the diaphragm. However, most clinicians use the diaphragm for chest examination because it is easier to use (see the box on pg. 99).

Choose a comfortable stethoscope. The tubes should be long enough to give the examiner some mobility, but excessively long tubes reduce sound transmission. About 22 to 26 inches from ear pieces to chest piece is about right. The tubing should be sufficiently thick to maintain the internal diameter without collapsing or narrowing at bends. The ear pieces should fit comfortably enough to be worn for several minutes. Soft ear pieces of a comfortable size may be used to replace uncomfortable ear pieces.

Subtle errors may trick the inexperienced examiner who is not able to identify extraneous sounds. Hair rubbing against the stethoscope or the tubing may mimic chest sounds. Occasionally, hairy chests need to have water applied to prevent this occurence. The rustling of a paper examination gown against a stethoscope tube may cause confusion. The constant muscle activity of tremors (e.g., either chills or parkinsonism) may lead to error. Similarly, patients who have shaking chills may have muscle noises, mimicking pulmonary crackles.

Normal sounds of breathing depend on where the stethoscope is placed during auscultation. *Tracheal breath sounds* are loud, harsh, and high pitched. They may be heard better while listening over the trachea in the neck than in the chest. These do not provide significant diagnostic information.

Bronchial breath sounds are loud and high pitched, with air swishing past. They are normally heard while auscultating over the midsternum. Bronchial breath sounds may be heard over the periphery of the lung, but sound as if the examiner were listening over the trachea or major bronchi.

Bronchovesicular sounds are a mixture of peripheral lung vesicular breath sounds and bronchial breath sounds and are heard near where the mainstream bronchi begin to branch. On the chest wall, they are heard by listening anteriorly over the first and second interspaces lateral to the sternum and posteriorly medial to the scapulas.

TABLE 3-11: Abnormal Sounds Heard During Chest Auscultation

Current Term	Older Term	Presumed Mechanism	Associated Diseases
Crackle (fine or course)	• Rale	• Fluid in airway	• Congestive heart failure, bronchitis, pneumonia
Wheeze	• Sibilant or musical rale	• Air moving rapidly past narrowed segment of airway	• Asthma
Rhonchus	• Sonorus (snoring) rhonchus	• Same as for wheeze	• Same as for wheeze
Pleural friction rub	• Pleural friction rub	• Parietal and visceral pleura roughened and rubbing with respirations	• Pneumonia, pulmonary infarction

Vesicular breath sounds are soft, low pitched, airy, and swishing as air rushes into the alveoli in most of the lung.

The abnormal absence of breath sounds may be caused by several disorders. Mucus plugging of a bronchus, pneumothorax, pleural effusion, or pulmonary emphysema may each prevent breath sounds from being heard in a particular portion of the chest.

Abnormal sounds (adventitious sounds) may be heard during auscultation of the lungs (Table 3-11). Because the nomenclature has changed during recent years, both the old and new terms are used. *Crackles* are soft, short, high-pitched fine sounds. These may be simulated by rubbing a lock of hair between the fingers near the ear. Another variety of crackle, the coarse crackle, is slightly longer and lower pitched. Older terms for crackles include *rales* and *crepitations* (rale means "noise"). The term rale was previously applied to fine crackles, but also to rhonchi and wheezes. Because these names were confusing, crackles became the term generally accepted as an alternative to rale. The *rhonchus* is a low-pitched sonorous (snoring) sound. The *wheeze* is sibilant (squeaking) and higher pitched. Both the low-pitched rhonchus and the high-pitched wheeze have a musical quality.

Crackles may be heard in normal lung bases posteriorly, but these clear, giving vesicular breath sounds after a few deep breaths or coughs. Persisting crackles indicate a pathologic process such as pneumonia, pulmonary edema, bronchitis, or bronchiectasis.

Rhonchi indicate fluid or mucus in the airways, trachea, or bronchi. Wheezes signify partial airway obstruction. Wheezes are usually loud and persist during exhalation. The pitch of the wheeze is determined by the velocity of the air passing the site of narrowing. Wheezes are found in patients with asthma, emphysema, or bronchitis. Occasionally, during asthmatic attacks, wheezes may be heard without a stethoscope.

The pleural friction rub is actually a special type of crackle. The *pleural friction rub* is a grating sound heard during breathing that stops when the breath is held. It is caused by friction of roughened visceral and parietal pleura. The pleural rub may be heard in pneumonia, pleural infarction, tumor of the pleura, or pleural

TABLE 3-12: Examination Techniques Used to Determine Underlying Lung Pathology

Pathologic Process	Inspection	Palpation Fremitus	Percussion Note	Auscultation
Consolidation in pneumonia	• Fever, tachypnea, splints one side of chest	• Increased tactile fremitus	• Dullness	• Crackles, E-to-A changes, or bronchophony
Pleural effusion	• Tachypnea • Trachea shifted away from involved side	• Decreased fremitus	• Dullness	• Absent breath sounds • E to A changes in compressed lung above effusion
Pneumothorax	• Tachypnea • Affected side may lag behind • Trachea may be shifted away from involved side	• Absent fremitus	• Hyperresonant	• Absent breath sounds
Atelectasis	• Tachypnea • May have affected side lag with respirations • Trachea may shift toward affected side	• Decreased fremitus	• Dullness	• Absent breath sounds

effusion. The development of a large effusion prevents continuing friction between the pleura and stops the rub.

Abnormal transmission of sounds may be heard over areas of lung consolidation caused by pneumonia or of lung compressed at the top of a pleural effusion. When a normal person whispers, "1, 2, 3" or "ninety-nine," the sound is not transmitted to the peripheral lung. Over areas of consolidation, the enhanced sound transmission is described by three phenomena: bronchophony, whispered pectoriloquy, and egophony.

Bronchophony is the increased transmission of the spoken word to the lung periphery as if listening over a bronchus. The examiner listens while the patient says, "ninety-nine" and he hears, "ninety-nine." Bronchophony indicates pulmonary consolidation.

Whispered pectoriloquy refers to the words being more clearly understood. When the patient whispers, "1, 2, 3" during auscultation, no sound is transmitted to the examiner. If the whispered word is transmitted and clearly understood, pulmonary consolidation is present. This sign may be observed even before pneumonia is apparent on the chest radiograph.

Egophony is a form of pectoriloquy in which the patient is instructed to say "E" but the examiner hears "A." This E-to-A change also can signify pulmonary consolidation or may mean lung compression caused by pleural effusion. The word "egophony" is derived from the Greek roots meaning "goat voice" because of the similarity of the sound to the bleating of the goat.

Solid, airless lung tissue allows sounds and vibrations from the larynx to be transmitted to the chest wall with less dampening than is normal. Normal lung tends to filter out high-pitched sounds more than low-pitched sounds.

Another special sound observed during auscultation is Hamman's sign. This is a crunching, crackling sound like walking in loose snow or the creaking of new leather. The crunch occurs in synchrony with the heart beat when mediastinal air is present. Free air in the mediastinum may follow chest or heart surgery, trauma, or rupture of the esophagus in Boerhaave's syndrome.

The examiner must use all of this information—inspection, palpation, percussion, and auscultation—to arrive at a diagnosis. Table 3-12 shows how these pieces of information fall together to form a working diagnosis for some common conditions.

History and Physical Findings in Selected Pulmonary Problems (Table 3-13)

Asthma

Between attacks of asthma, a patient may be well with normal chest examination findings or may have a few wheezes. An attack begins with cough, rapidly progressive dyspnea, and tachypnea. The patient assumes a sitting position, may lean forward, and becomes anxious. Inspection may show an anxious patient with labored breathing and occasionally one who sweats profusely. The respiratory rate is usually not increased, but the exhalation phase is prolonged. Fremitus shows the diaphragm to be depressed and the thorax to be held in full expansion through most of the respiratory cycle. Percussion reveals a hyperresonant chest with depressed diaphragms. On auscultation, wheezing is apparent during the exhalation phase and indeed may be apparent without the use of a stethoscope. Breath sounds may temporarily disappear from areas of the chest if bronchial mucus plugging occurs.

The differential diagnosis includes extrinsic asthma precipitated by allergens, respiratory infection, exercise, or cold exposure. Intrinsic asthma may be precipitated by unknown factors. Other disorders that cause wheezing resembling asthma include pulmonary edema, multiple small pulmonary emboli, or left-sided cardiac failure.

Atelectasis

Atelectasis occurs when something obstructs an air passage into a pulmonary segment, as when bronchial secretions are tenacious and form a plug. The volume of the involved lung decreases, and the airless, more dense lung mass is pulled toward the chest wall by the negative pressure. Inspection may show tracheal deviation toward the side involved if the atelectatic segment is sufficiently large. The patient may have fever. Tactile fremitus is decreased to absent. The percussion note is dull in the involved area. Breath sounds are decreased or absent. Usually, crackles are not caused by atelectasis alone.

The differential diagnosis besides bronchial plug includes obstruction to the airway by an aspirated foreign body, extrinsic compression of the bronchus by tumor growth, or loss of elastic recoil of the lung after thoracic or abdominal surgical procedures.

Bronchiectasis

Bronchiectasis indicates dilated bronchi or bronchioles related to frequent pulmonary infections. The history is one of coughing up large amounts of purulent sputum. The onset of bronchiectasis may not be clear or may relate to

TABLE 3-13: Key Elements in Diagnosis of Selected Pulmonary Conditions

Key Elements from History	Key Elements from Physical	Key Diagnostic Studies
I. Asthma—airway irritability stimulated by cause specific for the patient 　A. Allergic—airborne allergen (e.g., feathers, dander, molds) 　B. Drug induced—aspirin, coloring additive as tartrazine, beta-adrenergic antagonists, sulfating agents 　C. Pollution—industrial air contaminants, especially with atmospheric inversions, cigarette smoke 　D. Occupational—Metal salts, wood and vegetable dusts, industrial chemicals and plastics, laundry detergents, animal and insect dusts 　E. Infectious—Respiratory viruses as RSV and parainfluenza in children, rhinovirus and influenza virus in older patients 　F. Exercise—Bronchospasm induced by exercise 　G. Emotional stress—Psychologic factors often interact with disease process 　H. Idiosyncratic—No personal or family history of any above; attack may worsen with URI, exposure to cold, exercise	• Key triad—dyspnea, wheezing, cough • Inspection—anxious patient, sitting up pale, cyanosis only in late severe disease, use of accessory muscles in breathing; small children may show retractions • Palpation—fremitus shows depressed diaphragms • Percussion—depressed diaphragms; hyperresonant chest • Auscultation—prolonged exhalation, wheezing, lack of breath sounds in areas of mucus plugging	• Pulmonary function studies abnormal 　FEV-1 reduced to 30% of predicted for the patient 　MMEF reduced to 20% predicted patient 　RV may be four times normal • When RV is twice predicted and FEV-1 is 50% of predicted, patient feels like attack has subsided • Arterial blood gases 　Reduced oxygen (P_{O_2}) 　Reduced carbon dioxide (P_{CO_2}) 　Increased pH (respiratory alkalosis) • ECG evidence of right ventricular hypertrophy with very severe symptoms
II. Atelectasis • Volume of lung segment or lobe reduced because of obstruction of bronchus; potentially reversible • Obstruction maybe caused by tenacious secretions, neoplasm, or aspirated foreign body, with appropriate history for each; may follow general anesthetic for an operation • Later becomes infected with signs and symptoms of pneumonia becoming prominent	• Fever, tachypnea • Inspection—tracheal deviation toward involved side caused by loss of volume • Palpation—tactile fremitus decreased or absent • Percussion—dull in involved area • Auscultation—decreased or absent breath sounds • Crackles if pneumonia supervenes	• Chest x-ray is more sensitive and specific than physical examination • Tomograms or CT scan are useful in demonstrating tumor or foreign body as cause • Fiberoptic bronchoscopy often diagnostic and therapeutic

TABLE 3-13: Key Elements in Diagnosis of Selected Pulmonary Conditions—cont'd

Key Elements from History	Key Elements from Physical	Key Diagnostic Studies
III. Bronchiectasis • Abnormally dilated bronchus • Necrosis of bronchial wall and supporting structures, caused by necrotizing infection or obstruction of bronchus • Chronic cough, sputum, hemoptysis; recurrent pneumonia; sinusitis is common	• Inspection—digital clubbing in far-advanced disease • Percussion—resonance or hyperresonance • Auscultation—crackles over involved areas • Sputum separates into 3 layers after sitting	• Chest x-ray film may show dilated bronchi or even air fluid levels. May show tram tracks, superimposed circular shadows • Bronchography is an older procedure to show dilated bronchi on x-ray • Thin-slice CT scanning is replacing bronchography for diagnosis
IV. Bronchitis—acute • Onset with cough • May occur during course of cold or influenzal illness • Sputum may be produced • Retrosternal pain with breathing or coughing • Etiologies include bacteria, viruses, mycoplasma	• Inspection—findings are those of underlying URI, rhinorrhea, pharyngitis • Palpation—normal tactile fremitus • Auscultation—coarse crackles or rhonchi	• Not usually helpful

V. Bronchitis
A. Chronic
• Definition: expectoration of sputum during at least 3 consecutive months in 2 consecutive years; no apparent cause
• If wheezing has been prominent, some call it asthmatic bronchitis
• Incessant cough
• Largest amount of sputum in morning, but persists all day
• Smoking history 1 pack per day, 25% incidence of bronchitis; 40 to 60 pack years, 50% incidence
• Differential diagnosis includes emphysema, bronchiectasis, and cystic fibrosis
	• Inspection—frequently overweight, plethoric, jugular venous distention if cor pulmonale
	• Percussion—normal to hyperresonant
	• Purulent sputum
	• Palpation—sustained lift along left sternal border caused by right ventricular hypertrophy
	• Auscultation—increased P2, crackles and wheezes throughout
		• Pulmonary function studies
		  FEV-1 is reduced
		  TLC is normal
		  RV is increased
		• Arterial blood gases may be normal, or Pa_{O_2} reduced to 45 to 60 torr
		  Pa_{CO_2} increased to 50 to 60 torr pH 7.38 to 7.43
		• Hematocrit—slight polycythemia in severe disease

B. Bronchiolitis • Patient age 2 or under • Onset with cough and coryza • Mild fever for few days • Cough gets deeper • Patient breathes faster and becomes restless • Patient anxious at physician visit	• Inspection—wheezing is audible; cyanosis, tachypnea, restlessness are present • Retraction of chest wall; Nasal alae flare with inspiration, grunting with breathing • Percussion—hyperresonant with air trapping • Auscultation—wheezing and crackles	• Chest x-ray study to look for pneumonia

Continued.

TABLE 3-13: Key Elements in Diagnosis of Selected Pulmonary Conditions — cont'd

Key Elements from History	Key Elements from Physical	Key Diagnostic Studies

C. Cancer of the lung (bronchogenic)
• History of cigarette smoking
• Symptoms of chronic bronchitis or emphysema with cough, sputum, and dyspnea
• Recent hemoptysis, weight loss, and night sweats
• Age over 40
	• Inspection
	  Often findings of COPD
	  Unilateral telangiectasia
	• Percussion
	  Dullness if large tumor is close to chest wall or with postobstructive pneumonia
	• Auscultation
	  Crackles and signs of consolidation present or absent
	  Wheeze or stridor
	  Rhonchus over large airway, which does not clear with cough
		• Chest x-ray film may show tumor(s), postobstructive pneumonia, pleural effusion; may be negative

VI. Cor pulmonale • Symptoms (dyspnea, cough, retrosternal chest pain) appear when blood flow is increased as in exercise, fever, lung infection	• Inspection — dyspnea, cyanosis • Palpation — cardiac thrust along left sternal border with RV enlargement • Second left interspace thrust of pulmonary hypertension • Auscultation — loud P2, S3 may be present	• Chest x-ray study shows changes of COPD • VQ lung scan and pulmonary arteriogram for emboli • Normal pulmonary wedge pressure (equals left atrial pressure) and pulmonary arterial hypertension on right heart catheterization • Blood gases show increased arterial CO_2 • ECG changes
VII. Croup syndrome • Occurs in children • Cough with barking quality, hoarseness	• Inspiratory stridor	

A. Acute laryngotracheobronchitis
    • Age 6 to 24 months
    • Onset with URI
    • Low-grade fever
	• Fever
	• Swallows easily
	• Epiglottis is normal
		• X-ray film of lateral neck is normal

B. Acute spasmodic croup
    • Age 1 to 3 years
    • Sudden onset in evening
    • No fever, no URI
    • Previous episodes, lasts for a few hours
	• Child nearly well at exam a few hours after onset
	• Pharynx looks normal	

C. Bacterial croup
    • URI prodrome
    • Sore throat, fever
    • Swallowing is painful
	• Tonsillar exudates	• Leukocytosis
		• Blood and throat cultures grow *Streptococcus*

D. Aspiration of foreign body
    • Choking or coughing while eating
    • Eating objects easily aspirated (e.g., nuts, candy, popcorn)
    • No fever, no URI
	• Wheezing
	• Occasionally hemoptysis
		• Chest x-ray film may show foreign body or hyperinflated lung caused by ball valve bronchial obstruction, particularly in children; film may be normal
		• Flexible bronchoscopy to visualize

TABLE 3-13: Key Elements in Diagnosis of Selected Pulmonary Conditions—cont'd

Key Elements from History	Key Elements from Physical	Key Diagnostic Studies
E. Retropharyngeal abscess • Age under 3 years usually (may occur in adults) • Fever • Drooling, refuses to swallow	• Sits up • Hyperextends neck • Cervical nodes prominent • Palpation using gloved finger may show fluctuant abscess (avoid palpation if epiglottitis is possible diagnosis)	• X-ray of lateral neck taken during inspiration shows soft-tissue bulge anterior to cervical spine
F. Acute epiglottitis • Usually age 2 to 5 years • Sudden onset of sore throat and hoarseness • Adults with epiglottitis complain of "object caught in throat" feeling without any history of that happening • Patient sits up, drools, refuses to swallow	• Drools, hurts to swallow • Febrile, toxic appearing • Examination of the throat is dangerous because epiglottis can suffocate the patient; if seen, epiglottis is burgundy red	• X-ray of lateral neck shows enlarged epiglottis • Blood and throat cultures may demonstrate bacteria such as *Hemophilus influenzae* type B in children and nontypable hemophilus or other microbes in adults
VIII. Cystic fibrosis • Autosomal recessive multisystem disorder of exocrine gland function • Pulmonary disease is most common cause of disability and death • Cough, wheezing, tenacious sputum, and recurrent pneumonia • Meconium ileus at birth • Steatorrhea later • Hepatobiliary disease • Often sterile • Retardation of bone age	• Clubbing of digits • Examination finding of COPD	• Sweat test most reliable for cystic fibrosis diagnosis • Sweat chloride usually exceeds 70 mmol/l; normal sweat chloride is under 50 mmol/l
IX. Pleural effusion • Normal pleura with transudates as in congestive heart failure • Nephrosis or cirrhosis with hypoalbuminemia • Abnormal pleura give exudates in pneumonia, cancer, tuberculosis, pulmonary emboli with infarction, rheumatoid arthritis, subphrenic abscess, pancreatitis • Small effusions often produce no symptoms • Dyspnea may be present • Pleuritic chest pain or a dull aching pain may be present	• Trachea deviates away from affected side • Superior margin of fluid level detected by fremitus and dullness to percussion • Decreased breath sounds over fluid • Compression of lung at upper border of effusion functions like pulmonary consolidation giving egophony	• Chest x-ray film shows obliteration of sharp costophrenic angle; smaller effusions may be seen better on lateral view than on effusion PA view • Sonography may help to localize effusion • CT scans the most sensitive and may show effusions not otherwise detectable • Diagnostically separated by laboratory analysis of fluid into transudate and exudates • Transudates have protein < 3 g/dl, low lactic dehydrogenase content • Exudates have protein > 3 g/dl, high lactic dehydrogenase content

Continued.

TABLE 3-13: Key Elements in Diagnosis of Selected Pulmonary Conditions—cont'd

Key Elements from History	Key Elements from Physical	Key Diagnostic Studies

X. Emphysema
• Often present with chronic bronchitis COPD
• Dyspnea, cough
• Scanty sputum compared with that in chronic bronchitis
• Infrequent bronchial infections
	• Hyperinflated chest
	• Barrel-shaped chest
	• Patient usually thin
	• Hyperresonance
	• Narrow mediastinum by percussion
	• Diaphragms lowered
	• Few crackles
	• Heart sounds heard best in epigastrium
		• Chest x-ray film shows hyperinflation with lowered diaphragms, narrow mediastinum with long, narrow cardiac silhouette, increased size of retrosternal lucency; may have bullous changes
		• Arterial blood gases
		  P_{O_2} 65 to 75 torr, reduced but less than with chronic bronchitis
		  P_{CO_2} 35 to 40 torr
		  Diffusing capacity of interalveolar gases is decreased

XI. Pneumothorax • Air present between pleura • Onset spontaneous between ages 20 and 40 • May be caused by trauma or mechanical ventilation • Tension pneumothorax indicates a one-way "ball-valve" leak with build-up of tension • Hemopneumothorax indicates blood and air in pleural space • Pleuritic chest pain and dyspnea most common symptoms of pneumothorax	• Tachypnea • Asymmetric chest expansion with breathing • Trachea shifted away from side of pneumothorax • Apex beat shifted away from affected side • Hyperresonance to percussion • Reduced breath sounds on affected side • Splashing sound (succussion splash) heard if air and fluid both in pleural cavity	• Chest x-ray film taken in full exhalation is best to show pneumothorax

XII. Pulmonary embolism
• Venous clot moves from pelvic or larger leg veins or right heart into distal pulmonary arteries
• Risk factors include prolonged bed rest, postpartum period, heart failure, leg fractures, venous insufficiency of legs, use of oral contraceptives, obesity, cancer, and following some orthopedic and gynecologic procedures
• Most patients do not notice symptoms
• Sudden onset of unexplained dyspnea is most common symptom
• Pleuritic chest pain and hemoptysis if infarction
• Cough, syncope, substernal oppressive discomfort
	• Deep venous thrombosis gives a clue, if present
	• Crackles in bases
	• Wheezing may be present
	• Friction rub if infarction has occurred
	• Cardiac examination
	  — Tachycardia
	  — Prominent *a* waves in jugular venous pulse
	  — Palpable "lift" along right sternal border
	  — S_3 (right ventricular gallop)
	  — Loud P_2
	  — Wide splitting of S_2
		• Rare predisposing conditions are deficiency of
		  Antithrombin III
		  Protein C
		  Protein S
		• ECG changes, peaked P waves, right shift of QRS axis
		• Chest x-ray film shows infiltrate if infarcted; arteriogram shows cut off of an artery, different sizes of pulmonary arteries on two sides
		• Arterial blood gases
		  P_{O_2} decreased
		  P_{CO_2} decreased
		• Ventilation perfusion lung-scan shows "mismatch" of defects

TABLE 3-13: Key Elements in Diagnosis of Selected Pulmonary Conditions—cont'd

Key Elements from History	Key Elements from Physical	Key Diagnostic Studies
XIII. Pneumonias A. Community-acquired pneumonia<ul><li>Underlying disease is common COPD, diabetes</li><li>Chill and fever at onset</li><li>Cough, pleuritic chest pain, and sputum production</li></ul>	<ul><li>Inspection—fever, tachypnea</li><li>Percussion and auscultation Early, decreased breath sounds, crackles may appear E-to-A changes or bronchophony if consolidation is present</li></ul>	<ul><li>Chest x-ray film shows lobar or bronchopneumonia</li><li>Sputum and blood cultures to define microbial etiology</li></ul>
B. Atypical pneumonia<ul><li>Also called "walking" pneumonia</li><li>Fever, malaise, and headache</li><li>Incessant cough, worse at night</li><li>Sputum may be present but scanty</li><li>Pleuritic chest pain occasionally</li></ul>	<ul><li>Inspection—fever</li><li>Auscultation—crackles</li></ul>	<ul><li>Chest x-ray film usually shows bronchial pneumonia</li><li>*Mycoplasma pneumoniae* complement-fixation titer</li><li>TWAR antibodies (*Chlamydia pneumoniae*) may be found as a cause of atypical pneumonia</li><li>Other causes are not identified until acute and convalescent titers are obtained</li></ul>
C. Aspiration pneumonia<ul><li>Alteration of swallowing mechanism or gag reflex reduced</li><li>Recent loss of consciousness, seizure, drunkenness, dental extraction</li><li>Cough, fetid (foul or fecal odor) sputum</li><li>Recent general anesthesia</li></ul>	<ul><li>Inspection—fever, weight loss, tachycardia, poor oral hygiene is common</li><li>Auscultation—crackles</li></ul>	<ul><li>Chest x-ray film shows bronchopneumonia or segmental consolidation</li><li>Cavitation possible</li><li>Culture of sputum—anaerobes and gram negative bacilli</li></ul>

repeated episodes of pneumonia. The patient may be asked to lie with the legs on the examining table and the thorax and head hanging toward the floor. The patient with bronchiectasis in this position will ordinarily expectorate a large amount of purulent sputum. Inspect the sputum itself after it has sat for several hours; it may show the characteristic two or three layers. Percussion of the chest shows resonance to hyperresonance. Auscultation characteristically shows crackles in the bases corresponding with the site of disease.

The differential diagnosis includes other causes of chronic production of purulent sputum including, chronic bronchitis or cystic fibrosis.

Bronchitis

Acute bronchitis is inflammation or infection of the bronchi (often also involving the trachea—tracheitis), which may be accompanied by fever and substernal chest pain with coughing. The cough may be productive or nonproductive of sputum. Inspection depends on the severity of the illness but may have normal results. Palpation shows normal tactile fremitus, and the percussion note is normal resonance. Auscultation shows normal breath sounds, but crackles may be present. Occasionally wheezes may also be present. The usual etiologies of acute bronchitis include hemophilus, pneumococcus, mycoplasma, and viruses such as rhinovirus, coronavirus, or influenza virus.

Chronic bronchitis, on the other hand, has the distinctive history of the patient producing sputum on most days during the week for 3 months in each of 2 consecutive years or for 6 months continually. The patient has often been exposed to tobacco smoke or other inhaled irritants. Inspection shows a plethoric-appearing person, often wheezing. The cough has a rattling sound. The laugh of such people often has a rattly or wheezing quality to it as well. Tactile fremitus may be normal or increased, and the percussion note is resonant to hyperresonant. Auscultation shows a prolonged expiratory phase, and crackles are usually present.

The differential diagnosis of COPD includes emphysema, bronchiectasis, and cystic fibrosis.

Bronchiolitis

Bronchiolitis is a rather common disease of infants and children usually under 6 months of age. Symptoms may begin with cough, low-grade fever or no fever, and rhinorrhea. Wheezing and tachypnea follow. Hyperinflation of the lungs on examination is characteristic. Prolonged exhalation is apparent on inspection. The infant appears anxious and tachypneic, with perioral cyanosis and generalized intercostal and abdominal retractions during breathing. Percussion may demonstrate hyperresonance. Auscultation may show wheezing, prolonged expiratory phase, and occasionally crackles.

The differential diagnosis includes respiratory syncytial virus or other viruses. Acute pneumonia also needs to be considered.

Cancer of the Lung

The history in bronchogenic carcinoma usually includes exposure to tobacco smoke. Most patients have in excess of 35 pack-years of cigarette smoking. Individuals ordinarily have chronic bronchitis or emphysema along with lung cancer. Inspection demonstrates the associated findings of COPD. Skin telangiectasia may be discovered on the chest wall. Depending on the size and location of the cancer and the amount of tissue consolidation, signs of consolidation may be present. These include increased tactile fremitus, dullness to percussion, bronchophony, and egophony with larger tumors or distal pneumonic consolidation. Crackles may be present.

The differential diagnosis includes chronic bronchitis, emphysema, atelectasis, and pneumonia.

Cor Pulmonale

Cor pulmonale is virtually synonymous with pulmonary hypertension. Historical clues include retrosternal chest pain, cough, and shortness of breath. Pulmonary causes include a history of multiple pulmonary infections or one suggesting pulmonary emboli. Inspection may show cyanosis. Palpation and percussion may show no abnormalities of the lungs, yet the cardiac examination may show a precordial thrust of the right ventricle. Auscultation may show crackles in the bases and a very accentuated P_2.

The differential diagnosis includes multiple pulmonary emboli, severe COPD, multiple pulmonary infections, mitral stenosis, left-to-right cardiac shunts, and pulmonary fibrosis.

Croup

Croup is a syndrome diagnosed from the history and inspection of the patient. It occurs in young children, ordinarily boys more often than girls, usually under age 3 years. A child awakens after going to sleep and has a hoarse, brassy cough likened to the bark of a seal. Labored breathing, retraction, and inspiratory stridor may be present. Fever is usually absent. Inspection may show the patient to be cyanotic and exhibit air hunger. The larynx looks normal in spasmodic croup, but in inflammatory croup actual laryngitis with edema may be present in the subepiglottic region. The examination of the chest may be normal unless the viral etiology has produced tracheitis or bronchiolitis as well.

The differential diagnosis is between inflammatory croup and spasmodic croup. The inflammatory disorder should alert the physician to the possible danger of asphyxia. Spasmodic croup may remit suddenly and completely.

Cystic Fibrosis

Cystic fibrosis is an autosomal recessive disorder of the exocrine glands, including the lungs, pancreas, and sweat glands. At one time people with cystic fibrosis died in infancy. Currently many are living beyond age 30. The history is of chronic cough, wheezing, and very tenacious sputum. The patient may have bulky, malodorous stools characteristic of malabsorption. Previous history may include fecal impactions and bronchitis. Inspection may show clubbing of the fingers, coughing, and wheezing. Tactile fremitus may be decreased because of concomitant emphysema. Chest percussion tends toward hyperresonance. Breath sounds are decreased with prolonged exhalation. Crackles are common.

Pleural Effusion

The history in the patient with pleural effusion varies with the underlying etiology: pneumonia, carcinoma, pulmonary emboli, tuberculosis, or intraabdominal processes such as ascites, pancreatitis, or subdiaphragmatic abscesses. Fremitus is decreased in the area of effusion. The percussion note is dull. Breath sounds are reduced. With small effusions, a pleural friction rub may be present with respirations.

Pleural thickening (residual fibrosis) may result from previous pleural fluid. The history and findings may be similar to those of pleural fluid.

Emphysema

Emphysema and chronic bronchitis are frequently concomitant problems. The air sacs beyond the terminal bronchioles have been dilated, causing permanent hyperinflation of the lung. The history is similar to that of persons with chronic bronchitis, usually with many pack-years of cigarette smoking. As differentiated from chronic bronchitis, sputum production tends to be less prominent. Inspection shows the tendency toward barrel-chest configuration. The patient is usually not cyanotic, as compared with the more frequent cyanosis in severe chronic bronchitis. Tactile fremitus is decreased. The percussion note is ordinarily hyperresonant, the diaphragm is lowered. The cardiac border is difficult to define by percussion. Breath sounds are decreased with a prolonged expiratory phase. Crackles may or may not be present.

Epiglottitis

Epiglottitis is an acute sudden onset of inflammation of the epiglottis and the supraglottic tissues, including the pharynx and sometimes the uvula. Children are more often affected than are adults. The patient appears anxious, is unable to swallow, and drools from the mouth. An older child or adult complains of something caught in the throat. Fever is usual. Inspection of the pharynx is dangerous because the swollen epiglottis may get caught and suffocate the patient. Thus epiglottitis is a medical emergency. Before inspecting the throat in suspected epiglottitis, be prepared to immediately perform endotracheal intubation or tracheostomy. The chest is otherwise normal on examination.

The differential diagnosis of the etiology of epiglottitis includes *Hemophilus influenzae* type B in children and nontypeable *Hemophilus influenzae* in adults. Other etiologic organisms include pneumococcus and viruses.

Pneumothorax

Pneumothorax may occur spontaneously without apparent cause, following chest trauma, after rupture of a pleural bleb, or after a puncture wound of the chest. If air is drawn into the pleural space during inspiration and does not leak out, a tension pneumothorax occurs, again a medical emergency. A small pneumothorax may not be detected on physical examination and may even be missed on chest x-ray films. With a larger pneumothorax, the patient becomes dyspneic and anxious. The trachea shifts to the opposite side. Tactile fremitus is decreased or absent over a large pneumothorax. The percussion note becomes hyperresonant. Breath sounds are decreased or absent.

Pulmonary Hypertension

Pulmonary hypertension was discussed under cor pulmonale. Patients with pulmonary hypertension may have only vague complaints of weakness, dyspnea, or fatigue, or they may complain of severe pain over the precordium. Intense fatigue or fainting may be present. Findings are similar to those of cor pulmonale.

Pulmonary Edema

Pulmonary edema is most often found in severe left-sided congestive heart failure. However, mild left-sided heart failure may not result in pulmonary edema. The patient may complain of wheezing resembling asthma, PND, and orthopnea. Frequently with pulmonary edema the patient complains of PND with coughing, wheezing, labored breathing, cyanosis, and frothy sputum, which is occasionally bloody. Tactile fremitus, resonance, and breath sounds may be normal. Crackles and sometimes wheezes are prominent in the bases and throughout the lung fields. In addition, jugular venous distension may be present if concomitant right-sided heart failure exists along with a prominent third heart sound.

The differential diagnosis includes asthma and other causes of pulmonary edema. Pulmonary edema may be caused by uremia, heroin intoxication, snake bite, or circulatory overload with intravenous fluids or blood transfusions, or occur spontaneously at high altitudes or in mitral stenosis.

Historical Clues to the Etiology of Pneumonia

Pneumonia may be caused by a variety of pathogens. Occasionally we are able to get a clue as to possible causes of pneumonia from the patient's history of onset, progression of disease, or place of exposure. Such history is soft data because patients from areas endemic for one kind of pneumonia may have other types of pneumonia also.

The classic history for patients with pneumococcal pneumonia was for the patient to have a single, shaking chill and rusty-colored sputum. Yet that history is relatively uncommon for patients who have pneumococcal disease. Patients who complain of incessant nonproductive cough with or without ear pain may have mycoplasma pneumonia, particularly if the patient is relatively young and not severely ill. In the newborn, the staccato cough with multiple short coughs from 5 to 20 in series is characteristic of *Chlamydia trachomatis* pneumonia.

Pneumonia in association with conjunctivitis raises the possibility of adenoviral pneumonia or chlamydial pneumonia. Persons having poor oral hygiene and pneumonia should be considered at risk of aspiration pneumonia involving oral anaerobic bacteria. Pneumonia with diarrhea is typical of *Legionella* pneumonia, but diarrhea occurs with other types as well.

Animal exposure may be important in the production of pneumonia. Persons who are exposed to the dust from droppings of starlings in the midwest or guano from bats in caves, or who clean out old-fashioned chicken coops may be exposed to *Histoplasma capsulatum*. These types of guano support the growth of histoplasma. The patient who has been exposed to the droppings from pigeons may have cryptococcal disease. Coccidioidomycosis may occur in the form of pneumonia with a flulike syndrome in persons exposed to desert dust in the southwest United States.

House birds such as parrots and parakeets may harbor the agents of psittacosis or ornithosis. On occasion the infected birds will have ruffled feathers and unusually liquid stools, but other birds harboring the microbe may appear perfectly normal. Exposure to cattle or sheep in the birthing process can spread Q fever with subsequent pneumonia.

Tuberculosis with lung cavities should be considered in elderly nursing home patients, southeast Asian immigrants, homeless people, or those with AIDS who have chronic cough and sputum production.

Persons who have traveled to southeastern Asia may acquire the organism causing melioidosis, which can mimic tuberculosis, which is also common in that part of the world. Dietary habits in southeast Asia may expose native peoples to the lung fluke *Paragonimus westermani* with associated hemoptysis.

Persons who have AIDS may develop bacterial pneumonia with *S. pneumoniae* or *H. influenzae,* fungal pneumonia with *Histoplasma capsulatum, Coccidioides immitis,* or *Cryptococcus neoformans,* and viral pneumonia with cytomegalovirus, in addition to *Pneumocystis carinii* pneumonia.

Both bronchopneumonia and consolidated lobar pneumonia may be community- or hospital-acquired and may be atypical pneumonia or caused by aspiration. The history depends on the etiologic agent as well as whether bronchopneumonia or lobar consolidation are present. In bronchopneumonia, patients present with fever, chills, and expectoration of sputum or bloody sputum, and they may have night sweats. Inspection may show an acutely ill patient. Tactile fremitus and percussion are normal because areas of consolidation tend to be around the bronchi, thus not giving peripheral findings. Auscultation usually demonstrates crackles.

The etiologic causes of bronchopneumonia include mycoplasma, influenza, and pneumococcus (*Hemophilus influenzae,* aspiration pneumonia, and *Legionella pneumophila*).

The history of consolidated pneumonia may be similar to that for bronchopneumonia or may be unique, depending on the etiology. Fever, sputum

| CASE 3-4 | Community-Acquired Pneumonia (Mycoplasma) |

A 34-year-old man sought treatment with complaints of cough and fatigue. He was previously in good health until 5 days before when he had had headache and a scratchy throat and had developed a dry cough. The cough had become nearly incessant at times, especially when he tried to sleep at night. He denied known exposure to sick people and animals and had not traveled recently. He did not smoke.

The examination showed an afebrile man, not acutely ill, coughing. The chest examination showed a few crackles in the right base, but no signs of consolidation. The chest x-ray film showed a patchy bronchopneumonia in the same area.

The diagnostic impression was that the patient had an atypical pneumonia, probably caused by *Mycoplasma pneumoniae*. An acute mycoplasma complement fixation titer was reported negative, but a follow-up titer 10 days later was positive at 1:512. Other possible considerations included influenza (if during an epidemic), or *Chlamydia pneumoniae* (TWAR).

production, chills, or night sweats are common. Inspection may show an acutely ill patient. Tactile fremitus and bronchophony are increased. The percussion note is dull over the involved lobe or pulmonary segments. Breath sounds in the involved area are bronchial, and crackles are expected.

The microbes responsible for consolidated lobar pneumonia include *Streptococcus pneumoniae*, *Hemophilus influenzae*, *Klebsiella pneumoniae*, *Legionella pneumophila*, oropharyngeal flora in aspiration pneumonia, and other pathogens. Other causes include aspiration of a foreign body, obstruction of airways by tumor, or mucus plugging with distal pneumonic consolidation.

| CASE 3-5 | Hospital-Acquired Pneumonia |

A 38-year-old man underwent cadaveric renal transplantation on June 28. He was making an uneventful recovery until 10 days later, when he began having a fever up to 39° C and developed a cough. The sputum had a few tinges of blood but had no clots, nor was it grossly bloody. He began having loose stools several times a day.

Examination showed an acutely ill man. His respiratory rate was 25/min. He had a pulse rate of 115/min.

There was reduced chest expansion on the left side. Tactile fremitus was reduced along the left chest posteriorly. He had dullness to percussion over the left lower chest area. Crackles were present bilaterally, with bronchophony and E-to-A changes in the left midlung field.

The diagnostic impression was consolidated pneumonia, probably with some pleural effusion on the left. Because this occurred in a patient who was in the hospital, immunosuppressed following transplantation, and experiencing both rapid progression and diarrhea, *Legionella* sp. pneumonia and other opportunistic pathogens became important considerations.

Summary

A summary checklist for the examination of the respiratory system is presented in the accompanying box.

Summary Checklist for the Examination of the Respiratory System

General Examination
- Vital signs
- Breath odor
- Fingers and nails
- Eyelids and sclera
- Neck nodes
- Jugular veins
- Skin rashes

Inspection
- Anterior chest wall configuration
  Pectus excavatum
  Pectus carinatum
- Posterior chest wall configuration
  Buffalo hump
- Vertebral column abnormalities
  Barrel chest
  Lordosis
  Kyphosis
  Scoliosis
- Respiratory rate
- Patterns of breathing
  Tachypnea
  Cheyne-Stokes respiration
  Biot's respiration
  Sleep apnea

Palpation
- Tietze's syndrome
- Subcutaneous emphysema
- Tracheal tug
- Trachea shifted to either side
- Tactile fremitus

Percussion
- Technique
- Resonant
- Hyperresonant
- Tympany
- Dullness
- Flatness

Auscultation
- Choice of stethoscope
- Normal sounds
- Vesicular breath sounds
- Bronchial breath sounds
- Bronchovesicular breath sounds

Abnormal Sounds
- Crackles (rales)
- Rhonchus
- Wheeze
- Pleural friction rub
- Bronchophony
- Whispered pectoriloquy
- Egophony
- E-to-A changes

Typical History and Physical Findings in Lung Diseases
- Asthma
- Atelectasis
- Bronchiectasis
- Bronchitis
- Bronchogenic carcinoma
- Cor pulmonale
- Croup
- Cystic fibrosis
- Pleural effusion
- Emphysema
- Epiglottitis
- Pneumothorax
- Pulmonary hypertension
- Pulmonary edema
- Pneumonia
  Community-acquired
  Hospital-acquired
  Aspiration
  Atypical
  Bronchopneumonia

Suggested readings

Santiago TJ, Williams AJ: A reappraisal of the causes of hemoptysis, *Arch Intern Med* 151:2449-2451, 1991. *Some 264 patients underwent bronchoscopy for hemoptysis at a veteran's hospital in California. The frequency of tuberculosis and bronchiectasis had decreased. Bronchogenic carcinoma and bronchitis were more common causes.*

Irwin RS, Corrao WM, Pratter MR: Chronic persistent cough in the adult: the spectrum and frequency of causes and successful outcome of specific therapy, *Am Rev Respir Dis* 123:413-417, 1981. *The cause of cough in 49 consecutive patients was determined. Postnasal drip, asthma, chronic bronchitis, and gastroesophageal reflux were most common.*

Baughman RP, Loudon RG: Stridor: differentiation from asthma or upper airway noise, *Am Rev Respir Dis* 139:1407-1409, 1989. *This sophisticated study showed that the sound of stridor is more intense over the neck, and the sound of asthma, over the chest. Musical sounds of stridor are more prominent during inspirations, whereas asthmatic sounds are prominent during the expiratory phase.*

CHAPTER FOUR

The Heart

CHAPTER OUTLINE

The Medical History
Chest pain
Dyspnea
Palpitations
Fatigue
Syncope
Hemoptysis
Edema
Cyanosis

Physical Examination
General examination
Blood pressure
Examination of the heart and great vessels

Summary

Heart diseases are common. Coronary artery atherosclerosis is a leading cause of death, especially among men. Some 700,000 people die from myocardial infarctions each year. Atheromatous plaques begin as early as the second or third decade of life and progress initially without symptoms. Later, acute or chronic heart disease occurs.

Hypertension affects one in five people. It produces no symptoms for most people but becomes a significant factor in coronary artery disease and strokes.

Patients and families justifiably have concerns about possible cardiac disease. They ask to have their blood pressures checked, just in case, knowing that a fatal illness may be averted.

Noninvasive cardiac techniques of study (defined as not using long intravascular or intracardiac catheters) are now available to clinicians to augment the standard history and physical examination. These studies, including the chest x-ray examination, ECG exercise testing, echocardiography, Doppler echocardiography, and radionuclide imaging, have given a refinement to the diagnosis of heart disease that was lacking when autopsy comparisons were required for diagnosis.

Recently some bedside examination techniques have been analyzed so that the advantages and limitations are now much clearer than they were formerly.

Nonetheless, even in the present era, the history and physical examination remain the cornerstone of diagnosis. The inexperienced clinician is tempted to move prematurely to cardiac auscultation, but a thoughtful history and detailed, complete general examination are important to establish the diagnosis and detect complications in most cardiac patients.

History Taking

The cardiovascular history is the richest source of diagnostic information. The quality of the history may help determine the quality of care. As you take the history, you establish a bond with the patient that is helpful later should the patient require an invasive diagnostic study, a surgical procedure, or a complex medical treatment regimen. Should the patient not have cardiac disease, the rapport established during the history taking may allow you to maintain the patient's confidence while evaluating and treating symptoms that mimic heart disease.

Begin the medical history by asking open-ended questions:

- *What is troubling you?*
- *Tell me about your discomfort.* Allow the patient to relate his experience in his own words. This is time consuming but worthwhile because it allows you to assess the patient's intelligence, emotional make-up, and interpretations of symptoms. Later, concentrate questions on the onset of illness, the time course of symptoms, their location, quality, and intensity, the precipitating, aggravating, and relieving factors, and the response to previous therapy. Later questions can take the form of these:
- *What makes the discomfort better? Worse?*
- *Do you notice any associated symptoms?*

After that, review the past history of symptoms or diseases that may be of cardiac origin, followed by the family history of heart and vascular disease, and then the social history of habits that might lead to heart disease.

Symptoms suggesting cardiovascular disease are listed in the accompanying box. Other symptoms that may suggest cardiac disease include cough, nocturia, polyuria, and squatting. Each may be caused by diseases other than cardiac disease. A reasoned history aims to determine whether a symptom is related to cardiac disease. Analyze each symptom in terms of anatomy, physiology, pathology, functional status, and prognosis.

Chest Pain

Chest pain is a common symptom of heart disease. But because site and severity of the pain do not necessarily correlate with seriousness of the cause, patients may be unable to distinguish between cardiac and noncardiac problems.

Key Symptoms in the Evaluation of the Cardiovascular System	
Chest pain	Syncope
Dyspnea	Hemoptysis
Palpitations	Edema
Fatigue	Cyanosis

Chest pain may originate from the heart, aorta, lungs, diaphragm, esophagus, mediastinum, pleura, pericardium, pulmonary artery, or the chest wall (Table 4-1). Pain may originate from subdiaphragmatic organs.

Questions to ask the patient regarding chest discomfort follow:

- *Tell me about your chest problems.*
- *When did you have a recent episode? Tell me all about that.* Use an open-ended question to start so the patient will give his story.
- *What is this discomfort like? When did it begin? How frequently do you experience it? Can you bring it on or stop it after it begins? How?* The term *discomfort* is used at first because it is a more general term than is *pain*.

TABLE 4-1: Symptom: Chest Pain

Cause	Key Elements in History	Key Elements in Physical Examination
I. Cardiac ischemia		
A. Stable typical angina	• Substernal chest pain • Precipitated by effort • Relieved by rest or nitroglycerine within 30 seconds to 10 minutes • Precipitating factors are predictable	• S_4 during attack • May have paradoxically split S_2 with left ventricular dysfunction • ECG changes during attack
B. Unstable angina	• Unexplained changes in angina pattern • New onset of rest angina • Minimal effort angina • Increasing frequency, severity, and duration	• Same as above
C. Variant angina (Prinzmetal's angina)	• Recurrent chest pain at rest or with usual activity • Cyclic episode of attacks of pain for days, weeks, or months • Asymptomatic between attacks • Pain may be relieved by exercise	• Characteristic ECG changes differ from typical angina (i.e., ST segment elevation rather than depression)
D. Myocardial infarction	• Chest pain onset at rest, occasionally with extreme exertion or stress • Pain radiates to neck, arms • Burning, dull-aching or sharp • Dyspnea, weakness, and nausea	• Pale, anxious, diaphoretic • Tachycardia • Increase in blood pressure • Rales or crackles • S_4, S_3, gallop • Soft S_1 • Paradoxic split S_2 may preceed ECG changes
II. Nonischemic cardiac pain		
A. Mitral valve prolapse	• Chest pain common • Different from angina (i.e., at rest, longer duration) • Sharp, sticking • Less severe than myocardial infarction • Relieved by lying down • Occasional palpitations	• Midsystolic click • Late systolic murmur

Continued.

TABLE 4-1: Symptom: Chest Pain—cont'd

Cause	Key Elements in History	Key Elements in Physical Examination
B. Acute pericarditis	• Precordial chest pain • Often pleuritic (brought on by respirations) • Relieved by sitting up, leaning forward, or shallow breathing • Many causes	• Triphasic friction rub • Often heard at apex
C. Dissecting aortic aneurysm	• Sudden onset, severe • Tearing sensation • Anterior chest pain radiating to back • Jaw, throat, and abdominal pain • Prolonged pain	• Prostration • Inequality of pulses and blood pressure differences in one arm versus other or arms compared to legs • Aortic regurgitation if aortic root involved • Neurologic signs and symptoms may occur simultaneously
III. Pulmonary chest pain (see also Chapter 3)		
A. Pulmonary embolism	• Dyspnea more common than chest pain • Anxiety • Pleuritic chest pain • Dull substernal heaviness or tightness • Many conditions associated with venous thrombi	• Pallor, cyanosis • Accentuated P_2 • Tachycardia
B. Acute pleurisy	• Pain made worse by taking deep breaths • Pneumonia, emboli, common associations	• Friction rub ceases with holding breath
C. Pulmonary hypertension	• Primary disease in women • Secondary to chronic lung disease in cigarette smoker • May be caused by recurrent pulmonary emboli • Symptoms of dyspnea, substernal chest discomfort, palpitations, syncope, weakness, and cold hands and feet • Pain may be tight and constricting across the chest, especially with exertion	• S_2 shock felt by palpation in pulmonary area • Accentuated P_2 • When right heart failure occurs, ankle edema and hepatic congestion • Narrow splitting of S_2
D. Pneumothorax	• Spontaneous up to age 40 • Follows chest trauma • Barotrauma, during mechanical ventilation • Catamenial, during menses • Asthma or emphysema may engender • Pleuritic chest pain • Dyspnea • AIDS victims infected with *Mycobacterium avium* complex	• Dyspnea, tachypnea • Respiratory distress • Reduced breath sounds on involved side • Trachea shifted away from involved side

TABLE 4-1: Symptom: Chest Pain—cont'd

Cause	Key Elements in History	Key Elements in Physical Examination
IV. GI causes		
A. Esophageal spasm	• Chest pain, especially with eating or during effort • Dysphagia, sensation of food sticking in chest • Relieved by nitroglycerin	• Perspiration, pallor • Tachycardia
B. Reflux esophagitis	• Repeated burning substernal pain • Increased by large meals • Spicy foods, coffee, tobacco, or alcohol may induce pain • Episodes prolonged unless something done for relief	
V. Chest wall pain		
A. Tietze's syndrome	• Pain at costochondral joint of ribs anteriorly • Onset may follow trauma to the chest joint	• Joint tenderness • Joint swollen
B. Herpes zoster	• Pain follows a single dermatome on one side of body • Pain may be severe • Can be difficult to diagnose before vesicles appear • Vesicles may disseminate and appear outside primary dermatome	• Vesicles on a red base, look like chickenpox • Confined to one or two dermatomes • May disseminate
C. DaCosta's syndrome	• Sharp chest pain, anxiety, and palpitation • Chronic, functional complaint	
D. Vertebral column disease		
1. Cervical disc disease	• Usually dull, aching • May be sharp and cutting • Pain usually is felt near spine and follows dermatome to arms or chest	• Sensory disturbances • Twitching fasciculations • Decreased reflexes
2. Thoracic outlet syndrome	• As above, but dermatomes involve chest and upper abdomen	

- *Does the discomfort (or pain) move anywhere? Do you associate any other symptoms with it?*

Finally move to specific questions brought up by the patient's history.

CARDIAC CAUSES OF CHEST PAIN CAUSED BY MYOCARDIAL ISCHEMIA

Ischemic chest pain may take one of several forms: typical angina, unstable angina, variant angina, or myocardial infarction. Risk factors for coronary atherosclerosis that predispose to myocardial chest pain include:

- Hypertension
- Diabetes mellitus

- Hypercholesterolemia
- Cigarette smoking
- Hypothyroidism
- Heart disease in first-degree relatives

The pathophysiology of myocardial ischemia involves several steps. The reduced blood supply to the myocardium reduces myocardial compliance, a decreased ability to expand to volume changes *(diastolic dysfunction)*. Decreased cardiac muscle contractility *(systolic dysfunction)* follows. The ventricular diastolic pressure rises, the ECG develops abnormal S-T segment changes, and the patient may experience angina pectoris.

Some patients experience acute dyspnea as the diastolic filling pressure increases. Others notice fatigue as the reduction in left ventricular contractility reduces the cardiac output.

The classic description of symptoms of angina pectoris was given by William Heberden in the 18th century. He wrote that those affected

"...are seized while they are walking (more especially if it be uphill, and soon after eating) with a painful and most disagreeable sensation, in the breast which seems as if it would extinguish life, if it were to increase or to continue; but the moment they stand still all this uneasiness vanishes... The pain is sometimes situated in the upper part, sometimes in the middle, sometimes at the bottom of the sternum, and more often inclined to the left than to the right side. It likewise very frequently extends from the breast to the middle of the left arm. Males are most liable to this disease, especially if they have passed their 50th year."

Stable (Typical) Angina

Angina literally means choking, not pain. Patients often describe the chest sensation as an unpleasant feeling (e.g., pressing, squeezing, strangling, constricting, bursting, burning, a band across the chest, a weight in the center of the chest). Holding a clenched fist in front of the sternum while describing the sensation is called Levine's sign, a nonverbal classic sign for myocardial ischemia (Fig. 4-1). A classification of angina is shown in Table 4-1.

Angina is usually substernal or slightly to the left of the sternum. It is not felt as a sharp pain just at the cardiac apex or below the left breast. The discomfort may radiate into the arms, more often on the left, and into the neck or jaws. If it radiates down the left arm, it may move into distribution of the ulnar nerve but usually not into the thumb. Angina may radiate into the back or to the epigastrium but is not usually felt in the abdomen alone.

The effort needed to induce angina varies from patient to patient and from one time to another. Angina may be induced by raising the arterial blood pressure or increasing the heart rate. Both increase myocardial oxygen demands. A recent meal, cold weather, emotional stress, mental activity, walking uphill or upstairs, a hot or cold shower, clenching the fist, or vigorous use of the arms may induce angina. Some patients say that after an attack of angina, repeating the same activity later in the day does not provoke an attack. This is termed the *second-wind phenomenon*. Other patients continue the same effort during an anginal attack. The discomfort subsides even though the patient does not stop to rest. This is called *walk-through angina*. Angina may be stopped by resting or by sublingual nitroglycerin in only a few minutes. Nitroglycerin is not specific for

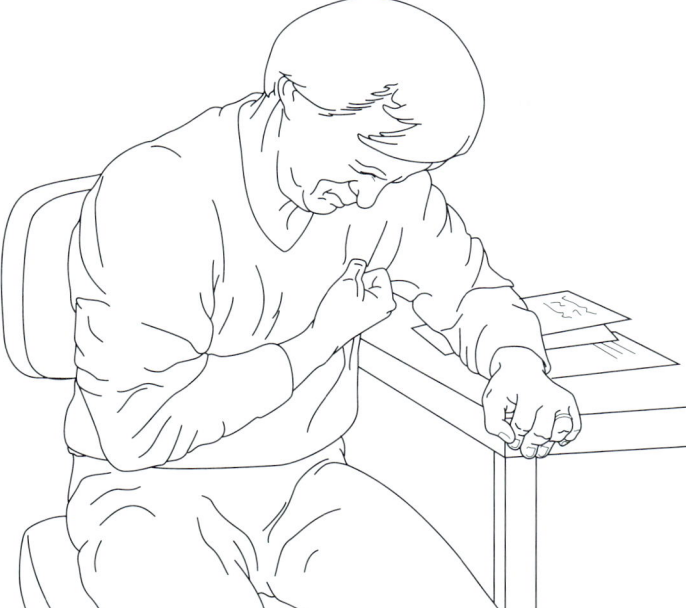

Fig. 4-1 Levine sign.

angina because smooth muscle spasm (e.g., esophageal spasm) may also be relieved.

Stable angina pectoris occurs for at least 60 days with predictable effort. Each episode of stable angina is of uniform severity. Duration of pain after activity lasts about the same length of time in stable angina.

Atypical Angina

Angina may be atypical in two ways: (1) inducing factors or (2) quality of the pain. The inducing factors may be typical (e.g., effort), but the quality of angina is not described in typical terms (e.g., sharp or stabbing). Alternatively, factors that effect it may be atypical (e.g., change in body position), but the discomfort is typical of angina.

Angina equivalents are symptoms other than angina caused by myocardial ischemia. Dyspnea or exhaustion may be angina equivalents. Sometimes even nausea, indigestion, gas and belching, dizziness, or profuse sweating may be angina equivalents. Another angina equivalent involves an atypical site of pain during effort; the pain may be localized to the left forearm, the lower jaw and teeth alone, the neck, or shoulders.

Unstable Angina

Depending on what is emphasized, unstable angina is called *preinfarction angina, crescendo angina, coronary insufficiency,* or *angina decubitus.* Angina is unstable when it has gotten worse or when the first episode has appeared during the past 60 days. Unstable angina, more than stable angina, is associated with an increased risk of acute myocardial infarction. Nearly 25% of patients develop myocardial infarction in 4 months.

CASE 4-1   Angina and Congestive Heart Failure

A 71-year-old man sought treatment for complaints of "no strength" and "can't breathe." He served as a minister to a small congregation and had to decrease the length of his sermons because of shortness of breath.

For 2 months he had had to sit up in a chair at night to sleep because of worsening breathing problems. He also had increasing ankle edema. During the past 3 weeks he had had nausea, which he treated with taking bicarbonate of soda. His exercise tolerance during the past week had gotten down to walking less than 50 feet before needing to rest.

Beginning 3 weeks previously, he had chest pressure and became quite short of breath when he exerted himself. He described this pressure as "squeezing or vicelike." This usually lasted 1 minute if he stopped immediately when the pressure came on. The day before seeking treatment he had an episode in which the pain lasted much longer and was accompanied by sweating. He refused to go to the hospital then because of some special obligation that he did not want to discuss.

The examination showed a cooperative man, sallow complexion, becoming short of breath during the history. The heart rate was 108 and regular, the respiratory rate was 22/min. Arteriolar narrowing was prominent on funduscopic examination. Jugular veins were distended. The chest examination showed crackles bilaterally. He had a grade II/VI systolic murmur at the apex that radiated to the left axillary line, and both third and fourth heart sounds. The liver span was 15 cm by percussion along the midclavicular line. He had 1+ pitting edema at the ankles and a trace at the knee.

This man had severe congestive heart failure manifested by orthopnea, fatigue (which he confused with weakness), and pedal edema. The intake of sodium for his nausea probably made the congestive symptoms worse. This chest pain sounds typical for angina at first. The most recent episode sounded as if he could have had a myocardial infarction. He needed to be admitted to the intensive care unit, an ECG tracing checked, and cardiac enzymes monitored.

The discomfort of unstable angina may occur while at rest or with minimal exertion. Less effort than usual is required to induce angina. Multivessel coronary artery stenosis is common. Fewer than 10% of patients with unstable angina have normal coronary vessels. Symptoms in persons with normal vessels have been attributed to arterial spasm, platelet aggregates, or thrombi.

Although the pain of unstable angina is more intense than that of stable angina, the location, character, and radiation are similar. Unstable angina may last several hours instead of minutes and is less often relieved by nitroglycerin than is stable angina.

When angina occurs at rest, it is called *angina decubitus.* Angina beginning during sleep awakens the patient. Other factors inducing angina decubitus include fever, anemia, or tachycardia.

Variant Angina

Variant angina, or *Prinzmetal's angina,* is paradoxic, beginning during rest instead of exercise. The pain resembles typical angina but may be more severe.

CASE 4-2 Myocardial Infarction

A 52-year-old man came to the emergency department at 8:30 AM with the chief complaint of severe chest pain.

He had felt a heaviness in his chest on awakening at 6:15 that morning. Although he did not feel like getting out of bed, he had gotten up, shaved, and showered. A few minutes later he developed severe pain in the midsternal area with pain down the left arm. He said it was so severe he had started to perspire.

Examination showed a diaphoretic, pale-gray man lying quietly, obviously in pain. His blood pressure was 170/95, heart rate was 110 and regular, and rate of respiration was 18/min. There was no jugular venous distention (JVD). The chest was clear to auscultation. He had an S_4 gallop and a grade II/VI systolic murmur along the left sternal border. There was no abdominal organomegaly and no peripheral edema.

The working diagnosis was acute myocardial infarction. A monitor was attached to the patient's chest, and an ECG tracing was obtained. The cardiology fellow was paged to see if the patient was a candidate for emergency cardiac catheterization and thrombolytic therapy.

Variant angina is caused by coronary artery spasm rather than by atherosclerosis, although the two may coexist. The majority of patients have right coronary artery spasm; a few have left main artery spasm. Variant angina is not benign because myocardial infarction may occur during the spasm. Characteristic ECG findings during the acute episode differentiate variant angina from typical angina.

Myocardial Infarction

The pain of acute myocardial infarction is similar to the pain of angina in location, radiation, and character, but it is more severe and lasts longer. Typically, pain is substernal pressure or squeezing, radiates into the neck or down the arms, and lasts longer than 15 minutes. A myocardial infarction often begins at rest, just as does Prinzmetal's angina. It is not relieved by nitroglycerin. The patient may have the feeling of impending death, usually lies quietly, and does not feel like engaging in activity requiring effort. Weakness, dyspnea, nausea, and profuse diaphoresis are commonly associated.

Myocardial infarctions may be "silent," with little pain in about 25% of patients. Alternatively, pain in myocardial infarction may be atypical in character: burning, dull and aching, or sharp, or atypical in location: arms or neck without chest pain.

A coronary arterial thrombus or arterial spasm is likely to be the cause of myocardial infarction. An embolus to a coronary artery is a less common cause.

CARDIAC CAUSES OF CHEST PAIN NOT CAUSED BY ISCHEMIA

Mitral Valve Prolapse

Mitral valve prolapse (MVP) is billowing of one or both mitral valve leaflets back into the left atrium during systole. It is the most common cardiac valve deformity. Most patients with MVP are symptom free. If pain is present, it is neither exertional nor effort induced, as is angina pectoris. Typical complaints of MVP are sharp, sticking, left precordial pain, lasting a few minutes but returning later. Sometimes it is prolonged. Lying down may give pain relief, which is not necessary in angina. Examination findings in MVP include a midsystolic click or late systolic murmur or both.

Pericarditis

Pericarditis (inflammation of the pericardium) caused by virus, bacteria, uremia, lupus, or neoplasm may cause precordial chest pain. The pain may be pleuritic or crushing in the retrosternal area. Often pain radiates to the shoulder. The patient gets relief by shallow breathing and by sitting up and leaning forward. For some the pain is relieved by kneeling on the hands and knees. If an enlarging pericardial effusion separates the visceral epicardium and parietal pericardium, the pain subsides. The characteristic pericardial friction rub has three components, but often only one or two components are heard. The pericardial rub remains present when the patient holds the breath (excluding a pleural friction rub) during auscultation. The sound is scratchy or creaky, resembling noise made with sandpaper.

Dissecting Aneurysm

A dissecting aneurysm begins with tearing of the arterial intima, separating layers of the artery wall. The pain of an aortic dissection begins suddenly with a tearing sensation. Pain in the chest and back moves, according to which arteries are dissecting, into the throat, jaw, back, or abdomen. The patient writhes in agony, or paces relentlessly in an effort to gain relief. Drenching sweats, apprehension, nausea, vomiting, and syncope are common. The patient appears to be in shock, but the blood pressure taken in the right arm may appear to be high. The blood pressure and pulses may be lost unequally in arms and legs. Neurologic abnormalities accompany cerebral artery involvement.

PULMONARY CAUSES OF CHEST PAIN

Pulmonary Embolism

Predisposing factors for emboli include:

- Oral contraceptives
- Malignancy
- Postpartum state
- Recent abdominal or pelvic surgical procedures
- Heart failure
- A long automobile ride punctuated with few exercise stops

Pulmonary embolism is often asymptomatic. Chest pain originating from pulmonary emboli may mimic myocardial ischemia. Cyanosis, tachycardia, and pallor may be found. Pain from large emboli is a dull substernal tightness. Small peripheral emboli create pulmonary infarction and later pleuritic chest pain. Dyspnea is a more common symptom than is chest pain.

Pleurisy

Pleuritic chest pain (made worse with breathing and subsiding with breath holding) may be caused by various disorders, including pulmonary emboli or by pneumonia when pleura are irritated or inflamed. Often pleural effusion is present. As the volume of effusion increases, the pleura no longer rub and the pain may stop.

Pulmonary Hypertension

Pulmonary hypertension signifies increased pulmonary artery pressure. It may occur secondary to chronic lung disease or pulmonary emboli. If no underlying cause is found, it is termed *primary pulmonary hypertension.* Dyspnea is a more common symptom. Pain is described as a discomfort (rather than pain), a nonradiating, tight-constricting band across the chest.

Pneumothorax

Air in the pleural cavity collapses the lung. Pneumothorax may occur spontaneously or may follow trauma. Dyspnea and chest pain in pneumothorax can be confused with pain of angina or myocardial infarction.

Mediastinal Emphysema

Mediastinal emphysema (free air in the mediastinum) produces chest tightness and dyspnea. A crunching sound may be heard synchronous with the heartbeat while auscultating over the precordium *(Hamman's sign).*

GASTROINTESTINAL CAUSES OF CHEST PAIN

Esophageal Spasm

Diffuse esophageal spasm is characterized by substernal chest pain and dysphagia. The pain may mimic angina and radiate to the arms or jaw, lasting several minutes.

Esophageal Reflux

Reflux esophagitis results from gastric contents refluxing into the esophagus. Substernal burning or cramping pain frequently radiates into the arms, neck, or jaw, mimicking angina pectoris. The pain may be relieved by milk or antacids (see the accompanying box).

Differentiating the Causes of Chest Pain

A patient who can point to the site of pain with one finger usually does not have angina pectoris.
The pain of myocardial infarction is typically accompanied by nausea, vomiting, and profuse sweating.
Pain of myocardial ischemia and pericarditis may radiate into the neck and jaw.
The pain of aortic dissection radiates to the back more commonly than to the anterior chest.
The pain of vertebral abnormality is radicular and is usually exacerbated by bending the spine.
The pain of esophageal spasm may be exacerbated by swallowing.
The pain of esophagitis may be substernal with epigastric burning, relieved by eating more than by antacids.
The pain of pericarditis may be accentuated by swallowing.
Coughing accentuates chest pain caused by pericarditis, bronchitis, pleurisy, or radicular pain.
Pneumothorax or pulmonary emboli are likely to have prominent dyspnea, but cardiac causes may also exhibit dyspnea.
Pulmonary embolism and infarction or lung tumor may be associated with chest pain and hemoptysis.
Fever accompanying chest pain suggests pneumonia or pericarditis, but low-grade fever may also be found after myocardial infarction.
Frequent sighing, anxiety or depression would be expected with functional pain.

Gallstone Colic

Cholelithiasis is usually associated with right upper quadrant (RUQ) pain, radiating to the back or right shoulder. Occasionally it may be confused with heart disease. Cholelithiasis, especially with an impacted stone in the cystic duct, can result in classic biliary colic.

CHEST WALL PAIN

Tietze's Syndrome

Tietze's syndrome (costochondritis) is characterized by tenderness and swelling over the costochondral rib joints. Point pressure over the involved areas alongside the sternum reproduces the patient's pain. Often the patient has not recognized this obvious association.

Herpes Zoster

Ordinarily, pain from herpes zoster precedes the rash. The pain follows a dermatome distribution that will later manifest the vesicular eruption. The pain of zoster may relent after vesicles have appeared, but in some cases the pain persists for months after the skin has healed. The clue that zoster is the etiology of chronic pain are the scars in the dermatome distribution of the previous vesicles.

DaCosta's Syndrome

DaCosta's syndrome, or neurocirculatory asthenia, is functional or psychogenic pain usually localized to the cardiac apex. The pain may be dull, aching, and persist for hours, but may alternate with sharp stabs for one or two seconds. It occurs with emotional strain or fatigue, not with exertion. The chest wall may be tender. Palpitations, hyperventilation, dyspnea, weakness, or depression coexist. The pain does not respond to rest or medication.

Vertebral Column Disease

Either cervical or thoracic vertebral disc disease may result in chest pain. Occasionally pain caused by these diseases may be confused with pain of cardiac origin.

Dyspnea

Dyspnea is shortness of breath, an uncomfortable awareness of breathing. Dyspnea feels smothering, causing an urgent need to take another breath, similar to the feeling one gets while holding the breath. Clues to the cause of dyspnea are shown in Table 4-2. Dyspnea caused by pulmonary disease is discussed in Chapter 3.

There are several questions to ask the patient who complains of shortness of breath:

- *Tell me about the shortness of breath you are experiencing. When did you have it most recently? What was that episode like?*
- *Did it occur with exercise? While you were at rest? During the night? Did it occur at once after you lay down?*
- *Can you predict what might bring it on?*
- *How do you get relief? What do you do for it? Do you sit up to breathe? Did you sit up the rest of the night during your last episode?*

TABLE 4-2: Symptom: Dyspnea

Cause	Key Elements in History	Key Elements in Physical Examination
I. Physical condition		
A. Lack of exercise (physiologic dyspnea)	• Dyspnea on exertion • No periods of effort in daily activities	• Strength normal • Dyspnea with stress testing
B. Reduction in exercise tolerance (may be pathologic)	• Regular periods of effort • Unable to perform previous effort without dyspnea now	• Strength normal • May not be dyspneic with usual stress testing • Subtle clues to cardiopulmonary disease
II. Heart diseases		
A. Valvular disease		
1. Mitral stenosis	• Dyspnea on exertion, later dyspnea at rest • Orthopnea • Rheumatic fever or known murmur • Pulmonary edema with lung infection, pregnancy, or atrial fibrillation	• Lung crackles or wheezes • Prominent *a* waves • Palpable P_2 • Loud S_1 • Opening snap, S_3 • Middiastolic rumble • Presystolic accentuation
2. Mitral regurgitation	• Recent myocardial infarction (papillary muscle dysfunction or chordae tendinae rupture) • Chronic regurgitation initially asymptomatic, later fatigue with dyspnea; progresses to orthopnea and PND	• Lung crackles or wheezes • Active precordium • S_3 and S_4 • Pansystolic (holosystolic) murmur
3. Aortic stenosis	• Angina and syncope are common • Dyspnea may occur early in young, active patients or later in older patients	• Delay in pulse upstroke • Narrow pulse pressure • Harsh systolic crescendo-decrescendo murmur, especially at aortic area, radiates to carotids and apex
4. Aortic regurgitation	• Usually without symptoms for years • Exertional dyspnea and fatigue occur later • Angina less common than in aortic stenosis	• Wide pulse pressure • PMI is displaced to the left and down • High-pitched diastolic blow along left sternal border • Acute regurgitation does not exhibit wide pulse pressure nor dilated LV
B. Other cardiac diseases		
1. Endocarditis	• Intravenous drug user • Fever or night sweats • Embolic episodes • Previous endocarditis • Dyspnea, orthopnea	• Lung crackles or wheezes • Murmurs variable depending on valve involved • Petechiae on conjunctivae, palate, nailbeds

Continued.

TABLE 4-2: Symptom: Dyspnea—cont'd

Cause	Key Elements in History	Key Elements in Physical Examination
B. Other cardiac diseases—cont'd 2. Congenital heart disease—tetralogy of Fallot	• Cyanosis by few months of age is common • Dyspnea with exertion is common • Squatting position to relieve dyspnea • Fainting episodes	• Clubbing if cyanosis has been present 3 months • Diamond-shaped murmur at left sternal border • Heart is quiet by palpation • Pulmonary stenosis murmur
C. Cardiomyopathy 1. Congestive cardiomyopathy	• Dyspnea at rest or with exercise • Orthopnea, paroxysmal nocturnal dyspnea • Chest pain, myocardial infarction, pulmonary emboli • Possible alcoholic or viral etiology	• Crackles in bases throughout • Elevated jugular venous pressure • Soft S_1 • S_3, often S_4 gallop • If biventricular failure, hepatomegaly and leg edema are seen
2. Hypertrophic cardiomyopathy	• Sudden death in family • Dyspnea on exertion • Chest pain, angina • Syncope • Palpitations	• Elevated jugular venous pressure • Loud S_4 • Presystolic precordial thrust followed by late systolic left ventricular impulse • Mid-to-late systolic murmur at apex and sternal border
D. Hypertension 1. Systemic hypertension	• Usually no symptoms of increased blood pressure • Symptoms if hypertension is caused by pheochromocytoma or chronic renal failure • Dyspnea if heart failure occurs	• Elevated systolic and diastolic pressure • Retinopathy • S_4, S_3, systolic ejection click, or systolic ejection murmur
2. Pulmonary hypertension (primary without identifiable cause, or secondary to pulmonary vascular obstruction)	• May be mild without respiratory symptoms • With increasing severity, dyspnea with fatigue • Chronic lung disease (if secondary pulmonary hypertension) • Respiratory tract infection may precipitate it in COPD	• Increase in AP diameter (if caused by chronic lung disease) • Elevated jugular venous pressure, prominent *a* or *v* waves • Holosystolic murmur of tricuspid regurgitation may be audible • Hepatomegaly
III. Lung diseases (see Table 3-2)		
IV. Metabolic causes (see Table 3-2)		
V. Functional dyspnea	• Sensation of inability to get enough air • Frequent sighing • Relieved by taking deep breaths • Brief stabbing pain near cardiac apex • Prolonged (over 2 hr) pain at apex, dull, relieved by exercise	• No examination findings to suggest other causes for dyspnea

- *Do you notice any associated symptoms such as cough, sputum, wheezing, fever, chest pain, or light headedness?*
- *How long has it been happening? What occurred to cause you to seek medical attention for it at this time?*

Observing the dyspneic patient, one may see *hyperpnea* (rapid, deep breathing). Normal people may feel dyspneic while performing unaccustomed exercise or when exercising at very high elevations. Thus one's physical condition, weight, and age are important in the sensation of dyspnea. A pregnant woman may become short of breath while climbing steps. If she does not *feel* uncomfortable, this would not be termed dyspnea.

Effort dyspnea is a common symptom of heart failure. The patient feels air hunger and often has a tight sensation in the chest. Coughing or wheezing may accompany dyspnea. Factors that bring on dyspnea include activities involving effort of arms or legs such as sweeping, making beds, climbing steps, or walking.

Excessive salt intake or a myocardial infarction, silent or symptomatic, may be occult reasons for dyspnea that require perceptive questioning on the part of the medical historian.

Dyspnea occurs at rest as well as with activity. Dyspnea at rest may signify lung diseases such as pulmonary embolism, pneumothorax, heart failure, end-stage COPD, or just anxiety. Dyspnea that occurs only at rest and disappears on exertion is almost always functional. Dyspnea associated with a brief, stabbing chest pain, relieved by sighing or deep breathing, is generally functional.

Dyspnea caused by anxiety occurs at rest, not with exertion. Normal breathing does not seem to satisfy the patient; only deep sighing breaths do. This deep breathing caused by anxiety may be part of the hyperventilation syndrome. Here, the patient breathes excessively, reducing the carbon dioxide content of the blood. The fingers and toes become numb and tingle. If hyperventilation continues, the fingers draw up into carpal spasm.

ORTHOPNEA

Orthopnea is dyspnea that occurs soon after the patient lies down and is relieved promptly by sitting up or standing up. Orthopnea is a manifestation of more severe heart failure than that seen in effort dyspnea. Patients who sleep on two or three pillows to elevate the head and chest to prevent dyspnea are said to have *two-pillow* or *three-pillow orthopnea*. Some patients with COPD also rest better with the head and thorax elevated on two or three pillows. Lying down shifts blood to the pulmonary circulation from the periphery. Pulmonary capillary pressure and lung stiffness are increased (decreased compliance). Pulmonary congestion decreases by the erect position, relieving symptoms.

PAROXYSMAL NOCTURNAL DYSPNEA

PND is also dyspnea after lying down. Unlike orthopnea, PND does not occur until the patient has been lying down for several minutes or hours. Typically, the patient goes to bed and falls asleep. Later, he awakens short of breath and sits up to breathe. Unlike orthopnea, PND is not relieved immediately after sitting up. Some patients open a window or walk around. Usually patients do return to bed and sleep. PND is a manifestation of early pulmonary edema and may be associated with chest pain or coughing. If the patient's symptoms are caused by

CASE 4-3 Paroxysmal Nocturnal Dyspnea

A 77-year-old woman presented in June with dyspnea, fatigue, and insomnia for 1 week. She felt that her weight had increased but was not certain by how much. Both ankles had begun to swell. Each night at 2 or 3 AM she awakened short of breath and had to sit up the rest of the night in a recliner.

She had been on vacation for 10 days before the onset of symptoms and volunteered that she had been unable to adhere to her usual low-salt diet.

Her past medical history included mitral valve replacement 1 year previously for severe mitral stenosis, atrial fibrillation with heart rate controlled with digoxin, and a previous episode of congestive heart failure.

The examination showed a thin white female with a blood pressure of 110/70 and a heart rate of 88 (irregularly irregular). The jugular veins were distended to 6 cm above the angle of Louis. There was increased fullness of jugulars with pressure of the examining hand over her liver (hepatojugular reflux). Bilateral basilar crackles were prominent. A grade II/VI early diastole murmur was heard at the lower left sternal border. A third heart sound was heard at the cardiac apex. She had 1+ pitting edema of the legs up to the mid-calves.

This patient had PND as a manifestation of heart failure. Her dietary intake of sodium, the atrial fibrillation, and probable prosthetic valve dysfunction combined to cause problems at this time.

---

left ventricular cardiac failure, he will usually sit on the side of the bed but not get up and walk around or do other activities that might make his symptoms worse.

PULMONARY EDEMA

Pulmonary edema may be a manifestation of advanced heart failure. The myocardium has reduced contractility. To maintain cardiac output, either the stroke volume or the heart rate is increased. As the diastolic volume of the left ventricle increases, filling pressure increases, resulting in pulmonary congestion and transudation into alveoli and interstitium.

Pulmonary edema may be a manifestation of left heart failure, whereas peripheral edema is typically a manifestation of right heart failure. Pulmonary edema is often preceded by orthopnea or PND. The patient with pulmonary edema is extremely anxious and dyspneic, frequently has cold sweats, exhibits moist, bubbling breathing sounds, pink (bloody) frothy sputum, and has a fear of impending death.

Cardiac causes of pulmonary edema include myocardial infarction and severe cardiomyopathy. Causes of dilated cardiomyopathy include ischemic heart disease, chronic alcoholism, and viral myocarditis.

Acute pulmonary edema may be caused by noncardiac causes, including narcotic abuse, pulmonary embolism, head injury, or high altitudes.

VALVULAR HEART DISEASE

Dyspnea is a principal symptom of mitral stenosis. It may occur late in the course of mitral regurgitation or aortic stenosis or regurgitation. As the functional obstruction to left ventricular outflow by valvular disease becomes more severe, the more likely the patient will experience dyspnea.

OTHER HEART DISEASES

Cyanotic congenital heart disease with shunting of venous blood into the systemic circulation results in a decreased arterial oxygen tension in *tetralogy of Fallot*. Dyspnea with exertion is common in children with this condition.

Infants with large *ventricular septal defects* develop heart failure during the first few months of life. Parents observe tachypnea and sweating with feedings. The infant becomes fatigued with just the work of sucking. The child is not cyanotic at first but becomes cyanotic as pulmonary vascular disease develops.

Hypertrophic cardiomyopathy (HC, or IHSS for idiopathic hypertrophic subaortic stenosis) refers to asymmetric septal hypertrophy that may obstruct the left ventricular outflow tract. Principal symptoms are dyspnea and chest pain, but fatigue, syncope, palpitations, and even sudden death are manifestations.

DIFFERENTIATING CARDIAC AND PULMONARY DYSPNEA

Differentiation between dyspnea of cardiac and pulmonary causes may be difficult, but certain clues are useful. Episodes of dyspnea associated with cough and sputum production are more likely to be caused by COPD. If expectoration relieves dyspnea, lung disease is more likely. Relief of dyspnea with sitting up is more typical of heart disease but is also seen in lung diseases. Dyspnea of COPD has a gradual onset over months to years, whereas dyspnea caused by asthma, pulmonary emboli, pneumothorax, or pneumonia begins abruptly. Dyspnea of heart failure ordinarily develops over a period of minutes to days.

OTHER CAUSES OF SHORTNESS OF BREATH

Patients with diabetic ketoacidosis demonstrate intense hyperventilation (Kussmaul respiration). This respiration is rapid deep breathing, but the patient does not complain of shortness of breath because of the CNS dysfunction in acidosis. Similar rapid breathing, although usually not so deep, may be seen after ingestion of an overdose of aspirin.

Palpitations

Palpitations are an unpleasant awareness of the heart beat. The unpleasantness depends on how sensitive the patient is, along with the variation in rate, rhythm, or force of contraction. Terms patients use to describe palpitations include pounding, fluttering, flopping, or skipping a beat. Some patients are aware of the heart beat with normal sinus rhythm or an occasional ectopic beat. Other patients have arrhythmias without even sensing palpitations. Questions to ask the patient that may give clues to the etiology of palpitations are found in Table 4-3.

In taking the history of palpitations, three questions to focus on are the following:

1. Was the onset gradual or sudden? Was a cardiac arrhythmia probable? If so, what? Answering this may require an ECG or a Holter monitor (provides a continuous ECG pattern for 24 hours).
2. What factors triggered the onset and cessation of the palpitations?
3. What associated symptoms were present (e.g., dizziness, syncope, or chest pain)?

TABLE 4-3: Clues to Etiology of Palpitations

Questions to Ask	Possible Diagnostic Significance
Does the rapid heartbeat begin and end abruptly?	• Paroxysmal tachycardia (e.g., PAT)
Do attacks develop gradually?	• Hypoglycemia, blood loss, medication use may be responsible
Are you aware of the heart beating when the rate is between 60 to 100 and the rhythm is regular?	• May be a manifestation of acute anxiety or cardiac neurosis
Are symptoms related to taking drugs or medications?	• Tobacco, caffeine, alcohol ingestion • Use of thyroid medication or adrenalin
Are you a menopausal woman with hot flashes and sweating?	• Menopausal syndrome
Does standing bring on the symptoms?	• Could mean postural hypotension with compensating tachycardia

Gradual acceleration of the heart rate may occur with the following:

- Exercise
- Anemia
- Sexual activity
- Postural hypotension
- Anxiety
- Use of stimulant drugs such as coffee, tea, tobacco, epinephrine, or amphetamines

On the other hand, paroxysmal atrial tachycardia (PAT) causes an instantaneous increased heart rate instead of gradual acceleration.

An instantaneous change in the regular heart rhythm may be caused by ectopic beats, extra systoles, and either premature atrial or ventricular contractions. A compensatory pause follows a premature ventricular contraction, allowing more filling of the ventricle with blood. The subsequent ventricular contraction feels stronger, giving the sensation of the heart beat. Rhythm disturbances are more common than rate disturbances in patients who complain of palpitations.

Some patients find relief from palpitations by vagal stimulation such as

CASE 4-4 Paroxysmal Atrial Fibrillation

A 27-year-old internal medicine resident was on call evaluating a new patient when the code-blue beeper sounded. He ran down the hall, down two flights of stairs, and jumped down the final four steps. When he did, he became acutely aware of rapid palpitations, and he felt too weak to continue walking to the code.

He had had episodes of paroxysmal atrial tachycardia previously and had had a "cardiac evaluation" without a disease process being identified. Each episode had lasted only a brief time, being stopped when he made himself gag or underwent carotid sinus massage with ECG monitoring in the emergency department.

performing Valsalva's maneuver or by gagging or vomiting. If such a maneuver stops palpitations, it implies a supraventricular arrhythmia was present. Syncope or seizures occurring with palpitations may mean asystole, bradycardia, or a Stokes-Adams attack. A Stokes-Adams attack is characterized by a slow or absent pulse, vertigo, syncope, and convulsions. After such a seizure, a patient may not recall preceding palpitations.

To evaluate palpitations, examine the radial pulse or carotid pulse for rate and rhythm. When the pulse alone is inconclusive, compare it to auscultation of the cardiac sounds. Observing the jugular venous pulse waves may show that atrial activity is not in synchrony with ventricular activity.

Fatigue

Of the symptoms related to heart disease, the subjective feeling of fatigue is the most difficult to evaluate. Fatigue may be caused by heart disease or may be a manifestation of many other illnesses (see the box on pg. 144). The diseases most commonly associated with fatigue in general practice are not heart disease, but rather depression, viral syndrome, and anxiety. Because patients confuse weakness and fatigue, ask whether the patient's muscle strength (weakness) or his endurance (fatigue) is affected.

FATIGUE CAUSED BY HEART DISEASE

Chronic fatigue may occur because of reduced cardiac output of chronic heart failure. Inadequate blood supply results in fatigue. Right or left heart failure with inadequate cardiac output or pulmonary failure with inadequate oxygenation may cause fatigue. Similarly, severe anemia also causes fatigue.

Of patients who have moderate-to-severe heart disease, fatigue commonly limits productivity and restricts activities. Early on, cardiac fatigue is uncommon for patients to experience in the early morning unless REM sleep has been disturbed. The patient may first notice unusual fatigue after what would previously have been normal activities. As heart disease progresses, the patient experiences fatigue earlier in the day. The patient may say the arms or legs feel heavy after the activity is completed, or he complains of unusual weakness or tiredness.

OTHER CAUSES OF FATIGUE

Neurologic and endocrine disease are less common causes of fatigue. Chronic infections and chronic liver or renal diseases commonly cause fatigue. Patients with cancer may experience fatigue for some time before the diagnosis of cancer is made. Psychologic and drug-induced fatigue are common. The chronic fatigue syndrome is a common cause of fatigue but remains of unknown etiology.

Syncope

Syncope refers to a transient loss of consciousness, commonly called a blackout or fainting episode. Syncope is rapid in onset and temporary in duration. The patient experiences dimming of vision, weakness, inability to stand, and the feeling of beginning to pass out. The face becomes pale, diaphoresis is common, and respirations become shallow. If the patient does not sit or lie down, he is likely to fall, slide, or slump down. Unlike epileptic seizures, syncope seldom results in injury. The patient is not likely to have fecal or urinary incontinence. After syncope, the patient quickly returns to normal, as compared with the postictal

Causes of Fatigue

I. Cardiopulmonary diseases
   A. Heart disease
      1. Right heart failure
      2. Left heart failure
      3. Da Costa's syndrome
         (a) Neurocirculatory asthenia
   B. Chronic obstructive pulmonary disease (COPD)
II. Neuropsychiatric disease
   A. Neurologic disease
      1. Eaton-Lambert syndrome
      2. Myasthenia gravis
      3. Amyotrophic lateral sclerosis
   B. Psychologic causes
      1. REM sleep deprivation
      2. Depression
III. Endocrine causes
   A. Thyroid disease
      1. Hypothyroidism
      2. Hyperthyroidism
   B. Addison's disease
   C. Cushing's syndrome
IV. Chronic diseases
   A. Infectious
      1. AIDS
      2. Bacterial and systemic fungal infections
   B. Organ dysfunction
      1. Kidney
      2. Liver
   C. Cancer
   D. Fibromyalgia
V. Drug-induced fatigue
   A. Electrolyte imbalance
      1. Diuretic-induced hyponatremia or hypokalemia
      2. Amphotericin B–induced hypokalemia and hypomagnesemia
   B. Adrenergic blockers
   C. Withdrawal from caffeine, alcohol, or sedatives
   D. Corticosteroids
VI. Idiopathic fatigue
   A. Chronic fatigue syndrome (CFS) or chronic fatigue immunodeficiency syndrome (CFIDS)

confusion and amnesia following a seizure. Table 4-4 shows the causes of syncope.

VASOVAGAL EPISODES

Simple vasovagal fainting is the most common cause of cardiac syncope. These may be precipitated by the sight of blood, by sudden stress, or by trauma, especially if the environment is hot and stuffy. Such syncope is believed to be

TABLE 4-4: Symptom: Syncope

Cause	Key Elements in History
I. Vasovagal episode (blackout or fainting)	• Causes majority of faints • Precipitated by sight of blood, sudden stress, severe trauma • More likely if patient hungry, in hot crowded room • Usually occurs when patient is standing or is tired
II. Cardiovascular causes A. Bradycardia, tachycardia, Stokes-Adams attacks	• Patient may be in any position • Patient may be aware of palpitations before passing out • Patient pale and pulseless and seems dead • Grand mal seizures occur
B. Cardiac outflow tract reduction (aortic stenosis, pulmonic stenosis, myxoma or thrombus of left heart, hypertrophic cardiomyopathy)	• Exertional syncope • History of heart murmur • With myxoma, syncope may be related to positions such as leaning forward
C. Myocardial ischemia	• As listed in Table 4-2 • Chest pain
D. Carotid sinus syncope	• Hypersensitivity of carotid sinus • Often elderly men • May occur with shaving or turning head
E. Impaired vasomotor reflexes (e.g., diabetic neuropathy, spinal cord injury, prolonged bed rest)	• Hypotension caused by peripheral venous pooling • Patient feels better lying down
F. Decreased blood volume	• Bleeding • Blood pressure decreases when patient sits or stands
III. Fluid removal A. Micturition syncope	• Fainting with urinating
B. Thoracentesis, paracentesis	• Rapid removal of large volume of fluid triggers vasovagal responses
IV. Posttussive syncope	• Middle-aged, short, stocky men with COPD
V. Psychogenic	• Seen in malingerers

vagally induced. In general, syncope caused by vagal stimulation occurs when the patient is standing.

CARDIOVASCULAR CAUSES

Arrhythmia

Syncope caused by cardiac arrhythmias may occur with the patient in any position. *Stokes-Adams syndrome* is a sudden, reversible loss of consciousness caused by reduction in cardiac output associated with an arrhythmia. Rapid or slow arrhythmias reduce the stroke volume, thereby reducing cardiac output and causing syncope. Bradycardia may occur without premonition; the patient appears pale and pulseless and seems dead. A grand mal seizure may occur with cardiac arrhythmias.

Cardiac Outflow Tract Obstruction

Aortic stenosis predisposes to syncope, as the valve orifice decreases to 0.5 cm^2 or less. Mitral valve prolapse is also associated with syncope, but no evidence for obstruction to flow is apparent. However, hypertrophic cardiomyopathy with septal hypertrophy does present cardiac outflow tract obstruction when the patient has fever or takes certain drugs such as digitalis or vasodilators. Such patients may experience fatigue and other symptoms.

Uncommonly, a left atrial myxoma may present with syncope. More often, findings may mimic endocarditis. Myxomas are usually attached to the atrial septum by a stalk that allows them to flop into or through the mitral ring, obstructing cardiac outflow. Intraventricular thrombi may similarly impede blood flow.

Tetralogy of Fallot is associated with fainting attacks. For unknown reasons, acute obstruction to pulmonary outflow occurs because of spasm of right ventricular muscle in the outflow tract. Desaturated blood is shunted through the ventricular septal defect (VSD) into the systemic circulation, and the patient becomes so hypoxic that syncope occurs.

Myocardial Ischemia

Syncope may be a component of ischemic heart disease:

- Angina pectoris
- Prinzmetal's angina
- Acute myocardial infarction

Carotid Sinus Syncope

Hypersensitivity of the carotid sinus occurs, especially in elderly men. Carotid sinus syncope during shaving is caused by pressure on the neck over the carotid sinus. Even a stiff collar is reported to have resulted in syncope.

Impaired Vasomotor Reflexes

Dilation of peripheral vessels occurs in baroreceptor failure. Changing from a supine to an upright position may cause syncope. Prolonged bed rest for several days, diabetic neuropathy, spinal cord injury, and tabes dorsalis are examples of impaired vasomotor responses that may result in syncope.

Decreased Blood Volume

Hypovolemia caused by bleeding, diarrhea, burns, or the use of diuretics can result in tachycardia, hypotension, light-headedness, and syncope.

FLUID REMOVAL

Several types of syncope are special cases of vasovagal stimulation. In micturition syncope, a healthy man rises from sleep to void. While standing at the toilet, syncope occurs during or after micturition. Syncope usually does not recur during the day, nor does it occur if he sits to urinate.

Rapid removal of pleural fluid or ascites may evoke vasovagal syncope. Syncope may occur with prostatic massage, eyeball pressure, or stimulation of the ear, pharynx, larynx, or soft palate.

POSTTUSSIVE SYNCOPE

Men who have COPD may be at risk of syncope during severe paroxysms of coughing even while sitting. The mechanism is believed to be similar to fainting in Valsalva's maneuver, with the high intrathoracic pressure impeding venous return.

Hemoptysis

Hemoptysis was discussed as a cardinal symptom of pulmonary disease in Chapter 3. Because hemoptysis by definition is expectoration of blood, cough is required for hemoptysis to occur.

The most common cause of hemoptysis as a cardiovascular symptom is mitral valve stenosis. Patients with mitral stenosis have a greater tendency to produce blood-streaked sputum in association with bronchitis than do noncardiac patients because of pulmonary venous congestion. A ruptured vessel or pulmonary infarction accounts for other causes of hemoptysis in mitral stenosis.

Pulmonary emboli with infarction is another cause of hemoptysis. Pulmonary edema, with its pink, actually bloody, frothy sputum, is another important cardiovascular cause of hemoptysis.

Edema

Edema is an excess accumulation of serous fluid in connective tissue interstitial spaces. Usually gradual swelling develops in both ankles and legs. Simultaneously, weight is gained as fluid is retained. Foot and ankle swelling decreases during the night when the patient is recumbent. During the day when the legs are dependent, swelling worsens.

When the examiner presses a finger against a swollen foot or leg, a pit remains from the finger pressure (Fig. 4-2). Chronic edema present for several years may no longer leave a pit following finger pressure.

The most common cause of pedal edema is congestive heart failure. If edema is allowed to progress untreated, the feet and legs remain swollen day and night. Bedridden patients without leg or foot swelling may have edema shown by pressing the finger against the sacrum (presacral edema). As edema progresses, the legs, thighs, back, and abdomen develop pitting edema. *Anasarca* refers to this generalized edema along with ascites. Anasarca is caused most often by severe heart failure, the nephrotic syndrome, or cirrhosis of the liver.

Edema may be classified according to etiologic cause: colloidal osmotic pressure, vascular pressure, and lymphatic pressure. Questions to ask the patient to assess increased hydrostatic pressure are as follows:

- *Does your leg swelling increase during the day and decrease at night?* This effect indicates edema caused by stasis (e.g., CHF, hypoalbuminemia, venous varicosities).

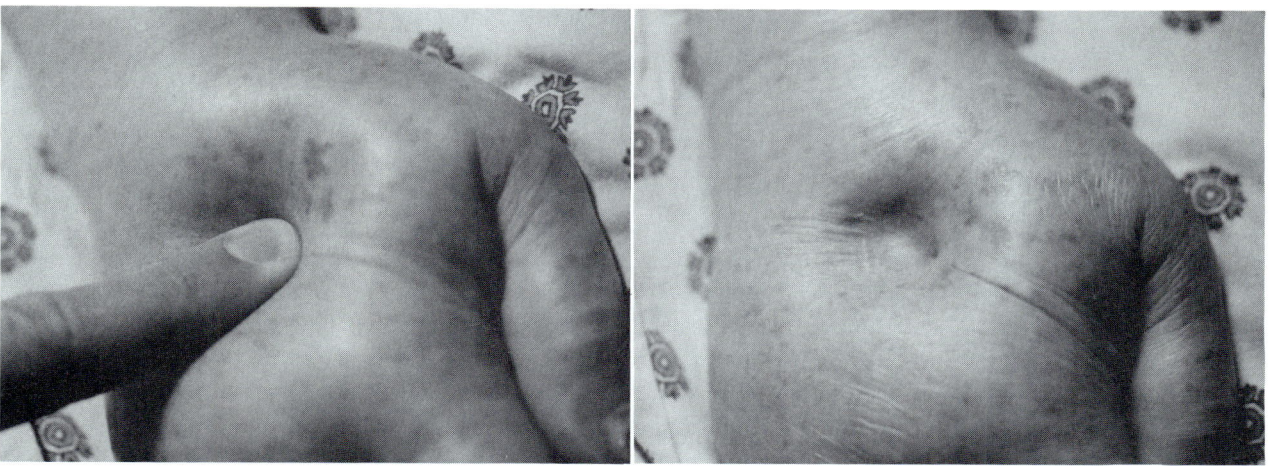

Fig. 4-2 Edema.

- *Do your legs or feet swell more after being up during the day?* Such edema is caused by increased capillary pressure (e.g., CHF, hypoalbuminemia, venous varicosities).

Reduced plasma oncotic pressure caused by decreased serum albumin is another cause of edema. Urinary protein loss (nephrotic syndrome) has no specific symptoms to indicate proteinuria. Decreased albumin synthesis occurs in liver disease or protein malnutrition. Protein loss can also occur from the GI tract (e.g., Ménétrier's disease) or the skin (severe third-degree burns). In some cases the capillary wall permeability to protein is abnormal, causing trauma or inflammation. Each of these may exhibit edema..

Lymphatic obstruction can lead to edema. To assess a mechanical obstruction, ask the patient about cancer, previous surgical procedures, parasites, or travel in Africa.

Right heart failure is frequently associated with peripheral edema. If left heart failure coexists, dyspnea appears. Physical findings include a third heart sound, jugular venous distention, and hepatomegaly.

Orthostatic edema of the feet and legs follows prolonged sitting or standing in persons with other risk factors for edema such as excessive salt intake or underlying heart disease.

Cyanosis

Cyanosis refers to a bluish gray discoloration of the skin and mucous membranes. The differential diagnosis for cyanosis has been presented (see Table 3-8). Here cardiac causes are considered.

Cyanosis becomes apparent when the concentration of reduced hemoglobin in the blood exceeds 5 g/dl. This is more oxygen desaturation than is present in venous blood of normal people. The concentration of hemoglobin can influence cyanosis. Cyanosis in a severely anemic person becomes impossible as the hemoglobin concentration approaches 5 g/dl. Thus serious hypoxia may be present without cyanosis. Conversely, in polycythemia with hemoglobin concentration above 18 g/dl, cyanosis may become apparent even when the blood has a high oxygen saturation.

Variant hemoglobins besides hemoglobin A may allow the cyanotic appearance without the patient being hypoxic. Hemoglobin Kansas is an example. Similarly, sulfhemoglobinemia and methemoglobinemia (in arc welders) give a cyanotic appearance.

Cyanosis is considered central (decreased pulmonary venous saturation) or peripheral (slow blood flow through capillaries). *Central cyanosis* may be caused by inadequate pulmonary oxygenation or venoarterial shunting in lungs or vessels. An example of a disease with central cyanosis is tetralogy of Fallot. Central cyanosis is observed in the conjunctivae, palate, tongue, inside of the lips, and cheeks. The skin is warm, and fingers and toes may exhibit clubbing.

Peripheral cyanosis or *acrocyanosis* occurs because of a decreased cardiac output or reduced rate of blood flow through capillaries and increased local extraction of oxygen. Diseases causing peripheral cyanosis include congestive heart failure, shock, and Raynaud's phenomenon. Peripheral cyanosis involves those parts of the body which turn blue on exposure to cold: fingers, ear lobes, cheeks, and the nose. Peripheral cyanosis may disappear with warming.

The age at which cyanosis appears may provide a clue to the etiologic cause.

Cyanosis in the newborn may be caused by cardiac, pulmonary, vasomotor, or metabolic disorders. Congenital heart lesions associated with cyanosis include:

- Large VSD
- Common single ventricle
- Hypoplastic left heart
- Transposition of the great vessels
- Tetralogy of Fallot
- Pulmonary stenosis or atresia with AV communications
- Epstein's anomaly

Septal defects may cause cyanosis at birth. Cyanosis beginning between 2 and 5 years is often caused by tetralogy of Fallot. Cyanosis caused by congenital heart disease that begins after age 5 most often results from Eisenmenger's syndrome.

Physical Examination of the Cardiovascular System

The physical examination begins at the introductory handshake by observing the sex, apparent age, face and hair, eye contact, body habitus, and grip effort. When evaluating cardiac symptoms:

1. Consider the effects of extracardiac diseases on the heart and circulation (see Table 4-5)
2. Look for effects of cardiovascular diseases on other systems
3. Consider other diseases as possible causes of symptoms in patients who have cardiac disease

General Examination

Diseases that are not primarily cardiovascular but that potentially cause a significant underlying cardiovascular abnormality may be apparent from the general physical examination. Table 4-5 lists disorders that have associated cardiovascular abnormalities. *Down's syndrome* is characterized by mental retardation, short stature, a small head, slanting eyes with prominent epicanthic folds, and protruding tongue. Septal defects or atrioventricular canal defects are possible cardiac abnormalities.

Patients with *Ehlers-Danlos syndrome* exhibit marked hyperextensibility of joints and excessive elasticity of the skin. The typical cardiac abnormality is mitral regurgitation. The patient with *Marfan syndrome* is often tall and slender. The finger-to-finger span of the outstretched arms span exceeds the person's height. The fingers are long (arachnodactyly), and finger length exceeds palm length. Skeletal abnormalities include scoliosis, kyphosis, pectus excavatum or carinatum, and a high arched palate. Cardiovascular associations include aortic insufficiency, aneurysm, and later dissecting aorta. Patients with *Friedreich's ataxia* are found to have thin, "storklike" lower legs, high arched feet (pes cavus), and kyphoscoliosis. Cardiomyopathy may develop. Scoliosis is common in children with congenital heart diseases such as tetralogy of Fallot. Kyphoscoliosis may result in cor pulmonale. A man with a dull expression, frontal balding, atrophy of temporal and sternocleidomastoid muscles, and atrophy of testes may have *myotonia dystrophica*. Arrhythmias and conduction block are possible cardiac abnormalities. A short female with hypertelorism, low-set ears, a broad

TABLE 4-5: Disorders with Associated Cardiovascular Abnormalities

Disorder	Associated Cardiovascular Findings
Hereditary and Congenital	
Down's syndrome	• Septal defects, atrioventricular canal defects
Ehlers-Danlos syndrome	• Rupture of arteries, atrial septal defect, tetralogy of Fallot
Fabry's disease	• Heart failure, conduction defects
Marfan's syndrome	• Aortic regurgitation, aortic aneurysm, dissecting aorta, septal defects
Hurler's syndrome	• Arrhythmia, valve disease, heart failure
Fredrick's ataxia	• Cardiomyopathy
Myotonia dystrophica	• Arrhythmias, coronary artery disease
Osteogenesis imperfecta	• Similar to Marfan's syndrome
Pseudoxanthoma elasticum	• Dilated aorta, dissection, regurgitation, coronary artery disease, pericarditis
Retinitis pigmentosa	• Conduction defects
Turner's syndrome	• Congenital heart defects, coarctation of aorta
Endocrine	
Acromegaly	• Myocardial hypertrophy accelerated coronary atherosclerosis
Cushing's syndrome	• Hypertension
Hyperthyroidism	• Heart failure, atrial fibrillation
Myxedema	• Pericardial effusion
Collagen diseases	
Ankylosing spondylitis	• Aortic valve disease
Lupus erythematosus	• Pericarditis, myocarditis, valvulitis
Polymyositis	• Arrhythmias, pericarditis, myocarditis
Raynaud's disease	• Pulmonary hypertension
Rheumatoid arthritis	• Mild aortic regurgitation
Scleroderma	• Pulmonary hypertension
Vasculitis	• Coronary arteritis and myocarditis
Other	
Chronic hemolytic anemia	• Cardiac dilation, myocarditis
Sarcoidosis	• Cardiomyopathy, arrhythmias

webbed neck, and a "shieldlike" chest with little breast development may have *Turner's syndrome*. Coarctation of the aorta is associated.

Cushing's syndrome is manifested by hirsutism, acne, truncal obesity, slender legs, plethoric and round moon face, buffalo hump, abdominal striae, and menstrual irregularities. Hypertension and weakness are common. Patients with *myxedema* exhibit a dull facial expression, large tongue, dry coarse hair, thin lateral eyebrows, and periorbital puffiness. Pericardial effusion may be present. The rigid spine of patients with *ankylosing spondylitis* is a clue to observe for signs of aortic regurgitation.

THE FACE

Facial clues to cardiovascular defects include puffiness of the face and eyes in myxedema (look for pericardial effusions). Plethoric puffiness is typical of superior vena cava syndrome, typically caused by obstruction of the superior vena cava by a neoplasm. Flushed cheeks are characteristic of mitral stenosis caused by rheumatic heart disease.

A diagonal crease across the earlobe has been associated with coronary artery disease.

THE EYES

Exophthalmos with a prominent stare along with tachycardia are found in hyperthyroidism. A staring gaze is occasionally found with heart failure.

Lid ptosis may occur in several diseases, including pulmonary stenosis and complete heart block. *Xanthelasma* (yellow, flat lipid-containing lesions around the eyes) in young people suggest possible coronary atherosclerosis.

The conjunctivae become pale in anemia. Conjunctival petechiae are characteristic of bacterial endocarditis. *Reiter's syndrome* (conjunctivitis, arthritis, and urethritis) may exhibit cardiac defects, including aortic regurgitation, pericarditis, or ECG abnormality (prolonged PR interval).

Blue-colored sclera are characteristic of osteogenesis imperfecta. Such patients may exhibit findings of aortic regurgitation.

Corneal arcus (arcus senilis) may be found in healthy persons, young or old, but in young people it suggests atherosclerosis. This association is considered more likely when corneal arcus is associated with xanthelasma of the eyelids.

Gray-white spots on the iris, *Brushfield's spots,* are found in Down's syndrome with the cardiac defects mentioned above. Iritis may occur alone or may be associated with sarcoidosis, rheumatoid arthritis, or Reiter's syndrome. The latter has the potential for the cardiac defects mentioned above.

Argyll Robertson pupils, which accommodate to distance but not to light, are a manifestation of CNS syphilis. Of course, tertiary syphilis does not necessarily manifest Argyll Robertson pupils. Cardiovascular syphilis, another manifestation of tertiary syphilis, includes aortic regurgitation, aneurysm of the ascending aorta, and coronary ostial stenosis.

The lens of the eye may be displaced (ectopia lentis), allowing the iris to flutter (iridodonesis) in a wavy motion in Marfan syndrome. Cataracts (opacity of lens) may be found in Down's syndrome, Cushing's syndrome, and diabetes mellitus. Rubella infection of the fetus in the first trimester can be manifested by cataracts, eighth cranial nerve deafness, and congenital heart disease.

Fundus examination allows visualization of small-vessel abnormalities in patients with hypertension or diabetes. In hypercholesterolemia the retinal artery may become beaded. Roth's spots in infective endocarditis are retinal hemorrhages with pale or white centers. Emboli may occlude the retinal arteries in atherosclerosis, rheumatic valvular disease, or left atrial myxoma.

THE MOUTH

Petechiae on the soft palate are found not only in infective endocarditis, but also in septicemia, scarlet fever, streptococcal pharyngitis, and infectious mononucleosis (see also Chapter 2). A high arched palate is typical of Marfan syndrome. Dark red, 1 to 2 mm dilated vessels on the lips, buccal mucosa, palate, or tongue suggest hereditary hemorrhagic telangiectasia *(Rendu-Osler-Weber syndrome).* These patients can bleed from pulmonary or GI arteriovenous fistulas.

Note the patient's oral hygiene, gingivitis, and any dental caries. Patients who have abnormal cardiac valves, a previous episode of endocarditis, or a prosthetic cardiac valve are at increased risk of developing endocarditis if dental cleaning or repair is not preceded by antibiotic prophylaxis.

THE SKIN

The color may be important. Cyanosis has been discussed.

Bronze pigmented skin of *hemochromatosis* is associated with deposition of iron in the skin and in the myocardium, causing cardiomyopathy.

Jaundice can result from cardiovascular causes, including large pulmonary infarctions, cardiac cirrhosis, and severe congestive heart failure.

Lentigines are small brown frecklelike lesions on the neck and trunk first appearing during childhood. Unlike freckles, lentigines are not increased by sun exposure. They are associated with hypertrophic cardiomyopathy or pulmonic stenosis.

Two skin lesions are characteristic of rheumatic fever. *Erythema marginatum* consists of large erythematous patches with serpentine margins and central clearing. These are found predominately on the trunk and may change appearance over a period of hours. *Subcutaneous nodules* are found in rheumatic fever over elbows, the skull, or the spine. Carditis, a prolonged P-R interval on an ECG tracing, valvulitis, and pericarditis, are cardiac manifestations.

Purplish red papules called *angiokeratomas* on the lower abdomen, groin, and scrotum in Fabry's disease are caused by hereditary glycolipid lipidosis. Cardiovascular associations include arrhythmias, heart failure, and renal failure. Angiokeratomas may be benign when found only under the tongue or on the scrotum.

Either neurofibromas or café-au-lait spots in a hypertensive patient should raise the suspicion of *von Recklinghausen's disease* (neurofibromatosis). Pheochromocytoma may be associated.

THE THORAX

In straight back syndrome, the normal thoracic kyphosis is replaced by a straight vertebral column. The anteroposterior diameter is also reduced. The heart may be displaced to the left, erroneously suggesting cardiomegaly. Atrial septal defect or mitral valve prolapse may be present. Scoliosis of the thoracic spine is common without associated cardiac abnormalities, but in patients with congenital cyanotic heart disease, scoliosis may also be found.

Inspect the anterior chest for a bulge along the upper left parasternum in atrial septal defect; along the lower left parasternum with ventricular septal defect; and along the right upper parasternal area for a pulsating aneurysm of the ascending aorta. Stenosis of the aortic valve can give pulsation in the second right interspace (aortic area), whereas neither hypertrophic cardiomyopathy nor supravalvular stenosis do so.

THE ABDOMEN

Findings on the abdominal examination that relate to cardiovascular problems more often result from effects of cardiac disease rather than direct causes. Exceptions are renal artery stenosis with epigastric bruits transmitted to the flanks, or palpably enlarged polycystic kidneys. Either of these may cause hypertension.

Hepatomegaly (large liver) commonly accompanies increased venous pressure in fairly severe right heart failure. The congested liver becomes tender, as the capsule is tense. Pulsations of the liver may be palpable in severe tricuspid insufficiency. However, apparent liver pulsations may be transmitted from a dilated aortic aneurysm.

THE EXTREMITIES

Clues to heart disease from examination of the hands include clubbing of the nails and cyanosis, characteristic of right-to-left shunts in septal disease or of pulmonary arteriovenous fistulas. Clubbing without cyanosis may be found in chronic infective endocarditis and in many noncardiac conditions. Clubbing may be familial, but only rarely.

Clubbing begins with swelling of the tissues proximal to the nailbed. Viewed from the side, the fingernail or toenail loses the normal obtuse angle with the proximal digit. The nail and proximal tissues become a continuous sweeping arc as the proximal attachment of the nail swells and the nail floats freely. Direct pressure over the proximal nail takes on a spongy feeling.

Besides clubbing, infective endocarditis may present with more common signs in the hands. *Osler's nodes* are tender erythematous nodules of the distal pads of the fingers. *Janeway lesions* are proximal erythematous nodules on the palms. These are nontender, raised, and palpable and caused by vasculitis. *Splinter hemorrhages* under the nailbeds are often more readily seen by shining a penlight through the tip of the finger. Splinter hemorrhages are not specific for endocarditis but may follow minor nail trauma. The hands in Down's syndrome are characterized by a single midpalmar transverse crease. Space between the fourth and fifth fingers is often increased, with the fifth finger short and curved inward. Several cardiac defects may be associated.

Raynaud's phenomenon is characterized by a three-fold color change after exposure of the hands to cold. Cold air or water may initiate the skin blanching to a chalky-white. Pain is common; often numbness occurs. As warming occurs, the fingers turn blue (cyanotic), and later red. Incomplete Raynaud's phenomenon lacks the three-color change. Associated disorders include pulmonary hypertension and collagen vascular disease.

An abnormal shape or number of fingers should suggest congenital heart disease. Marfan syndrome is associated with abnormally long fingers, termed arachnodactyly. A test for this syndrome is to make a fist over one's own clenched thumb. Normally, the thumb does not extend beyond the ulnar side of the clenched hand. In patients with Marfan syndrome the thumb does so. Another test is to have the patient encircle his own wrist using the thumb and little finger of the opposite hand. The finger and thumb overlap by 1 cm or more in most people with Marfan syndrome, but rarely does this phenomenon occur in others.

Blood Pressure

Initial blood pressure measurements are usually taken casually, without regard to previous activity. If the blood pressure is higher than normal, repeat the measurement after the patient has rested in a quiet room for 15 to 30 minutes. Emotions or stress may elevate blood pressure. The rush to arrive on time for an appointment may cause a spuriously high reading. Seeing a new physician or contemplating the physical examination can be stressful. Some patients with stress-induced high blood pressure exhibit normal blood pressure when readings are repeated at home.

Fig. 4-3 **A**, Systolic blood pressure is first determined by palpation of the brachial artery. **B**, Pressure is then determined by auscultation.

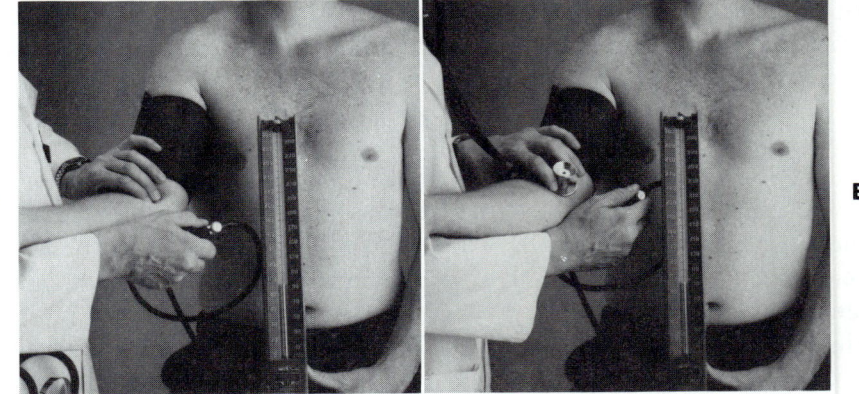

EQUIPMENT

The choice of sphygmomanometer cuff size should be determined by the arm size. The cuff should fit snugly around the upper arm, with the lower cuff edge 1 inch above the antecubital fossa (see Fig. 4-3) Palpate the brachial artery by applying firm pressure medial to insertion on the biceps tendon at the antecubital fossa. The diaphragm of the stethoscope is then placed near the edge of the cuff over the brachial artery.

The standard adult cuff size is 5 inches (12.5 cm) wide. The inflatable bladder encircles at least 70% to 80% of the circumference of the arm. For infants the cuff width is ½ inch; for ages 2 to 5 years, 3 inches; for obese adults, 8 inches. In obese patients, when an 8-inch wide cuff is not available, blood pressure may be determined by using a standard adult cuff around the forearm and recording the blood pressure measurements using the radial artery.

The standard position for blood pressure measurement is to position the artery being observed near the level of the heart to avoid the effect of gravity. Position the patient sitting with the elbow and forearm slightly supported on a desk or table. The arm is not to be hanging at the patient's side, nor held up by the patient's own muscles during blood pressure determination because these may falsely elevate the reading.

PALPATION

The blood pressure is first checked by palpation (Fig. 4-3, *A*). Snugly secure the cuff around the arm. Pump the pressure in the cuff higher than the expected systolic pressure while palpating the brachial artery. After pulsations are obliterated, slowly (2 mm/beat) but continuously decrease the cuff pressure while palpating the brachial artery for pulsations. The initial pulsations indicate the systolic pressure by palpation. Then completely deflate the cuff before filling it again.

AUSCULTATION

Next recheck the pressure by auscultation over the brachial artery with the patient in the same position (Fig. 4-3, *B*). Five phases of sounds called *Korotkoff sounds* are heard as the cuff pressure is gradually decreased (Fig. 4-4). At *phase 1*, clear tapping sounds appear first. These represent the systolic pressure by auscultation. *Phase 2* sounds are softer tones that appear as the cuff pressure is further decreased. *Phase 3* sounds are louder. *Phase 4* sounds are muffled tones.

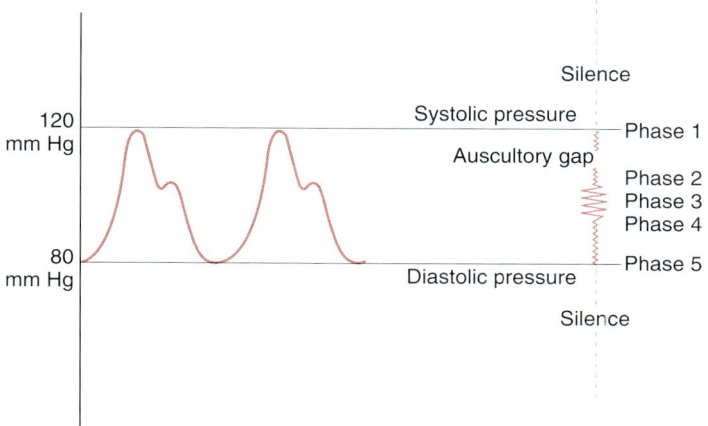

Fig. 4-4 Arterial pulse tracing and the Korotkoff sounds.

At *phase 5* the sounds disappear. Intraarterial pressure readings show that phase 5 sounds closely approximate diastolic arterial pressure. In some hypertensive patients, the phase 5 sound may be spuriously higher by 10 to 18 mm Hg than intraarterial pressures.

Blood pressures depend on many factors, including the patient's age (lower in children), time of day (lower early in morning), diet (lower with habitually lower sodium intake), and race (lower in white than in black persons). Normal ranges are shown in Table 4-6.

In infants, the standard cuff blood pressure may be difficult to measure. The "flush" method can be used as an alternative. Place a uninflated small cuff on the infant's forearm. Hold the arm high and massage it to produce blanching. With the blanched arm elevated, inflate the cuff above anticipated systolic pressure. Then lower the arm to the level of the heart and slowly deflate the cuff. The pressure at which the blanched extremity flushes approximates the mean blood pressure.

INTERPRETING THE RESULTS

Errors in Blood Pressure Measurements

Errors in blood pressure measurements can occur through several mechanisms. An *auscultatory gap* is a silent period occasionally occurring between phase 1 and

TABLE 4-6: Normal Ranges for Blood Pressures by Patient Age

	Age	Systolic		Diastolic	
		Maximum	Minimum	Maximum	Minimum
Children	3 to 6	116	80	76	50
	6 to 9	122	85	78	55
Young adults	10 to 13	126	90	82	55
	14 to 19	142	90	86	60
Adults	20 to 60	150	90	90	60
	60+	160	90	95	60

Data from Blumenthal S: Report of the Task Force on Blood Pressure Control in Children, Pediatrics 59(suppl):797, 1977; and the 1988 Report of the Joint National Committee on Detection, Evaluation, and Treatment of High Blood Pressure, Arch Intern Med 148:1023-1038, 1988.

phase 2 Korotkoff sounds. An auscultatory gap may be caused by venous distention or severe aortic stenosis (see Fig. 4-4). If the cuff pressure is not pumped above the systolic pressure, but to a point in the range of the auscultatory gap, the recorded systolic blood pressure could be falsely low. Avoid this by palpating the radial or brachial artery while inflating the cuff. After the palpable pulse disappears, the auscultatory gap, if present, has been passed. If a gap is found, record the beginning and ending of the gap as follows: auscultatory gap between 105 and 95 mm Hg.

A second potential error in blood pressure measurement involving the auscultatory gap is to call the disappearance of tones (at the auscultatory gap) the diastolic pressure. Palpation of pressure first and then listening for each phase of the Korotkoff sounds prevents this mistake.

Another potential error in measuring blood pressure occurs in patients with prosthetic aortic valves. Falsely high readings can result from transmitted prosthetic valve sounds, giving the impression of Korotkoff sounds.

A fourth potential error concerns arteriosclerosis. Cuff measurements of diastolic pressure in the elderly can be up to 40 mm Hg higher than intraarterial pressures because of inelastic arteries, or "stiff pipes." Stiff pipes may be detected by Osler's maneuver. Inflate the cuff above systolic pressure. Roll the brachial and radial arteries under the palpating finger. If the artery remains palpable without blood pressure, the patient has pseudohypertension of the elderly. Patients may have both stiff pipes and hypertension, which can be confusing and requires the use of intraarterial pressure measurement.

When a patient arrives for a complete physical examination or when a patient has hypertension, it is usual to measure the blood pressure in both arms. The pressures should be similar, with the difference between arms being less than 15 mm Hg. Arterial obstruction or supravalvular aortic stenosis may cause greater differences. Similarly, blood pressures should be measured in the legs when hypertension is present or when pressures are unequal in the arms.

Orthostatic Hypotension

When blood pressure is being measured in hypertensive patients who are receiving blood pressure medications or in patients who complain of lightheadedness, measurements should be made with the patient supine, sitting, and standing. When changing from supine to standing, systolic pressure normally decreases no more than 5 to 15 mm Hg, whereas diastolic pressure rises slightly. The heart rate increases up to 10 beats/min, causing mean blood pressure to remain slightly higher when the patient is sitting or standing.

If the blood pressure falls with the changes in position, postural or orthostatic changes are present. When this occurs, the patient normally develops an even more pronounced increase in heart rate.

Orthostatic hypotension may be caused by vascular volume loss from hemorrhage, diarrhea, vomiting, dehydration, or excessive diuresis. Similarly, redistribution of blood volume because of antihypertensives, antidepressants, alcohol, or nitrates occasionally produces orthostatic hypotension. Prolonged bed rest, simple vasovagal fainting, autonomic nervous system dysfunction in diabetic neuropathy, or adrenal insufficiency may yield similar findings.

The Obese Patient

The technique for taking the blood pressure when Korotkoff sounds are faint in the obese patient is similar to that used in the infant. After placing the large cuff snugly around the patient's arm, ask the patient to elevate the arm and pump the fist a few times. This allows venous and capillary emptying. Inflate the cuff pressure above systolic pressure while the arm remains elevated. Lower the arm, support it so the patient's muscles are relaxed, and the Korotkoff sounds become audible.

Hypertension

Hypertensive patients should have the blood pressure measured in both arms and one leg. The systolic leg pressure may be as much as 20 mm Hg higher than in the arms, but diastolic pressures should be similar. Intraarterial measurements show systolic, diastolic, and mean pressures in the femoral artery to be similar to those in the brachial artery.

When the thigh diastolic pressure is much higher than that in the arm, the cuff may be too small. Either use a larger leg cuff or place the cuff about the calf and auscultate over the dorsalis pedis or posterior tibial artery.

In coarctation of the aorta, the systolic pressure is lower in the thigh than in the arm, but the diastolic pressures remain similar. This is a rare but potentially treatable cause of hypertension, which is the reason that blood pressure in the leg should be measured in the initial evaluation of every hypertensive person.

Most hypertensive patients have essential hypertension, signifying no detectable cause. Of those who have identifiable causes, renal diseases, adrenal disorders, and oral contraceptives are uncommon causes.

Complications of hypertension may be caused by the elevated blood pressure or may be related to atherosclerosis accelerated by hypertension. Direct effects of hypertension include:

- Renal failure
- Hemorrhagic stroke
- Congestive heart failure
- Retinopathy
- Dissecting aneurysm

Accelerated atherosclerosis may be responsible for acute myocardial infarction, thrombotic cerebral infarction, and intermittent claudication.

The funduscopic examination may show changes related to hypertension or to atherosclerosis. It may be difficult to differentiate the findings of these two processes because they often occur concomitantly, and changes of each appear similar on examination.

Comparison of funduscopic findings for hypertension and atherosclerosis are shown in Table 4-7.

Examination of the Heart and Great Vessels

The findings on cardiac examination can indicate abnormal structure or function of the cardiovascular system. Fig. 4-5 shows the circulation of blood through the heart. The sequence of opening and closing of heart valves in the cardiac cycle is shown in Fig. 4-6. The cardiovascular examination will be discussed first with attention to veins, then arteries, and finally the heart itself:

1. Jugular venous pulse
2. Arterial pulses
3. The precordium
4. The stethoscope

TABLE 4-7: Comparison of Retinal Changes in Hypertension and Atherosclerosis

Atherosclerosis	Grade	Hypertension
• Arteriole to venous diameter ratio is 2:3 to 3:5	0 (Normal)	• Same ratio; vessels curve gently
• Light reflected from arterioles is red-brown (called copper wiring) • Slight AV crossing defects	I	• Focal or diffuse narrowing of arterioles, reversible if caused by spasm
• Light reflected from arterioles is whitish (called silver wiring) because of thickening of vessel walls • The AV crossing defects are more prominent	II	• Copper wiring and AV crossing defects • Arteriole diameter is about 50% of normal
• As above; may have hemorrhages always near optic nerve, especially in elderly • Vein invisible when it crosses arteriole	III	• Silver wiring; more prominent AV crossing defects • Flame-shaped retinal hemorrhages may not be near optic nerve • Soft white cotton-wool exudates (fluid exudate); hard exudates (ischemic infarcts) around; may have star shape
• Veins obstructed, arterioles obliterated or very narrow	IV	• Papilledema present (increased ICP) along with findings

Data from Kirkendall WM, Armstrong ML: Vascular changes in the eye of the treated and untreated patient with essential hypertension, Am J Cardiol pp 663-668; May 1962; and Keith NM, Wagener HP, Barker NW: Some different types of essential hypertension: their course and prognosis, Am J Med Science 197:332-343, 1939.

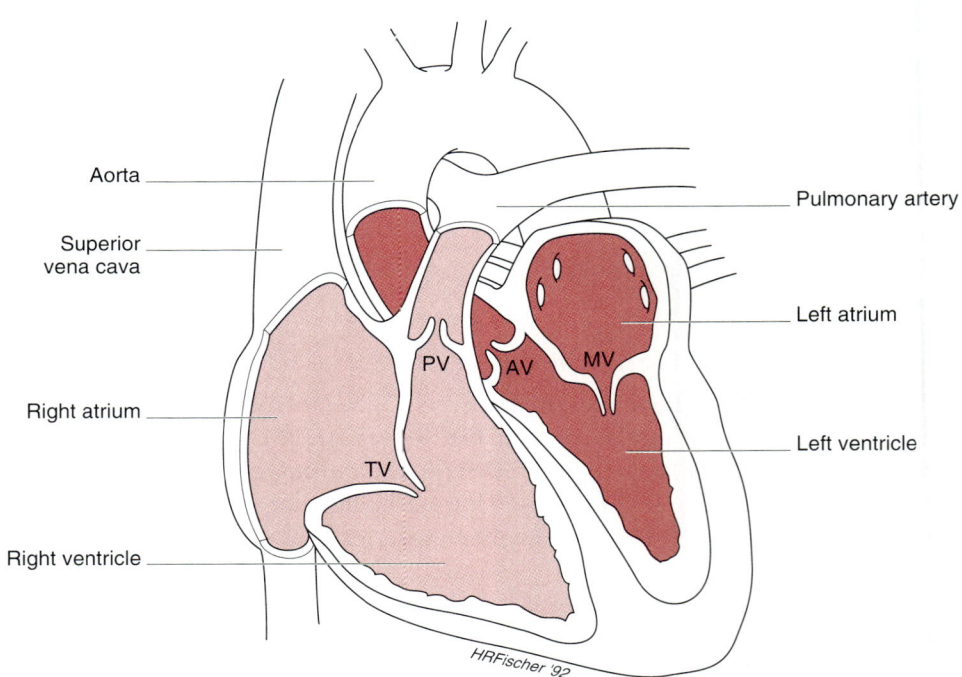

Fig. 4-5 Anatomy of the heart.

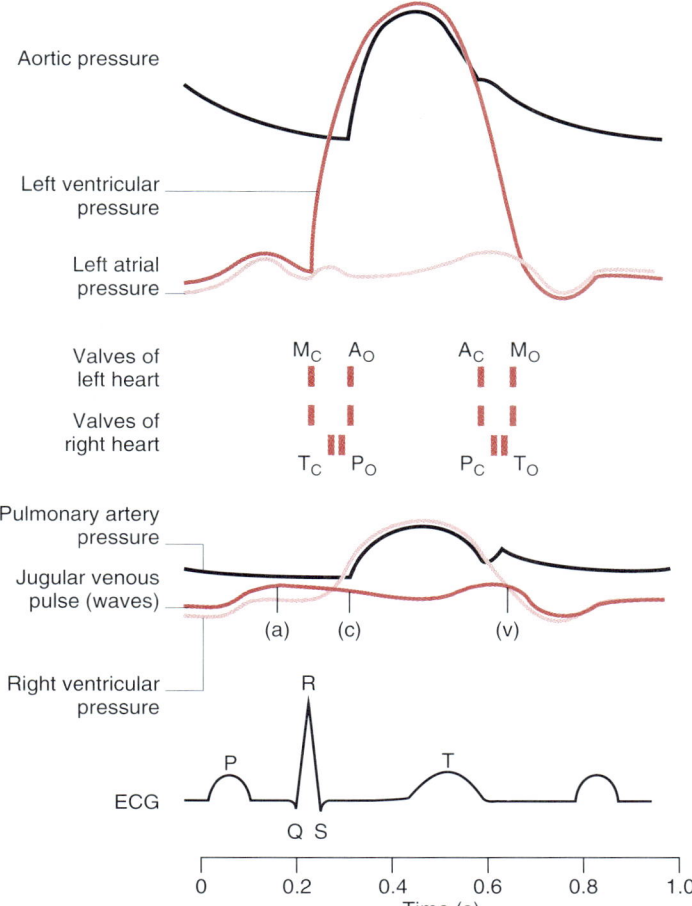

Fig. 4-6 The cardiac cycle. The sequence of cardiac valves opening ($_o$) and closing ($_c$) is shown with pressures. M, mitral; P, pulmonic; A, aortic; T, tricuspid; a, left atrial; A, aortic; Ra, right atrial; JVP, jugular venous pressure. The normal valve sequence is $M_c T_c P_o A_o A_c P_c T_o M_o$ (i.e., the closing of valves is the reverse sequence of opening).

5. Special techniques to improve cardiac examination
6. Cardiac sounds
7. Systolic clicks
8. Pericardial rubs
9. Prosthetic valve sounds
10. Cardiac murmurs
11. Examples of systolic murmurs
12. Examples of diastolic murmurs

The examination of the jugular venous pulse is by inspection, whereas the carotid pulse is examined by palpation and auscultation. Percussion is of limited usefulness in cardiovascular examination, but it may be useful in determining the approximate heart size.

JUGULAR VENOUS PULSE

Examination of jugular venous pulsations is often poorly done, for two reasons. First, the terminology of the venous waves and descents may be confusing. Second, line drawings of jugular pulse tracings may be difficult to correlate with pulsations seen at the bedside. Nonetheless, examination of the

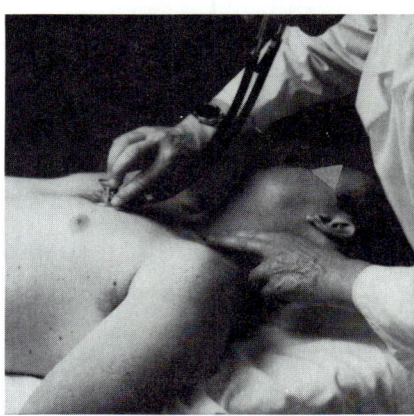

Fig. 4-7 Gentle palpation of the carotid artery while observing the jugular vein and listening to cardiac sounds.

jugular venous pulse and jugular venous pressures can be important for three reasons:

1. Jugular venous pressure gives information concerning body fluid volume and can indicate the presence of congestive heart failure.
2. Jugular venous pulses may indicate abnormal right heart structure or function that would otherwise be difficult to diagnose at the bedside.
3. Jugular venous pulses often give bedside clues about cardiac arrhythmias that are otherwise difficult to diagnose.

Examine the right jugular veins, internal and external, from the patient's right side. The internal jugular vein is located deep in the neck within the carotid sheath. Pulse waves are not seen directly, but pulsations are transmitted to the overlying skin. Shining a light tangentially across the neck enhances visibility of jugular pulse waves. Positioning of the patient is of utmost importance. The patient's head and trunk should be elevated to show maximum pulsations in the right internal jugular, usually 30 to 45 degrees from the horizontal. Extremely high jugular venous pressures may require positioning the patient at 60 or 90 degrees. For low venous pressures, less than 30 degrees is desirable. Seeing pulsations with very low venous pressures may require the patient's thorax to be horizontal and the patient's legs elevated.

Palpate the left carotid gently with your left index and middle fingers while visualizing the patient's right external and internal jugular veins (Fig. 4-7). Right-sided jugular pulsations are viewed because the right jugular is straighter than is the left. These transmit pressures from the right atrium and right ventricle because no valves are present in the internal jugular. The right external jugular may not be pulsatile because of the presence of valves. Although observations of the right external jugular are considered less accurate, these may give information about mean right atrial pressure.

To find the jugular venous pressure, estimate how far the top of the column of blood in the jugular vein is above the level of the right atrium. When the patient sits up, the clavicles are about 10 cm above the right atrium. Because normal central venous pressure is ordinarily less than 8 cm, the jugular veins normally are not seen above the clavicles. If the jugular veins were distended to the angle of the patient's jaw when the patient was sitting, the central venous pressure would be about 20 cm. (Calculations: 10 cm from right atrium to clavicles + 10 cm

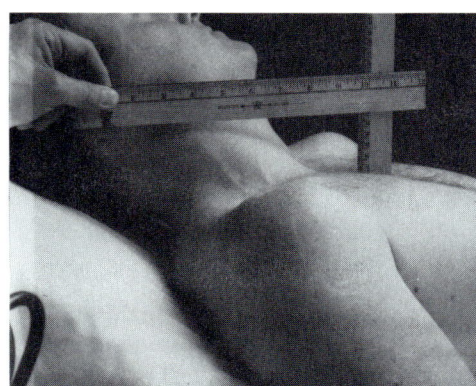

Fig. 4-8 Vertical measurement from sternal angle of Louis to top of column of blood in jugular vein. For estimate of jugular venous pressure, add 5 cm (right atrium to sternal angle distance) to measured column.

jugular venous distension above clavicles = 20 cm jugular venous pressure.)

When the patient is supine with the thorax elevated to 30 degrees, the reference point is the sternal angle of Louis, about 5 cm above the right atrium. When the patient's thorax is positioned at 30 degrees, jugular venous distension is normally visible to 3 cm above the sternal angle (total 8 cm). The technique of vertical measurement from the sternal angle of Louis to the top of the column of blood in the jugular vein is shown in Fig. 4-8.

Respiration affects jugular venous pressure. During inspiration, intrathoracic pressure decreases and the flow from peripheral venous return to the vena cava increases, decreasing the internal jugular pressure. When inspiration stops, intrathoracic pressure increases, which increases jugular venous pressures. If one performs Valsalva's maneuver, the intrathoracic pressure is artificially increased, filling the jugular veins.

Kussmaul's sign is the phenomenon of paradoxic filling of the jugular veins. Jugular veins become distended instead of emptying during inspiration. Kussmaul's sign is caused by a restriction in diastolic filling of the right ventricle by diseases such as pericardial effusion.

In *superior vena cava syndrome*, compression of the superior vena cava causes the jugular veins to remain distended continuously, without the pulsations of venous waves discussed below.

A useful adjunct in evaluating increased central venous pressure is the *hepatojugular reflux*. This may be elicited when the patient is lying with the thorax elevated at 30 degrees. While observing the jugular venous distension with the patient breathing normally, exert pressure over the RUQ, especially over a distended liver. The hand must be warm, the pressure gentle. Maintain compression of the upper quadrant for 30 to 60 seconds. The response in normal people is a transient increase in the initial jugular venous distension, even though pressure on the abdomen is maintained. In right-sided congestive heart failure, the increase in jugular venous pressure is maintained throughout.

An Alternative to Jugular Venous Pressure

The jugular veins may be difficult to visualize in the patient who has a short, stocky neck. Here an estimate of venous pressure may be made using the veins of the right arm. Ask the patient to drop his arm to the side, allowing the veins to become distended. Then slowly raise the patient's arm out to the patient's side,

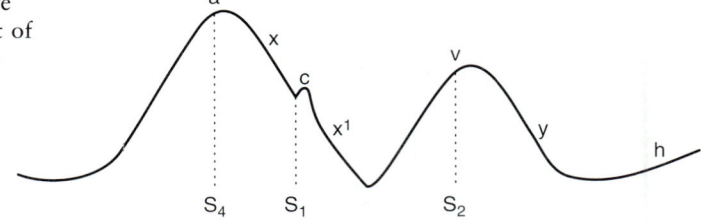

Fig. 4-9 Venous pressure as shown by the amount of distention in the jugular vein.

keeping the elbow straight. The level at which the hand veins collapse is measured in relationship to centimeters above the sternal angle of Louis. This is added to 5 cm to obtain an estimate of the peripheral venous pressure. By this technique the venous pressure should be less than 10 cm.

Jugular Venous Waves

The three waves of the jugular venous pulse waves are termed the *a* wave, *c* wave, and *v* wave. Three descents, one after each wave, are named *x* descent, x^1 (x prime) descent, and y descent. Finally, the h (slow-filling) wave precedes the *a* wave of the next venous cycle (Fig. 4-9).

The *a* wave corresponds to the peak filling of the jugular vein produced by right atrial contraction. The *x* descent is the decrease in filling that follows the *a* wave as the atrium relaxes. The *c* wave, usually not seen at the bedside, signals contraction of the ventricles, causing a slight tricuspid bulge back up into the atrium. The "c" stood for carotid because the "c" wave was synchronous with the carotid artery pulse.

The *v* wave occurs because of passive atrial filling during ventricular contraction. The tricuspid valve ("v" for valve) remains closed during ventricular contraction. The tricuspid valve opens at the peak of the *v* wave. At the bedside, the *v* wave cannot normally be seen by most clinicians. The slight *y* descent is caused by the brief decreases in atrial pressure after the tricuspid valve opens. Following the *y* descent, the right jugular pressure rises slowly in the *h* wave, or *h* ascent (named by Hirschfelder). Then the jugular venous pressure cycle repeats, beginning with the *a* wave.

To the eye, these waves are seen as a series of crests and troughs. It is usually easiest to see the *a* wave followed by the *x* descent. Timing of the *a* wave and the *x* descent is done by palpating the left carotid pulse and watching the right jugular. The carotid pulse occurs just after the *a* wave during the *x* descent, actually at the *invisible c* wave. Because the *v* wave and *y* descent normally are much smaller than are the *a* wave and *x* descent, they are difficult to see. If one auscultates the heart while watching jugular venous pulses, the first heart sound occurs during the *x* descent. The second heart sound occurs just before the peak of the *v* wave.

Abnormal *a* or *v* waves (unusually large *a* waves), or abnormal *x* or *y* descent patterns can suggest right heart abnormality or an arrhythmia (see the accompanying box). Large *a* waves occur when the column of blood refluxes into the jugulars in anatomic or functional tricuspid valve narrowing. Large *a* waves are characteristic of tricuspid stenosis, insufficiency, decreased compliance in right ventricular hypertrophy, pulmonic stenosis, or pulmonary hypertension (Fig. 4-10). In tetralogy of Fallot a large *a* wave is not expected because the ventricular septal defect decompresses the right ventricle.

Diagnosis Suggested by Abnormal Jugular Venous Pulse Waves	

Large *a* waves
  Tricuspid stenosis
  Atrial septal defect
  Pulmonary hypertension
  Pulmonic stenosis
Giant *a* waves
  Complete heart block
  Cardiac pacemaker
  Premature ventricular contractions
  Junctional rhythm
	No *a* waves
	  Atrial fibrillation
	Large *v* waves
	  Tricuspid insufficiency
	Large *a* and *v* waves
	  Atrial septal defect
	  Anomalous pulmonary venous drainage
	No waves
	  Superior vena cava obstruction
	  Low venous volume
	  Positioning of patient needed

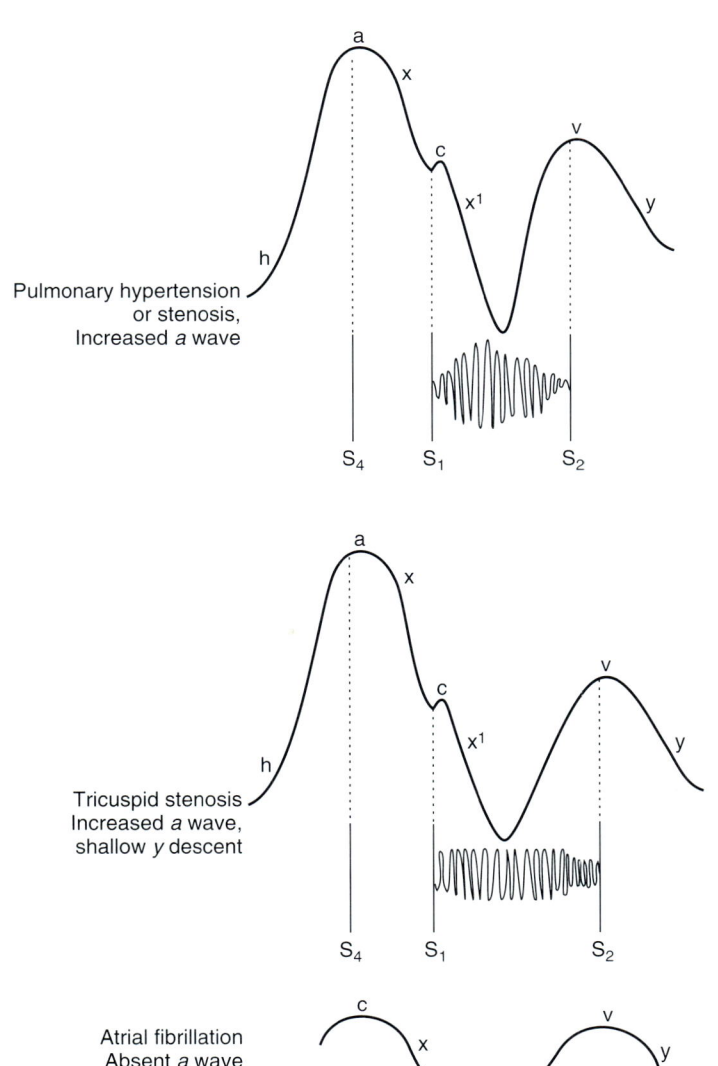

Fig. 4-10 Jugular venous pulses in select conditions.

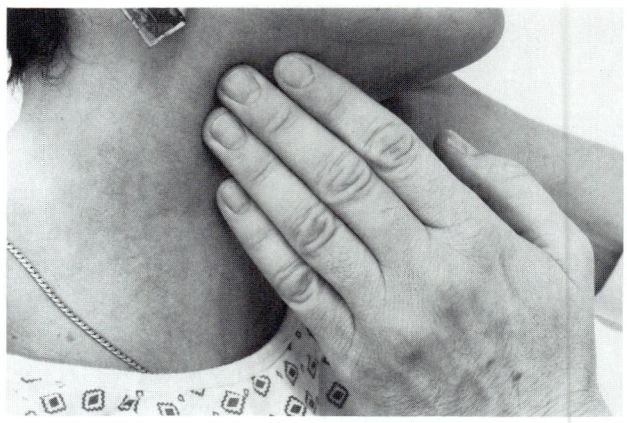

Fig. 4-11 Palpation of the carotid artery.

Very large *a* waves, called giant or cannon *a* waves, can suggest arrhythmias. Giant *a* waves occur when the atria contract during ventricular contraction. The ventricular pressure keeps the tricuspid valve closed despite the increase in atrial pressure. This causes blood to be pumped back into the jugulars. Giant *a* waves may even be palpable. Premature atrial contractions, cardiac pacemaker rhythms, and atrioventricular dissociation (ECG diagnoses) may show giant *a* waves.

In contrast, *a* waves may be small in atrial flutter or absent in atrial fibrillation. Unless the jugular pulse waves are clearly visible, one must not assume that an absence of visible *a* waves indicates an abnormal cardiac rhythm.

The *v* wave may be visible in certain situations. Normally blood enters the jugulars constantly from the venous system. After the atrium and superior vena cava fill, the jugulars begin to fill. When the tricuspid valve opens at the end of ventricular systole, the *y* descent of the *v* wave begins. Increased flow into the right atrium during systole increases the height of the *v* wave (e.g., atrial septal defect with left-to-right shunt). Tricuspid valve incompetence with regurgitation into the right atrium during systole also increases the *v* wave. In severe tricuspid insufficiency, the *v* wave may even be palpable in the swollen liver. In atrial fibrillation, the *v* wave is seen, but the *a* wave is absent.

ARTERIAL PULSES

The extent of examination of arterial pulses depends on the patient's age and problems. Selected pulses are routinely evaluated during a general examination. Inspection, palpation, and auscultation are the applicable techniques.

In infants, examine the brachial and femoral arteries. In children and adults, the carotid vessels should be included routinely. For patients over age 55, the examination of pulses includes carotid, brachial, radial, femoral, popliteal, dorsalis pedis, and posterior tibial arteries and the abdominal aorta.

When palpating the carotids, locate the common carotid near the base of the neck. The carotid should not be compressed significantly, and only one carotid at a time is palpated to avoid risk to the patient (Fig. 4-11). Vigorous carotid palpation, especially if the other carotid is obstructed, has the potential to reduce cerebral blood flow and produce syncope. Compression of the carotid bulb can produce vagally mediated bradycardia.

Palpate the radial artery to evaluate pulse rate and rhythm. Place the first, second, and third finger tips over the vessel just proximal to the styloid process

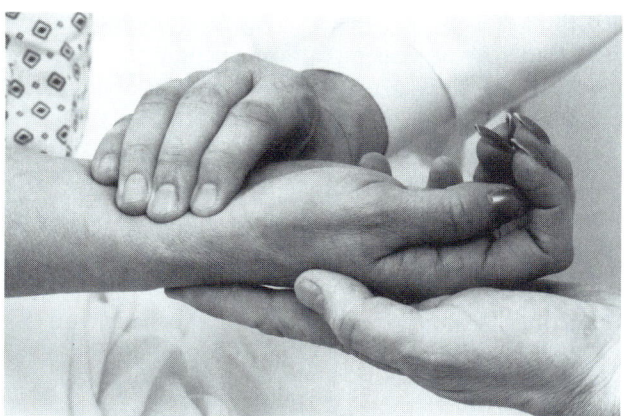

Fig. 4-12 Palpation of the radial artery.

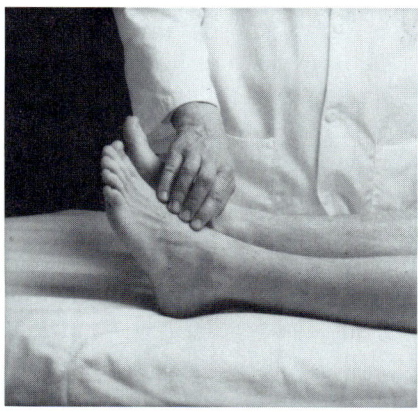

Fig. 4-13 Palpation of the dorsalis pedis pulse.

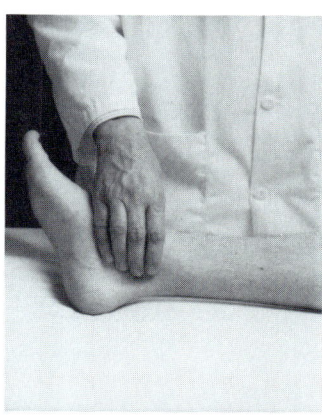

Fig. 4-14 Palpation of posterior tibial pulse.

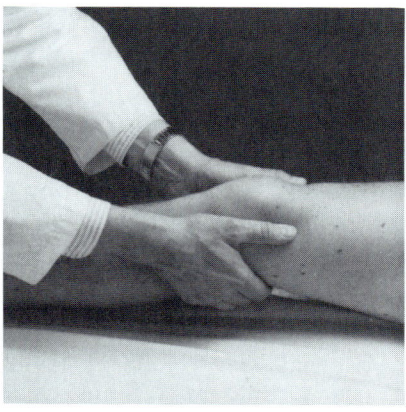
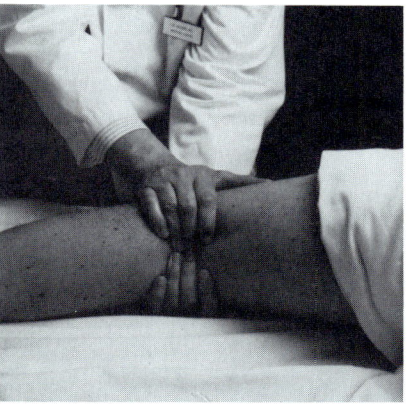

Fig. 4-15 **A,** Palpation of popliteal pulse. Posterior view **(B)** shows position of fingers.

of the radius (see Fig. 4-11). Compare the right and left radial arteries and other arteries for symmetric equality. Then palpate the brachial arteries (Fig. 4-12).

Palpate the femoral pulses below the inguinal ligaments, using the second and third fingers. The dorsalis pedis pulse (Fig. 4-13) is most often found between the tendons of the great and second toe. The posterior tibial pulses (Fig. 4-14) are located slightly posterior to the medial malleolus.

Popliteal pulses are more difficult to palpate (Fig. 4-15). These are best located when the patient is supine with the knee slightly flexed. Cup the fingers of each hand around the posterior knee, gradually increasing and releasing pressure until you feel the pulse. The position of the popliteal artery varies so that you may need to examine the popliteal fossa extensively to locate it.

Examine the abdominal aorta with the patient supine. Abdominal wall relaxation is enhanced by having the patient flex the knees. Normally, the abdominal aorta is palpable above the umbilicus. Palpate below and to the left of the umbilicus to identify an abdominal aortic aneurysm. The lateral margins of the aorta or aneurysm are identified by palpating with the fingers of each hand simultaneously. Bimanual palpation allows approximation of the width of the aorta. If the width by palpation appears to be greater than 6 centimeters, obtain ultrasound measurements to look for aneurysm.

Arterial Pulse Rate

The radial pulse is usually palpated to determine the cardiac rate and rhythm. Count the number of beats in 30 seconds; if an irregular rhythm is present, counting for a minute may be more accurate. The normal adult heart rate is 60 to 99 beats/min. Rates of 100 or more are termed *tachycardia*. Rates less than 60 beats/min, termed *bradycardia*, may be normal in athletes.

Normal rates in the child vary with age. For the newborn, 140 beats/min is normal. By 1 year the rate is 115 beats/min.

Arterial Pulse Rhythms

Arrhythmias are readily suspected but seldom precisely identified by using the arterial pulse alone. The pulse rhythm is first identified as regular or irregular. If irregular, the pattern, if one is present, is identified. An ECG may be needed to firmly identify a particular rhythm. Examples of arterial pulse rhythms are shown in Fig. 4-16.

Sinus arrhythmia Sinus arrhythmia is a variation in the heart rate with respiration. The heart rate accelerates with inspiration. To abolish sinus arrhythmia during examination, the cooperative patient can hold the breath in midcycle. Patients usually are not aware of having sinus arrhythmia.

Premature contractions Premature beats caused by atrial premature contractions (APCs) do not interrupt the overall cardiac rhythm except for that single APC. In contrast, ventricular premature contractions (VPCs) are followed by a compensatory pause. Thus a new rhythm is established. Patients may be aware of either APCs or VPCs. The ventricular beat following the prematurity is usually stronger because of increased ventricular filling.

Atrial fibrillation The rhythm of atrial fibrillation is termed *irregularly irregular*: there is no necessary pattern to the irregular beating. Bedside observation may show sequences of beats that seem to be regular. Thus atrial fibrillation may resemble a sinus rhythm with multiple VPCs, unless an *a* wave can be seen in the jugular pulse or an S4 heard. Either of these would be caused by atrial contraction and exclude atrial fibrillation.

In atrial fibrillation with tachycardia, the radial pulse rate may not equal the cardiac apical pulse rate. Two beats in rapid succession fail to allow sufficient ventricular filling to generate a peripheral pulse wave. The difference between the apical and peripheral pulse rates is called the *pulse deficit*. Large pulse deficits indicate poor control of the ventricular response.

Some patients with atrial fibrillation have no symptoms. Others experience

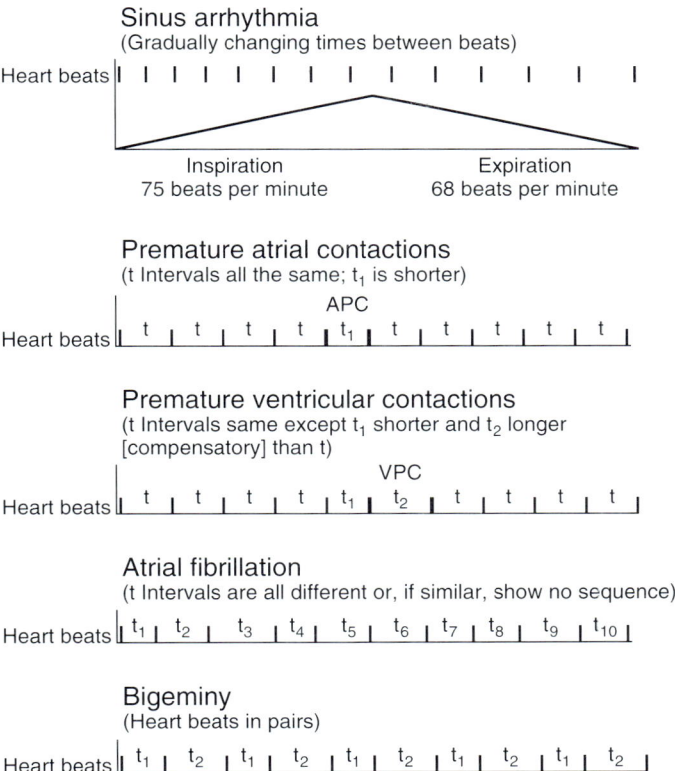

Fig. 4-16 Arterial pulse rhythms in select conditions.

palpitations. Patients with large pulse deficits are more likely to experience symptoms. In those who have chronic atrial fibrillation, exercise may aggravate symptoms of rapid or irregular heart beats.

Bigeminal pulse Pulsus bigeminus indicates two consecutive heart beats closely coupled, with a subsequent delay before the next beat. Bigeminy may occur because of premature atrial or ventricular contractions.

Arterial Pulse Volume

The volume of the arterial pulse (pulse pressure = systolic − diastolic pressure) and the pulse duration have been traditionally used to describe the pulse. Some of these descriptions may be difficult to identify at the bedside.

One fairly characteristic pulse is the hyperkinetic pulse, which has a quick upstroke and a full volume. Examples of this type of pulse are found in hypertension, anxiety, anemia, or thyrotoxicosis.

Corrigan's pulse Corrigan's, or water-hammer, pulse (Fig. 4-17) is found in aortic regurgitation. Because the diastolic back flow through the aortic valve is large, the pulse is brisk with a large volume that collapses. A water hammer was a 19th-century child's toy in which water was sealed in a closed vacuum tube. When the tube was inverted, the water dropped to the other end. A synonym is the collapsing pulse (see below). When the bell of the stethoscope is used to auscultate and compress the femoral artery, *Duroziez's murmur* (a to-and-fro bruit) becomes apparent in patients who have Corrigan's pulse.

Quincke's pulse Another physical sign of aortic insufficiency is Quincke's pulse, visible capillary pulsations in the nailbeds. Place a penlight under the distal

Fig. 4-17 Peripheral arterial pulse (radial) rhythms in select conditions.

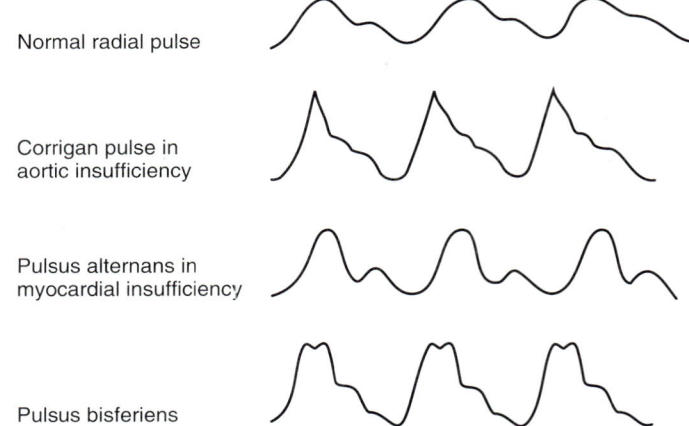

fingernail to enhance this phenomenon. The pinkish vascular filling of the nailbed moves distally and proximally with each heartbeat.

Pulsus bisferiens Pulsus bisferiens (bifid pulse) has two distinct impulses with each heartbeat. This is best felt in the carotid artery in aortic regurgitation or hypertrophic cardiomyopathy (idiopathic hypertrophic subaortic stenosis).

Pulsus alternans Pulsus alternans is a variation of pulse volume or force with successive beats (see Fig. 4-17). One pulse feels full, the next, small. Pulsus alternans signifies that every other pulsation is weaker, usually because of decreased myocardial contractility. Pulsus alternans carries a poor prognosis.

Pulsus paradoxus Pulsus paradoxus refers to weakening of the pulse with inspiration. During normal inspiration the systolic pressure usually decreases less than 10 mm Hg. In pulsus paradoxus the decrease is 10 mm Hg or more. Diseases of the pericardium, pericardial effusion, and constrictive pericarditis are causes of paradoxic pulse.

To check for paradoxic pulse, inflate the blood pressure cuff above systolic pressure while the patient is supine. Deflate the cuff so that the initial Korotkoff sounds are heard during slow exhalation. Next, recheck the peak systolic pressure during inspiration. Pressure differences greater than 10 mm Hg signify a paradoxic pulse.

GRADING PULSES

Describe the amplitude and volume of pulses, and compare vessels for symmetry. The pulses are usually graded 0 to 4+.

    0   Absent pulse
    1+ Markedly reduced
    2+ Slightly reduced
    3+ Normal pulse
    4+ Bounding pulse

Pulses may be absent or reduced for many reasons, including arterial embolus, atherosclerosis, or diabetes mellitus. Bounding pulses may be found in thyrotoxicosis, aortic regurgitation, or anemia.

Atherosclerosis

Gradual reduction of peripheral pulses in the legs is typical of atherosclerosis and diabetes mellitus. Usually the pulses in the dorsalis pedis or posterior tibials,

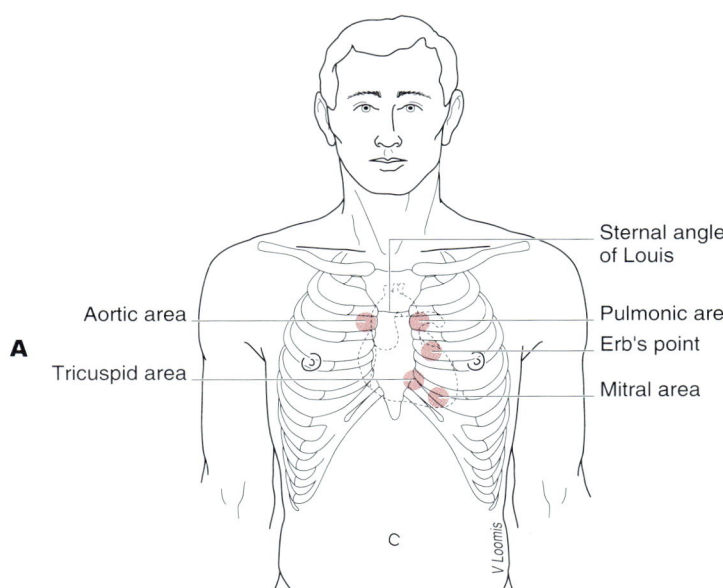
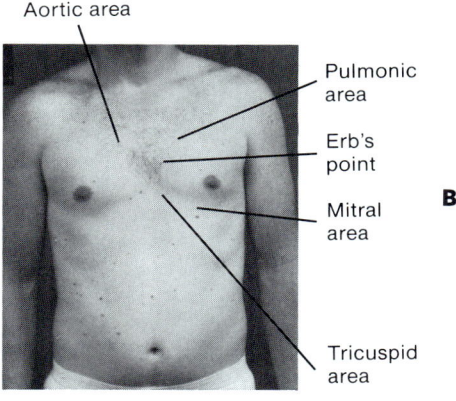

Fig. 4-18 Site on chest where cardiac auscultation is routinely performed. **A,** Drawing of underlying structures. **B,** Surface anatomy.

and later the popliteals, are reduced. Because the dorsalis pedis pulse may be absent in 5% of healthy persons, use care in drawing conclusions. Even smaller digital artery disease is common in diabetic persons, and it is often associated with neuropathy and foot ulcers.

Carotid arteries may be involved, giving transient cerebral ischemic attacks or strokes. At other times, atheromatous plaques involve large vessels such as the iliac or femoral arteries.

Intermittent Claudication

Intermittent claudication occurs in patients with arterial insufficiency, usually of the legs. Calf or thigh tightness progressively increases during exercise. When the patient stops, the discomfort quickly subsides.

Leriche's Syndrome

Leriche's syndrome involves atherosclerosis of the aorta and iliac arteries at the bifurcation, reducing flow. Intermittent claudication of the legs, hips, or buttocks is often associated with erectile dysfunction of the penis.

Takayasu's Disease

Takayasu's (or pulseless) disease is an uncommon disorder generally exhibiting absent arm pulses. This is a progressive obliterative arteritis of vessels arising from the aortic arch, involving young women.

THE PRECORDIUM

With the clinician at the patient's right side, inspection and palpation of the precordium are performed together. The aortic valve area (second right interspace), pulmonic area (second left interspace), Erb's point (third left interspace), tricuspid valve area (lower parasternum), mitral valve area (apex), midprecordium, and epigastrium are each inspected and palpated (Fig. 4-18).

Palpation is used to find and evaluate the apical impulse, other pulsations or shocks, heaves or lifts, and thrills.

The Apical Impulse

Although clinicians often palpate with the patient sitting, the supine position is usually preferred. The apical impulse of the left ventricle, also called the *point of maximal impulse (PMI)*, may feel more forceful when the patient is sitting. The fingertips are used to palpate for the PMI, normally medial to the midclavicular line at the fifth intercostal space. An alternative to enable finding the PMI is to ask the supine patient to roll toward the left decubitus position. The apical impulse is palpable in 40% to 50% of patients, usually over a 2 cm diameter.

A shift in PMI laterally or down is typical of an enlarged left ventricle. The PMI may be felt in the fourth intercostal space in patients with a thin, long chest and a normal heart. Patients who have COPD may have the PMI shifted medially and down, toward the epigastrium.

Right ventricular hypertrophy can shift the PMI produced by the left ventricle posteriorly, making it difficult to palpate.

A faint PMI may be found in obesity because of a thick chest wall or in severe mitral stenosis because of underloading of the left ventricle.

Finding the apical impulse to be more than 10 cm lateral to the midsternal line (instead of the midclavicular line) is both sensitive and specific in showing cardiomegaly.

Precordial Pulsations and Shocks

When a precordial pulsation is palpated, it must be correlated with other cardiac findings to determine its significance. At times the significance may be difficult to establish.

A shock is an impulse of a heart sound transmitted to the examining hand. An example would be an S_4 shock in which an apical impulse coincides with atrial contraction, and a fourth heart sound could be auscultated shortly before the systolic apical impulse.

Especially prominent heart sounds may be felt. Mitral valve disease with an especially loud first heart sound can produce a tapping impulse at the apex. In pulmonary hypertension, the P_2 may be palpable at the second left intercostal space. This is called a pulmonic valve shock, or P_2 shock.

Generally, palpation of higher frequency sounds (discussed later under auscultation) such as S_1, S_2, or ejection sounds, an opening snap of mitral stenosis, and thrills are best felt by pressing firmly with the fingers. Movements of the ventricles are diffuse and usually felt better by gentle pressure of the pads of the fingers or the flat hand. Sometimes applying several fingers to the interspaces between ribs allows more to be detected. In contrast, the fingertips are best to define localized impulses (Fig. 4-19).

Heaves or Lifts

A heave is a forceful, usually systolic, thrust that moves the palpating hand little. The heave produces a sustained lifting movement not obliterated by the palpating fingers. The heave may be at the PMI, as in left ventricular hypertrophy.

A parasternal lift along the fourth to fifth interspaces is common in right ventricular enlargement or hypertrophy. If the patient has this, and the PMI is also shifted laterally and down, consider biventricular hypertrophy or enlargement as possible.

Heaves and lifts may be better felt with the palm or with the fingers between the ribs.

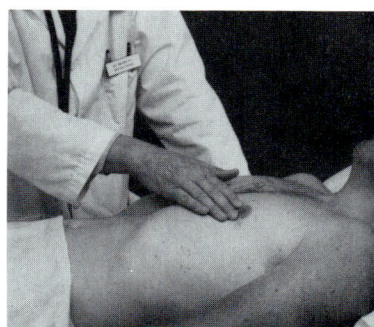

Fig. 4-19 Palpation of the cardiac apex (point of maximum impulse).

Thrills

Thrills are vibrations, palpable manifestations of heart murmurs. These vibrations are high in frequency and sustained. If a vibration is palpated but no murmur is later auscultated, the vibration is not termed a thrill. Murmurs associated with thrills nearly always have an organic cause.

Percussion of the Precordium

In patients in whom an apical impulse cannot be palpated, the use of light percussion can be useful in demonstrating cardiomegaly. In this case, percuss the cardiac border in the fifth intercostal space with the patient supine. Lay the middle finger of the left hand between the ribs so the distal and proximal interphalangeal joints touch the skin. The tip of the middle finger of the right hand is used to strike the distal interphalangeal joint. Begin percussion at the axillary line and move medially by 0.5 to 1 cm increments while remaining in the rib interspace.

Using this technique, percussion dullness of greater than 10.5 cm to the left of the midsternal line has excellent sensitivity and specificity for cardiomegaly. Percussion in other interspaces or to the right of the sternum is generally less reliable.

CHOICE OF STETHOSCOPE

Sound vibrations are produced as blood moves through the heart and vessels. These vibrations may be heard as they set into motion the column of air in the stethoscope applied to the skin of the chest.

Characteristics of Clinical Sounds

Cardiac sounds are described by loudness *(intensity)*, pitch *(frequency)*, and quality *(timber* or *harmonics)*. Normally the ear can distinguish sounds between 20 and 20,000 hertz (Hz) (Hz = vibrations/sec). The lowest note on the piano keyboard is 30 Hz and the highest, 5000 Hz. As we age or sustain acoustic trauma from loud sounds (such as rock music or firing shotguns) or from aminoglycoside ototoxicity, the higher tones are not heard so well. Because the pitch of most heart tones is relatively low, older clinicians usually maintain perception of cardiac sounds.

Patient Characteristics Influencing Sound Transmission

Intensity (loudness) of heart sounds depends on chest wall thickness and the distance of the heart from the surface, the sequence of electrical activity of the heart, the force of contractions, and the integrity of the valves.

Heart sounds seem louder in persons with thin chest walls, pediatric patients, and cachectic patients. Sounds seem softer with obese chest walls or with hypertrophied pectoral muscles. If auscultation is through the breast tissue of a woman, the intensity of sounds may be similarly diminished. The patient who has COPD with a barrel chest has greater distance between the heart and skin because of the enlarged air-filled lung spaces. This, along with a more vertically positioned heart, reduces intensity of heart sounds at the usual sites for auscultation.

The sequence of electrical activity and pump mechanics determines the position of valve leaflets at the time of valve closing. Valves that are wide apart when systole occurs may produce a loud closure sound when compared with that of valve leaflets that are nearly closed already.

Narrowed valve orifices *(stenosis)* generally cause softer heart sounds but may cause loud murmurs. Thickened valves may give loud heart sounds.

Sounds may take on a musical quality if a tone and overtones are present. When unrelated tonal frequencies are present, sounds are termed harsh or blowing.

The distinction between heart sounds and murmurs is based on duration (heart sounds are brief, murmurs longer), timing in the cardiac cycle (e.g., for valve closure, S_1, S_2) and the presumed mechanism (closing of valve leaflets).

Characteristics of Stethoscopes

To enhance auscultation of cardiac sounds and murmurs, consider the following points in the choice of stethoscope (Fig. 4-20):

1. More effective stethoscopes have shorter tubes (28 to 30 inches from chest piece to earpiece). Long tubes tend to reduce the intensity of high-frequency sounds. Sound transmission decreases according to the inverse square law.
2. Thick tubing is better than is thin in reducing extraneous room noises. Larger internal tube diameters transmit more effectively than do thin. A separate tube from the chest to each ear reduces loss of high-frequency vibrations. Some newer stethoscopes have two tubes constructed to appear single.
3. The ability to collect sound vibrations from the chest wall depends on the diameter of the chest piece. Using the largest bell and diaphragm available is ideal. A smaller bell and diaphragm are useful for pediatric patients or malnourished patients with prominent ribs. These pieces should be easy to change between patients if necessary.
4. The tubing, earpieces, and chest pieces should be free from holes or defects, which might impair sound transmission.

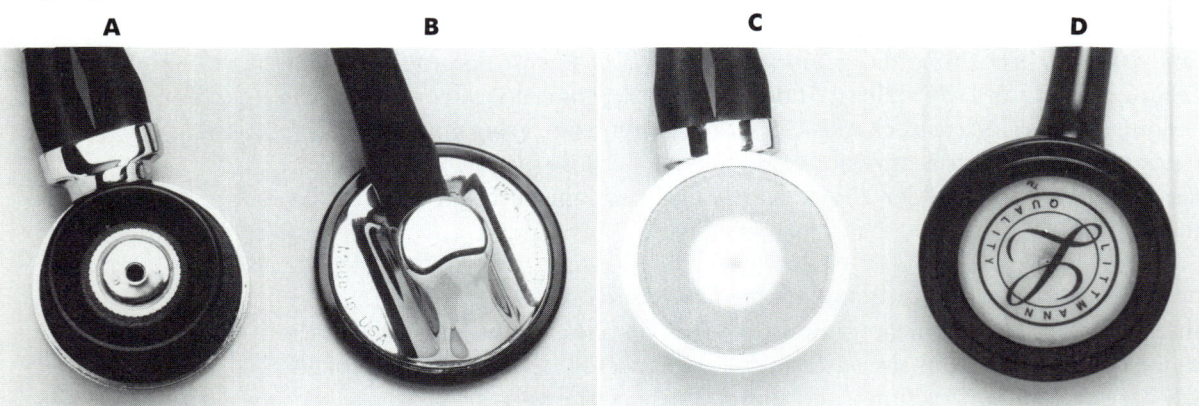

Fig. 4-20 The stethoscope. A, Bell. B, Top side of stethoscope. C, Diaphragm. D, Diaphragm appearance (with both bell and diaphragm functions).

5. The bell is better for low-frequency sounds, and the diaphragm for high-frequency sounds.
6. A corrugated-disc diaphragm is better than is a smooth-disc diaphragm because it will amplify faint sounds and murmurs.
7. Some newer stethoscopes have both functions in a chest piece that looks like a diaphragm alone. Light pressure makes use of a bell function; firm pressure allows for diaphragm function (Fig. 4-20, *B* and *D*).
8. Earpieces that will fit comfortably should be chosen. Soft rubber earpieces that conform to the ear are available. Making sure the earpiece tips are aligned correctly with the ear canal (earpieces point slightly forward) will enhance comfort. The earpieces should seal so that pressing the diaphragm causes pressure on the clinician's tympanic membranes.

Proper use of the stethoscope bell and diaphragm is important. For the diaphragm to properly amplify higher frequency sounds, it should be pressed firmly against the chest wall. Examples of higher frequency heart sounds are S_1 and S_2.

To properly hear lower frequencies, the bell should just touch the skin around the entire rim. When the bell is moved, no indentation should be left on the skin. If the bell is pressed too firmly, the skin under it is stretched tightly, causing the bell to function like a diaphragm. When not pressed firmly enough, a seal is not made with the skin. An example of a low-pitched sound best heard with the bell is the S_3.

TECHNIQUES TO IMPROVE CARDIAC EXAMINATION

Improved recognition of heart sounds and murmurs may be enhanced by attention to the environmental surroundings. When possible, use a quiet room with minimal background noise. Turn off the television, radio, piped-in music, fans, or noisy air conditioners. Visitors may be asked politely to refrain from talking aloud or to leave the room for a few minutes.

To be certain heart sounds are heard appropriately, routinely place the patient in three positions for the cardiac examination: supine, left lateral decubitus, and sitting (Fig. 4-21). Less commonly, two additional positions are used: standing on the feet or kneeling on elbows and knees.

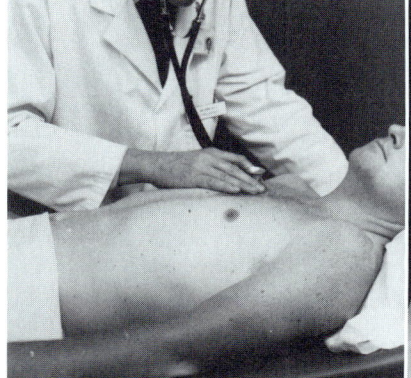
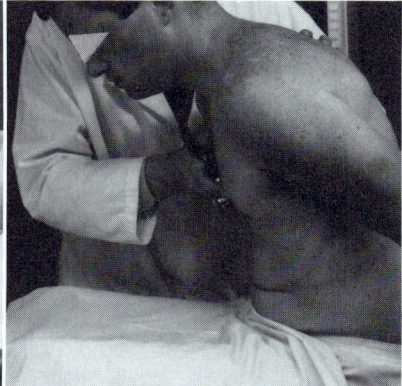
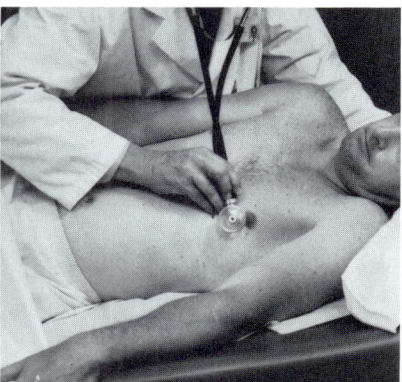

Fig. 4-21 Auscultation of the heart with the patient in three standard positions: **A**, supine, **B**, sitting (leaning forward and exhaling), and **C**, left lateral decubitus position. Sitting position allows murmurs of aortic regurgitation to the heart. Left lateral decubitus position enhances recognition of third heart sounds and diastolic murmurs of mitral stenosis.

A **B** **C**

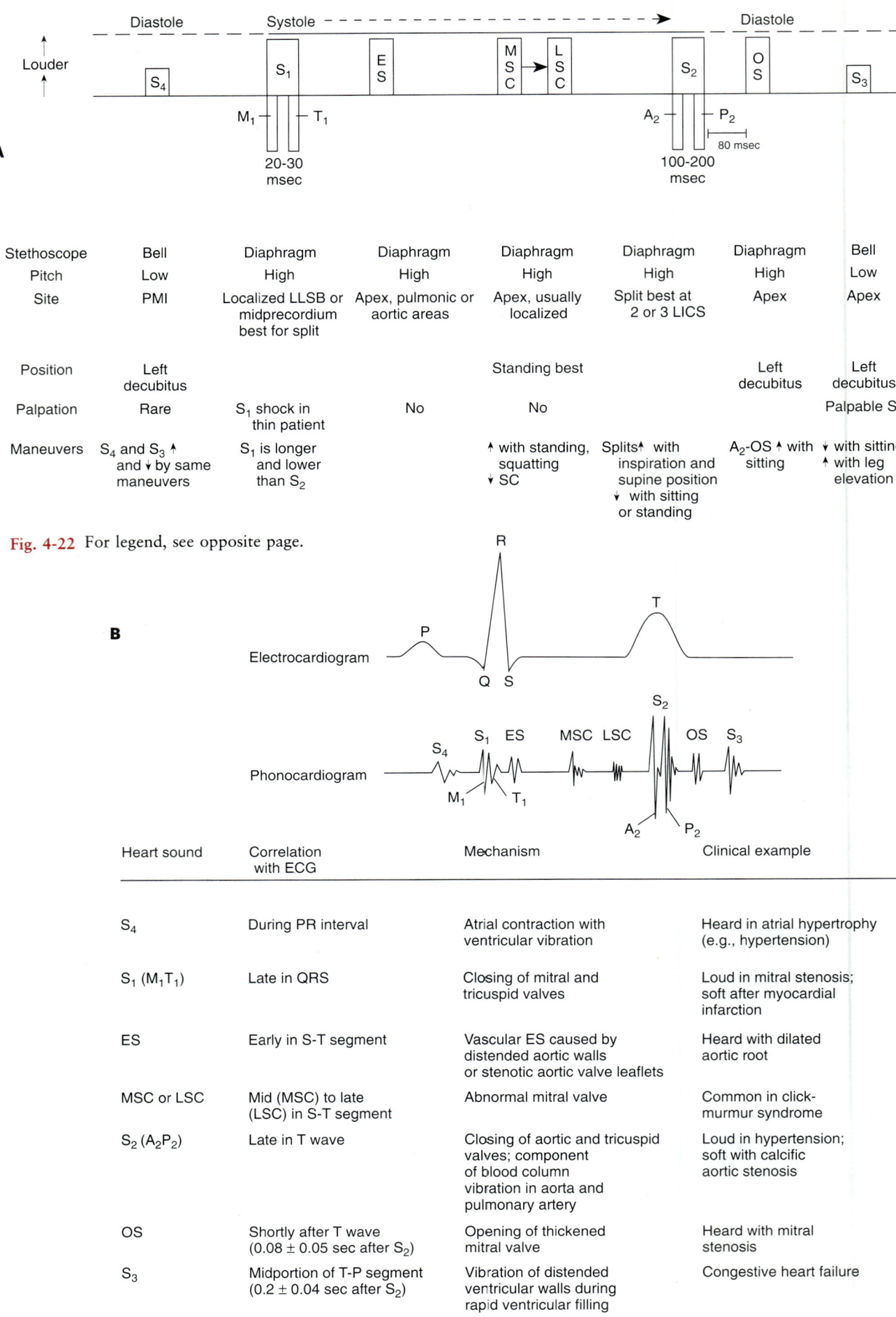

Fig. 4-22 For legend, see opposite page.

First, auscultate the heart with the patient in the supine position from the patient's right side. Elevate the patient's head 30 to 45 degrees from horizontal. Carefully examine the five areas for cardiac auscultation (see Fig. 4-18, *B*): aortic (second right parasternal interspace), pulmonic (second left parasternal interspace), tricuspid (lower left parasternal area), mitral (lower parasternal area, moving toward apex and the anterior axillary line), and the precordium. First use the diaphragm in each area, followed by the bell. Use of the bell in the tricuspid and mitral areas potentially may give more information than use of the bell in aortic or pulmonic areas because of the murmurs likely at each site. Pulmonic and tricuspid murmurs are best heard with the patient supine.

Next ask the patient to assume the left lateral decubitus position. Use the bell to auscultate at the apex (PMI) to look for the low-pitched diastolic rumble of mitral stenosis and for S_3 gallop rhythms.

With the patient sitting, listen for the soft, high-pitched blowing murmur of aortic regurgitation or pulmonic regurgitation. Press the diaphragm firmly, first at the aortic area, then move it little by little (called "inching") toward the third left parasternal interspace (Erb's point), then down along the left sternal border for the diastolic decrescendo murmur of aortic regurgitation. Continue listening out toward the apex (changing to the bell) for an S_3 gallop or a diastolic rumble of regurgitant mitral murmur. If a murmur is not apparent, ask the patient to lean forward, exhale, and hold the breath in exhalation while you use the diaphragm to auscultate in the aortic areas for a diastolic blowing murmur.

Then use the diaphragm to listen at the left second interspace for the murmurs of pulmonic stenosis and regurgitation. The splitting of S_2 with respirations may be heard best there also.

The standing position may enhance the distant heart sounds in pulmonary emphysema. Sometimes in patients with emphysema, heart sounds are heard better over the epigastrium.

A pericardial friction rub may be most apparent with the patient on elbows and knees. As pericardial effusions form between the heart and pericardial sac, the pericardial rub is abolished.

Finally, listen over the midprecordium, the back, the right chest, and the vessels at the base of the neck for murmurs, bruits, and other sounds. Auscultate above the sternoclavicular joints for a venous hum.

Inching, or moving the chest piece short distances, allows the examiner to find sites where sounds are heard best. Often when sounds are most intense, timing is easier in relationship to other heart sounds. The pericardial friction rub is an example of a sound that may be heard in only a very small site on the chest wall.

CARDIAC SOUNDS

Follow a systematic plan in cardiac auscultation. That is, auscultate at each of the six anatomic sites. Examine the patient in the standard positions—supine, sitting, and standing. Finally, listen to the first heart sound and then the second sound at each site (Fig. 4-22, *A*).

Fig. 4-22 **A,** Cardiac sounds: timing, intensity, pitch, and site at which they are heard best. *ES,* Ejection sound (systolic); *MSC,* midsystolic click; *LSC,* late systolic click; *OS,* opening snap of mitral stenosis; *LLSB,* lower left sternal border; *LICS,* left intercostal space; *SC,* systolic click M_1 mitral valve; T_1, tricuspid valve; A_2, aortic valve; P_2, pulmonic valve. **B,** Timing and mechanisms of cardiac sounds related to components of the ECG.

Fig. 4-23 **A,** Electrical conducting system in the heart. **B,** Position of heart valves on chest x-ray film.

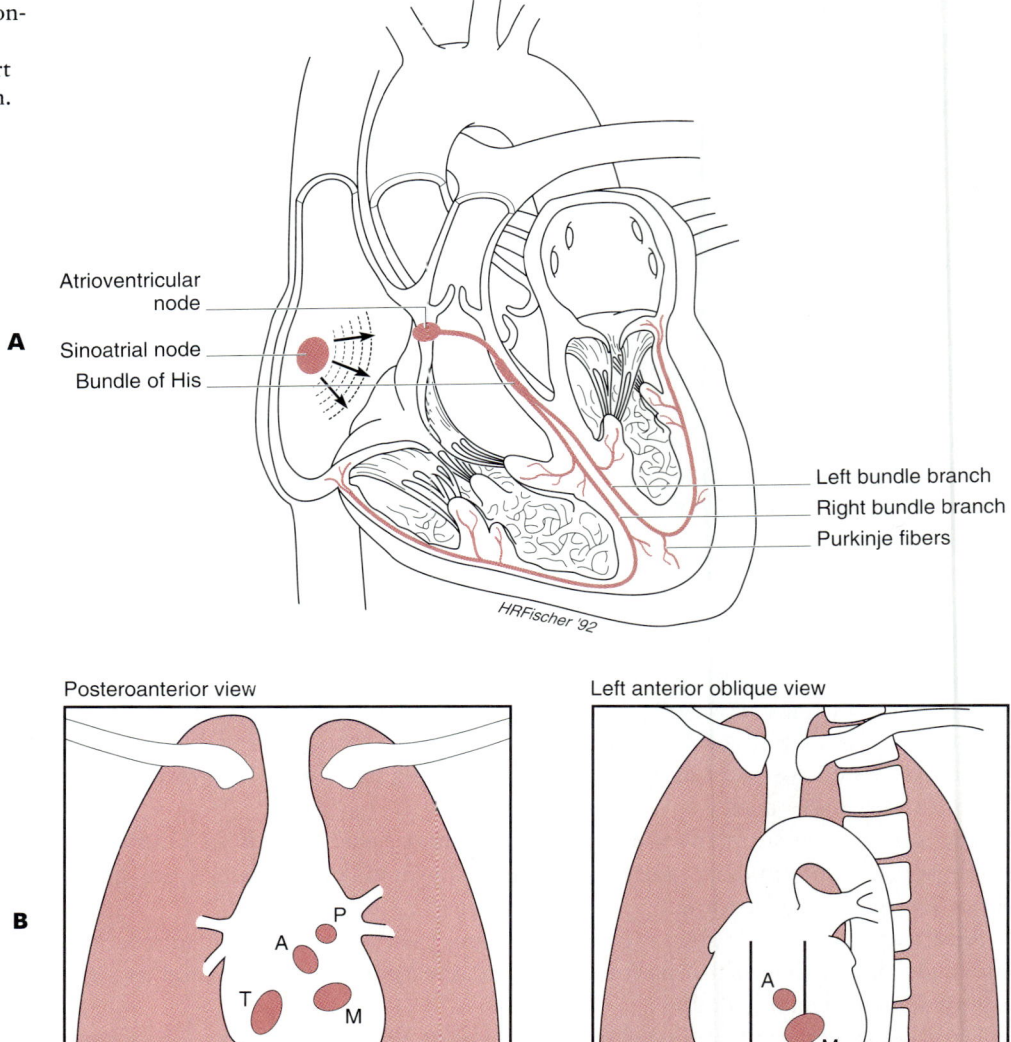

Position of heart valves on chest x-ray

The examiner generally cannot identify specific characteristics of first (S_1) and second (S_2) heart sounds simultaneously. Instead, concentrate first on S_1 and then on S_2 sounds. If you need to discern which is S_1, palpate the carotid artery during auscultation. Then look for splitting of S_1 and S_2.

Next listen for any additional sounds and determine whether each occurs in early, mid, or late systole or in diastole. Finally, listen first with the diaphragm, then with the bell. High-pitched systolic clicks and murmurs are heard best with the diaphragm, whereas the low-pitched sounds (S_3 and S_4) are best heard with the bell.

Heart sounds, correlation with ECG tracings, the putative mechanism of sounds, and clinical examples are shown in Fig. 4-22, *B*.

The electrical depolarization is useful in explaining the components of cardiac sounds (Fig. 4-23). The sinus node, located in the right atrium, spontaneously initiates the stimulus for contraction. The discharge passes to the atrioventricular node, to the bundle of His, and splits along the right and left bundle branches. The left ventricle begins to contract first, and the mitral valve (M_1) closes before the tricuspid valve (T_1). However, because the pulmonary artery pressure is less than aortic pressure, ejection of blood begins slightly earlier from the right ventricle. Finally, ejection from the left ventricle ends first, again because of higher pressure in the aorta, allowing aortic (A_2) closure to precede pulmonic (P_2).

The First Heart Sound

When beginning the cardiac examination, initially identify the first (S_1) heart sound. The S_1 has two components, the M_1 component of the first sound and the T_1 component. These sounds are attributed to valve closure with the sudden change in blood velocity. Three components may be responsible for A_2: (1) vibrations in the left ventricle, (2) opening of the aortic valve, and (3) vibrations of the aorta.

The S_1 is best heard near the cardiac apex or PMI. S_1 has a lower tone or pitch and longer duration than the shorter, higher pitched S_2. Thus the term "lubb-dupp" closely approximates actual sounds. Because S_1 and S_2 have moderately high pitch, they are heard better with the diaphragm.

Components of S_1 When auscultating along the lower left sternal border, the examiner can identify two components, M_1 and T_1. The two occur quite close together, with M_1 preceding T_1 by 0.02 to 0.03 sec. Most beginning students need repeated attempts to hear two components.

Intensity of S_1 The loudness of S_1 depends on how open the valve leaflets are at ventricular contraction and the strength of ventricular contraction. This sound has been compared to noise made by closing a door. Using the same closing force, a wide open door makes more noise than one already nearly closed. A gentle push gives a softer sound than a hard slam.

Factors that close the valve from an open wide position with a loud S_1 include a short PR interval, tachycardia, and mitral stenosis. Vigorous ventricular contractions in the high cardiac output of fever, exercise, or thyrotoxicosis may result in a loud S_1.

Impaired myocardial contraction with a soft S_1 is found in myocardial infarction and myocarditis. A soft S_1 is found when mitral valve leaflets are calcified, immobile, or open only partially, as in mitral regurgitation.

The Second Heart Sound

Just as M_1 and T_1 refer to mitral and tricuspid components of the first sound, A_2 and P_2 refer to the aortic and pulmonic components of the second sound.

Components of S_2 The second heart sound has been called "the key to auscultation of the heart." The normal closure sequence is A_2 followed by P_2. Ordinarily S_2 splits into A_2 and P_2 during inspiration (0.02 to 0.06 sec apart). The two components become single, or nearly so, during exhalation. Although S_2 is generally heard throughout the precordium, P_2 is heard best at the second left parasternal interspace or at Erb's point. Splitting of S_2 cannot be identified away from this area in the normal examination.

The mechanism of physiologic splitting of S_2 during inspiration has been attributed to increased venous return, thus increasing right ventricular stroke volume and resulting in longer ejection time. As a result, the closure of the pulmonary valve is delayed.

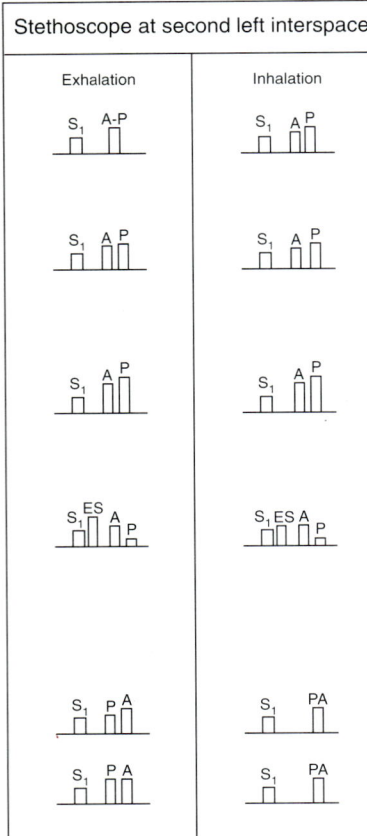

Fig. 4-24 Splitting of the second heart sound.

Normally split S_2
Single sound heard in exhalation, but split in inspiration so that two components are heard

Persistently split S_2
Split during inspiration and exhalation, but duration of split increases during inspiration (e.g., right bundle branch block)

Fixed split S_2
S_2 has a wide fixed split, giving little or no perception of respiratory variation (A_2 to P_2 at least 30 msec with respiratory variation no greater than 15 msec):
Atrial septal defect: split is abnormal in exhalation, no change in inspiration

Inability of right ventricle to change stroke volume; wide split, but P_2 soft; pulmonic ejection sound common in pulmonic stenosis

Paradoxic split S_2
S2 splits with exhalation and becomes single with inspiration:

Left ventricular depolarization is delayed (e.g., left bundle branch block)

Prolonged left ventricular emptying time (e.g., severe outflow obstruction in aortic stenosis)

S_2 may be persistently but variably split, may have a fixed split, or may be split paradoxically. Because of the variety of diseases associated with abnormalities of S_2, splitting of the second sound may be useful diagnostically (Fig. 4-24).

Intensity of S_2 Either component of S_2 may be soft, which gives the impression of a single S_2. A markedly soft A_2 (aortic stenosis or regurgitation) or soft P_2 (pulmonic stenosis or tetralogy of Fallot) are examples. Inability to hear P_2 is the more common reason for hearing a single S_2.

A loud A_2 is most commonly caused by hypertension. When A_2 is accentuated, a palpable A_2 may be observed in the second right interspace. A loud A_2 may also be found in advanced atherosclerosis and in children who have a thin chest wall.

A soft A_2 is commonly caused by a thick chest wall in obesity or by large breasts. The left breast should be moved during auscultation so that the stethoscope is placed on the chest wall. Aortic stenosis and significant aortic regurgitation both result in a soft A_2.

The Third Heart Sound

The third heart sound may be physiologic in children and teen-agers, but after age 35 an S_3 is considered abnormal.

The S_3 is a low-pitched sound that occurs between 0.10 to 0.20 sec (usually 0.12 to 0.16 sec) after A_2. To get a feel for the time sequence of S_1, S_2, and S_3, say the word Kentucky (Ken-tuc-ky). The syllables give the relative timing of the three sounds.

An S_3 may arise from the right or left ventricle. The mechanism of sound production may be caused by either of two factors: (1) abnormally large diastolic blood flow into a normal ventricle, or (2) normal volume of flow into a ventricle with abnormal myocardial compliance. These both result in vibrations perceived as S_3 because of sudden deceleration of blood flow when the ventricular chamber has reached maximal distension.

Left ventricular S_3 is best heard with the patient in the left lateral decubitus position. Right ventricular S_3 is heard best along the lower left sternal border with the patient supine. Cor pulmonale is often the cause of right ventricular S_3. To distinguish a left-sided from a right-sided S_3, the site where it is heard best is one clue. Also, right-sided S_3 increases in intensity with inspiration.

A gallop rhythm refers to an S_3 or S_4 creating the cadence of a galloping horse, especially when tachycardia is present. An S_3 or S_4 that does not resemble a gallop is just referred to as S_3 or S_4.

The S_3 gallop usually suggests ventricular dysfunction and cardiac failure. The louder an S_3, the more important it tends to be as an indicator of disease.

Diseases that cause excessive ventricular volume, such as mitral or aortic regurgitation even in the absence of heart failure, produce an S_3. In contrast, in patients with mitral stenosis and small left ventricular volume, an S_3 would be unusual. If an S_3 were found in mitral stenosis, either mitral regurgitation is greater than expected or the S_3 originates from the right side of the heart.

The Fourth Heart Sound

Normally a fourth heart sound is not present. The S_4 as well as the S_3 occurs during diastole. S_4 occurs after S_2 but shortly before the next S_1. The timing can be approximated by repeating the word Tennessee (Ten-nes-see for S_4, S_1, and S_2). Both the S_3 and the S_4 are low pitched, best heard with the bell, and often better felt than heard. The S_4 and S_3 are best heard at the apex with the patient turned to the left side. S_4 may be better heard during expiration. An S_4 may originate from either the right or left side of the heart. An S_4 is always considered to be abnormal, even in children.

The S_4 is caused by atrial contraction, thus an S_4 disappears in atrial fibrillation. The sound itself does not originate from ventricular filling. The most prominent S_4 is heard when the ventricles are pumping against resistance and there is decreased left ventricular compliance.

A left-sided S_4 may be audible in hypertension, aortic stenosis, or angina pectoris. A right-sided S_4 may be found in pulmonary hypertension or pulmonic stenosis (Fig. 4-25).

In hypertension the S_4 may appear early. An S_4 may be especially loud in acute myocardial infarction. If it persists during recovery, an akinetic segment of the myocardium should be suspected.

Summation Gallop

When there is tachycardia with S_3 and S_4, the S_3 and S_4 sounds fuse in the summation gallop (see Fig. 4-25). Patients with chronic hypertension or myocardial hypertrophy who develop congestive heart failure may show a summation gallop. To differentiate S_3 and S_4 in a summation gallop from a similar sounding middiastolic murmur, clinicians like to slow the heart rate. Careful carotid sinus massage has been used, but should not be tried by the student without expert supervision.

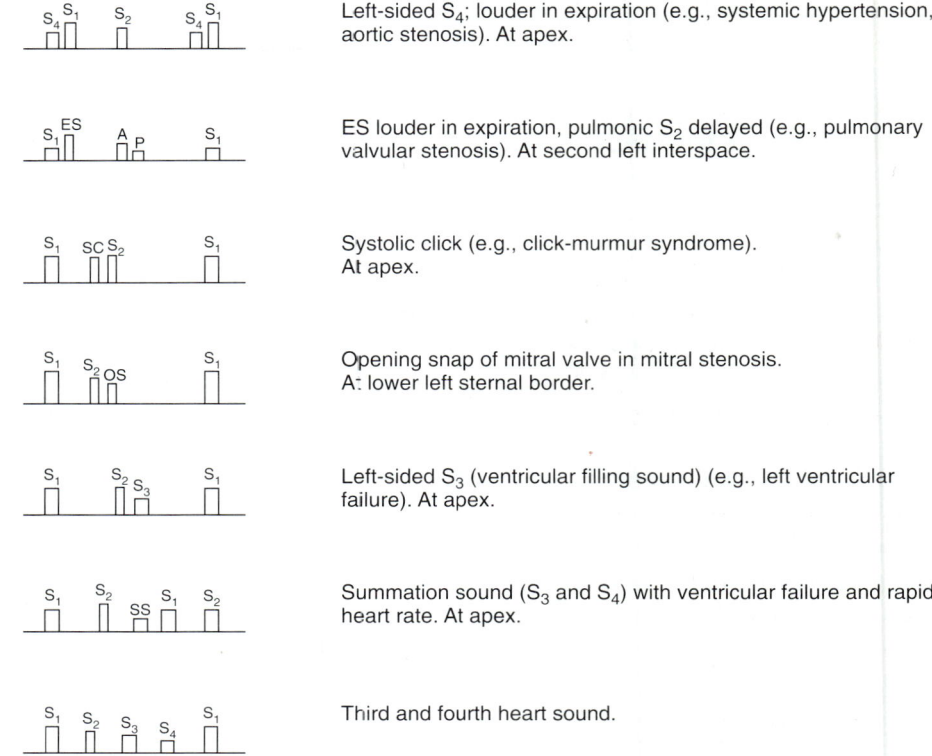

Fig. 4-25 Interpretation of extra sounds. *A,* Aortic valve; *P,* pulmonic valve; *LIS,* left intercostal space; *LSB,* left sternal border.

Opening Snap

The opening snap (OS) of mitral stenosis is another abnormal diastolic sound (see Fig. 4-25). This is a brief, high-pitched sound best heard with the diaphragm over the midprecordium. It occurs 0.03 to 0.14 sec (usually about 0.08 to 0.10 sec) after the S_2. The S_2-OS time is shorter with more stenotic mitral valves. These times are found when the patient is examined in the supine position. If the patient is examined in the standing position, the S_2-OS interval tends to be longer because gravity delays venous return to the heart. The left atrial pressure is lower, which delays opening of the mitral valve, giving a longer interval.

SYSTOLIC SOUNDS AND CLICKS

Between the first and second heart sounds, early ejection sounds and clicks may be present. Clicks occur in early, middle, or late systole (see Fig. 4-25). Usually only one click is heard, but clicks may be multiple. Ejection sounds and clicks are high pitched and best heard with the diaphragm. Aortic ejection sounds or clicks are best heard at the base but are usually present over the precordium. In contrast, pulmonic ejection sounds are best heard in the pulmonic area or at Erb's point and are not well transmitted.

Ejection Sounds

The sounds that occur in early systole (about 0.02 to 0.06 sec after S_1) are called systolic ejection sounds. Click has been used for these, but click is now avoided to prevent confusion with mid and late systolic clicks. These early ejection sounds are caused by abnormal aortic or pulmonic valves or a dilated aorta or pulmonary artery. A pulmonic ejection sound may vary considerably with respirations.

TABLE 4-8: Auscultatory Clues to Differentiate Certain Sounds

	Late Systolic Click	Split S_2	Opening Snap of Mitral Stenosis	S_3
Exam site	Apex	Second or third left interspace	Second left interspace to apex	Apex
Diaphragm versus bell	Diaphragm	Diaphragm	Diaphragm	Bell
Standing	Louder	No change	Longer S_2 - OS time	Softer

Mitral Valve Prolapse

Mid and late systolic clicks in MVP are caused by ballooning of the posterior mitral leaflet back into the atrium during left ventricular contraction. This is a very common cardiac abnormality, especially in young women. Such clicks may occur alone (more commonly) or be followed by a systolic murmur of mitral regurgitation.

Clicks in MVP are high pitched and best heard with the diaphragm at the apex. Clicks may be heard intermittently. Changing the position of the patient may change audibility. Having the patient stand reduces venous return, produces a smaller left ventricle, and increases MVP. This accentuates the click or murmur. In contrast, if the patient squats or does an isometric handgrip, venous return and afterload increase. The click becomes softer, later in systole, or inaudible.

Timing of a late systolic click may be difficult. If the click is mistaken for an S_2, the S_2 may be mistaken for an OS. Table 4-8 lists factors that differentiate a click from a split S_2, an opening snap, and an S_3.

PERICARDIAL KNOCK

Pericardial knock is heard at some time in the majority of patients who have constrictive pericarditis. It is high pitched and best heard during diastole with the diaphragm. The best auscultatory site for the pericardial knock is over the right internal jugular at the base of the neck. The pericardial knock is caused by the thickened pericardium limiting expansion of the ventricle during the rapid filling phase of diastole. The pericardial knock is heard better during inspiration and is accentuated by squatting.

PERICARDIAL FRICTION RUBS

Pericardial friction rubs may be confused with heart sounds, clicks, or heart murmurs. Rubs are attributed to friction of roughened epicardium against pericardium as the heart beats. The sound is high pitched and best heard with the diaphragm. Rubs are usually best heard in the left parasternal space, often limited to a very small area. To exclude pleural friction rub, ask the patient to hold his breath during auscultation. The unusual position of the patient on knees and elbows brings the visceral and parietal pericardium into opposition and may enhance a pericardial rub.

A three-component friction rub is most indicative of a rub being pericardial in origin. At times a biphasic- or even a single-component rub may be pericardial in origin but is less diagnostic. Pericardial rubs wax and wane, so listen repeatedly over the entire precordium when a rub is anticipated.

Disorders that produce pericardial effusions or inflammation of the pericardium may result in rubs. Pericardial effusion is not required to produce a rub. Large effusions often cause a rub to disappear as the epicardium and pericardium are separated. Trauma, uremia, collagen disease, coxsackievirus infection, and tuberculosis are a few causes of pericarditis and rubs.

PROSTHETIC VALVE SOUNDS

Four types of artificial heart valves are used: a ball in a cage (Starr-Edwards), a floating or tilting disc (Bjork-Shiley), bileaflet valves, and biologic valves (porcine valves). Each of these makes distinctive sounds. The ball and the disc valves often make opening and closing sounds. Generally, the position at which the sound is heard best is the same as the usual site for auscultation of the valve that was replaced. Sounds made by mechanical valves are often quite loud and heard over the entire precordium. Some may be heard without the stethoscope being applied to the chest.

HEART MURMURS

By identifying the first and second heart sounds, the clinician establishes timing so that murmurs can be analyzed. While listening for murmurs, examine each patient in the three standard positions, sitting, supine, and left lateral decubitus. Less frequently other positions will be needed.

A *murmur* is defined as a series of sound vibrations that may be heard, recorded with the phonocardiogram, and occasionally palpated. Murmurs may be generated by abnormal blood flow patterns under certain conditions:

1. An increased rate of blood flow through a normal valve
2. Forward blood flow through a narrow valve
3. Flow into a dilated vessel
4. Backward flow (regurgitation) through an incompetent valve
5. Flow through an abnormal communication between heart chambers or arteries

Murmurs are characterized according to the following findings:

1. Timing of murmurs relate them to heart sounds S_1 and S_2, systole and diastole.
2. Location designates the chest site where the murmur is best heard.
3. Transmission or radiation designates anatomic sites where the murmur is heard other than the primary (loudest) site.
4. Configuration of murmur designates both timing and intensity. This is also called the shape of the murmur.
5. Duration refers to timing, when the murmur begins and ends.
6. Intensity, or loudness, is characterized by a grade system.
7. Frequency of vibrations is the tonal pitch.
8. Quality is closely related to pitch but describes tone as a musical term.

Characteristics

Timing The most important feature used to identify a heart murmur is the timing, its beginning and ending in relation to S_1 and S_2. This establishes it as one of the following:

- Systolic murmur positioned between S_1 and S_2
- Diastolic murmur positioned between S_2 and S_1

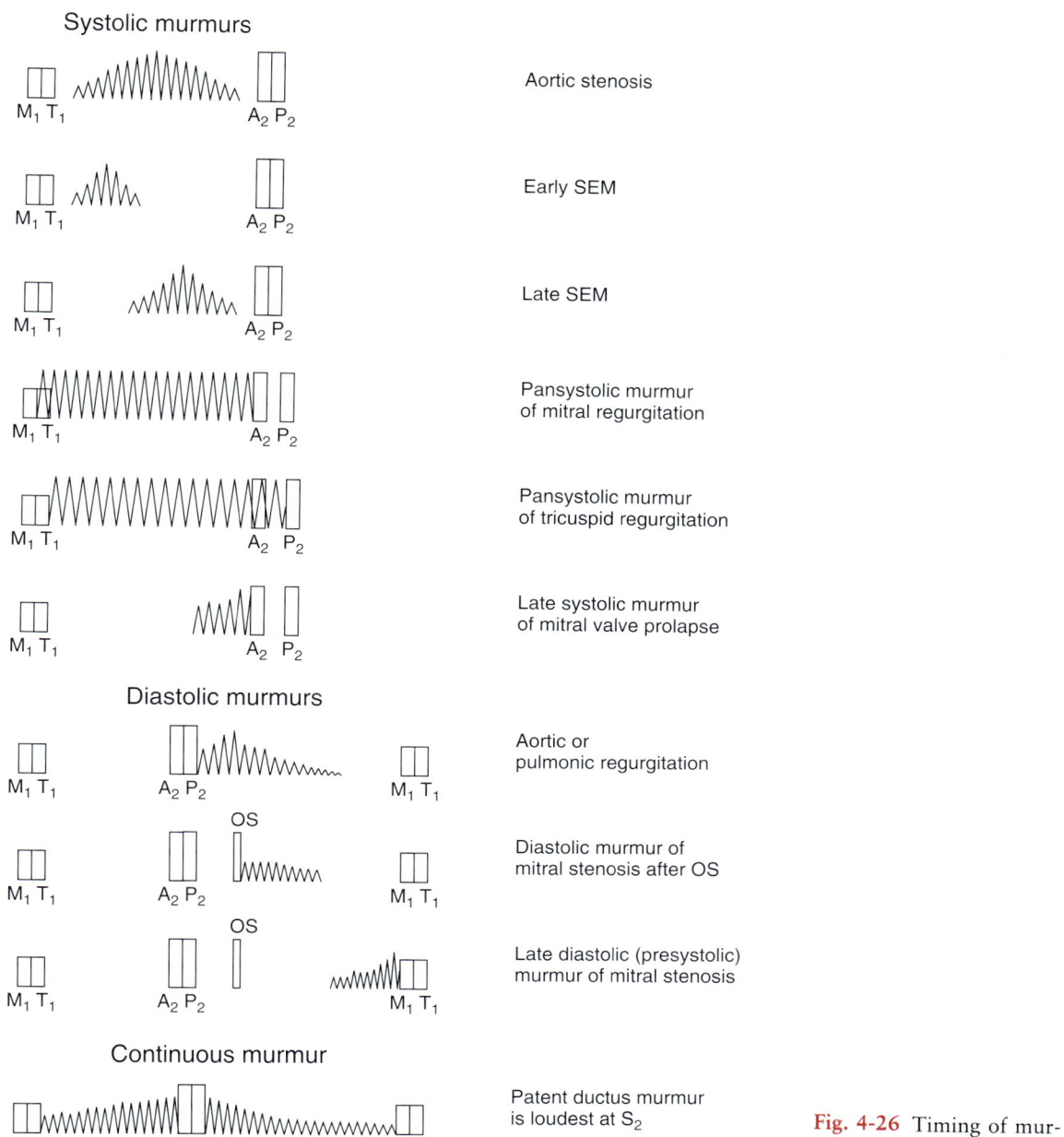

Fig. 4-26 Timing of murmurs.

To help establish timing, use clues about the first and second heart sounds. S_1 is a longer sound and lower in pitch than is S_2. Systole is shorter than diastole. S_1 is louder than S_2 at the apex, but S_2 is louder than S_1 at the second right and left intercostal spaces. Simultaneously auscultate the heart and palpate either the carotid pulse or the apical impulse to identify S_1.

Next identify the beginning and ending of each murmur. Systolic murmurs most often are either ejection type or are holosystolic (pansystolic).

Systolic ejection murmurs (SEMs) begin after S_1 and end before S_2. An early SEM begins shortly after S_1 and ends in midsystole. A midsystolic ejection murmur clearly begins after S_1, increases in intensity to midsystole, and decreases and ends before S_2. A late SEM begins in midsystole and ends close to S_2. Examples are shown in Fig. 4-26.

> **Locations Where Murmurs are Characteristically Heard**
>
> Apex (PMI)
>   Holosystolic (pansystolic) murmur of mitral regurgitation
>   *Diastolic murmur of mitral stenosis, and the presystolic accentuation*
> Aortic area (second right interspace)
>   Systolic ejection murmur of aortic stenosis
>   *Diastolic blowing murmur of aortic regurgitation*
> Pulmonic area (second left interspace)
>   Systolic ejection murmur of pulmonic stenosis
>   Systolic murmur of atrial septal defect (ASD)
>   *Diastolic murmur of pulmonic regurgitation*
> Erb's point
>   *Diastolic murmur of aortic regurgitation*
> Tricuspid area (lower left sternal border)
>   *Diastolic murmur of tricuspid stenosis*
> Other areas
>   Systolic murmur of coarctation of aorta in the midback along the left side of the spine

A holosystolic murmur begins with S_1 and continues to the respective component of S_2, either A_2 or P_2, for left-sided or right-sided pathologic condition. Examples are mitral or tricuspid regurgitation.

A late systolic murmur may begin in midsystole and end with S_2 (A_2). An example would be mild mitral regurgitation in MVP.

Diastolic murmurs may also be early, mid or late diastolic. An early diastolic murmur begins with A_2 or P_2. Examples are aortic or pulmonic regurgitation.

Middiastolic murmurs clearly begin after S_2 (A_2 or P_2), as in mitral or tricuspid stenosis.

A late diastolic murmur is also called a presystolic murmur because it just precedes S_1 and systole. These begin or become prominent after the middle of diastole. Mitral stenosis is an example.

Location Listen for systolic and diastolic murmurs in each site during auscultation. A soft murmur may be heard in only a small area, whereas a loud murmur may be prominent over most of the precordium. The site where a murmur is loudest is called its location.

When describing location of murmurs, use reference to aortic, pulmonic, tricuspid, or mitral area or second right interspace, second left interspace, Erb's point, and so on. Saying a systolic murmur is best heard in the aortic area does not necessarily mean that the source of the murmur is of aortic valve origin.

Certain murmurs are characteristically loudest in certain sites (see the accompanying box).

Transmission Transmission, or radiation, refers to the ability to readily hear the murmur in sites other than the primary, or loudest, site. Transmission is caused by several factors, including loudness of murmur, pitch of the murmur, and anatomic relationships to structures that can transmit the sound. Transmission is so characteristic that it may be diagnostically useful.

Examples of transmission include the following:

- The systolic ejection murmur of aortic stenosis is best heard at the aortic area and transmitted to the carotids.
- The systolic murmur of pulmonic stenosis radiates from the second left interspace to the suprasternal notch. The systolic murmur of atrial septal defect is localized to the pulmonic area but does not radiate.
- The diastolic murmur of aortic regurgitation is best heard at the second right interspace (aortic area) and is transmitted to Erb's point and the apex.

Configuration The shape of the murmur refers to changes in loudness. A murmur that progressively gets louder is termed *crescendo*. An example would be mitral stenosis; the late diastolic (presystolic) crescendo murmur ends with S_1.

A murmur that decreases progressively is decrescendo. An example is aortic regurgitation, in which the diastolic decrescendo blowing murmur begins louder and fades into inaudibility (as when one blows out a match). Another type is a combined *crescendo-decrescendo*, also called *diamond shaped*. This is the configuration of the systolic ejection murmur that gets louder, then softer. Finally, the *sustained*, or *plateau shaped*, murmur maintains constant loudness. A holosystolic murmur of mitral regurgitation is plateau shaped.

Duration This describes the duration of a murmur in either systole or diastole. A sustained murmur would continue throughout much of either systole or diastole.

Intensity Just as heart sounds are louder in thin people and softer in the obese, so heart murmurs are likewise influenced. Factors important in intensity include blood flow and the pathologic condition present.

Loudness of murmurs is graded from one to six, and written as I/VI, II/VI, and so on. The denominator shows that a six-point scale was used.

- *Grade I.* A faint murmur that can only be heard with special effort. Inexperienced observers often miss these.
- *Grade II.* A soft murmur that can be heard by the experienced clinician as soon as auscultation is begun. Students usually hear these.
- *Grade III.* A moderately loud murmur without a palpable thrill.
- *Grade IV.* A loud murmur with a palpable thrill.
- *Grade V.* A very loud murmur but requires use of a stethoscope to be audible. A thrill is present.
- *Grade VI.* A murmur so loud that it can be heard without the stethoscope making complete contact with the chest. A thrill is also present.

A thrill is the palpable vibrations of the murmur, felt by the hand on the chest. A rather loud murmur is produced by vibrations that are prominent enough to be palpable.

Grading the intensity of a heart murmur allows the clinician to assess changes in intensity between examinations. It allows clinicians to compare findings, and it allows assessment of the importance of a murmur. A grade I/VI to II/VI systolic ejection murmur is common in normal people. A grade III or greater intensity murmur is more likely to be significant.

Frequency Frequency or pitch refers to the tone as high (best heard with the diaphragm) or low (best heard with the bell). Systolic murmurs are usually high or medium pitched. Diastolic murmurs may be high pitched in aortic regurgitation or low pitched in mitral stenosis.

Fig. 4-27 Aortic stenosis.

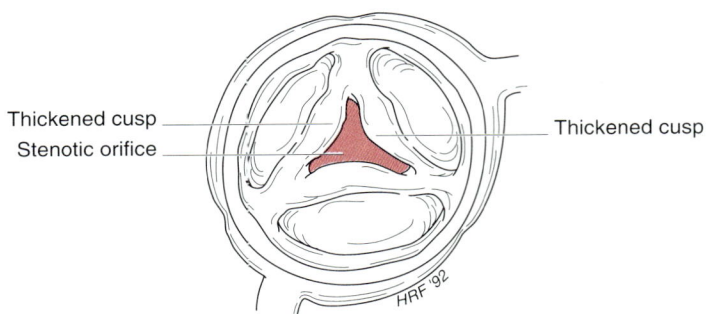

Quality The quality of a murmur refers to overall sound. The quality may be harsh and nonmusical. Others are musical, squeaking, honking, rumbling, or blowing.

Systolic Murmurs

Generally, finding a systolic murmur is less likely to be significant than is finding a diastolic murmur under certain conditions:

Systolic murmurs of the ejection type without an associated thrill are common without a significant underlying cardiac pathologic condition. These are usually midsystolic and have been attributed to several mechanisms, including vibrations of pulmonic leaflets, of the pulmonary trunk, or of the systemic arteries. In older adults, vibrations of aortic cusps may create an innocent systolic murmur.

No innocent diastolic murmurs are recognized, although a venous hum or a mammary souffle (described below) may have both systolic and diastolic components in a continuous murmur.

Several systolic murmurs are associated with characteristic history, physical findings, and pathologic conditions. This section will consider some of the important causes of systolic murmurs (see Fig. 4-26).

Aortic stenosis The etiologic cause of aortic stenosis may be congenital, degenerative, or rheumatic (Fig. 4-27). Congenital aortic stenosis with a bicuspid aortic valve may or may not impede blood flow but produce a systolic ejection murmur anyway. With a bicuspid valve, a systolic ejection sound may be heard at the apex. Of degenerative valve diseases, calcific aortic stenosis is important. A similar-sounding systolic ejection murmur also occurs with coarctation of the aorta and even aneurysm of the ascending aorta.

The murmur of aortic valvular stenosis follows S_1 after a brief interval after M_1 because there is an interval between mitral closure and the beginning of ejection of blood through the aortic valve. (Pressure in the aorta is higher than is the pressure in the left atrium.) Blood flow slows before aortic valve closure, so the murmur of aortic stenosis stops before S_2 (actually A_2).

The murmur of aortic stenosis is typically loud, high pitched, and harsh. Maximal intensity is in the second right intercostal space (Fig. 4-28). Such murmurs transmit well into the carotids and may be heard well at the apex, but they do not radiate to the axilla. Severe aortic stenosis often gives a narrow split S_2 because of delay in aortic closure (A_2). Calcified or scarred aortic valve cusps result in a soft A_2 that may not be heard. Palpate the carotid pulse for additional

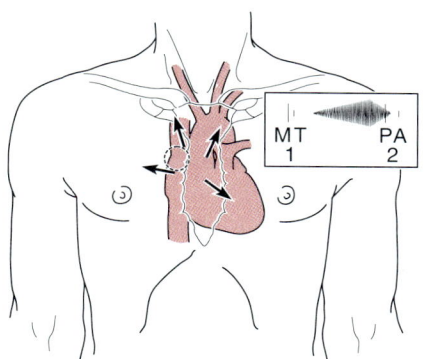
Severe aortic valve stenosis

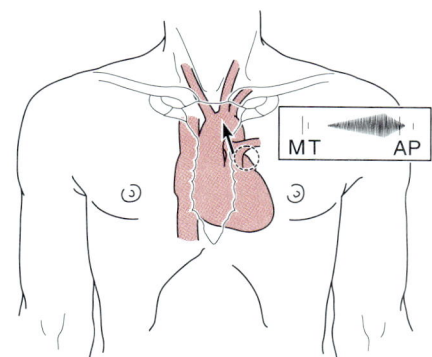
Severe pulmonary valve stenosis

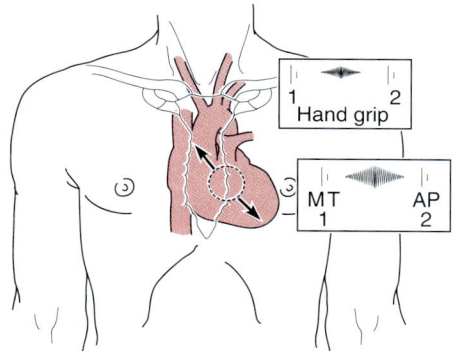
Hypertrophic cardiomyopathy

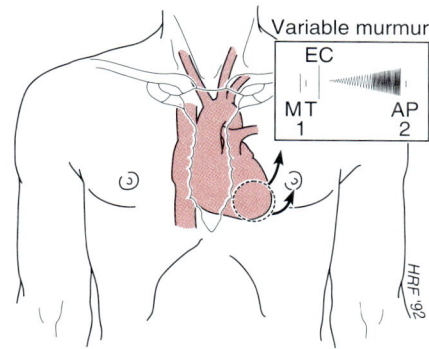
Mitral valve prolapse and regurgitation

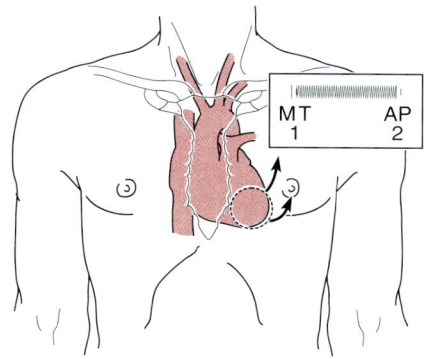
Mitral regurgitation

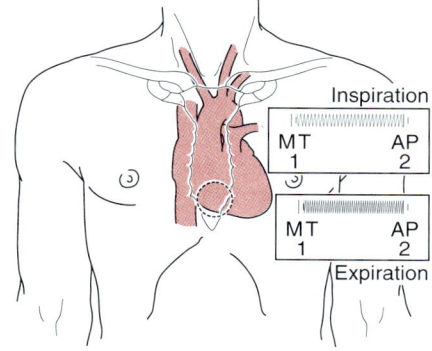
Tricuspid regurgitation

Fig. 4-28 Sites for auscultation of murmurs.

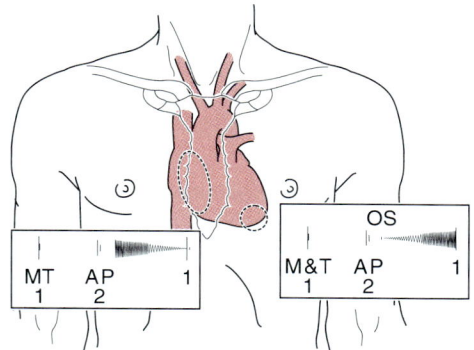
Diastolic murmurs

Mitral stenosis: loud first sound, opening snap; presystolic accentuation

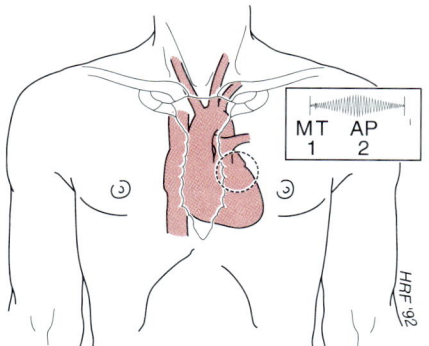
Continuous murmurs

Patent ductus arteriosus

evidence that aortic stenosis is the cause of a systolic ejection murmur. In significant stenosis, the carotid pulse is small and has a delayed upstroke *(pulsus parvus et tardus)*. So if A_2 splits normally and the apex beat is normal, aortic stenosis is likely to be mild. Severe aortic stenosis may result in left ventricular thickening and poststenotic dilation of the aorta.

If aortic stenosis and regurgitation are combined, the high-pitched decrescendo diastolic murmur is also heard. In aortic regurgitation without significant aortic stenosis, a systolic ejection murmur may be present because of increased flow back across the aortic valve. This leads to an increased stroke volume and the murmur. It may be difficult to determine from the examination whether a systolic murmur is caused by significant aortic stenosis in a patient with aortic insufficiency, or if the murmur is caused by increased flow resulting from the regurgitation.

Pulmonic stenosis The murmur of pulmonic stenosis is similar in configuration to that of aortic stenosis but is best heard in the second or third left parasternal interspace. It may be heard in the suprasternal notch but is not transmitted to the carotids, thus helping to differentiate from aortic stenosis. The murmur of pulmonic stenosis extends beyond A_2, which occurs first, but stops before P_2. This murmur is also diamond shaped and increases in intensity with inspiration. A late peak in intensity or a softer (inaudible) P_2 both correlate with more severe stenosis (see Fig. 4-28).

Hypertrophic obstructive (and nonobstructive) cardiomyopathy The obstructive form of hypertrophic cardiomyopathy is called *idiopathic hypertrophic subaortic stenosis (IHSS)*. This may have dominant inheritance or a sporadic occurrence.

The cardinal features include the following: (1) the septal region of the left ventricular outflow tract is thickened asymmetrically; (2) the left ventricle becomes hypertrophied; (3) during systole the septum causes abnormal anterior motion of the anterior leaflet of the mitral valve; (4) there is impaired relaxation of the left ventricle during diastole; and (5) sudden death may follow exertion.

Patients with hypertrophic cardiomyopathy seek treatment for dyspnea, chest pain, or a heart murmur. Other symptoms include fatigue, dizziness, and palpitations or syncope. On examination there is a bifid carotid pulse and a bifid apical impulse. The systolic murmur begins early in systole as the abnormal septum begins to obstruct left ventricular outflow. A harsh systolic ejection murmur is transmitted to the left lower sternal border. The murmur is heard in the aortic area along the sternum and extends toward the apex (PMI) but not into the carotids. An S_3 and S_4 are common.

Murmurs of aortic stenosis or mitral regurgitation may be confused with those of hypertrophic cardiomyopathy. Techniques that increase the volume of the left ventricle reduce the amount of obstruction caused by the septal hypertrophy combined with the anterior mitral leaflet. Thus the murmur is decreased by isometric exercise (handgrip), by going from a standing to a squatting position, and by passively elevating both legs (see Fig. 4-28).

Late systolic murmurs may be caused by hypertrophic cardiomyopathy, mild mitral regurgitation, or MVP.

Mitral valve prolapse MVP with the midsystolic click–late systolic murmur may actually have a click, a murmur, or both. The click is caused by prolapse or ballooning of the posterior leaflet of the mitral valve. The click is produced when the posterior leaflet is suddenly snapped to a stop, like air snapping into a parachute. If the mitral valve allows regurgitation back into the left atrium, the late systolic murmur is heard after the click (see Fig. 4-28).

The murmur of MVP is high pitched, best heard at the apex with the diaphragm, and continues through A_2. The murmur can have a honking or whooping quality.

Examination techniques that reduce left ventricular volume cause an earlier click and, just as for hypertrophic cardiomyopathy, a louder murmur. When the ventricle has less blood volume, ventricular walls move closer together. The mitral valve leaflets balloon earlier and regurgitate more. Having the patient stand or inhale amyl nitrite enhances these findings of MVP.

Holosystolic murmurs These are plateau-shaped murmurs, so called because of their constant intensity throughout systole. A synonym is *pansystolic murmur*. *Regurgitant murmurs* has also been used, but calling holosystolic murmurs regurgitant murmurs is not invariably correct because VSD may cause a holosystolic murmur without mitral regurgitation.

Holosystolic murmurs indicate blood is flowing from a higher pressure to a lower pressure, as from the left heart to the right heart, or from ventricles to atria. Important examples are mitral regurgitation, tricuspid regurgitation, ventriculoseptal defect, and the systolic component of the continuous murmur of patent ductus arteriosus, aortopulmonary window, or coronary arteriovenous fistula.

Mitral regurgitation The most common cause for a holosystolic murmur is mitral regurgitation. Regurgitation occurs when the mitral valve becomes incompetent because of any of the following:

- MVP
- Rupture or dysfunction of papillary muscles after myocardial infarction
- Shortened chordae tendinea caused by rheumatic fever
- Perforation of a valve in infective endocarditis
- Rupture of chordae tendinea normally connecting papillary muscles and valve cusps

The holosystolic murmur of mitral regurgitation is high pitched (use the diaphragm), harsh, and blowing. The murmur radiates to the left (axilla), and the louder the murmur, generally the more likely it will radiate. Murmurs caused by ruptured chordae of the anterior leaflet may be heard up and down the spine. Rupture of chordae from the posterior leaflet may be heard over the anterior precordium. Papillary muscle dysfunction pansystolic murmurs may be best heard at the apex using the diaphragm. Rupture of a papillary muscle may produce a murmur similar to that of ruptured chordae.

These holosystolic murmurs begin with S_1. As soon as the mitral valve closes, regurgitation begins, so the murmur may obscure S_1. The murmur ends with or shortly after A_2. Because aortic pressure is higher than left atrial pressure, after aortic valve closure left ventricular pressure may briefly continue to allow regurgitation across the mitral valve (see Fig. 4-28).

More severe mitral regurgitation characteristically has several features:

1. The apex beat (PMI) is shifted downward and to the left because of left ventricular hypertrophy and dilation.
2. An S_3 gallop becomes prominent at the apex.
3. The murmur may be grade III/VI or louder and have an associated thrill.
4. Left atrial enlargement is caused by regurgitation back into the left atrium (Fig. 4-29).
5. The mitral valve ring may become calcified (a chest x-ray film finding).

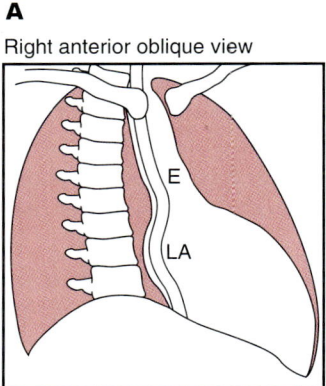
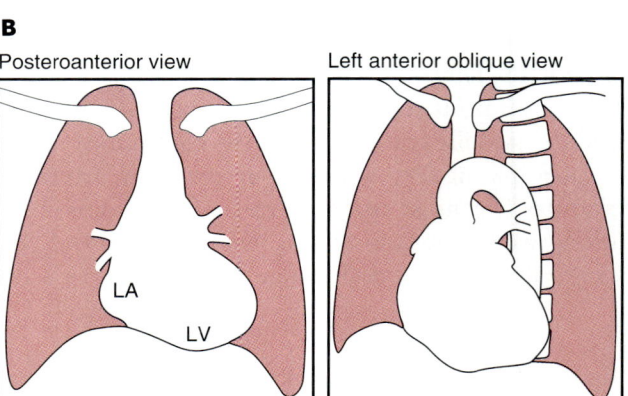

Fig. 4-29 Change in left atrium size in mitral regurgitation. *E,* Esophagus; *LA,* left atruim; *LV,* left ventricle.

Mitral regurgitation may begin acutely in endocarditis. Ischemic inferior wall of the myocardium can result in papillary muscle dysfunction and a new murmur of mitral regurgitation.

Ventricular septal defect The size of a VSD has little bearing on the murmur. A small VSD may produce a loud murmur, and a large VSD, a soft murmur. The VSD murmur is of medium pitch, best heard at the lower left parasternal border. The VSD murmur, like the murmur of mitral regurgitation, radiates to the left chest, but unlike mitral regurgitation not to the left axilla. As pulmonary hypertension occurs, P_2 becomes accentuated, even becoming louder than A_2.

Often VSD murmurs are confused with pulmonic stenosis or with mitral regurgitation. The reasons for this confusion is the increased flow from the left ventricle into the right ventricle because of the higher left ventricle pressure. The resulting increased right ventricle stroke volume produces the pulmonic ejection murmur.

Aortic valve regurgitation may be present with VSD. The two together can produce a nearly continuous murmur.

Murmurs of mitral regurgitation, hypertrophic cardiomyopathy, and VSD may be confusing. All three exhibit long pansystolic murmurs and each may have an S_3 and left ventricular prominence. Severe left ventricular hypertrophy (seen on ECG tracing) is more characteristic of obstructive cardiomyopathy.

Tricuspid regurgitation Tricuspid regurgitation may result from endocarditis in intravenous drug abuse, rheumatic heart disease, or mitral disease with increased pulmonary vascular resistance. The tricuspid murmur is holosystolic, usually best heard with the diaphragm positioned at the lower left sternal border or below the xiphoid (see Fig. 4-28). The murmur increases in intensity with

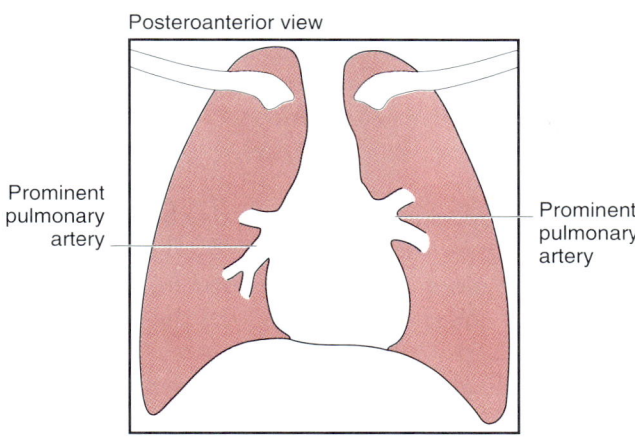

Fig. 4-30 Increased pulmonary blood flow in atrial septal defect.

inhalation and may be transmitted toward the apex but not beyond it toward the axilla. Large v waves appear in the jugular venous pulse.

Other systolic murmurs The murmur of atrial septal defect is a systolic ejection–type murmur with a wide split S_2. Atrial septal defect itself does not cause the murmur, but the blood flow from the left atrium to the right atrium increases the volume across the pulmonic valve, giving the murmur of pulmonic stenosis (relative stenosis caused by the volume) at the pulmonic area or Erb's point (Fig. 4-30).

The increased right-sided flow caused by the left-to-right atrial shunt delays P_2 closure to much later after A_2. The two never come together, even during exhalation (fixed split of the second sound).

Straight back syndrome The straight back syndrome is found in slender persons who lack the normal thoracic vertebral kyphosis and have reduced anterior-to-posterior dimension. A systolic ejection murmur best heard in the pulmonic area is common, often with an associated widely split S_2. Close observation shows the S_2 does become single. Dilation of the pulmonary artery is thought to be the cause of the murmur.

Innocent murmurs An innocent murmur is any murmur found on examination in which the patient has a normal cardiovascular system and has been examined at rest. Innocent murmurs are more common in younger patients. These are usually systolic, diamond-shaped ejection murmurs in midsystole. Innocent murmurs are best heard along the left sternal border and are usually grade I/VI or II/VI. These frequently disappear when the patient stands.

Venous hum The venous hum is a continuous bruit heard over the base of the heart or above the clavicles in normal individuals. The sound continues throughout the cardiac cycle. Turning the patient's head or occluding the cervical veins may reduce or stop the venous hum. Having the patient sit or stand may increase venous return and accentuate the murmur.

Mammary souffle The mammary souffle is a high-pitched continuous flow murmur heard over the base of the heart and the upper breasts during pregnancy. Pressure over the chest wall may obliterate the mammary souffle.

Diastolic Murmurs

Unlike systolic murmurs, which may be innocent murmurs, diastolic murmurs are nearly always caused by a significant pathologic condition. Diastolic murmurs occur in early, mid, or late diastole. They may be regurgitant (aortic, tricuspid) or be filling murmurs with middiastolic or presystolic murmurs (mitral stenosis).

Aortic regurgitation An important early diastolic murmur is aortic regurgitation. Causes of aortic regurgitation include bicuspid aortic valve, calcific aortic stenosis, chronic rheumatic fever, infective endocarditis, dissecting aortic aneurysm, previous syphilitic aortitis, Reiter's syndrome, ankylosing spondylitis, or degeneration of valve leaflets.

The regurgitant flow from the aorta back across the aortic valve begins at valve closure so that the murmur is continuous with A_2. Generally, the longer the murmur continues during diastole, the more severe the valvular incompetence. If cardiac output decreases because of congestive heart failure, the murmur of aortic regurgitation becomes softer.

The diastolic high-pitched (use diaphragm) blowing murmur of aortic regurgitation is best heard at the aortic area, Erb's point, and is transmitted toward the apex.

An associated murmur, the Austin Flint murmur is a low-pitched (use bell) diastolic rumble occurring simultaneous with the high-pitched regurgitant murmur. The regurgitant flow across the aortic valve displaces the anterior leaflet of the mitral valve, narrowing the orifice for blood flow from the left atrium into the ventricle. This causes a functional mitral stenosis (without an opening snap) diastolic rumble.

The murmur of aortic regurgitation is termed blowing or decrescendo, and it fades out before S_1. The murmur may be heard along the right sternal border if the aortic root is dilated. In contrast, the murmur of pulmonary regurgitation is not found there. With aortic regurgitation, an aortic ejection sound is heard at the second right interspace. If the ejection sound is heard at the apex, a bicuspid valve is suspected.

The technique of auscultation for aortic regurgitation is to have the patient sitting, leaning forward, and holding the breath in complete exhalation. This procedure is helpful when the diastolic blow cannot be heard with the patient supine. To increase the intensity of the aortic insufficiency murmur, examine the patient squatting or doing an isometric handgrip. Squatting compresses femoral arteries, reduces flow to legs, and raises blood pressure. The murmur becomes louder and longer.

Besides the characteristic murmur, several associated physical findings are characteristic of aortic regurgitation.

1. *Corrigan's water hammer pulse* hits the palpating fingers in a bolus like the toy water hammer. Very little upstroke or downstroke is felt with this type of pulse.
2. *de Musset's sign* is to-and-fro head movement synchronous with the heartbeat.
3. *Quincke's pulse* refers to capillary pulsation in the fingertips, especially visible in the nailbeds.
4. *Duroziez's sign* refers to systolic and diastolic bruits auscultated with the stethoscope partially compressing the femoral artery.
5. *Hill's sign* refers to blood pressure in the legs being higher than that in the arms. Normally this difference is 10 to 20 mm Hg. In aortic insufficiency the difference may be 60 to 100 mm Hg.

Pulmonic regurgitation Two diastolic regurgitant murmurs are related to pulmonic regurgitation. One is called Graham Steell's murmur, caused by dilation of the pulmonic annulus secondary to pulmonary hypertension. The second murmur is caused by pulmonic regurgitation without pulmonary hypertension.

Graham Steell's murmur has certain characteristics that separate it from ordinary pulmonic regurgitation. These findings are caused by pulmonary hypertension. The jugular venous pulse has a giant *a* wave characteristic of pulmonary hypertension.

The right ventricle becomes enlarged, and the heart is displaced clockwise so the PMI becomes a diffuse precordial heave.

Abnormal splitting of S_2 occurs, with P_2 being first and accentuated. Continuous with P_2 is the high-pitched diastolic decrescendo murmur best heard along the left sternal border and at the pulmonic area. In contrast to aortic regurgitation, the murmur of pulmonic regurgitation is not widely heard over the precordium, neither along the right parasternal space, nor at the apex. The pulmonic murmur may become louder with inspiration.

The murmur of pulmonic regurgitation with normal pulmonary artery pressure is less common. It is heard at Erb's point and is pitched medium to low. The P_2 is soft, and the murmur tends to be middiastolic crescendo-decrescendo.

Middiastolic murmurs Either middiastolic or late diastolic murmurs most often are caused by mitral or tricuspid stenosis.

These murmurs do not occur at once after A_2 or P_2 because a brief time of isovolumic relaxation is required after S_2 before either the mitral or tricuspid valve opens. The opening is marked by the opening snap of mitral stenosis (an opening snap of tricuspid stenosis rarely occurs). The typical time lapse between S_2 and OS is 0.08 sec. Shorter times signify more stenotic (narrower) valves.

If the middiastolic murmur is caused by a large flow across the valve rather than by stenosis, the murmur is usually preceded by an S_3 from that ventricle (e.g., severe mitral regurgitation).

Mitral stenosis The most common cause of mitral stenosis is chronic rheumatic valvular disease. The murmur may be simulated by the rare left atrial myxoma on a long stalk that flops into the valve ring to cause a narrowed orifice. An opening snap is absent with an atrial myxoma.

The pitch of mitral stenosis murmurs is low, and intensity is soft. The murmur has a rumbling quality. With atrial contraction a presystolic (late diastolic) increase in intensity of the murmur occurs. The presystolic accentuation ceases if atrial fibrillation occurs. Loudness of the murmur is related to flow velocity, a function of volume and pressure. A lower cardiac output reduces the intensity of the murmur.

The optimal technique to hear the murmur of mitral stenosis is to exercise the patient (a few sit-ups) to increase flow. Then auscultate with the bell midway between the sternum and apex and inch toward the apex. Turn the patient to the left lateral decubitus position, palpate, and listen at the PMI to hear optimally. The M_1 is often loud, an opening snap follows S_2, and both are heard over the precordium. The middiastolic low-pitched rumble and the presystolic (crescendo) accentuation that follow the opening snap are heard only at the apex (see Fig. 4-28). If mitral regurgitation is combined with mitral stenosis, a high-pitched holosystolic murmur is also present.

Tricuspid stenosis The murmur of tricuspid stenosis is also low pitched, diastolic, and heard best with the bell at the lower left sternal border. It does not radiate widely and is not heard better in the decubitus position. It may be heard at the apex if the right ventricle is dilated. Inspiration often intensifies it.

The jugular venous pulse shows a large *a* wave when tricuspid stenosis is present or when pulmonary hypertension accompanies mitral stenosis.

TABLE 4-9: Use of Bedside Techniques in Cardiac Diagnosis

	Right-sided Murmur	Aortic Stenosis	Hypertrophic Obstructive Cardiomyopathy	Mitral Regurgitation	Ventricular Septal Defect
Inspiration	↑	↓	↓	↓	↓
Exhalation	↓	↑	↑	↑	↑
Müller's maneuver	↓ NC*	↓	↓	↓ NC	↓
Valsalva's maneuver	↓	↑	↑ ↓	↓	↓
Stand to squat	↑ NC	↑	↓	↑ ↓ NC	↑ NC
Squat to stand	↓ NC	↓	↑	↑ ↓ NC	↓ NC
Leg elevation	↑ ↓ NC	↑ NC	↓	↑ NC	↑ NC
Handgrip	↑ ↓ NC	↓ NC	↓	↑	↑
Arterial occlusion	NC	NC	NC	↑	↑
Amyl nitrite	↑	↑ NC	↑	↓	↓

From Lembo NJ, et al: Bedside diagnosis of systolic murmurs, New Engl J Med 318:1572-1578, 1988.
*NC = No change.

Other diastolic murmurs The *Carey Coombs murmur* occurs with acute rheumatic fever. Valvitis causing valve deformity but no obstruction causes a soft middiastolic rumble. No opening snap is present, but S_1 may be accentuated. This murmur may be present one day, disappear the next, and reappear later.

Continuous Murmurs

Heart murmurs caused by combinations of defects are not continuous. Systolic and diastolic murmurs may be caused by defects of a single valve or by multiple lesions. An interval usually exists between systolic and diastolic murmurs.

Continuous murmurs are produced by blood flowing from higher to lower pressure continuously throughout systole and diastole. This may be caused by patent ductus arteriosus between the aorta and left pulmonary artery. Peripheral arteriovenous fistulas may make a similar continuous bruit. The venous hum and mammary souffle, both discussed above, can also do this.

The murmur of patent ductus arteriosus is louder and coarser when the shunt is large. It is often best heard along the left sternal border but is usually obvious over the entire precordium (see Fig. 4-28). The murmur is referred to as a machinery murmur when its quality resembles the roar of machines.

If a patent ductus goes uncorrected surgically, pulmonary hypertension develops. The diastolic murmur first decreases, later followed by reduced intensity of the systolic murmur.

Enhancing Diagnosis During Auscultation

Ten cardiac diagnostic maneuvers have been used at the bedside to enhance diagnosis in cardiac auscultation (Table 4-9).

Inspiration During inspiration, the outward expansion of the chest wall and the depression of the diaphragm reduce the intrathoracic pressure. Venous return increases. Pulmonary vascular resistance decreases, and P_2 occurs later, moving away from A_2, which normally occurs first in the cardiac cycle. Normal splitting of the second sound is increased during inspiration.

If A_2 occurs abnormally late after P_2, as in left bundle branch block, inspiration

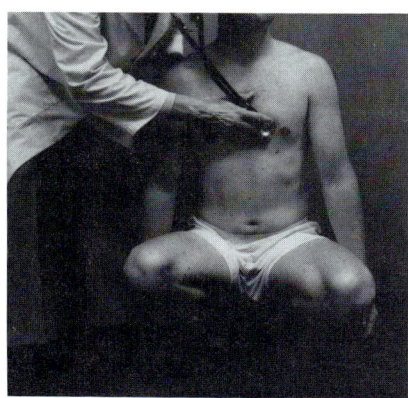

Fig. 4-31 Auscultation of the heart with the patient squatting increases left ventricular volume and decreases the murmur of hypertrophic obstructive cardiomyopathy.

would move P_2 (later) toward A_2. This is called paradoxic splitting because the splitting is decreased with inspiration.

All right-sided murmurs caused by either tricuspid regurgitation or pulmonic stenosis increase during inspiration because of the increased flow *(the Carvallo sign)*. Murmurs from the left side of the heart usually decrease during inspiration. An occasional patient with hypertrophic obstructive cardiomyopathy or MVP will show inspiration-accentuated murmur.

Exhalation Exhalation results in decreased intensity of most right-sided murmurs such as tricuspid regurgitation or pulmonic stenosis. Most left-sided murmurs do not change.

Müller's maneuver Müller's maneuver is performed by having the patient pinch the nostrils shut with one hand and suck hard on a finger of the other hand. This produces a prolonged negative intrathoracic pressure and prolongs the types of changes found in inspiration. At the same time, it prevents annoying breathing sounds. Unfortunately, Müller's maneuver does not appear to be useful in differentiating right-sided from left-sided murmurs.

Valsalva's maneuver Valsalva's maneuver is performed by asking the patient to hold the breath and bear down for 20 seconds as if having a bowel movement. Alternatively, ask the patient to blow into a manometer to a pressure of 40 mm Hg. As the intrathoracic pressure rises, the blood return is reduced to the right heart. For a few beats, the increased intrathoracic pressure increases venous return to the left heart, which increases left ventricular stroke volume. Most left-sided murmurs are intensified during the initial 5 to 10 seconds. Continuing Valsalva's maneuver keeps intrathoracic pressure high, reduces venous return from the lungs, and reduces the left ventricular stroke volume, pulse pressure, and heart rate. Most murmurs grow softer because of the decreased flow across left-sided valve lesions. However, a murmur of hypertrophic obstructive cardiomyopathy usually increases or may be heard for the first time. The murmurs of MVP may increase. The patient should not be expected to hold the breath longer than 20 to 30 seconds. The first and second heart sounds usually become single. An exception is a split S_2 caused by atrial septal defect. Also, in a right bundle branch block the S_1 remains widely split. After breathing is resumed, left-sided systolic murmurs increase for a few beats while the murmur of hypertrophic obstructive cardiomyopathy decreases.

Standing to squatting Instruct the patient to squat, but to breathe normally and to avoid performing Valsalva's maneuver (Fig. 4-31). Squatting increases left

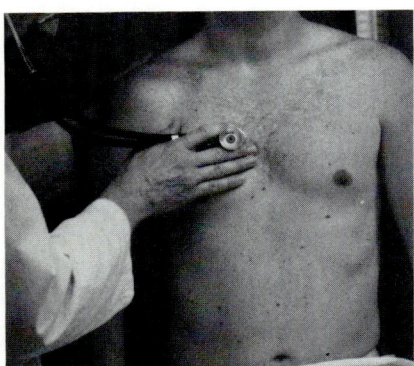

Fig. 4-32 After 30 seconds of squatting, the patient stands. The murmur of hypertrophic obstructive cardiomyopathy usually increases, and that of mitral regurgitation may increase.

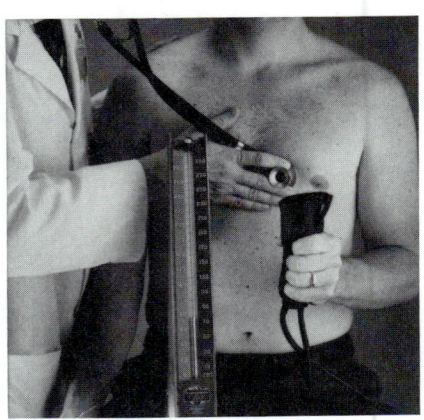

Fig. 4-33 This patient is squeezing a partially inflated blood pressure cuff in an isometric handgrip. The murmur of hypertrophic obstructive cardiomyopathy would be reduced because of increased resistance. Avoid this maneuver in patients who have unstable angina or ventricular arrhythmias.

ventricular volume. The murmur of hypertrophic obstructive cardiomyopathy decreases immediately. Mitral regurgitation murmurs occasionally decrease. Most others increase or do not change. Squatting moves the click and murmur of MVP later in systole toward S_2. Squatting may intensify aortic regurgitation.

Squatting to standing After the patient has been squatting for 30 seconds or longer, ask him to stand (Fig. 4-32). Observe changes in cardiac sounds during the next 20 seconds. The murmur of hypertrophic obstructive cardiomyopathy nearly always increases. Mitral regurgitation increases in about a third of patients. Most other murmurs decrease or do not change. Standing moves the click and murmur of MVP earlier in systole toward S_1.

Passive leg elevation With the patient supine, keep the legs straight and elevate them to 45 degrees. Note changes in murmurs for 20 seconds. A decrease in the murmur of hypertrophic obstructive cardiomyopathy is the most consistent finding. This is caused by increased venous return and an enlarged left ventricle.

Isometric handgrip The patient sustains a tight handgrip for 1 minute (Fig. 4-33). This increases the peripheral vascular resistance (the *afterload*). The murmur of hypertrophic obstructive cardiomyopathy decreases, but the murmur of aortic stenosis decreases in only 30%. Some right-sided murmurs decrease or increase, whereas murmurs of aortic or mitral regurgitation and VSD increase. Thus this characteristic helps distinguish murmurs of mitral regurgitation and VSD from aortic stenosis and hypertrophic obstructive cardiomyopathy. Avoid the isometric handgrip in acute myocardial infarction, unstable angina, or ventricular arrhythmia.

Transient arterial occlusion Place a blood pressure cuff around both of the patient's arms and inflate to 20 mm Hg above systolic pressure. Twenty seconds later observe changes in murmurs. Murmurs of mitral regurgitation and VSD increase in 80% of patients. As with handgrip, murmurs of mitral regurgitation and VSD are not differentiated on the basis of this maneuver. Most other murmurs do not change or decrease.

Amyl nitrite inhalation Instruct the patient to take three rapid, deep breaths from a broken ampule of 0.3 ml amyl nitrite. Note murmur intensity 15 and 30 seconds later. The murmur of VSD nearly always decreases, and the murmur of mitral regurgitation usually decreases. Right-sided murmurs, aortic stenosis, and hypertrophic obstructive cardiomyopathy increase.

Spontaneous premature ventricular contractions may also be useful in differentiating murmurs. After a premature ventricular contraction, ventricular filling time is longer during the compensatory pause. Aortic blood pressure drops lower than usual. Ejection and forward flow murmurs are generally louder after the compensatory pause. In contrast, murmurs of mitral regurgitation, except those caused by papillary muscle dysfunction, tend to be softer.

Summary

A summary checklist for the examination of the cardiovascular system is included in the box below.

Summary Checklist for Examination of the Heart

Symptoms that May Show Examination Findings
- Angina
- MVP
- Pericarditis
- Dissecting aneurysm
- Dyspnea
- Orthopnea
- PND
- Palpitations
- Fatigue
- Carotid sinus syncope
- Hemoptysis
- Edema
- Cyanosis

Blood Pressure
- Korotkoff sounds
- Orthostatic hypotension
- Hypertension

Jugular Venous Pulse

Arterial Pulses
- Sinus arrhythmia
- Premature contractions
- Atrial fibrillation
- Bigeminal pulse
- Corrigan's pulse
- Quincke's pulse
- Collapsing pulse
- Pulsus bisferiens
- Pulsus alternans
- Pulsus paradoxus
- Intermittent claudication
- Leriche's syndrome
- Takayasu's disease

Cardiac Sounds
- Components of S1
- Components of S2
- The third heart sound
- The fourth heart sound
- Summation gallop
- Opening snap
- Ejection sounds
- MVP
- Pericardial knock
- Pericardial rubs

Heart Murmurs
- Systolic murmurs
- Aortic stenosis
- Hypertrophic cardiomyopathy
- MVP
- Mitral regurgitation
- Innocent murmurs
- Venous hum
- Mammary souffle
- Diastolic murmurs
- Aortic regurgitation
- Mitral stenosis
- Continuous murmurs

Suggested readings

Enselberg CD: Measurement of diastolic blood pressure by palpation, *New Engl J Med* 265:272-274, 1961. *This shows a relatively little-used method to detect diastolic blood pressure by palpation.*

Frank MJ, Alvarez-Mena SC, Abdulla AM: *Cardiovascular physical diagnosis,* ed 2, St. Louis, 1983, Mosby-Year Book. *A thorough but brief summary of important components of the cardiovascular examination.*

Hurst JW: The examination of the heart: the importance of initial screening, *Dis Mon* 36:247-313, 1990. *This is an outstanding review of the cardiovascular examination by a master of the subject.*

Keith NM, Wagener HP, Barker NW: Some different types of essential hypertension: their course and prognosis, *Am J Med Sci* pp 332-343, 1939.

Kirkendall WM, Armstrong ML: Vascular changes in the eye of the treated and untreated patient with essential hypertension, *Am J Cardiol* May, pp 663-668, 1962.

Lembo NJ, et al: Bedside diagnosis of systolic murmurs, *New Engl J Med* 318:1572-1578, 1988. *Bedside maneuvers were evaluated and compared for accuracy in diagnosis of 50 patients with systolic murmurs.*

McCutcheon EP, Rushmer, RF: Korotkoff sounds. An experimental critique, *Circ Res* 20:149-161, 1967. *Korotkoff sounds are experimentally evaluated.*

O'Neill TW, et al: Diagnostic value of the apex beat, *Lancet* 1:410-411, 1989. *The apex beat was evaluated in 100 patients to determine its diagnostic value in cardiomegaly. Sensitivity and specificity values were calculated.*

Perloff JK: Physical examination of the heart and circulation, Philadelphia, 1982, WB Saunders. *An excellent, small paperback volume on the cardiac examination.*

Perloff JK, Child JS, Edwards JE: New guidelines for the clinical diagnosis of mitral valve prolapse, *Am J Cardiol* 57:1124-1129, 1986. *Distinguishes pathologic mitral valve prolapse from normal superior systolic displacements of the mitral valve leaflets. These authors have proposed criteria to help distinguish normal from abnormal.*

Phillip SJ, et al: A community blood pressure survey: Rochester, Minnesota, 1986, *Mayo Clin Proc* 63:691-699, 1988. *Results of a community-based blood pressure survey.*

The 1988 Report of the Joint National Committee on detection, evaluation, and treatment of high blood pressure, *Arch Intern Med* 148:1023-1040, 1988.

CHAPTER FIVE

The Abdomen

CHAPTER OUTLINE

History Taking
Abdominal pain
Anorexia and related symptoms of appetite disturbance
Nausea and vomiting
Dysphagia
Diarrhea
Constipation
Hematemesis
Hematochezia and melena

Physical Examination of the Abdomen
General considerations
Inspection
Percussion
Auscultation
Palpation
Special considerations in the physical examination of the patient with abdominal pain
Evaluation of the patient with jaundice

Abdominal Pain Syndromes
Acute abdominal pain
Chronic abdominal pain

Summary

GI disorders are extremely common and are a leading cause of patient visits to physicians. Approximately 35% of the population develops intermittent indigestion, 50% have intermittent symptoms of diarrhea and/or constipation, 10% of the adult male population is affected by peptic ulcer disease (PUD), and 10% of the population over age 50 develop diverticular disease of the colon. A thorough clinical history is frequently reliable in directing the clinician's attention to appropriate diagnostic considerations of patients with GI symptoms. All of the cardinal methods of physical examination are helpful in evaluating a patient with GI symptoms. As noted above, the most common complaints include abdominal pain, alterations in bowel habit, and indigestion.

To illustrate further the magnitude of GI problems, note that approximately 135,000 new cases of colonic carcinoma are diagnosed yearly, over 500,000 patients develop viral hepatitis each year, and over 40,000 patients die because of cirrhosis of the liver. In this chapter we discuss the cardinal symptoms and physical findings indicative of GI and liver diseases and the correlation of the history and physical examination in suggesting the correct diagnosis.

History Taking

Abdominal Pain

Abdominal pain is one of the most common complaints physicians must evaluate. Taking a careful, orderly history is essential, as it may not only alert the examiner to key elements of the physical examination to check in detail or to investigations to order, but it often leads to the correct diagnosis. In questioning a patient with abdominal pain, the examiner should obtain specific information on each point listed below:

- Character of the pain
- Location of the pain
- Radiation of the pain
- Factors precipitating and relieving pain
- The patient's assessment of the severity of the pain
- Comparison with other types of abdominal pain or discomfort
- Whether other symptoms described below are present when pain is experienced

These points are discussed in detail below.

CHARACTER OF THE PAIN

Ask the patient to describe, in his own words, the character of the pain. If he has difficulty doing so, provide suitable descriptive terms and ask the patient to use terms that best characterize the pain. Thus pain can be dull, aching, cramping, sharp, burning, gnawing, stabbing, knifelike, colicky (you should explain this term), pressurelike, and caused by bloating or distention. Furthermore, determine whether the pain is persistent, intermittent, or recurrent with or without a pattern, and whether it occurs at specific times of the day, month, or season.

The discomfort of PUD illustrates the above concepts. Classically, the pain is burning or gnawing in character, epigastric in location, occasionally radiating to the back, and is precipitated by skipping meals or long periods without oral intake. Thus patients with PUD frequently have early morning pain that is relieved by ingestion of food or antacids; pain recurs and is especially prevalent in spring and fall. The pain of PUD illustrates the concepts of rhythmicity, periodicity, and chronicity (see section below). Another classic example is the discomfort caused by gastroesophageal reflux. Typically, this pain is described as burning in character, epigastric and xiphisternal in location, radiating retrosternally, and associated with a bitter or water brash taste in the pharynx. The pain is precipitated by overeating, bending over, or reclining (the latter facilitating reflux) and is relieved by antacids.

Key Symptoms in the Evaluation of Gastrointestinal Disorders

- Abdominal pain
- Anorexia and related symptoms of appetite disturbance
- Nausea and vomiting
- Dysphagia
- Diarrhea
- Constipation
- Hematemesis
- Hematochezia and melena

LOCATION OF THE PAIN

Pain originating in specific viscera is often referred to specific sites in the abdomen (Fig. 5-1). Esophageal pain is usually retrosternal, xiphisternal, or epigastric in location. Gastric pain is typically epigastric in location or in the LUQ, whereas gallbladder pain is classically in the RUQ. In approximately 15% of patients, gallbladder pain is epigastric in location or in the LUQ. Small bowel pain

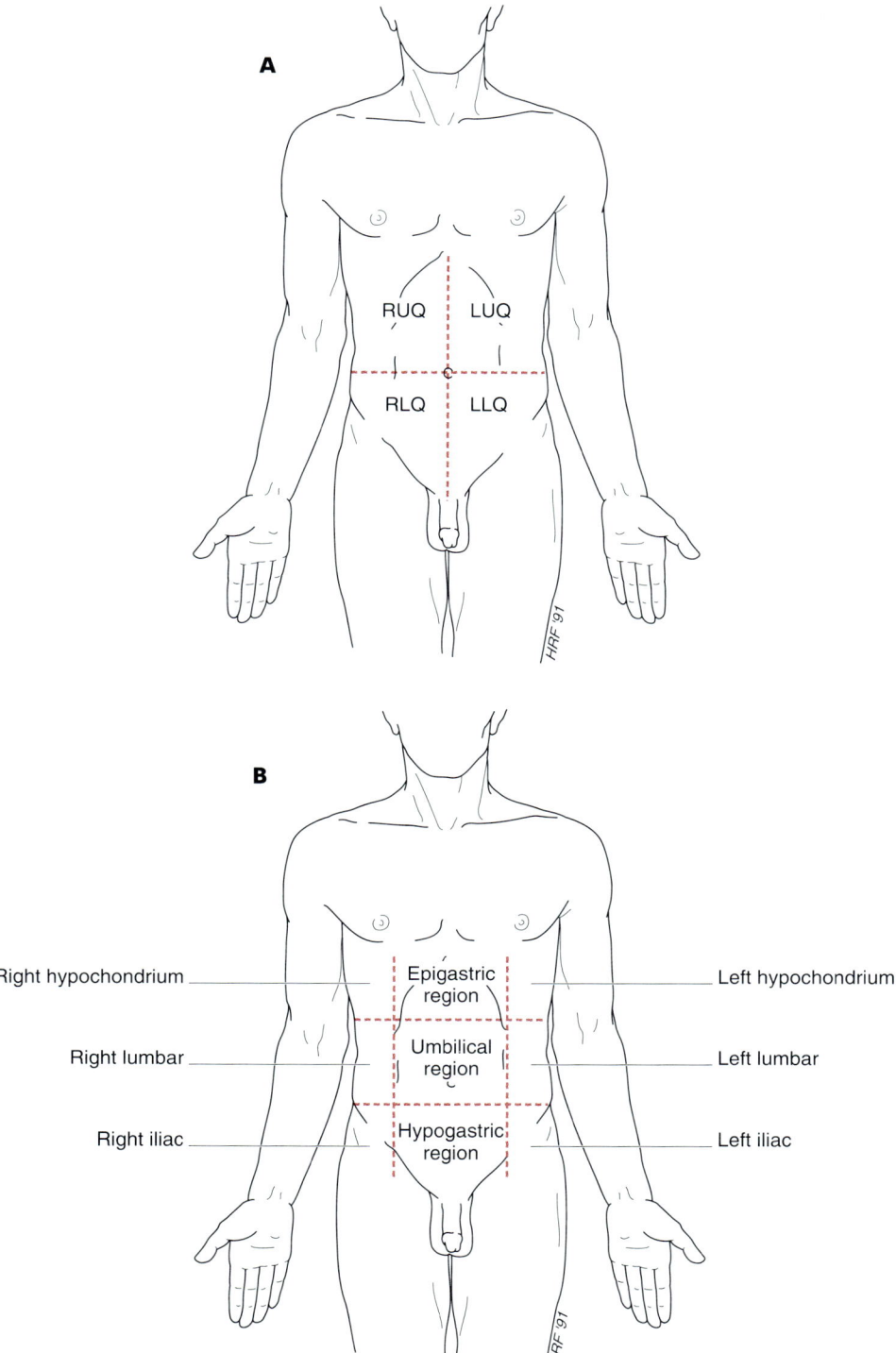

Fig. 5-1 A, The four quadrants of the abdomen. B, The nine regions of the abdomen.

Continued.

Fig. 5-1, cont'd C, The abdomen and chest depicting the location of the liver and the spleen as outlined by percussion. Note that the liver descends 1 to 3 cm with inspiration, which is reflected by a change in liver dullness. **D**, Location of areas of referred pain from specific organs, and illustrative disorders responsible for the radiation of pain.
(*D* Redrawn from Welch CE: *Intestinal obstruction,* Chicago, 1958, Mosby–Year Book.)

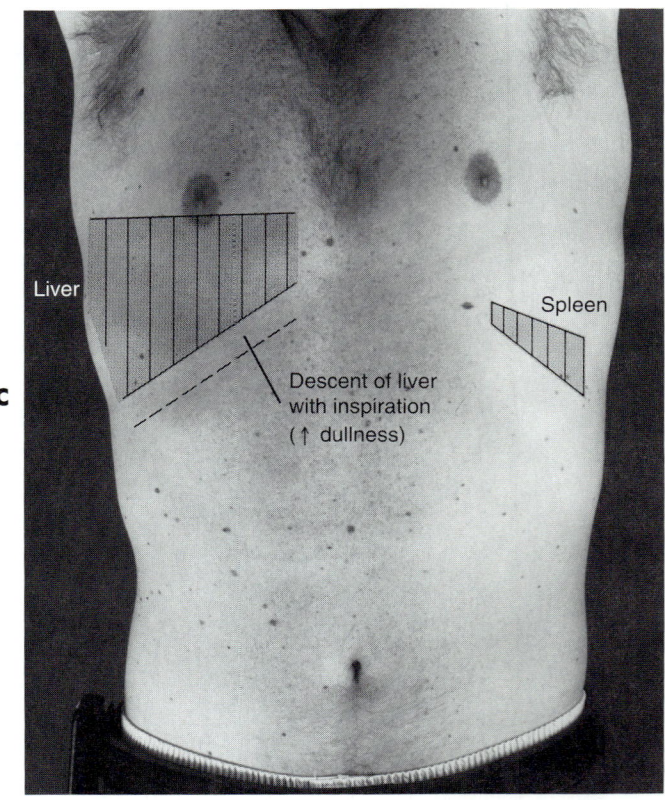

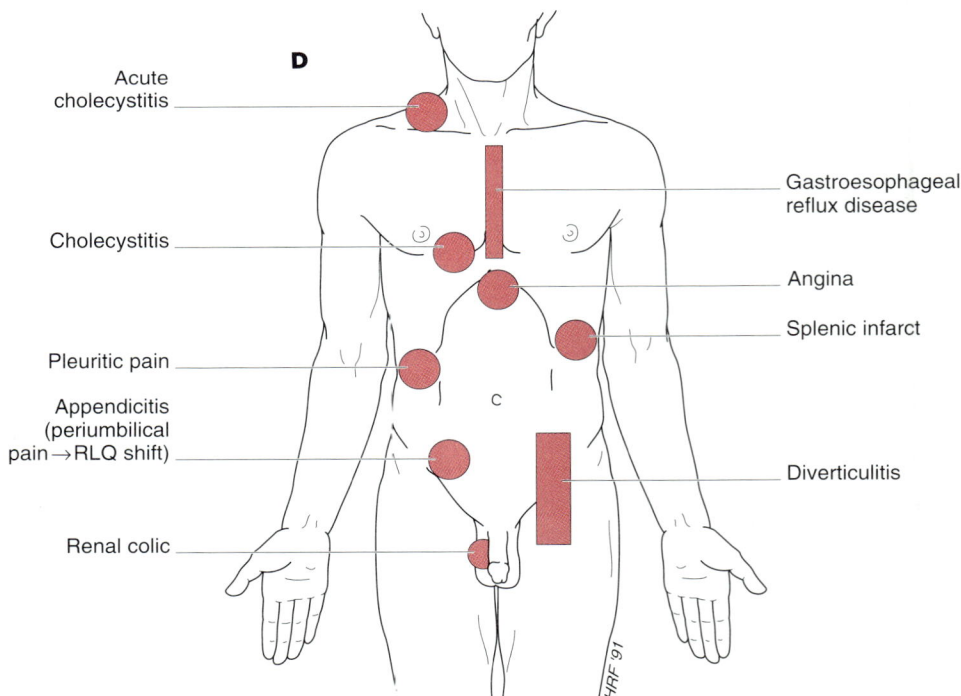

is often referred to the periumbilical area, whereas ileal pain is often in the RLQ. Colonic pain is most frequently referred to the LLQ and RLQ. Pancreatic pain, as may occur in pancreatitis or carcinoma, is typically epigastric or periumbilical in location or in the LUQ, often radiating to the back. The pain of renal colic is often felt in the back and loin and radiates to the groin. The pain of acute pyelonephritis can be felt in the costovertebral angle, loin, and both RUQ and LUQ, the latter two locations simulating a GI-tract origin of discomfort. Understandably, splenic pain is in the LUQ and hepatic pain is in the RUQ, but in both settings back pain may be present as well.

The pain of distended small or large bowel often does not conform to the classic pain locations noted above. Thus pain from dilation of the cecum or sigmoid colon can be referred to the upper abdomen.

RADIATION OF THE PAIN

The radiation of pain may be an important clue to the diagnosis. As noted above, some examples are the pain associated with renal colic that often radiates to the groin, pancreatic pain radiating to the back, gallbladder pain radiating to the scapula and right shoulder, and splenic pain radiating to the back (see Fig. 5-1, D).

FACTORS PRECIPITATING AND RELIEVING ABDOMINAL PAIN

A detailed inquiry into factors precipitating and ameliorating abdominal pain may give important clues useful in the diagnosis of PUD, reflux esophagitis, acute and chronic pancreatitis, cholelithiasis and chronic cholecystitis, disorders causing delayed gastric emptying, irritable bowel syndrome, milk intolerance, and intestinal angina among many others. Disorders are discussed in more detail below in the differential diagnosis of acute and chronic abdominal pain.

PATIENT ASSESSMENT OF PAIN SEVERITY

Asking the patient to assess the severity of the pain on an objective scale is useful for several reasons. The patient should rate the pain on a scale from O to 10, where 0 represents no pain and 10 represents the most severe pain ever experienced; labor pain and renal colic are typical examples of pain that rates a 10. The examiner gains an important clue if a patient who is instructed in the use of this scale rates his pain as 11 or higher. This obvious attempt to emphasize the pain, especially if the patient shows no obvious signs of discomfort, often indicates that the pain is psychophysiologic or functional in origin. Another use of this pain scale is that it permits the physician to evaluate the efficacy of a treatment regimen in alleviating the patient's discomfort. Further, in some disorders such as renal colic, acute pancreatitis, and biliary colic, one can gauge improvement in the patient with symptomatic therapy. Not infrequently, merely hospitalizing a patient and the resultant "tincture of time" in a different setting results in spontaneous improvement in pain. The above applications indicate that a scale of this type can be quite useful, provided the patient can understand what is being asked.

COMPARISON WITH OTHER TYPES OF PAIN

In evaluating a patient with upper abdominal pain, ask the patient to compare the character, location, and severity of the current pain with other abdominal pain he may have experienced. This is illustrated by the following two examples:

- A 48-year-old woman who underwent cholecystectomy 10 years earlier now complains of vague epigastric and RUQ pain. Ask such a patient specifically, *Is the current discomfort identical with, similar to, or different from the pain experienced before the cholecystectomy?* Pain described as identical would obviously focus attention on the biliary tract. However, pain that is totally different in character and severity and occurring with other symptoms such as early satiety and postprandial distention suggests delayed gastric emptying.
- A 55-year-old man complains of a steady epigastric pain and despite careful coaxing is unable to clearly describe it. The examiner might then ask, *Have you ever experienced 'heartburn?'* If he answers yes, the next question might be, *Have you used antacids? Did they alleviate the pain?* If the answers to both questions are yes, then ask, *Is the current pain identical to, similar to, or different from the 'heartburn' pain you have experienced in the past?* If the discomforts are identical, then attention can now be directed to the possibilities of acid peptic disease, reflux esophagitis, and other conditions.

CASE 5-1 Peptic Ulcer with Pyloric Obstruction

A 50-year-old-man with known duodenal ulcer disease presents with a tetrad of complaints of epigastric pain, nausea, emesis, and postprandial distention. He is also found to have a succussion splash. These findings clearly point to pyloric outlet obstruction secondary to duodenal ulcer disease.

OTHER SYMPTOMS IN ASSOCIATION WITH PAIN

Clinicians often recognize disease entities by a constellation or grouping of symptoms or signs. Accordingly, in any patient with abdominal pain, inquire about other symptoms such as anorexia, nausea, vomiting, abdominal distention, early satiety, and diarrhea. The accompanying two case vignettes illustrate this principle.

Finally, in patients with puzzling abdominal pain, repeating the history on more than one occasion and also interviewing family members is often necessary. Further information will indicate whether the history is consistent and also may provide clues to the correct diagnosis.

CASE 5-2 Irritable Bowel Syndrome

A 50-year-old woman complains of long-standing (years) intermittent LLQ pain. The pain often precedes a bowel motion and is relieved by defecation. She has no nocturnal discomfort. She usually has two or three fairly loose bowel motions in the morning after breakfast but has a feeling of incomplete evacuation. She has no systemic symptoms (i.e., anorexia, fever, weight loss) or signs (i.e., anemia), and a stool specimen is negative for occult blood. This symptom complex is most likely caused by irritable bowel syndrome or colonic diverticular disease.

Anorexia and Related Symptoms of Appetite Disturbance

Anorexia, or loss of appetite, is a most important, albeit nonspecific symptom. Anorexia is frequently present with the following:

- Neoplastic disorders
- Depression
- Anorexia nervosa and other eating disorders such as bulimia
- Chronic renal failure
- Acute viral hepatitis
- Chronic parenchymal liver disease(s)
- Chronic infections (e.g., tuberculosis)
- Medications (e.g., metronidazole, iron preparations, and sulfasalazine)
- Chronic debilitating conditions (e.g., cerebrovascular disease, parkinsonism, and demyelinating diseases such as multiple sclerosis)
- Concurrent total parenteral nutrition
- The first trimester of pregnancy

Ask not only the patient but also family members about decreased appetite, as many patients may not be fully aware of their anorexia. Anorexia nervosa is a complex psychiatric disorder characterized by the following (see also Chapter 7):

- Marked weight loss of ~ 25% of ideal body weight
- Distorted implacable attitudes towards eating food and weight loss
- Desired body image of extreme thinness
- Denial of illness with failure to recognize nutritional needs
- No known medical illness to account for anorexia and weight loss

Amenorrhea, over-activity, and bulimia with induced vomiting are often present.

Polyphagia refers to an excessive appetite. The combined symptoms of weight loss in the face of polyphagia are found in only a few disorders, including diabetes mellitus with glycosuria, hyperthyroidism, and malabsorption, especially with pancreatic exocrine insufficiency. Other causes of polyphagia include treatment with corticosteroids, fad diets with periods of sharply reduced food intake, increased nervousness, and patients who by their personality are destined to become morbidly obese (e.g., people who react to stress by eating).

Relatively few disorders result in significant weight loss, which is arbitrarily defined as a weight loss of > 10 lbs. or > 5% of body weight without obvious cause such as diet modification. The box on pg. 206 lists some important diagnostic considerations in approaching the patient with a significant weight loss.

Nausea and Vomiting

Nausea is defined as the unpleasant feeling or sensation that one is about to vomit; the discomfort is experienced in the upper abdomen, epigastrium, or throat. Vomiting is defined as the forceful oral expulsion of gastric contents. Retching often precedes vomiting and consists of spasmodic and abortive respiratory movements against a closed glottis and gastric cardia. Because vomiting is usually preceded by nausea they are considered together.

Nausea is frequently associated with disorders of the stomach and duodenum and is quite common with conditions causing delayed gastric emptying (see boxes on pp. 206-207). Altered autonomic nervous system activity often accompanies

Causes of Weight Loss

I. GI disorders
   A. Malnutrition
   B. Malabsorption
II. Metabolic disorders
   A. Diabetes mellitus
   B. Hyperthyroidism
   C. Adrenal insufficiency
   D. Hypopituitarism
III. Neoplastic disorders
IV. Infectious diseases
   A. Tuberculosis
   B. Fungal disorders
   C. Infectious disease in immunocompromised hosts
      1. AIDS
      2. Immunosuppressive drugs (e.g., corticosteroids, azathioprine)
V. Psychiatric disorders
   A. Depression
   B. Eating disorders
      1. Anorexia nervosa
      2. Bulimia
      3. Anorexia nervosa/bulimia
VI. Chronic renal failure
VII. Connective tissue disorders
   A. Vasculitis (e.g., SLE, polyarteritis, leukocyte disease)
   B. Scleroderma
VIII. Inflammatory conditions
   A. Inflammatory bowel disease
      1. Ulcerative colitis
      2. Regional enteritis

Disorders Causing Chronic Gastric Retention and Delayed Gastric Emptying

I. Disorders causing pyloric outlet obstruction
   A. Chronic duodenal ulcer disease
   B. Idiopathic hypertrophic pyloric stenosis
   C. Crohn's disease (regional enteritis) of the stomach and/or duodenum
   D. Eosinophilic gastroenteritis
   E. Carcinoma of the stomach or duodenum
   F. Carcinoma of the pancreas
II. Neural and smooth muscle disorders
   A. Idiopathic intestinal pseudo-obstruction
   B. Progressive systemic sclerosis (scleroderma)
   C. Vagotomy with previous gastric surgery
   D. Demyelinating diseases (multiple sclerosis)
   E. Bulbar poliomyelitis
   F. Brain tumor

Causes of Nausea and Vomiting

I. CNS disorders
   A. Intracranial mass lesion (tumor, abscess, hematoma)
   B. Inflammatory conditions (meningitis, encephalitis)
   C. Hydrocephalus
   D. Labyrinthine disorders (Ménière's syndrome, labyrinthitis)
II. Endocrine and hormonal disorders
   A. Diabetic ketoacidosis
   B. Adrenal insufficiency
   C. Myxedema
   D. Early pregnancy
III. Disorders causing acute abdominal pain (see box on pg. 246)
   A. Consider especially disorders described in boxes on pp. 247 to 259
IV. Disorders causing delayed gastric emptying (see box below)
V. Peptic ulcer disease
VI. Acute infections of the GI tract
   A. Viral, bacteria, fungal, protozoal
VII. Systemic infections
   A. Sepsis
   B. Acute pyelonephritis
VIII. Drugs and toxins (some examples follow)
   A. Anticholinergics
   B. Mucosal irritants (nonsterodial antiinflammatory drugs)
   C. Iron preparations
   D. Digitalis glycosides, meperidine and other opiates
   E. Food poisoning
IX. Psychiatric
   A. Eating disorders (bulimia; psychogenic vomiting)
X. Miscellaneous
   A. Acute myocardial infarction

III. Metabolic disorders
   A. Diabetes mellitus
   B. Hypothyroidism
IV. Drugs
   A. Anticholinergics
   B. Opiates (e.g., codeine, morphine)
   C. Ganglionic blockers
   D. Aluminum-containing antacids
V. Psychiatric disorders
   A. Anorexia nervosa
VI. Miscellaneous
   A. Antecedent viral illness (may result in gastroparesis for up to 6 months)

nausea, as evidenced by increased perspiration, increased salivation, skin pallor, and vagal discharge that may cause bradycardia and hypotension.

Vomiting is an involuntary act of integrated movements. During nausea, gastric tone is reduced and peristalsis in the stomach is diminished or absent. Duodenal and jejunal tone are increased, and reflux of duodenal contents into the stomach occurs. Retching may supervene, and inspiratory movements of chest wall and diaphragm are countered by expiratory abdominal muscular contractions. The distal antrum and pylorus contract, and the fundus relaxes. The diaphragm then descends. The gastric cardia elevates and opens, the distal stomach contracts, the abdominal muscles contract forcefully, and gastric contents are ejected through the esophagus and out the mouth. The entire act of vomiting occurs as a result of stimulation of the emetic center, which is situated in the floor of the fourth ventricle. Furthermore, a chemoreceptor trigger zone lies close by in the brainstem. Projectile vomiting is a particularly forceful type, unique in lacking antecedent nausea and of special significance in that it often denotes increased ICP.

Nausea and vomiting are common manifestations of several disorders; these are summarized in the box on pg. 207. The reader is also referred to several boxes as noted. Persistent nausea and vomiting should prompt a detailed history, physical examination, and appropriate diagnostic studies. A distinction should also be made between vomiting and *regurgitation*. The latter refers to the passage of food into the esophagus and frequently through the mouth as well, *without* nausea or vomiting. Regurgitation implies obstruction in the distal esophagus (achalasia), an esophageal diverticulum, an over-filled stomach, or an autonomic or functional cause of delayed gastric emptying. Reflux of gastric contents into the upper esophagus often gives rise to the sensation of a water brash or bitter taste in the oropharynx. This occurs frequently in patients with a decreased lower esophageal sphincter pressure.

Rumination is an unusual symptom characterized by regurgitation of food into the mouth that is then swallowed again. Rumination usually occurs shortly after meals, although some patients can ruminate at will. Recent studies have identified an unique abnormality in GI motility in such patients.

Finally, it should be reemphasized that several drugs and gastric mucosal irritants frequently cause nausea.

Dysphagia

Dysphagia is broadly defined as difficulty in swallowing. Odynophagia refers to difficulty in swallowing that is painful. The new onset of dysphagia, especially if such dysphagia persists, mandates an explanation. The disorders causing dysphagia are listed in the accompanying box. In approaching the patient with dysphagia, the examiner should ask several questions:

- *Does food seem to 'hang up' in a particular area during the swallowing process?*
- *Is swallowing painful?* New onset of odynophagia is common in candida and herpetic infections of the esophagus and in drug-induced ulceration of the esophagus, as may occur with tetracycline.
- *Do you have difficulty in swallowing both liquids and solids, or just solids?* The former should suggest a motor disorder of the esophagus, whereas the latter suggests an obstructive lesion.
- *Has dysphagia become progressively more severe?* This also suggests an

Causes of Dysphagia

I. Neurologic and muscular diseases
   A. Cerebrovascular disease*
   B. Pseudobulbar palsy
   C. Multiple sclerosis
   D. Amyotrophic lateral sclerosis
   E. Bulbar poliomyelitis
   F. Parkinsonism*
   G. Myasthenia gravis
II. Obstructive lesions
   A. Intrinsic
      1. Tumors* (esophageal carcinoma, benign tumors)
      2. Esophageal stricture
         a. Reflux esophagitis*
         b. Corrosive
      3. Esophageal rings and web
         a. Mucosal (Schatzki ring)*
         b. Muscular
      4. Diverticulum (Zenker's, traction)
      5. Foreign body
   B. Extrinsic compression
      1. Intrathoracic tumor (carcinoma lung, lymphoma)
      2. Aortic aneurysm
      3. Enlarged left atrium (mitral stenosis)
III. Primary esophageal motility disorders
   A. Achalasia*
   B. Diffuse esophageal spasm*
   C. Variants of achalasia and diffuse esophageal spasm
IV. Secondary esophageal motility disorders
   A. Connective tissue diseases
      1. Scleroderma*
      2. SLE
      3. Raynaud's disease
      4. Polymyositis, dermatomyositis
   B. Metabolic
      1. Diabetes mellitus
      2. Myxedema
      3. Thyrotoxicosis
V. Infections
   A. Candidiasis* (causes odynophagia)
   B. Herpes
   C. Diptheria
   D. Botulism
   E. Tetanus
VI. Medications
   A. Anticholinergics
   B. Ca^{++} channel blockers
VII. Psychiatric
   A. Globus hystericus

*Most important

obstructive lesion; if significant weight loss has also occurred, the differential diagnosis must include carcinoma of the esophagus.
- *Is dysphagia accompanied by regurgitation?* This suggests a motor disorder of the esophagus such as achalasia, an esophageal diverticulum, or an over-filled stomach.
- *Are symptoms intermittent?* This should suggest Schatzki's or a mucosal ring, and a seeming difficulty in swallowing that is merely a feeling of a lump in the throat or an obstruction without any actual difficulty in swallowing suggests *globus hystericus.*

As noted in the box on pg. 209, the most common causes of dysphagia include cerebrovascular accidents, parkinsonism, reflux esophagitis, mucosal rings, esophageal tumors, motor disorders of the esophagus, and infections such as candidiasis.

Diarrhea

Although *diarrhea* is often defined as the defecation of watery or loose stools, such a definition is incomplete. Patients often erroneously conclude that passage of one or two loose bowel movements per day constitutes diarrhea. In essence, diarrhea reflects impaired colonic absorption of water and electrolytes and can be quantitatively defined as the excretion of > 300 g of stool/day on the typical Western diet. The number of daily bowel movements per se may not represent diarrhea. In this regard, extensive studies have revealed a wide range of "normality" for bowel movements, anywhere from 2 to 21 stools/week, or up to 3/day. Similarly, the passage of a loose bowel movement may merely reflect subtle alterations in diet with ingestion of food known to have laxative effects (e.g., foods containing bran, lactose, or sorbitol and brassica vegetables). Therefore, when the examiner asks patients about their bowel habits, they should describe number, consistency, and whether defecation is accompanied by pain or relieves pain if it is present. More importantly, ask whether any recent changes in bowel habits have occurred and whether such changes have persisted.

Diarrhea is a cardinal symptom of several types of disorders. Diarrhea can be categorized as *acute* or *chronic*. The acute onset of diarrhea raises questions of the following types of disorders:

- Acute infectious enteritis (viral, bacterial, protozoal)
- Ingestion of contaminated food (e.g., *Staphylococcus, Bacillus cereus, Salmonella, Shigella, Campylobacter* sp.)
- Food intolerance (lactose intolerance caused by lactase deficiency or ingestion of inordinate amounts of foods with laxative effects)
- Antibiotic-associated diarrhea (the abrupt onset of diarrhea is well documented during or after a course of antibiotics)
- Acute onset of inflammatory bowel disease (e.g., ulcerative colitis)
- Disorders such as systemic infections and gram-negative sepsis

Accordingly, ask the patient with abrupt onset of diarrhea in detail about recent travel, contact with other persons known to have developed diarrhea, ingestion of all foods within the previous 48 hours and where such meals were taken, recent (within the previous 8 weeks) receipt of antibiotics, and whether other family members are ill. In addition, ask about hematochezia, rectal tenesmus (rectal pain with defecation) and systemic symptoms (fever, anorexia, weight loss). The constellation of fever, musculoskeletal complaints, chills, nausea and vomiting, cramping abdominal pain, and diarrhea strongly suggests a diagnosis of acute infectious enteritis. The presence of hematochezia means a break is present in the colonic mucosa; suspect *Campylobacter, Shigella,* and *Salmonella* sp. and invasive *E.coli*. The next step is to try and identify the putative infectious agent by appropriate cultures and serologic tests.

Table 5-1 provides a useful classification of chronic diarrheal disorders and lists some of the key elements in establishing the correct diagnosis. An important part of the history, often given short shrift, is the dietary history, which is particularly relevant in patients with a chronic or recurrent diarrheal disorder. The examiner should inquire specifically about ingestion of coffee, tea, cola beverages (especially ones that contain large amounts of fructose), simple sugars, lactose- and sorbitol-containing foods, cookies, candies, pastries, and so-called "dietetic" or "diabetic" foods and low-calorie mints (all of which may contain sorbitol, a potent laxative food component). Not infrequently, merely discontinuing some of these foods may result in amelioration of diarrhea.

Another important question to ask all patients complaining of diarrhea is whether they are ever incontinent of stool (i.e., whether they defecate involuntarily in their underclothing before they can reach a toilet). Patients are often embarrassed and reluctant to tell physicians they are actually incontinent and they may opt to describe this as "diarrhea." If a patient is incontinent of stool, the differential diagnosis is quite limited. Recurrent incontinence is usually related to diabetes mellitus with anal sphincter dysfunction, previous hemorrhoidal, rectal, or perirectal surgery with damage to the anal sphincter, or an errant episiotomy or traumatic childbirth, also with damage to the anal sphincter.

Constipation

Recent studies have suggested that approximately 4% of normal individuals have less than two bowel movements per week. Many patients, however, cannot accept the fact that two or three bowel movements per week is normal, and cling to the old folklore that states good health requires at least one bowel movement per day. This belief has resulted in a countless number of patients using laxatives

TABLE 5-1: Symptom: Chronic Diarrhea

Cause	Examples	Key Elements in Diagnosis
Iatrogenic dietary factors	• Excess tea, coffee, cola beverages, simple sugars, sorbitol, fructose, and lactose-containing foods	• Careful history
Infectious enteritis	• Amebiasis • Giardiasis	• Demonstrate leukoyctes in stool • Identify trophozoites or cysts in stool and duodenal aspirate (giardiasis)
Inflammatory bowel disease	• Ulcerative colitis • Regional enteritis	• History: diarrhea, abdominal pain, rectal bleeding, physical examination, colonoscopy, barium enema, UGI and small bowel series

From Greenberger NJ, et al: The medical book of lists: a primer of differential diagnosis in internal medicine, ed 3, Chicago, 1990, Mosby–Year Book.
Mnemonic to remember the classification: I, I, I, I, I, I, L, L, D, D, M, M, M, N, P.

Continued.

TABLE 5-1: Symptom: Chronic Diarrhea—cont'd

Cause	Examples	Key Elements in Diagnosis
Irritable bowel syndrome	• (See text)	
Incontinence	• Diabetes • Rectal surgery • Errant episiotomy	• Careful history • Rectal exam • Anorectal motility
Idiopathic secretory diarrhea	• Zollinger-Ellison syndrome • Pancreatic tumors with vasoactive intestinal peptide (VIP)	• Stool output >1.0 L/24 hr • No decrease in stool volume with fasting • Stool osmolality gap ≤40 mosm/kg
Lactose intolerance	• Milk intolerance; ice cream, cheese, etc Also important to note that patients may also have irritable bowel syndrome	• Milk → abdominal pain, diarrhea, gas, bloating • Cessation of milk drinking → amelioration of symptoms • Lactose load (1 g/kg) → exacerbation of symptoms and breath H_2
Laxative abuse		• Add few drops of NaOH to stool—because most laxatives contain phenolphthalein, the stool will turn red
Drug-induced	• Antacids, antibiotics (clindamycin, lincomycin, ampicillin, penicillin), colchicine, lactulose, sorbitol	• Careful history and review of medication
Diverticular and prediverticular disease		• History: intermittent symptoms • PE: palpable left colon • Barium enema: diverticulosis and/or muscle hypertrophy
Malabsorptive disease	• Sprue • Pancreatic insufficiency	• UGI plus small-bowel x-ray films; tests of intestinal absorption function: D-xylose, stool fat, Schilling test, serum carotenes, calcium, albumin, cholesterol, iron, prothrombin time
Metabolic	• Diabetes mellitus • Hyperthyroidism • Adrenal insufficiency	• Abnormal blood glucose levels • ↑ T4, ↑ RAI uptake • ↓ Plasma cortisol, ↓ response to synthetic ACTH
Mechanical	• Fecal impaction	• Rectal exam
Neoplastic	• Carcinoma of the pancreas • Carcinoid syndrome • Villous adenoma • Medullary carcinoma of the thyroid • Tumors producing VIP • Gastrinoma	• Suspect the diagnosis
Postoperative	• After gastric surgery • After cholecystectomy • After bowel resection	• History

on a regular basis. In patients with a lifelong history of infrequent bowel movements, little need be done unless they become uncomfortable because of abdominal distention. On the other hand, the *recent* development of frank constipation (< two stools/week) or a definite reduction in stool frequency should prompt a detailed evaluation. The most common causes of new-onset constipation include the following:

- Decreased food intake
- Decreased fluid intake
- Medications (e.g., anticholinergics, antispasmodics, antidepressants, tricyclics, opiates, calcium channel blockers, sucralfate)
- Hypothyroidism
- Hyperparathyroidism
- Fecal impaction (more likely if first three conditions noted above occur)
- Chronic debilitating disease (e.g., post cerebrovascular accident)

Hirschsprung's disease, or *aganglionic megacolon,* is an unusual disorder characterized by the following:

- Lifelong constipation
- Occasional passage of enormous stools
- Absence or marked diminution in ganglion cells in rectal tissue
- Marked colonic dilation

Increasing constipation, especially if a history of a decrease in stool calibre is also elicited, should raise the question of a colonic carcinoma. Elderly debilitated patients may become constipated because of rectal dyskinesia, in that they do not heed the normal call to defecate. Consequently, bowel movements become infrequent, and the stools are *scybalous* (like marbles).

Increased attention has been devoted to colonic transit and anorectal motility in chronic idiopathic constipation. One series of studies has revealed that women may have an incoordination of the pelvic floor muscles; these women appear to experience *contraction* rather than *relaxation* of the striated muscles of the pelvic floor on attempted defecation. A useful means of assessing colonic transit is to give the patient 20 radiopaque small cylindric markers by mouth and determine the length of time required for these markers to be excreted. This can be done by obtaining a plain film of the abdomen on the first and fifth days. Markedly delayed colonic transit is characterized by retention of markers in the colon after 5 days. Thus patients with idiopathic intractable constipation may have a colonic transit defect or a pelvic floor muscle abnormality. These are but two possible explanations for failure to respond to laxatives or a high-fiber diet.

Hematemesis

Hematemesis is defined as the vomiting of blood that is usually derived from sites in the esophagus, stomach, or duodenum. Less frequently, swallowed blood from epistaxis, hemoptysis, and a bleeding mouth or gums is vomited. If blood is vomited soon after hemorrhage, it is bright red. However, if blood is retained in the stomach, it is broken down to a brown material that has the appearance of coffee grounds. If patients complain of vomiting dark-colored emesis, check such materials promptly for the presence of occult blood.

Hematemesis is an urgent and often a life-threatening problem. Accordingly, the cause of hematemesis must be diagnosed with dispatch. The major causes of hematemesis are PUD, erosive gastritis, Mallory-Weiss tear of the esophagus at the cardio-esophageal junction, and esophageal and gastric varices. Table 5-2 details key elements in the history and physical examination and key diagnostic tests in the evaluation of patients with hematemesis.

Hematochezia and Melena

Hematochezia is defined as the passage of bright red blood in the stool. *Melena* refers to the passage of black or very dark stool that is often tarry and reflects the conversion of hemoglobin to various breakdown products. The presence of occult

TABLE 5-2: Symptom: Hematemesis

Major Causes	Key Elements in History	Key Elements in Physical Exam	Key Diagnostic Tests
Peptic ulcer disease (duodenal, gastric)	• Recurrent dyspepsia and nocturnal pain • Frequent antacid use with partial relief of symptoms • Rhythmicity, periodicity, and chronicity of pain (see text) • History of black tarry stools, nausea, dizziness preceding or following hematemesis • 10% patients have few or no symptoms	• Signs: volume depletion, ↓ blood pressure, ↑ heart rate, orthostatic changes • Epigastric tenderness may be present	• UGI endoscopy will confirm the diagnosis in greater than 90% of cases • Consider arteriography if UGI endoscopy negative
Erosive gastritis	• Use of ulcerogenic drugs (nonsteroidals, antiinflammatory agents, salicylates), alcoholic debauch, postoperative state, burns, multiple systems trauma	• Signs: volume depletion, as noted above	• UGI endoscopy
Mallory Weiss tear at cardioesophageal junction	• Predominantly males • Recent heavy alcohol use • Nausea, vomiting, retching before hematemesis	• Signs: volume depletion	• UGI endoscopy
Esophageal-gastric varices	• Previous documentation of chronic liver disease • Prior alcoholism or viral hepatitis • Abdominal pain, epigastric pain • Hematemesis may be painless	• Peripheral stigmata; chronic parenchymal liver disease (see text) • Splenomegaly • Ascites (may be present) • Increased abdominal collateral veins (may be present)	• UGI endoscopy
Other causes of hematemesis (esophagitis, gastric cancer, gram-negative sepsis, blood dyscrasias)			

blood in the stool can be checked by several tests, the most widely used being the Hemoccult® test, which gives a distinct blue color if occult blood is present. Substances other than blood breakdown products can cause the stool to become black; these include iron-containing medications, bismuth-containing medications (Pepto Bismol®), charcoal, and ingestion of very large amounts of black cherries.

The complaint of hematochezia always warrants a detailed evaluation. The major causes of hematochezia include the following:

- Hemorrhoids
- Colorectal carcinoma
- Colonic polyps
- Chronic diverticular disease
- Inflammatory bowel disease
- Angiodysplasia of the colon
- Acute infectious enteritis
- Infectious proctitis
- Ischemic colitis

Table 5-3 details the key elements in the history and physical examination and the key diagnostic tests in the evaluation of patients with hematochezia. A common error is, after visualizing hemorrhoids in a patient with hematochezia, then assuming that rectal bleeding is caused by hemorrhoids. Similarly, rectal bleeding in a patient with known colonic diverticular disease should not be ascribed to diverticular disease without a thorough workup, including a colonoscopy.

Table 5-3 also refers to the passage of maroon-colored stools. Maroon-colored stools usually indicate massive bleeding; in this setting an upper GI-tract source, such as a bleeding duodenal ulcer, must be excluded. Finally, many of the disorders that cause hematochezia can also result in melena.

TABLE 5-3: Symptom: Lower Gastrointestinal Bleeding (Hematochezia)

Major Causes	Key Elements in History	Key Elements in Physical Exam	Key Diagnostic Tests
Hemorrhoids	• Pruritus ani • Painless defecation frequent • Constipation, hard stools • Blood *on* toilet tissue • Blood *on* stools but not mixed with stools • Patient can feel hemorrhoids	• Visualization of external and internal hemorrhoids • Stool in rectal vault often negative for occult blood	• Anoscopy → hemorrhoids • Proctosigmoidoscopy reveals no other lesion • See text for discussion of need for additional tests
Carcinoma of rectum or colon	• Risk factors for colon cancer checked for (see text) • Change in bowel habits (constipation, diarrhea)	• Careful digital rectal exam with test for occult blood • Careful palpation of RLQ and LLQ for masses	• Colonoscopy *or* flexible sigmoidoscopy with double-contrast barium enema; colonoscopy is preferable

Continued.

TABLE 5-3: Symptom: Lower Gastrointestinal Bleeding—cont'd

Major Causes	Key Elements in History	Key Elements in Physical Exam	Key Diagnostic Tests
Carcinoma of rectum or colon —cont'd	• Change in calibre of stools (smaller) • Systemic symptoms may be present (anorexia, weight loss, symptoms of anemia)	• Check for hepatomegaly • Check for lymphadenopathy (supraclavicular) • Check for periumbilical lymph nodes	• CT scan of abdomen to check for occult liver metastasis • Check for stigmata of iron-deficiency anemia, which, if present, indicates *chronic* blood loss
Colonic polyps	• Recurrent rectal bleeding • Previous history of polyps or colon cancer • Check for colonic polyposis syndromes (see text)	• Same as for carcinoma • Check for incisional lesions and osteomas (Gardner's syndrome)	• Colonoscopy *or* flexible sigmoidoscopy with double-contrast barium enema
Diverticular disease of colon	• Painless hematochezia • Previous intermittent LLQ pain with or without diarrhea • Documented colonic diverticular disease	• Check for volume depletion • May feel thickened sigmoid colon (myochosis) in LLQ	• Colonoscopy after cessation of hematochezia
Inflammatory bowel disease (idiopathic ulcerative colitis, regional enteritis)	• Symptoms: crampy abdominal pain, diarrhea, and rectal bleeding that have persisted • Systemic symptoms: fever, weight loss, symptoms of anemia, arthritis/arthalgia, aphthous ulcer, skin lesions, eye pain (uveitis), history of kidney stones, gallstones (both increased in regional enteritis) • Family history positive for inflammatory bowel disease	• Check vital signs for fever, tachycardia, signs of toxicity or sepsis • Look for extraintestinal signs of inflammatory bowel disease (e.g., arthritis, uveitis, skin lesions, aphthous ulcers of the mouth) • LLQ tenderness (LF colon) • RLQ tenderness (palpable bowel) • Check for perirectal disease (fissure, perirectal abscess)—if present, they suggest Crohn's disease	• Flexible sigmoidoscopy if scope can be passed until normal mucosa is visualized • Colonoscopy • Small-bowel x-ray films if Crohn's disease suspected • Biopsy of affected colon and/or review of surgical specimens
Angiodysplasia of the colon	• Painless rectal bleeding • Elderly patient (> age 60) • Previous conventional workup for bleeding nondiagnostic (negative sigmoidoscopy, barium enema, UGI x-ray films, endoscopy, small-bowel x-ray films)	• Check for signs of volume depletion • PE may be entirely normal • May hear murmur of aortic stenosis	• Colonoscopy • Selective mesenteric angiography NOTE: both of the above tests may be negative

TABLE 5-3: Symptom: Lower Gastrointestinal Bleeding—cont'd

Major Causes	Key Elements in History	Key Elements in Physical Exam	Key Diagnostic Tests
Acute infectious enteritis • *Shigella* • *Salmonella* • *Campylobacter* • Invasive *Escherichia coli* • *Amebiasis* • *Yersinia*	• Abrupt onset of abdominal pain and diarrhea with hematochezia, often with fever; check for putative foods, contacts with similar and concurrent symptoms, recent travel, contact with animals	• Check for volume depletion	• Culture stool for enteric pathogens; serologic tests
Proctitis in homosexuals practicing anal-receptive intercourse may be caused by several infections such as those resulting from *Salmonella* and *Shigella* organisms and Mycobacterium avium-intracellulare or by infections such as syphilis, amebiasis, gonorrhea, herpes, histoplasmosis, cytomegalovirus, chlamydia, campylobacter, and candidiasis	• Sexual practices • Partner with similar recent illness	• Careful proctoscopic sigmoidoscopic examination	• Culture stools for pathogens listed • Biopsy any ulcerating or mass lesion
Ischemic colitis	• Is known cardiac disease present? Congestive heart failure? Digitalis glycosides? Cardiac arrhythmias? Use of oral contraceptives?	• Check cardiac examination • Check for signs of volume depletion	• Flexible sigmoidoscopy • Barium enema (may show "thumbprinting", which is characteristic of submucosal edema and hemorrhage)
Maroon-colored Stools			
Massive bleeding that may be *colonic* in origin (see items above) or may be of the *distal small bowel* Meckel's diverticulum, angiodysplasia, or UGI; that is, peptic ulcer disease	• See items above • Check for history of peptic ulcer disease	• Patients with maroon-colored stools resulting from UGI bleeding, as in peptic ulcer disease, have sustained a massive blood loss (2 to 3 units of blood) and will invariably have unstable vital signs (and BP, ↑ HR, and orthostatic changes)	• Do UGI endoscopy first if there is any question of acid peptic disease; otherwise proceed as for workup of hematochezia

Continued.

TABLE 5-3: Symptom: Lower Gastrointestinal Bleeding—cont'd

Major Causes	Key Elements in History	Key Elements in Physical Exam	Key Diagnostic Tests
Melena			
Although the causes listed above may cause melena, it is more frequently a sign of UGI bleeding, especially of peptic ulcer disease	• See above • See Table 5-2	• See above • See Table 5-2	• See above • See Table 5-2
Ingestion of iron-containing medications may result in black stools	• Inquire whether patient is taking iron or a multivitamin preparation • If patient has stigmata of iron deficiency anemia, the site and cause of blood loss must be determined		

Physical Examination of the Abdomen

General Considerations

The abdomen contains several organs that can be the sites of disease. These include *solid organs,* such as the liver, spleen, kidneys, pancreas, adrenals, ovaries, and uterus; *fluid-filled structures,* such as the aorta, gallbladder, and urinary bladder; and predominantly air-filled *hollow viscera,* such as the stomach, small bowel, and colon. Conventionally, the abdomen can be divided into four quadrants or nine regions (see Fig. 5-1). As noted above, localization and characterization of pain to specific areas of the abdomen often provide clues as to the organ involved and the specific disease.

To ensure an accurate examination of the abdomen, you should observe the following conditions. The room should be well-lit and warm and the patient adequately covered so as not to shiver and tense the abdomen. The patient should be resting comfortably on his or her back with a pillow under the head. Expose the entire abdomen from the xiphoid to the pubic symphysis, but with a sheet or drape covering the genitalia and a gown covering the breasts. Stand at the right side of the patient and make sure your hands and the stethoscope are warm.

The methods of physical examination are usually employed in the following sequence: (1) inspection; (2) percussion; (3) auscultation; and (4) palpation. However, many physicians reserve auscultation for last.

Inspection

The important procedure of inspection, too often omitted or slighted, often gives vital clues to the nature of an intraabdominal disease process. Physicians should discipline themselves to inspect the abdomen in a careful manner before palpating. For example, ask the patient to take a deep breath. Deep inspiration may reveal enlargement of the liver or spleen, enhance recognition of abdominal masses, and even permit visualization of a distended gallbladder. Further, asking the patient to cough may make abdominal hernias more obvious or help localize pain from an inflamed organ (e.g., appendicitis).

By the time the abdomen is examined, the observer should have noted whether the patient is malnourished, dehydrated, or hyperpigmented. Next, inspect the abdomen for scars, striae, dilated veins, visible pulsations, and visible peristalsis. Scars may confirm the history of previous surgical procedures. Scar tissue that becomes unusually dense is termed a *keloid*. *Striae* may be pink, blue, or silvery and are often seen in pregnancy and in women who have borne children. They are also seen in obesity, ascites, Cushing's syndrome, and intraabdominal tumors. Striae result from stretch-induced rupture of the elastic fibers in the skin. Visible pulsations may be seen in patients with aortic aneurysms, a tortuous aorta, or with solid masses overlying the aorta, and they are more likely to be noted in thin individuals. Visible peristalsis may occasionally be appreciated in thin individuals. Importantly, however, visible peristalsis is often caused by a mechanical obstruction of the small bowel or colon. Early in the course of pyloric outlet obstruction, before the stomach dilates, vigorous gastric peristalsis is often evident.

Dilated or engorged veins on the anterior abdominal wall are common in patients with portal hypertension. Indeed, the triad of findings of splenomegaly, ascites, and prominent abdominal wall veins is virtually diagnostic of portal hypertension. Other causes of dilated abdominal veins include obstruction of the superior or inferior vena cava and marked emaciation. Obstruction of the inferior vena cava should be considered in any patient with large venous collateral vessels over the trunk and back. *Diastasis recti* is the term used to describe separation of the two abdominal rectus muscles; this is often quite obvious when the patient raises his head from the pillow. Diastasis recti can occur after abdominal surgery, after pregnancy, and also without any obvious precipitating factor.

PROTUBERANT OR DISTENDED ABDOMEN

The abdomen may appear protuberant or distended for several reasons:

- Internal obstruction
- Obesity
- Organomegaly
- Pregnancy
- Cysts
- Increased gas or air within the bowel
- Increased free air in the peritoneal cavity
- Neoplasms
- Ascites

When inspecting a distended abdomen, note carefully whether the distention is diffuse over the entire abdomen or limited to a portion of it, such as the upper or epigastric region. The detection of a mass or the visible outline of the intestine, such as the colon in congenital aganglionic megacolon, is also important. Intestinal movement or activity is rarely seen in the distended abdomen, but vigorous peristaltic movements of the intestine are virtually diagnostic of partial small bowel obstruction. Obesity of the abdomen often appears as folds or aprons of fat, especially in the suprapubic and flank areas. In such patients, generalized obesity is obvious, and the examiner must exclude other causes of abdominal distention, particularly if the patient complains of abdominal pain. Organomegaly, such as enlargement of the liver, spleen, kidneys (as in polycystic kidney disease), or uterus (pregnancy) can cause abdominal distention. Palpation will confirm these findings. There is an interesting condition termed *pseudocyesis,* or *pseudopregnancy,* in which a patient either imagines or wishes herself pregnant; this is associated with marked enlargement of the abdomen. Several kinds of cysts cause abdominal distention, including ovarian and mesenteric cysts and pancreatic pseudocysts. Ultrasound examination of the abdomen will confirm the above three diagnoses and permit clear differentiation from ascites. Chapter 8 discusses the examination of the pregnant patient.

Increased gas or air in the bowel causing abdominal distention can occur for several reasons:

- Intestinal obstruction caused by mechanical factors such as adhesions from previous surgery, incarcerated hernia, neoplasms of the small or large bowel, foreign bodies, volvulus, intussusception, and stenosis of the gut as in regional enteritis
- Adynamic or paralytic ileus, which is characterized by decreased or absent bowel sounds and which can occur after surgical operations in the abdomen; perforated viscus causing peritonitis; acute pancreatitis; mesenteric vascular disease causing gut infarction; metabolic disorders such as diabetic ketoacidosis (DKA), hypokalemia, and uremia; and drugs causing hypomotility, such as anticholinergics
- Intestinal pseudo-obstruction in which the gut is dilated with the seeming clinical picture of mechanical obstruction but no obstruction can be identified

Intestinal pseudo-obstruction can occur as a result of infiltrative disorders such as scleroderma and amyloidosis; metabolic disorders such as hypothyroidism and diabetes with associated visceral autonomic neuropathy; drugs such as anticholinergics, tricyclics, and ganglionic blockers; and finally as the idiopathic (often familial) varieties associated with either a hollow visceral neuropathy or hollow visceral myopathy, as discussed in detail below under auscultation. Abdominal distention with tympany and hyperactive peristaltic sounds should suggest mechanical obstruction, whereas distention and tympany with diminished or absent sounds should suggest either adynamic ileus or intestinal pseudo-obstruction.

Free air in the peritoneal cavity causing abdominal distention and tympany can occur with several disorders, including the following:

- Perforated viscera (duodenal or gastric ulcer, colonic diverticulum, gastric or colonic neoplasms, sharp foreign bodies)
- Traumatic rupture
- Therapeutic pneumoperitoneum
- After laparoscopy and rupture of gas-filled cysts as in pneumatosis cystoides intestinalis

The most common neoplastic causes of abdominal distention include primary and metastatic tumors of the liver, gastric carcinoma, pancreatic carcinoma, colon carcinoma, and intraabdominal lymphoma.

Ascites

Ascites, or free fluid within the peritoneal cavity, is an important cause of abdominal distention, and the most common cause of ascites is cirrhosis of the

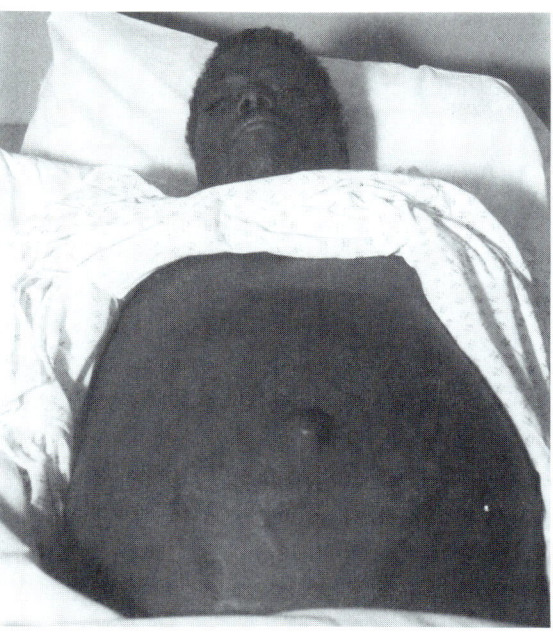

Fig. 5-2 A 40-year-old man with biopsy-proven cirrhosis of the liver caused by excessive consumption of alcohol over a 20-year period. Note the markedly protuberant abdomen. With diuretic therapy the patient lost 20 kg (44 lb), and his abdominal girth decreased from 125 to 95 cm.

liver. The physical findings characteristic of ascites include protuberant abdomen, bulging flanks, positive fluid wave, shifting dullness, and puddle sign, all of which are discussed in detail below (Fig. 5-2). In addition, an umbilical hernia may be present. The differential diagnosis of ascites is detailed in the box on pg. 222. *Chylous ascites* is characterized by a milky look to the ascitic fluid, which results from markedly increased concentrations of triglycerides in ascitic fluid. The diagnosis of chylous ascites is confirmed by demonstrating that triglyceride levels in peritoneal fluid exceed that of plasma. Triglycerides deriving from the intestinal absorption of lipid traverse the gut lymphatics and ultimately drain into the thoracic duct. Any disease process that either obstructs the major intraabdominal lymphatics or causes their rupture can be expected to result in chylous ascites. Thus, intraabdominal lymphomas, Hodgkin's disease, inadvertent incision of major lymphatics in the porta hepatis during portal systemic shunt surgery, and intestinal lymphangiectasia with hypoplastic intraabdominal lymphatics are all causes of chylous ascites.

JAUNDICE

The terms *jaundice* and *icterus* are used to designate yellow-appearing skin and eyes resulting from retention and deposition of bilirubin pigments (bilirubin diglucuronide and monoglucuronide). Although bilirubin stains all tissues, jaundice is most evident in the sclerae, face, and trunk. Jaundice is most commonly caused by parenchymal liver diseases such as viral hepatitis or cirrhosis, obstruction of the extrahepatic biliary tree as in choledocholithiasis and carcinoma of the pancreas, and less commonly by disorders associated with brisk hemolysis such as sickle cell anemia. The key elements of the history and physical examination of the jaundiced patient and the differential diagnosis of jaundice are discussed in a later section (see below).

Ecchymoses localized to the abdomen and flanks occur in only a few conditions. Such discolorations may appear bluish, blue-purple, blue-red,

Differential Diagnosis of Ascites

I. Transudative effusions
   A. Cirrhosis of the liver*
   B. Congestive heart failure*
   C. Constrictive pericarditis*
   D. Obstruction to the hepatic veins (Budd-Chiari syndrome)*
      1. Associated with tumors (hepatoma, hypernephroma, cancer of pancreas)
      2. Associated with hematologic disorders (myeloproliferative disease, polycythemia vera, myeloid metaplasia)
      3. Caused by infections (pyelophlebitis)
   E. Obstruction to the inferior vena cava
   F. Nephrotic syndrome
   G. Viral hepatitis with submassive or massive hepatic necrosis
   H. Meigs' syndrome
   I. Myelofibrosis
II. Exudative effusions
   A. Neoplastic diseases involving the peritoneum*
      1. Peritoneal carcinomatosis
      2. Lymphomatous disorders
   B. Tuberculous peritonitis*
   C. Pancreatitis* (also leaking pseudocyst and disrupted main pancreatic duct)
   D. Talc or starch powder peritonitis following surgery
   E. Transected lymphatics following portal-caval shunt surgery
   F. Myxedema
   G. Sarcoidosis
   H. Lymphatic obstruction
      1. Intestinal lymphangiectasia
      2. Lymphomas
   I. Pseudomyxoma peritonei
   J. Struma ovarii
   K. Amyloidosis
   L. Previous abdominal trauma with ruptured lymphatics
   M. Nephrogenic ascites†
III. Disorders simulating ascites
   A. Pancreatic pseudocyst
   B. Hydronephrosis
   C. Ovarian cyst
   D. Mesenteric cyst
   E. Obesity

*Most common disorders.
†Occurs in patients with renal failure on maintenance hemodialysis.
From Greenberger NJ: *Gastrointestinal disorders: a pathophysiological approach,* ed 4, Chicago, 1989, Mosby–Year Book, p 367.

blue-green, or green-brown, depending on the degree of hemoglobin degradation on the tissues. When associated with severe acute pancreatitis, such discoloration of the abdomen is termed Grey Turner's sign; the finding implies increased likelihood of mortality. Other less common causes of ecchymoses include rhabdomyolysis, muscle infarction, mesenteric thrombosis or strangulated bowel with extensive gut infarction, and massive intraperitoneal bleeding.

ABDOMINAL HERNIAS

External hernias are protrusions of a part of the abdominal cavity within a peritoneal sac through a weak point in the abdominal wall into an extraabdominal space. The several types of hernias include:

- Inguinal hernias
- Femoral hernias
- Obturator hernias
- Richter's hernia
- Umbilical hernias
- Spigelian hernias
- Incisional hernias (Fig. 5-3)

Gas in a herniated loop may cause peristaltic sounds. If the contents of the hernial sac can be easily replaced, the hernia is said to be *reducible;* if they cannot, the hernia is *irreducible* or *incarcerated.* When the blood supply of the incarcerated contents is interrupted, the hernia is strangulated, and gangrene may quickly ensue.

Inguinal hernias are often described as indirect or direct. Knowledge of basic anatomy is important to understand such hernias. The inguinal ligament extends between the anterosuperior iliac space and the pubis. Above and parallel to the

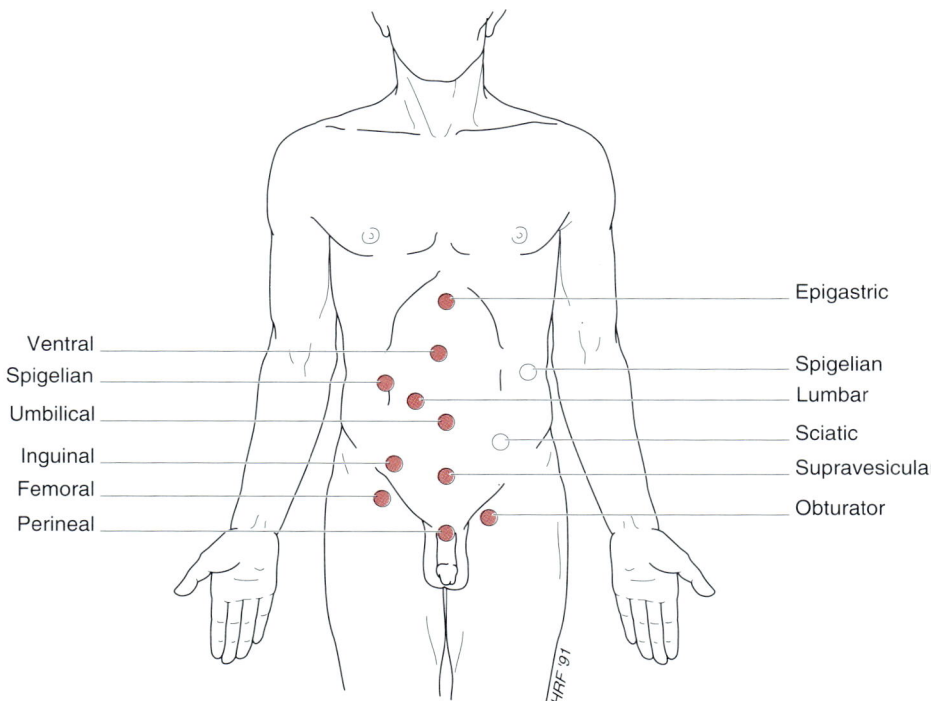

Fig. 5-3 The typical location of various hernias. Open circles indicate posterior. For details, see text.

inguinal ligament is the inguinal canal. The lateral end of the canal is the internal inguinal ring. The spermatic cord in males exits the abdominal cavity through the internal inguinal ring, enters the inguinal canal, and emerges from the subcutaneous or external ring just lateral to the pubis and passes over the inguinal ligament into the scrotum. An inguinal hernia follows the course of the spermatic cord in males and may traverse all or a part of the inguinal canal and actually descend into the scrotal sac (see Figs. 5-3 and 6-7). In females, the inguinal canal contains the round ligament, and an inguinal hernia follows the same course. Thus an indirect inguinal hernia produces a bulge over the midpoint of the inguinal ligament. A hernia through the posterior wall of the inguinal canal is termed direct. This usually produces a bulge *above* the inguinal ligament and often medial to the site of the bulge for an indirect hernia. With large inguinal hernias, the distinction between direct and indirect becomes academic.

To determine whether an inguinal hernia is present, place the tip of the index finger at the uppermost part of the scrotum and insert it gently into the subcutaneous or external inguinal ring (see Fig. 6-6). The patient should then cough or strain; a hernia causes an impulse felt on the fingertips. Large hernias feel like a mass in the inguinal canal or above the inguinal ligament. In males, the presence of bowel in the scrotal sac can be confirmed by listening for and detecting peristaltic bowel sounds over the scrotum.

Femoral hernias represent about 5% of hernias but, importantly, 20% incarcerate because of the narrow neck of the hernia sac. The femoral canal lies about 2 to 3 cm medial to both the femoral artery and femoral vein. *Obturator hernias* are unusual and usually affect elderly, thin, emaciated women. Such hernias are characterized by protrusion of a peritoneal sac through the obturator foramen, causing a fullness or mass on the femoral triangle. Because the hernia contents often press on the femoral nerve, pain or paresthesias running down the anteromedial thigh are characteristic. A tender mass can be palpated by rectal or vaginal examination. *Richter's hernia* describes a variant in which only a portion of the bowel circumference is incarcerated in the hernia sac. The most frequent sites of involvement are the femoral and inguinal regions.

Umbilical hernias occur in obese multiparous women with long-standing ascites and in those with prolonged increase in intrathoracic pressures such as in patients with asthma and chronic bronchitis. Patients with ascites are at increased risk of hernia rupture, strangulation, and ulceration.

Spigelian hernias are unusual anterior abdominal wall hernias that usually occur below the umbilicus but well above the inguinal ligament. Such hernias occur between the muscle fiber and aponeurosis of the transversus abdominis muscle when a peritoneal sac with extraperitoneal fat perforates the semilunaris to actually lie within the abdominal wall; they are covered by skin, subcutaneous fat, and the aponeurosis of the abdominal oblique muscle. One can suspect this diagnosis when the patient has a painful bulge in the anterior abdominal wall that is accentuated by standing and coughing.

Incisional hernias are characterized by bulges adjacent to scar tissue. Having the patient flex the neck and perform Valsalva's maneuver or cough often accentuates the hernia.

Percussion

Percussion of the abdomen is important for several reasons. First, the size of solid organs such as the liver and spleen can be evaluated by percussion. One can

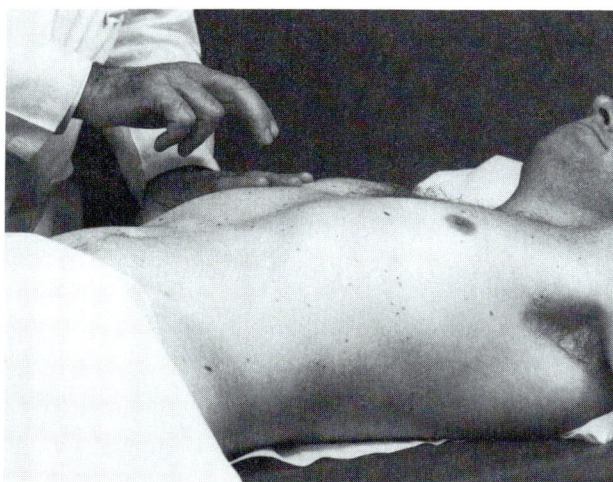

Fig. 5-4 Determination of liver size by percussion over the lower right anterior chest and the RUQ of the abdomen.

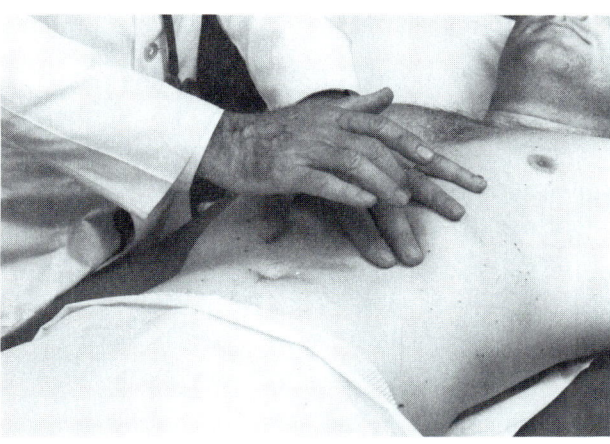

Fig. 5-5 Technique for percussion of the spleen. If splenomegaly is present, the percussion note will be dull, and with inspiration the spleen moves downward and medially and the percussion note changes accordingly.

often determine whether an increased amount of intraperitoneal fluid (i.e., ascites) is present. Furthermore, the finding of generalized or sharply localized increased tympany frequently indicates the presence of dilated bowel and possible intestinal obstruction. Lastly, unexpected dullness over an area may indicate a mass.

Assess the upper and lower border of liver dullness by percussion along the right midclavicular line from the mid-chest to the mid-abdomen (Fig. 5-4). The liver size can be further assessed by having the patient inspire and noting the descent of the liver (see Fig. 5-1, C). The lower border of liver dullness alerts the examiner to the site where the liver edge should be palpable. The liver span, as judged by liver dullness, measures between 10 to 12 cm in men and 8 to 11 cm in women. A sudden *decrease* in liver dullness can occur in several conditions, such as viral hepatitis with the development of submassive or massive liver cell necrosis, localized dilation of the transverse colon (as in toxic megacolon associated with ulcerative colitis), and ileus associated with peritonitis or a perforated viscus (e.g., duodenal ulcer, ruptured diverticulum).

Normally the spleen is not palpable, but percussion over the spleen reveals an area of dullness extending from the tenth rib posteriorly at the midaxillary line to the left anterior chest (Fig. 5-5). If the patient inspires, the area of splenic

Fig. 5-6 Technique for eliciting a fluid wave. The examiner's left hand is placed on the right lateral abdomen and the right hand taps the left flank or loin while a second examiner or the patient's hand compresses the abdomen in the midline. For further details, see text.

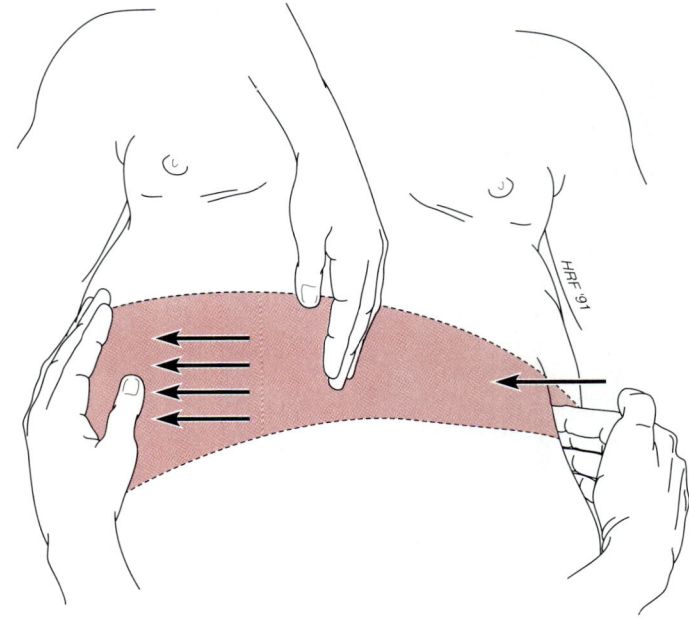

dullness moves inferiorly and to the right. Percussion of splenic dullness is important for three reasons:

1. It may indicate splenic enlargement before the spleen can actually be palpated.
2. It alerts the examiner to the site where the spleen might be palpated.
3. Increasing dullness in the left flank may be a valuable clue to the diagnosis of a traumatic rupture of the spleen or a subcapsular hematoma.

Assessment of shifting dullness is often used to determine whether ascites is present. When free fluid is present in the abdomen, such fluid gravitates to the flanks, and the intestines float upward when the patient lies on his back. Percussion with the patient in this position will disclose tympany over the anterior abdomen and dullness over the flanks. However, if the patient is now turned on one side, the dullness shifts, and the percussion noted on the side that is uppermost becomes tympanic, as that area is now occupied by gas-filled intestine.

Another physical finding pointing to a diagnosis of ascites is the *fluid wave*. A fluid wave is demonstrated by tapping the left flank sharply with the right hand while the left hand is placed against the opposite flank (Fig. 5-6). In addition, either the patient or a second examiner must place the ulnar surface of his hand along the midline of the abdomen. A positive test is one in which an impulse on the opposite flank is percussed after tapping the right flank. Both the test for shifting dullness and a fluid wave will not uniformly detect modest amounts of ascitic fluid (< 1000 ml). Indeed, both tests have a sensitivity of only about 60%; furthermore, the tests can be spuriously positive in obese patients.

A third test, bulging flanks, while often noted in ascites, is frequently present in obese subjects as well. A fourth test of ascites is the puddle sign. In this test the patient lies prone for a few minutes, then is positioned on hands and knees. The diaphragm of the stethoscope is placed over the most dependent part of the abdomen, where puddling would be expected to occur. The examiner then repeatedly flicks the near flank of the abdomen while moving the stethoscope

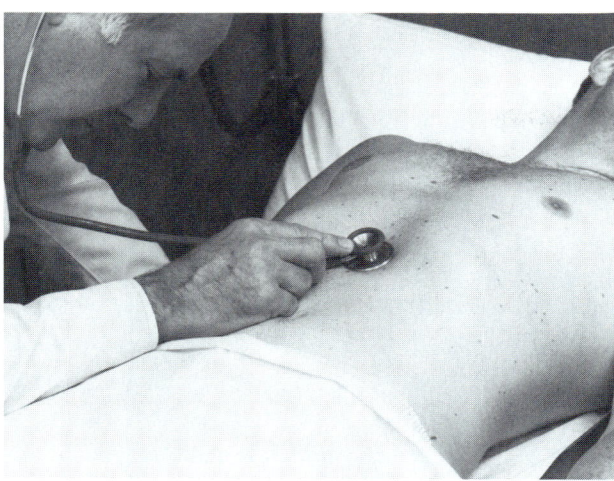

Fig. 5-7 Technique for auscultation of the abdomen. The examiner should use both the diaphragm and the bell of the stethoscope and listen over the lower spleen, kidneys, and aorta for bruits. For further details, see text and Table 5-4.

toward the opposite flank. A positive test consists of a definite change in the intensity and character of the percussion note as the stethoscope is moved.

The presence or absence of ascites can be confirmed most reliably by imaging procedures such as ultrasound or CT scans.

Finally, the urinary bladder is often percussed in the hypogastrium, especially if urinary retention is present.

Auscultation

Although often omitted from the physical examination, auscultation of the abdomen can elicit valuable signs. The technique for auscultation of the abdomen is depicted in Fig. 5-7. Interpretation of bowel sounds requires a fundamental knowledge of the causes of such sounds and continued practice. Peristaltic sounds require that both fluid and air be present in the lumen of the bowel; it is their movement in the intestine that produces normal sounds. Thus a normal peristaltic wave produces audible sounds of air and fluid moving along a tube. It is preferable, although not essential, that auscultation be done before percussion or palpation, as stimulating the viscera may obscure vascular murmurs or bruits.

PERISTALTIC SOUNDS

Place the bell or diaphragm of the stethoscope to either the right or left of the umbilicus and note the frequency and character of the sounds. Ordinarily, two to three gurgling-type sounds are heard per minute. If no sounds are apparent, listen in all four quadrants for 1 to 2 minutes. Bowel sounds can sometimes be stimulated by flicking the abdominal wall with the fingers.

Two types of abnormal peristaltic sounds can be heard: absence of bowel sounds, and increased or abnormal bowel sounds. Absence of bowel sounds occurs when motility of the bowel is inhibited, as with ileus resulting from peritonitis, inflammation as in acute pancreatitis, reflex ileus as in pneumonia, anticholinergic drugs, mesenteric thrombosis, gangrenous bowel, hypothyroidism, frank uremia, or spinal cord injury.

Conversely, increased activity can occur with brisk diarrhea as in gastroenteritis and with disorders such as intestinal obstruction or pyloric outlet obstruction. High-pitched bowel sounds that are often loud and associated with

TABLE 5-4: Abdominal Bruits: Diagnostic Considerations

Location of Bruits	Diagnostic Considerations	Comment
Liver	• Alcoholic hepatitis • Hepatoma • Surgically created • Portal-systemic shunt • Hepatic artery aneurysm • Hepatic AV fistula (trauma)	• Bruits may change day to day • Suspect in decompensated cirrhotics with a disproportionately raised serum alkaline phosphatase
Spleen	• Splenic artery aneurysm • Splenorenal shunt • Splenic AV fistula	• May see calcification in LUQ on plain films of the abdomen
Aorta	• Calcified aorta • Aortic aneurysm • Celiac axis compression • Celiac/superior mesenteric; artery disease (atheroma; thrombi)	 • Bruits common in thin individuals, especially after meals • Intestinal angina characterized by triad of (1) bruit, (2) weight loss, and (3) postprandial abdominal pain
LF upper quadrant	• Pancreatic cancer (body/tail)	• Bruit is caused by encasement of splenic artery or vein by tumor; present in 25% of cases
Umbilicus	• Cruveilhier-Baumgarten syndrome	• Bruits is caused by increased flow through umbilical veins secondary to portal hypertension
Kidneys	• Renal artery stenosis (atheroma; emboli) • Renal artery fibromuscular hyperplasia • Renal artery aneurysm	• Bruits may be unilateral or bilateral

rushes are termed *borborygmi*. These are particularly significant as they indicate possible mechanical obstruction. Such loud gurgling and tinkling sounds are caused by exaggerated peristalsis attempting to push fluid and air against an obstruction. The tetrad of findings of cramping abdominal pain, vomiting, abdominal distention, and borborygmi is virtually diagnostic of small bowel obstruction.

SUCCUSSION SPLASH

The presence of increased amounts of fluid in the stomach, as occurs after a meal, frequently produces a splashing sound when the stethoscope is placed over the stomach and the patient is rocked from side to side. However, if a succussion splash is audible after an overnight fast or after 12 to 24 hours of taking nothing by mouth, pyloric outlet obstruction is likely present. The causes of pyloric outlet obstruction include PUD with pyloroduodenal scarring, regional enteritis, tumors (gastric, pancreatic, duodenal), acute pancreatitis, and foreign bodies.

ABDOMINAL BRUITS

Bruits are systolic sounds usually created by the turbulence of blood flowing through diseased or compressed blood vessels. The many causes of abdominal bruits are listed in Table 5-4. The most common causes of such bruits include

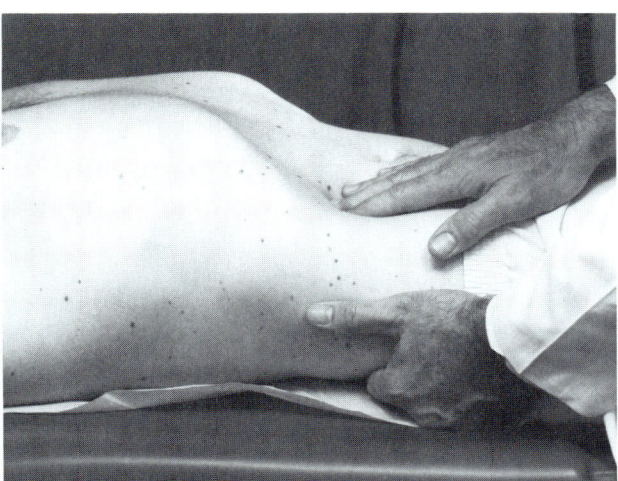

Fig. 5-8 Technique for palpation of the liver. For details, see text.

calcification of the aorta, celiac axis compression, and alcoholic hepatitis. An epigastric bruit can be appreciated in 20% of healthy thin young adults, especially if auscultation is carried out after a meal. Such bruits are usually caused by compression of the celiac axis artery by muscle fibers compressing the crus of the diaphragm. Abdominal bruits are often important clues leading to the diagnosis of hepatoma, renal artery stenosis, fibromuscular hyperplasia of the renal arteries, intestinal angina, aortic aneurysm, and pancreatic cancer.

PERITONEAL FRICTION RUBS

A friction rub heard over the liver should suggest the diagnosis of liver metastases or primary hepatocellular carcinoma. Other causes of hepatic friction rubs include infarction of the liver (as in sickle cell anemia and polyarteritis nodosa), liver abscess, and following needle biopsy of the liver. A transient friction rub caused by a hematoma around the puncture site is common after liver biopsy but is usually no longer audible 4 to 6 hours after biopsy.

Palpation

The most important procedure in the physical examination of the abdomen is palpation, especially when the patient's chief complaint is abdominal pain. One important feature of palpation is to confirm and amplify the findings obtained from the history and inspection, percussion, and auscultation of the abdomen. Thus, as an example, a mass that is barely visible on inspection may be firm or soft, fixed or movable, smooth or irregular, tender, or cystic. Importantly, a mass that may not be visible can often be felt on palpation.

All quadrants of the abdomen must be palpated in an orderly fashion. When palpating the abdomen, make sure the hand is warm and the entire palm and extended fingers of the right hand are placed flat and held parallel to the surface of the abdomen (Fig. 5-8). Use the pads of the fingers together to perform a light general palpation. Use light palpation of the abdomen first and, as tense muscles relax, then try deeper palpation. Avoid quick, jabbing movements. Note any areas of tenderness or increased muscular resistance and examine them in detail.

Having the patient clearly discriminate between the sensation of pain versus pressure of the palpating hand is useful. Press firmly on a nontender area such as the shoulder or anterior chest and indicate to the patient that he should perceive

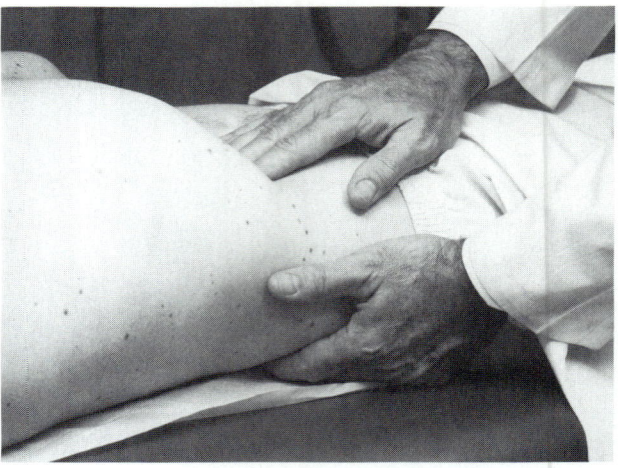

Fig. 5-9 Technique for palpation of the liver. For details, see text.

this as pressure. After light palpation, place the index finger firmly in each of nine areas (see Fig. 5-1, *B*) two or three times and determine whether this elicits a sensation of pain or pressure. In this manner, the examiner can determine whether the patient's discomfort is reproducibly localized to a specific area of the abdomen. This approach will also help the examiner determine whether the patient is unduly sensitive to discomfort (i.e., hyperpathic). If no region of the abdomen is suspected of harboring pathology, palpation should begin in both iliac fossae and work upward to the costal margins. In this manner, a markedly enlarged liver or spleen, that might otherwise be missed because the edge is not felt, can be appreciated.

LIVER

As noted above, percussion should have alerted the examiner to the approximate size and lower edge of the liver. Beginning at the right iliac fossa, move the right hand gradually upward until the edge of the liver is appreciated (Fig. 5-9). The patient can also be asked to take a deep breath slowly; the descent of the diaphragm carries the liver down, which facilitates palpation of the liver edge. The edge of the liver can be felt in the majority of normal subjects if the patient's anterior abdominal wall muscles are relaxed and he takes a slow deep breath. Occasionally, in normal subjects, a fairly low-lying thin segment of liver can be palpated in the RUQ; this is termed *Riedel's lobe* of the liver. An alternative approach to feeling the liver edge is to gently curl the fingers of the right hand below the costal margin in the suspected vicinity of the liver edge and ask the patient to inspire slowly (Fig. 5-10). In this manner the liver edge will descend and be appreciated by the finger tips. This method is important in delineating minimal enlargement of the liver or a liver palpable only in the epigastrium, as may occur in advanced cirrhosis.

The examiner should describe whether the liver is soft or firm and hard or irregular, whether the edge rounded or sharp, whether or not discrete masses are present, and whether the left lobe is palpable across the midline. Further, note the size of the liver as judged by the location of the edge below the right midclavicular line and the xiphoid. Normally, the liver edge is sharp, smooth, and not hard, and the left lobe is not palpable. A rounded edge suggests liver disease. A palpable left lobe suggests either chronic, infiltrative, or neoplastic liver disease. Modest

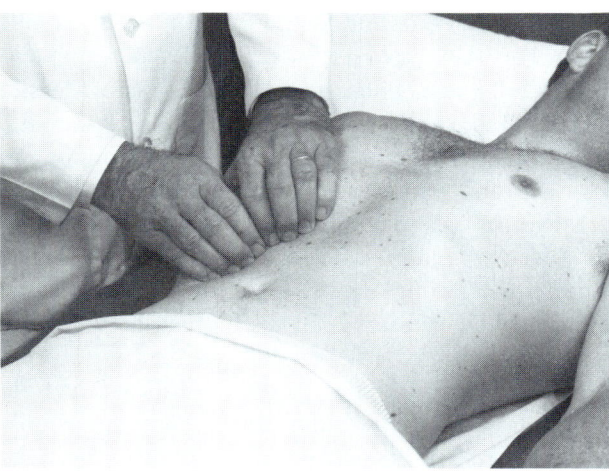

Fig. 5-10 Alternative technique for palpation of the liver. The best results are obtained with gentle pressure of the curled fingers on the anterior abdominal wall. For further details, see text.

enlargement of the liver occurs in several disorders, most notably viral hepatitis, chronic active liver disease, cirrhosis, choledocholithiasis, and extrahepatic biliary tract obstruction, but not in metastatic liver disease as in early stages of pancreatic carcinoma. Marked enlargement of the liver (edge > 10 cm below the costal margin) occurs in relatively few disorders:

- Primary and metastatic tumors of the liver, including lymphomas
- Alcoholic liver disease (fatty liver, alcoholic hepatitis, cirrhosis)
- Severe congestive heart failure
- Infiltrative diseases of the liver such as amyloidosis and myelofibrosis
- Chronic myelogenous leukemia

Finally, a pulsatile liver should raise the question of tricuspid regurgitation, which may occur with advanced mitral stenosis or following endocarditis of the tricuspid valve.

SPLEEN

As noted above, percussion of the LUQ may have alerted the examiner to the presence of an enlarged spleen. Palpation for the spleen should begin in the left iliac fossa and move upward to the left costal margin (Fig. 5-11). If the spleen is

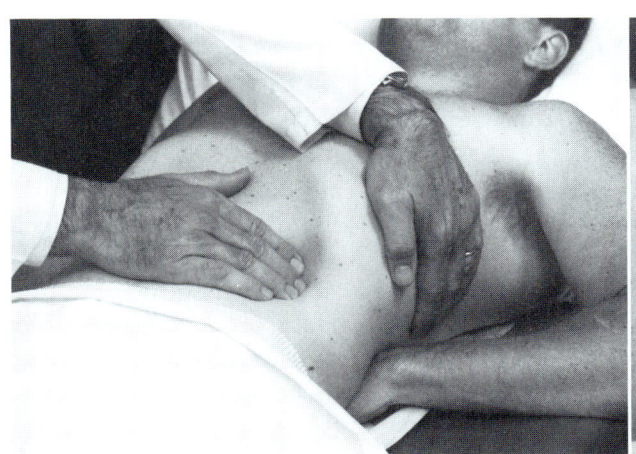
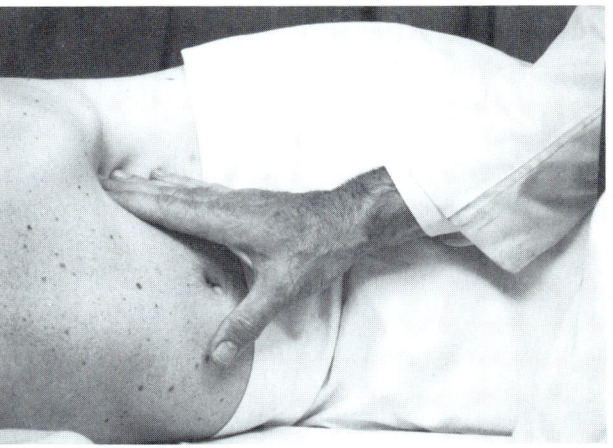

Fig. 5-11 A and B, Techniques for palpation of the spleen. Palpation with the patient in the right lateral decubitus position should be carried out in all patients with suspected splenomegaly if the spleen is not felt with the patient in the supine position.

not felt while the patient is supine, the patient should roll over on the right side so the examiner can again examine the LUQ (see Fig. 5-11, *B*). This method takes advantage of the fact that when the spleen enlarges, it becomes more easily palpable inferiorly and medially. This enlargement is better appreciated when the patient is in the right lateral decubitus position. Alternatively, the examiner can stand at the patient's left side with the patient's left hand placed under the eleventh rib so as to elevate the thorax. The examiner then curls the fingers of either one or both hands below the costal margin and asks the patient to inspire. The splenic margin may then be felt by the fingertips.

A common problem in evaluating LUQ masses is to distinguish between the spleen and the left kidney. Palpation of a notch on the medial surface suggests that the organ being palpated is the spleen. Differentiation of the left lobe of the liver from the spleen may be difficult if massive hepatomegaly exists. One can usually discern a space or open area between the two organs. Common causes of splenomegaly include the following:

- Portal hypertension caused by cirrhosis of the liver
- Infections (viral, bacterial, fungal)
- Leukemias, lymphomas, and Hodgkin's disease
- Connective-tissue diseases (e.g., SLE and rheumatoid arthritis)
- Infiltrative disorders (e.g., amyloidosis and sarcoidosis)
- Hemolytic disorders
- Myelofibrosis

GALLBLADDER

The gallbladder, when enlarged, can often be palpated in the RUQ at the angle formed by the lateral border of the rectus abdominis muscle and the right costal margin (see Fig. 5-1). The gallbladder is palpable in approximately 25% of cases of carcinoma of the head of the pancreas *(Courvoisier's law)* because of painless distension of the gallbladder. The gallbladder is also palpable in about 30% of patients with acute cholecystitis, often because of stones impacted in the neck of the gallbladder. In acute cholecystitis, often rather marked RUQ tenderness is present and palpation may be difficult because of intense involuntary spasm of the abdominal muscles. Percussion over the right lower anterior chest and RUQ often elicits pain.

Another sign pointing to acute cholecystitis is RUQ pain aggravated by inspiration *(Murphy's sign)*. The patient is asked to inspire after the examining fingers are placed high in the RUQ; inspiration causes the gallbladder to descend and come in contact with the extended fingers, causing pain and inspiratory arrest.

KIDNEYS

The kidneys are normally about 11 to 12 cm in length and about 5 cm in width; the right kidney is in front of the twelfth rib and the left kidney a bit higher, between the eleventh and twelfth rib. Normally the kidneys cannot be palpated. When a kidney enlarges, it is bordered superiorly by the twelfth rib and posteriorly by the psoas muscle; consequently, most enlargement occurs downward and anteriorly. Bimanual palpation (one hand anterior just under the costal margin and the other posterior under the lower thorax) may be necessary to discern an enlarged kidney. The most common causes of enlarged kidneys include polycystic kidney disease, hypernephroma, renal cysts, and hydronephrosis. Infrequently, a normal-sized kidney is displaced from its normal position to sites inferiorly; this is termed a *ptotic kidney*.

AORTA

The aorta is frequently palpable in normal individuals (especially if they are thin) just to the left of the midline; the approximate diameter of the aorta by palpation is usually less than 3 to 4 cm. A diameter greater than 6 cm indicates an aortic aneurysm. A mass with expansive pulsations suggests an aortic aneurysm. Systolic bruits are often present with both aortic aneurysms and heavily calcified aortas. A mass associated with the pulsation is most likely a transmitted pulsation through a pancreatic or gastric tumor, cyst, or pseudocyst.

MASSES AND BOWEL LOOPS

Palpable masses are characterized by location and size, and whether they are hard or soft, movable or fixed, regular or irregular, cystic or fluctuant, and tender or nontender. Not infrequently, masses are better appreciated by light rather than by deep palpation. If it is not clear that a mass is present, simultaneously palpate the contralateral area of the abdomen to try and discern a difference between the two areas of the abdomen. RLQ masses may represent the following:

- Cecal or right colon carcinomas
- Appendiceal abscess
- Thickened ileum and/or right colon that feels "sausagelike" as occurs in Crohn's disease
- Cysts (mesenteric, ovarian)
- Hernias
- Feces in the right colon

LLQ masses may represent the following:

- Colon carcinoma
- Colonic diverticular disease with a markedly thickened colonic musculature, which is termed *myochosis*
- Pericolic abscess
- Thickened colon as in Crohn's colitis
- Ovarian cyst
- Feces in the left colon
- Hernias

RUQ masses may represent the following:

- Hepatomegaly with or without additional lesions
- The right kidney
- An enlarged gallbladder
- An inflamed and enlarged pancreas or pancreatic pseudocyst

LUQ masses may represent the following:

- The spleen; the stomach
- The left kidney
- An inflamed and enlarged pancreas or pancreatic pseudocyst
- An aortic aneurysm or splenic artery aneurysm

Epigastric masses may represent lesions in the stomach, omentum, left lobe of the liver, pancreas, gallbladder, or transverse colon.

Hypogastric masses may reflect the following:

- An enlarged uterus (pregnancy, uterine carcinoma, uterine fibromyomata)
- An enlarged bladder
- An aortic aneurysm
- A hematoma of the rectus abdominis muscle
- An ovarian cyst

The umbilical and periumbilical area should be palpated carefully; a hard periumbilical lymph node (Sister Joseph nodule) suggests metastatic disease from a GI tract, pelvic, or breast primary tumor. A distended bladder can usually be percussed and palpated, with disappearance of both abnormal physical findings after the bladder is emptied by voiding or catheterization.

FEMORAL PULSES AND DISTAL AORTA

The aorta divides about 2 to 3 cm below the umbilicus, giving rise to the common iliac arteries, which in turn give rise to the femoral arteries. A decreased or absent femoral pulse may be a vital clue to the diagnosis of the following:

- Severe atherosclerotic peripheral vascular disease
- Thrombosis of the common iliac artery
- Dissecting aortic aneurysm
- Coarctation of the aorta
- Thrombosis or saddle embolus at the aortic bifurcation (Leriche's syndrome)

A tetrad of findings, absent femoral pulses, intermittent claudication, gluteal pain, and impotence, strongly suggest the diagnosis of Leriche's syndrome.

RECTAL EXAMINATION

Examination of the rectum and perirectal structure is a vital part of the general physical examination and should never be omitted. Initially, examine the perirectal area by spreading the cheeks of the buttocks widely and looking for evidence of anal fistulas, hemorrhoids, perirectal inflammation, or anal fissures. Next, insert the lubricated index finger of the gloved hand into the rectum of the male in either the lateral decubitus or lithotomy position (Fig. 5-12). The prostate gland and seminal vesicles are felt anteriorly. Anterior and superior is the rectovesical pouch of the peritoneum, although the actual pouch is usually not palpable. Not infrequently, intraabdominal metastatic deposits occur in this area, producing the feeling of a hard shelf on rectal exam; this is termed a Blumer's shelf.

Because the average index finger is 8 to 10 cm in length, the distal rectum can be carefully examined for mass lesions by rotating the index finger slowly through a 360-degree arc. Rectal masses palpated in this manner may reflect the following:

- Carcinoma
- Melanoma (may be amelanotic)
- Lymphoma (rare)
- Perirectal abscesses (usually fluctuant and tender)
- Pelvic abscesses
- A normal cervix
- Appendiceal abscess

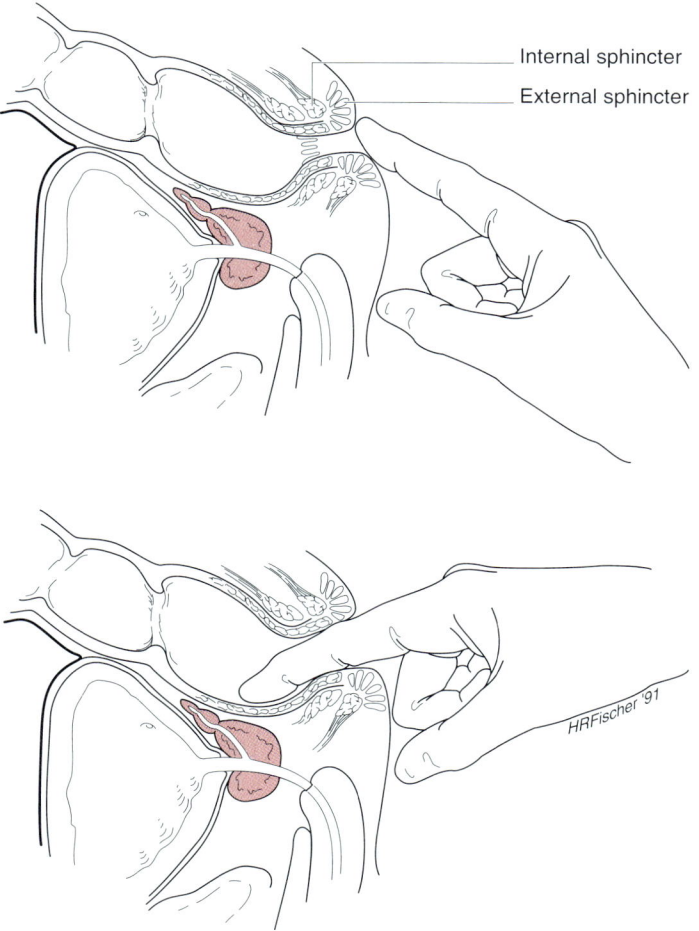

Fig. 5-12 Technique for examining the rectum. The prostate is in color. For further details, see text.

- Tubo-ovarian abscess
- Uterine lesions

For further details, see the chapters on examination of the male and female genitalia.

PELVIC EXAMINATION

This topic is discussed in Chapter 7.

Special Considerations in the Physical Examination of the Patient with Abdominal Pain

Attention is again called to the section on history taking in the patient with abdominal pain and the section concerning the patient and his discriminating between pain and pressure and the reproducibility of pain. The examiner must devote special attention to those areas of the abdomen identified as the site(s) of pain.

LOCALIZING PAIN TO INTRAABDOMINAL SITES

A useful maneuver to confirm that abdominal pain is of peritoneal or intraabdominal origin rather than of the anterior abdominal wall is to have the patient raise his head off the pillow, thus tensing the abdominal wall muscles. The increased tone of the abdominal wall muscles, in essence, insulates the underlying viscera from the pressure of the palpating hand and results in decreased pain. Conversely, if the site of abdominal pain is the anterior abdominal wall (as may occur in a hematoma or scar pain resulting from a neuroma), this maneuver will result in increased pain.

INVOLUNTARY GUARDING AND MUSCLE RIGIDITY

The detection and perception of abdominal rigidity and tenderness is important in evaluating the severity of intraperitoneal disease. Voluntary muscle guarding should be recognized and eliminated by reassuring the patient, by using firm but nontickling motions, and by warming the hands. When the examiner gains the patient's confidence and relaxation, one can usually detect involuntary guarding and various degrees of muscle rigidity. Persistence of rigidity proves it is involuntary. When such abdominal rigidity is diffuse, the peritoneal cavity is generally involved with an infectious, inflammatory, or neoplastic process. For example, rigidity is present in acute pancreatitis, acute mesenteric vascular occlusion, and generalized peritonitis. The most severe degree of abdominal rigidity, the "boardlike" abdomen, is felt in acute perforation of a viscus with free spillage of air or GI contents into the peritoneal cavity. This occurs with perforation of a peptic ulcer of the anterior duodenum, stomach, or jejunum, from perforated bowel in ulcerative colitis or regional ileitis, or from a ruptured colonic diverticulum. When perforations occur in patients receiving corticosteroid therapy, the intensity of the pain and the rigidity and tenderness are ameliorated so much that detection of these findings may be very difficult indeed. When local or generalized rigidity of the abdomen is present, detailed evaluation of abdominal tenderness is absolutely essential.

DIRECT AND INDIRECT TENDERNESS

Direct tenderness may be caused by localized inflammation of the abdominal wall, the peritoneum, or a viscus. However, pain resulting from palpation is most often caused by the stretching of the visceral peritoneum over an abdominal organ. Similarly, a solid organ may be tender when its capsule is distended (i.e. the liver in congestive heart failure). Rebound tenderness is tested for by pressing the tips of the fingers gently into the abdominal wall, both at a site where palpation previously elicited pain and also a site remote from it, and then suddenly withdrawing them from contact. The transient feeling of intense pain developing after withdrawal of pressure is termed *rebound tenderness;* it results from the sudden stretching of the involved parietal peritoneum on release of the hand. Rebound tenderness is all the more significant when pressure and release at a site remote from the area of direct tenderness elicits pain. Rebound tenderness is a reliable sign of peritoneal irritation and is usually, but not invariably, accompanied by diffuse tenderness.

"Jar" tenderness is also a reliable sign of peritoneal irritation. Many variations of this maneuver exist: the patient may indicate that the ride into the hospital by automobile, with stops and starts and bumps in the road, all jarring to him, caused increased abdominal pain. Similarly, if the examiner shakes the bed itself and jars the patient, it often results in pain. The examiner may ask the patient to move his body to and fro as if doing a hula dance, with resulting movement eliciting pain. If the patient can cooperate, his hopping on one leg will evoke pain. The latter test is especially helpful in evaluating children with abdominal pain and suspected

acute appendicitis. The above signs are often positive in patients with peritoneal irritation (e.g., acute pancreatitis) and often subside as the patient improves. Conversely, if all the above signs are negative, it argues against a diagnosis of peritoneal inflammation.

Evaluation of the Patient with Jaundice

Jaundice is common in patients with liver and biliary tract diseases. The important questions to ask patients with jaundice are summarized in the accompanying box, and the key elements in the physical examination are listed

History Taking in the Patient with Jaundice

General or Systemic Symptoms

- Anorexia
- Weight loss
- Chills and fever
- Arthritis and/or arthralgias
- Skin lesions
- Abdominal pain
- Other major illnesses

Specific Questions to Ask Patients with Jaundice

- Medications used; ask about over-the-counter medications (e.g., laxatives)
- Illicit or illegal drug use; needle injections
- Sexual practices (homosexuality; anal-receptive intercourse)
- Exposure to and contact with jaundiced persons
- Blood transfusions
- Occupational history; exposure to hepatotoxins
- Foreign travel
- Previous history of jaundice
- Family history of jaundice
- Previous history of gallbladder disease: gallbladder surgery; cholecystography; symptoms suggestive of cholecystitis
- Evolution of jaundice; sequential changes in color of urine and stool
- Pruritis
- Ingestion of raw shellfish
- Changes in smell: decreased sense of smell (hyposmia); unpleasant smells (dysosmia)
- Changes in taste: decreased sense of taste (hypogeusia); unpleasant tastes (dysgeusia)
- History of anemia: sickle cell disease; other hemoglobinopathies
- History of inflammatory bowel disease or protracted diarrhea
- History of alcohol ingestion
  - Obtain detailed quantitative history of both recent and previous use of alcohol
  - Evidence of withdrawal symptoms
  - Evidence of tolerance
  - History of alcohol-associated illnesses: erosive gastritis with upper GI bleeding; pancreatitis; peripheral neuropathy; organic brain syndrome
  - Psychosocial factors
- Recent change in menstrual cycles; amenorrhea

in the box below. The differential diagnosis of jaundice is listed in the box on the opposite page. In the adult patient presenting with jaundice, the odds are over 90% that the patient will have 1 of the disorders on the opposite page:

Physical Examination of the Jaundiced Patient

General Inspection

- Scleral icterus
- Pallor
- Wasting
- Needle tracks
- Evidence of skin excoriations
- Ecchymoses or petechiae
- Muscle tenderness and weakness
- Lymphadenopathy
- Evidence of pneumonia
- Evidence of congestive heart failure

Peripheral Stigmata of Liver Disease

- Spider angiomata
- Palmar erythema
- Gynecomastia*
- Dupuytren's contracture*
- Parotid enlargement*
- Testicular atrophy
- Paucity of axillary and pubic hair
- Eye signs mimicking hyperthyroidism

Abdominal Examination

- Hepatomegaly
- Splenomegaly
- Ascites
- Prominent abdominal collateral veins
- Bruits and rubs
- Abdominal masses
- Palpable gallbladder

Signs of "Decompensated" Hepatocellular Disease

- Jaundice
- Ascites
- Oliguric hepatic failure
- Hepatic encephalopathy
  - Fetor hepaticus
  - Asterixis
  - Behavioral alterations (confusion, disorientation, failure to complete simple mental tasks)

*The triad of physical findings of gynecomastia, Dupuytren's contracture, and parotid enlargement, if present, strongly suggests the diagnosis of alcoholic liver disease.

- Viral hepatitis
- Alcoholic liver disease
- Drug-induced jaundice
- Chronic active liver disease
- Choledocholithiasis
- Cancer of the pancreas
- Metastatic liver disease

Differential Diagnosis of Jaundice

I. Common causes
   A. Viral hepatitis
   B. Alcoholic liver disease
   C. Drug-induced liver disease
   D. Chronic active liver disease
   E. Choledocholithiasis, cholecystitis
   F. Carcinoma of the pancreas
   G. Metastatic liver disease
II. Less common causes
   A. Primary biliary cirrhosis
   B. Primary sclerosing cholangitis
   C. Gilbert syndrome
   D. Sickle cell anemia
   E. Hodgkin's disease and non-Hodgkin's lymphoma
III. Causes and presumed sites of intrahepatic cholestasis
   A. Liver cell (hepatocellular)
      - Viral hepatitis
      - Alcoholic liver disease
      - Chronic active liver disease
      - α-1-Antitrypsin deficiency
   B. Hepatocanalicular
      - Drugs (androgens, phenothiazines)
      - Sepsis
      - Postoperative
      - Total parenteral nutrition
      - Hodgkin's and non-Hodgkin's lymphoma
      - Amyloidosis
      - Sickle cell anemia
      - Toxic shock syndrome
   C. Ductular
      - Sarcoidosis
      - Primary biliary cirrhosis
   D. Bile ducts
      - Intrahepatic biliary atresia
      - Intrahepatic sclerosing cholangitis
      - Caroli's disease
      - Cholangiocarcinoma
   E. Recurrent cholestasis
      - Benign recurrent intrahepatic cholestasis
      - Recurrent jaundice pregnancy
      - Dubin-Johnson syndrome

If primary biliary cirrhosis, primary sclerosing cholangitis, Gilbert syndrome, sickle cell anemia, and Hodgkin's disease and non-Hodgkin's lymphoma are added to the lists, the odds increase to 98% to 99%.

A suggested diagnostic approach to the patient with jaundice is presented in Table 5-5. The key elements in the history and physical examinations are integrated with standard liver tests and special diagnostic procedures. A carefully obtained history and physical examination will provide the correct diagnosis in about 85% of jaundiced patients.

TABLE 5-5: Symptom: Jaundice

Cause of Jaundice	History	Physical Examination	Liver Test Abnormalities	Imaging/Invasive Procedures and Comment
Viral hepatis (hepatitis A, hepatitis B, hepatitis C)	• Anorexia • Exposure to jaundiced persons • Transfusion of blood products • Homosexual contacts • IV drug abuse • Systemic symptoms (see box on pg. 237) • Foreign travel	• Hepatomegaly (modest increase) • Splenomegaly (< 25% cases) • Absence of stigmata of chronic liver disease except spider angiomata may be present	• (+) Hepatitis serology • Hepatitis A antibody (HAV) with IgM fraction (+) • Hepatitis B surface antigen (HB$_c$Ag) and/or hepatitis B core antibody (HB$_c$Ab) (+) • Serum AST/ALT values increased • Prothrombin time usually normal; prolongation > 4 sec should raise questions of submassive hepatic necrosis	• Imaging procedures are not indicated for typical viral hepatitis • Ultrasonography and cholestatic liver test abnormalities to exclude dilated intrahepatic ducts should be considered in patients with protracted jaundice (> 1 mo). Cholestasis can occur with hepatitis, especially type A
Alcoholic liver disease • Fatty liver • Alcoholic hepatitis • Cirrhosis	• Alcohol abuse (see box on pg. 251) • > 40 g/day • Be sure to check with family members concerning alcohol intake • Amenorrhea • ↓ Libido/impotence • Abdominal distention • Weakness	• Peripheral stigmata or chronic liver disease (see Table 7-11) • Hepatomegaly (check for LF lobe) • Stigmata of portal hypertension • Splenomegaly • Ascites • ↑ Abdominal collateral veins • Malnutrition • Muscle weakness	• Markers of chronic alcoholism • ↑ MCV • ↑ AST (SGOT) • ↑ AST: ALT ratio > 3:1 • ↑ GGIP • ↓ Serum albumin • ↓ Serum cholesterol • ↑ (Prolonged) prothrombin time • AST/ALT usually < 300 units	• Presence of two physical findings (ascites and encephalopathy) and two laboratory findings (↓ albumin, ↑ prothrombin time) strongly suggests cirrhosis • If three stigmata of portal hypertension present, esophageal varices

TABLE 5-5: Symptom: Jaundice—cont'd

Cause of Jaundice	History	Physical Examination	Liver Test Abnormalities	Imaging/Invasive Procedures and Comment
	• Fatigue	• RUQ bruits • Edema • Signs of hepatic encephalopathy (see text and box on pg. 238)	• Alkaline phosphatase usually only modestly ↑ (< 3+ units) • Hepatitis B markers usually (−)	are likely; if three laboratory tests (albumin, cholesterol, prothrombin time) are abnormal, this indicates markedly impaired hepatocellular synthetic function • With cholestatic liver tests, ultrasound should be considered to exclude dilated intrahepatic ducts

Drug-induced	• A careful drug history is mandatory in all patients with jaundice; be sure to also inquire about over-the-counter preparations, especially acetaminophen-containing medication as well as antibiotics, diuretics, isoniazid, sulfonamides, anticonvulsants, oral hypoglycemics, tranquilizers, and androgen preparations	• Liver is usually minimally enlarged if at all
		• Spleen is not enlarged
		• Stigmata of chronic parenchymal liver disease are absent
			• Either a cholestatic or hepatocellular injury pattern may be present
			• Cholestatic
			  • AST/ALT < 300
			  • Alkaline phosphatase ↑ > 3 × NL
			  • Serum proteins NL
			  • Prothrombin time NL
			• Hepatocellular
			  • AST/ALT > 300
			  • Alkaline phosphatase ↑ < 3 × NL
			  • Serum proteins normal or abnormal
			• Studies for viral hepatitis A and B are negative
				• The following tetrad of findings (fever, arthritis, rash, and eosinophilia) strongly suggests drug-induced jaundice
				• In cases with protracted jaundice (>1 mo) and persistent cholestatic liver test abnormalities, an ultrasound examination of the liver should be considered

Chronic active liver disease (CALD) • Chronic active hepatitis without cirrhosis	• Previous hepatitis B • Previous hepatitis C • Transfusions of blood products	• Check for Kayser-Fleischer rings • Hepatomegaly (check for LF lobe)	• AST/ALT usually ↑ > 5 × NL • Reversed albumin globulin ratio, often with serum globulin > 4.0 gm/dl	• Diagnosis of CALD is established by liver biopsy

Continued.

TABLE 5-5: Symptom: Jaundice—cont'd

Cause of Jaundice	History	Physical Examination	Liver Test Abnormalities	Imaging/Invasive Procedures and Comment

Chronic active hepatitis with cirrhosis	• Homosexuality; rectal intercourse
	• History of
	  • Fever ⎱
	  • Arthritis ⎰ >3 months
	  • Fatigue ⎱
	• History of
	  • Anemia
	  • Colitis
	  • Neurologic abnormalities
	• History of drug use especially methyldopa, isoniazid, nitrofurantoin
		• Splenomegaly
		• Peripheral stigmata and chronic liver disease may be present (see box on pg. 238)
		• Stigmata portal hypertension
		• Hypertension (see above)
		• Edema
		• Striae, hirsutism may be present with autoimmune CALD (see above)
			• Serum antinuclear antibodies (ANA) and/or smooth muscle antibody (SMA) (+) in ~85% cases of autoimmune chronic active hepatitis
			• May see cholestatic features
			• Must exclude Wilson's disease and α-1-antitrypsin deficiency in all CALD patients < 35 years of age; check urine copper serum ceruloplasmin and for Kayser-Fleischer rings	

Choledocholithiasis	• RUQ pain • Previous episodes of biliary colic • Factors predisposing to gallstones • (+) Family history • Female • Obese • Ethnic background • Medications (oral contraceptives, clofibrate) • Ileal disease/resection • Short bowel syndrome • On total parenteral nutrition	• Hepatomegaly (tender) • Palpable gallbladder (33% of cases) • (+) Murphy's sign • (+) RUQ pouch tenderness • Absence of peripheral stigmata of chronic liver disease • Fever, tachycardia, tachypnea should suggest diagnosis of ascending cholangitis with sepsis, especially if brisk leukocytosis and hypotension are also present	• Primarily cholestatic changes with ↑ serum alkaline phosphatase • AST/ALT ↑ but < 300 units (NOTE: 10% of patients will have transient [i.e., 48 to 72] increases in AST/ALT >300 units) • Normal serum proteins • Prothrombin time usually NL: if not, vitamin K → normalization of prothrombin time	• Ultrasound has > 90% sensitivity in demonstrating gallstones • Ultrasound has > 90% sensitivity and specificity in demonstrating dilated intrahepatic ducts if serum bilirubin ≥ 10 mg/dl for > 2 weeks • HIDA/PIPIDA scans have > 90% sensitivity in confirming diagnosis of acute cholecystitis • If ultrasound shows dilated ducts, the next procedure is either endoscopic retrograde cholangiopancreatography (ERCP) or percutaneous transhepatic cholangiography (PTC) (see Fig. 5-14)

TABLE 5-5: Symptom: Jaundice—cont'd

Cause of Jaundice	History	Physical Examination	Liver Test Abnormalities	Imaging/Invasive Procedures and Comment
Carcinoma of the pancreas	• New onset of persistent and unexplained abdominal or back pain • Painless jaundice • Weight loss • Anorexia • New onset of unexplained diarrhea • New onset of diabetes mellitus after age 50 without a reason (i.e., no family history, obesity, or diabetogenic drugs such as corticosteroids or thiazide diuretics)	• Lymphadenopathy • Hepatomegaly • Splenomegaly (splenic vein thrombosis) • Palpable gallbladder (25% cases) • Epigastric/LUQ mass • LUQ bruit • Ascites	• Cholestatic changes • 40% of cases have evidence of carbohydrate intolerance • Negative tests for viral hepatitis	• CT scan will be abnormal in > 80% of cases (see Fig. 5-15) • If CT scan shows a mass in the pancreas plus dilated intrahepatic ducts, the choices are to proceed to either laparatomy or ultrasound-guided diagnosis of the pancreatic mass or carry out ERCP or PTC to visualize the extrahepatic biliary tract. Either of the latter two procedures are clearly indicated if stenting the common bile duct is contemplated
Carcinoma of the pancreas —cont'd	• Stigmata of pancreatic exocrine insufficiency • Onset of acute pancreatitis after age 50 without obvious reason			

Primary biliary cirrhosis	• Predominantly women (9:1)
	• Pruritus
	• Asymptomatic patient with a disproportionately raised serum alkaline phosphatase
		• Skin excoriations
		• Xanthomas
		• Hepatomegaly
		• Splenomegaly
		• Peripheral neuropathy fairly common
		• Ascites and encephalopathy are late manifestations
		• Sjögren's syndrome may also be present
		• May see Kayser-Fleischer rings
			• Cholestatic liver tests with ↑↑ serum alkaline phosphatase
			• (+) Antimitochondrial antibody or AMA (> 95% cases)
			• ↑ Serum IgM
			• ↑ Serum cholesterol
			• Synthetic function well preserved until late stage of the disease
			• Negative tests for viral hepatitis
			• AST/ALT < 300
				• Liver biopsy and (+) test for AMA establish the diagnosis
				• Usually not necessary to prove patency of extrahepatic biliary tree by ERCP or PTC
				• Usual sequence of disease progression
				  • ↑ Serum alkaline, phosphatase
				  • Pruritus
				  • Hepatomegaly
				  • Hyperbilirubinemia
				  • Xanthomas
				  • Splenomegaly
				  • GI bleeding
				  • Ascites
				  • Encephalopathy

Continued.

TABLE 5-5: Symptom: Jaundice—cont'd

Cause of Jaundice	History	Physical Examination	Liver Test Abnormalities	Imaging/Invasive Procedures and Comment
Primary sclerosing cholangitis	• Predominantly men (3:1) • 50% to 75% have a history of inflammatory bowel disease, especially ulcerative colitis • Pruritus • Asymptomatic patient with ↑↑ serum alkaline phosphatase	• Hepatomegaly • Splenomegaly	• Cholestatic liver test with ↑↑ serum alkaline phosphatase • (-) tests for AMA and viral hepatitis • AST/ALT < 300 • Synthetic function usually well preserved until late stage of the disease	• ERCP or PTC shows classic beading/stricturing of extrahepatic biliary tree • Liver biopsy confirms ERCP/PTC findings

Gilbert syndrome (chronic idiopathic unconjugated hyperbilirubinemia)	• Mild jaundice noted intermittently after events such as
	  • Strenuous exertion
	  • Fasting
	  • Febrile illnesses
	  • Excess alcohol ingestion
	  • Trauma
		• Entirely normal except for scleral icterus; specifically, no hepatomegaly or splenomegaly	• CBC and reticulocyte count normal
			• Only abnormality is increased total serum bilirubin to values between 2.0 and 5.0 mg/dl but with normal direct-reacting (conjugated) bilirubinemia; AST, ALT, alkaline phosphatase, serum proteins, and prothrombin time all normal
				• Not indicated; patient should be reassured condition is benign

Metastatic liver disease	• Usually a history of systemic symptoms, weight loss, anorexia, and abdominal pain	• Obvious hepatomegaly with a markedly enlarged, firm, hard liver • Cachexia and obvious weight loss	• ↑↑ Alkaline phosphatase • AST/ALT usually < 300	• If jaundice is caused by metastatic liver disease, the liver is usually almost totally replaced by tumor (see Fig. 5-15) • In rare cases of Hodgkin's disease or non-Hodgkin's lymphoma, jaundice is caused by intrahepatic cholestasis

Abdominal Pain Syndromes

As emphasized before, abdominal pain is a cardinal symptom in leading to a specific diagnosis in diseases of the abdomen. Also, as discussed previously in detail, the examiner should inquire in detail concerning the character, location, radiation, precipitating factors, ameliorating factors, chronicity, and time sequence of abdominal pain (see first section). In this section, attention is directed to two types of abdominal pain: acute abdominal pain and chronic abdominal pain.

Acute Abdominal Pain

The abrupt onset of severe acute abdominal pain creates a situation that is commonly termed the "acute abdomen." The accompanying box summarizes some important dictums in the approach to such a patient. The box on pg. 246 summarizes the most important disorders to consider in the differential diagnosis of acute abdominal pain. The boxes on pp. 247–259 contain detailed information on the relevant history, physical examination, and pertinent investigations for several of these disorders.

Several nonsurgical conditions may simulate acute abdominal pain; these are listed separately in the box on pg. 246. Patients with metabolic disorders such as DKA, porphyria, abrupt onset of hypokalemia and hypercalcemia, and hyperthyroidism may all complain of abdominal pain. In patients with DKA and hypokalemia, the abdominal pain is often caused, at least in part, by delayed gastric emptying. In patients with vasculitis, abdominal pain often results from gut ischemia, which not infrequently results in frank infarction. However, in such patients abdominal pain may also result from pancreatitis and cholecystitis. The work-up in such patients should include the investigations summarized in the boxes on pp. 250 and 251. Patients with lower lobe pneumonias may have associated pleuritis with or without an effusion and often have pain referred to the RUQ or LUQ. Accordingly, a chest film should be obtained on all patients with new onset of severe abdominal pain.

Dictums in the Evaluation of the Patient with Acute Abdominal Pain

1. An orderly, painstakingly detailed history is vital, especially the chronologic sequence of events.
2. The location, quality, intensity, temporal aspects, and factors aggravating or ameliorating pain should be elicited.
3. Careful pelvic and rectal examinations are mandatory on every patient with abdominal pain.
4. Possibility of an intrathoracic lesion must be considered in every patient with abdominal pain, especially if pain is in the upper abdomen.
5. Laboratory studies may be of considerable value, but with few exceptions, they rarely establish the diagnosis (example: ↑ WBC count).
6. Sometimes, even under the best of circumstances, a definitive diagnosis cannot be established at the time of the initial examination.

Differential Diagnosis of Acute Abdominal Pain

I. Inflammatory conditions
   A. Acute appendicitis
   B. Acute cholecystitis
   C. Acute pancreatitis
   D. Alcoholic hepatitis
   E. Crohn's disease
   F. Acute infectious enteritis
   G. Acute diverticulitis

II. Perforations of the GI tract
   A. Peptic ulcer (duodenal, gastric)
   B. Diverticular disease of the colon
   C. Trauma

III. Obstruction of various viscera
   A. Renal colic (kidney, ureter, bladder calculi)
   B. Biliary colic (impacted cystic duct stone)
   C. Choledocholithiasis
   D. Mechanical obstruction small bowel or colon
      1. Adhesions
      2. Incarcerated hernia
      3. Volvulus
      4. Intussusception
      5. Foreign body
      6. Neoplasms
      7. Stenosis (Crohn's disease)

IV. Gynecologic
   A. Pelvic inflammatory disease
   B. Ectopic pregnancy
   C. Twisted ovarian cyst
   D. Mittelschmerz

V. Miscellaneous
   A. Dissecting aneurysm aorta
   B. Acute pyelonephritis
   C. Splenic infarction/splenic rupture
   D. Acute mesenteric vascular occlusion and variants thereof

VI. Nonsurgical conditions simulating acute abdominal pain
   A. Metabolic
      1. Diabetes mellitus, especially with ketoacidosis
      2. Hyperthyroidism
      3. Acute intermittent porphyria
      4. Hypercalcemia
      5. Hyperkalemia
      6. Familial Mediterranean fever
   B. Connective tissue disorders
      1. Vasculitis (polyarteritis, systemic lupus)
   C. Miscellaneous
      1. Pneumonia
      2. Sickle cell crisis
      3. Papillary necrosis of the kidney
      4. Herpes zoster
      5. Hemolytic uremic syndrome
      6. Henoch-Schölein purpura

Acute Appendicitis

I. History and physical examination
   A. Abdominal pain — almost invariably the initial symptom
      1. Frequently poorly localized to epigastrium and periumbilical area
      2. Reaches peak of intensity 4 to 6 hours, then may subside
      3. Reappears in RLQ as progressively severe steady pain aggravated by motion or cough
   B. Anorexia, nausea, vomiting (1 of these symptoms present in 90% cases)
      1. Presence of hunger distinctly unusual
   C. Abdominal tenderness found in locations corresponding to location of appendix (abdomen, flank, pelvis)
      1. RLQ tenderness (especially at McBurney's point)
      2. Percussion, rebound tenderness, referred rebound tenderness, jar tenderness — signs of peritoneal irritation
   D. Low-grade fever (99-101° F) common
   E. If chronic symptoms, weight loss > 10 lbs or anemia — consider Crohn's disease
II. Laboratory studies
   A. Modest leukocytosis (12,000 to 16,000 WBC/mm^3)
   B. Appendolithiasis seen on plain film of the abdomen (15% of cases)
   C. Ultrasound examination showing a thickened appendix (positive in 65% to 70% of cases)
III. Diagnosis of Appendicitis in the Elderly
   A. Diagnosis is often overlooked because symptoms and signs mild and diagnosis is not considered
   B. Pain is often minimal or even absent
   C. Shift of pain to RLQ occurs in only 20%
   D. Temperature may be elevated only slightly
   E. Abdominal tenderness may be deceptively mild
   F. Can present with a painless mass (appendiceal mass)
IV. Differential diagnosis
   A. Most common conditions discovered at operation when acute appendicitis is erroneously diagnosed
      1. Mesenteric lymphadenitis (? viral, Yersinia)
      2. Acute pelvic inflammatory disease
      3. Mittelschmerz (rupture of an ovarian follicle)
      4. Twisted ovarian cyst
      5. Regional enteritis
      6. Ruptured ectopic pregnancy
   B. Other disorders presenting diagnostic difficulties
      1. Cholecystitis, pancreatitis, diverticulitis, ureteral calculus, Meckel's diverticulitis, perforated ulcer

Patients with sickle cell anemia in crisis often complain of abdominal pain, which may be related to the crisis per se or other disorders such as cholecystitis, renal papillary necrosis, gut ischemia, or pancreatitis. In addition to sickle cell disease, the causes of renal papillary necrosis include obstructive uropathy as in benign prostatic hypertrophy, analgesic nephropathy, and severe acute pyelonephritis as may occur in a diabetic patient. Puzzling acute abdominal and lower pain

Acute Cholecystitis/Biliary Colic

I. History and physical examination
   A. RUQ pain and tenderness may be similar to previous episodes
   B. Nausea is common, vomiting less so
   C. Murphy's sign (increased tenderness during inspiration with RUQ palpation)
   D. Abdominal findings range from mild to severe RUQ pain and tenderness
   E. Gallbladder palpable 33% of cases; jaundice (serum bilirubin < 4.0 mg/dl) present in 20% of cases
   F. Low-grade fever (38° F)
   G. *Key point:* sudden onset of pain and tenderness in the RUQ should always suggest the diagnosis of acute cholecystitis or biliary colic
II. Laboratory findings
   A. Modest ↑ WBC (10,000 to 16,000)
   B. Mild-to-moderate ↑ SGOT/SGPT usually present
   C. Gallstones seen in plain film of abdomen in 15% of cases
   D. Ultrasound may suggest diagnosis if gallstones clearly demonstrated (Fig. 5-13)
   E. PIPIDA/HIDA scans positive in 90% of cases; infrequent false positive
III. Differential diagnosis
   A. Acute appendicitis
   B. Acute pancreatitis—serum amylase ↑ 20% to 30%
   C. Alcoholic hepatitis—10% of patients with acute cholecystitis have AST/ALT > 300 units
   D. Gonococcal perihepatitis
   E. Pneumonitis
   F. Hepatic tumors
   G. Perforated peptic ulcer—usually produces more striking findings
IV. Choledocholithiasis
   A. Diagnosis proven by
      1. Endoscopic retrograde cholangiopancreatography (ERCP) showing stone(s) in common bile duct (Fig. 5-14)
      2. Percutaneous transhepatic cholangiogram showing stone(s) in common bile duct

often heralds the onset of herpes zoster. This diagnosis should be considered in patients having new-onset abdominal and/or lower pain and having a disorder known to predispose to herpes zoster (e.g., immunocompromised host, corticosteroid therapy, underlying leukemia, lymphoma or Hodgkin's disease). Acute abdominal pain is a frequent complaint in patients with hemolytic uremic syndrome and Schönlein-Henoch purpura.

Chronic Abdominal Pain

The most important consideration in evaluating the patient with chronic abdominal pain is a thorough history, which often leads to the correct diagnosis. In this section, the salient characteristics of the history are detailed for several common disorders causing chronic abdominal pain.

PEPTIC ULCER DISEASE

The pain of PUD is similar in gastric and duodenal ulcer disease. The pain classically is described as gnawing, burning, or aching in character, epigastric xiphisternal or upper abdominal in location, frequently most severe when the stomach is empty (early morning hours or when meals are skipped), and relieved or at least partially ameliorated by ingestion of food or antacids. Thus classic PUD is characterized by what has been termed "the icities": *chronicity, rhythmicity,* and *periodicity.* However, ulcer symptoms are often atypical, especially in adolescents and young adults. Thus, in patients with predisposing factors to acid peptic disease or mucosal ulceration (positive family history, cigarette smoking, use of nonsteroidal antiinflammatory drugs), any persistent epigastric discomfort should raise the question of acid peptic disease. Similarly, the occurrence of nocturnal pain awakening the patient from sleep and partially relieved by antacids strongly suggests acid peptic disease.

CHOLELITHIASIS AND BILIARY COLIC

Biliary colic is characterized by paroxysms of sharp pain that are RUQ and/or epigastric in location, often radiating to the back or right mid-abdomen and less frequently to the shoulder. The pain is severe, never fleeting, and usually changes from a colicky pain to an aching, nagging discomfort that persists for 1 to 6 hours. Whereas biliary tract pain is more likely to occur after meals and especially after large meals, postprandial pain per se is not a discriminating indicator of biliary tract disease. Similarly, intolerance to greasy foods, fried foods, and brassica vegetables, although common in patients with gallbladder disease, also occurs in up to 20% of normal healthy adults. In patients with chronic upper abdominal pain, and especially if factors known to predispose to cholelithiasis are present within them (positive family history, obesity, regional enteritis, short bowel syndrome, oral contraceptive use, and sickle cell anemia), an ultrasound examination should be obtained. It is the best screening test for cholelithiasis, with a sensitivity of greater than 90% (Figs. 5-13 and 5-14).

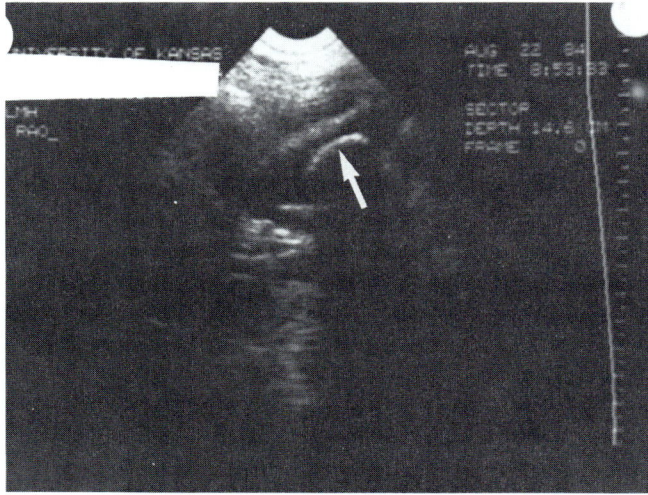

Fig. 5-13 Ultrasound examination showing gallstones.

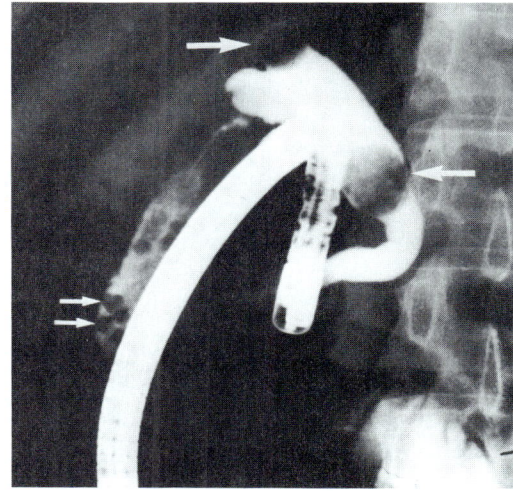

Fig. 5-14 Endoscopic retrograde cholangiogram showing a dilated common bile duct and a common duct stone (choledocholithiasis).

> **Acute Pancreatitis**
>
> I. History and physical examination
>   A. Causes of acute pancreatitis
>   1. Alcohol ingestion
>   2. Cholelithiasis
>   3. Drugs—diuretics, estrogens, tetracycline, valproic acid, sulfas, azathioprine
>   4. Postoperative
>   5. Hypertriglyceridemia
>   6. Hyperparathyroidism
>   7. Abdominal trauma
>   8. Vasculitis/connective tissue diseases
>   9. Viral infections
>   10. Pancreatic carcinoma
>   B. Physical examination
>   1. Tenderness, often diffuse
>   2. Signs of peritoneal irritation
>   3. Ileus (decreased-to-absent bowel sounds)
>   4. Cullen's discoloration of flanks or Grey Turner sign
>   C. Nonspecific indicators of an inflammatory response (fever, tachycardia, leukocytosis)
> II. Laboratory studies (any one of the following)
>   A. Serum amylase increased greater than 2× over normal
>   B. Serum lipase, serum trypsinogen, or serum pancreatic isoamylase increased above normal
> III. Radiographic abnormalities
>   A. Abnormal pancreas on abdominal ultrasound or CT examinations
> IV. Diagnosis
>   A. Definite diagnosis
>   1. Etiologic insult identified
>   2. Compatible physical examination
>   3. Nonspecific indicators of an inflammatory response (fever, tachycardia, leukocytosis) are present
>   4. Biochemical confirmation and/or radiographic abnormalities (ultrasound or CT examination) are present
>   B. Probable diagnosis
>   1. Etiologic insult identified
>   2. Compatible physical examination
>   3. Nonspecific indicators of an inflammatory response (fever, tachycardia, leukocytosis) are present
>   C. Possible diagnosis
>   1. Etiologic insult identified
>   2. Compatible physical examination

DELAYED GASTRIC EMPTYING

Several disorders may result in delayed gastric emptying (see box on pp. 206-207). Delayed gastric emptying should be considered in any patient with abdominal pain, especially if it is accompanied by nausea, emesis, and early satiety

Alcoholic Hepatitis

I. History and physical examination
   A. History of chronic alcoholism
      1. Intake > 40 g/day
      2. "CAGE" criteria
         C = Concerned about drinking; unable to cut back
         A = Angry about questions concerning drinking
         G = Guilty about drinking
         E = Eye opener or drink needed in early morning
   B. Abdominal pain, especially RUQ
   C. Hepatomegaly, especially if LF lobe is palpable
   D. Jaundice
   E. Peripheral stigmata of chronic parenchymal liver disease, but especially
      1. Parotid enlargement
      2. Gynecomastia
      3. Dupuytren's contracture
   F. Stigmata of portal hypertension (may be absent)
      1. Splenomegaly
      2. Ascites
      3. ↑ Abdominal collateral veins
   G. Stigmata of portal systemic encephalopathy (may be absent)
II. Laboratory studies
   A. Laboratory markers of chronic alcoholism
      1. MCV ↑ > 100 μm
      2. SGOT ↑ > 100 units
      3. SGOT:SGPT (AST:ALT) ratio ≥ 3:1
      4. GGTP ↑
   B. Abnormal tests of liver synthetic function (*note:* these abnormalities are more likely to be found in patients with active cirrhosis)
      1. ↓ Serum albumin
      2. ↓ Serum cholesterol
      3. ↑ (Prolonged) prothrombin time
   C. Liver biopsy findings of alcoholic hepatitis
      1. Absolute criteria
         a. Hepatocellular necrosis
         b. Polymorphonuclear leukocyte infiltration
      2. Generally accepted criteria
         a. Mallory alcoholic hyaline
      3. Often present but not required for diagnosis
         a. Fatty infiltration of the liver
         b. Fibrosis
         c. Cirrhosis

and is more marked postprandially. Physical examination may reveal abdominal distention as well as a succussion splash that persists for several hours after a meal. Further, this disorder must be suspected in such patients if radiologic (upper GI tract series) or endoscopic (upper GI tract) procedures have not identified a

> **Diverticulitis of the Colon: History, Physical Examination, and Investigations**
>
>   I. Diverticulitis is a disease of variable severity characterized by lower abdominal pain and tenderness
> II. Diverticulitis occurs more commonly in men and is 3 to 4 times more frequent in the left versus right colon
> III. History of previous attacks of diverticulitis is helpful
> IV. Colonic obstruction symptoms or signs mandate that carcinoma of the colon be excluded
>   V. Acute diverticulitis without free perforation
>   A. Lower abdominal pain and tenderness, especially in LLQ
>   B. Signs of peritoneal irritation (i.e., muscle spasm, guarding, rebound tenderness, referred tenderness)
>   C. Plain film of the abdomen suggesting obstruction (no bowel gas below left middescending colon)
>   D. Fever
>   E. Leukocytosis
> VI. Acute diverticulitis with free perforation
>   A. Symptoms and signs noted
>   B. Boardlike, rigid abdomen with involuntary guarding
>   C. Free air under the diaphragm on plain film abdomen

specific lesion to account for the above symptoms or physical findings. In this setting, a radionuclide gastric emptying study should be carried out to confirm the diagnosis of gastroparesis.

CHRONIC PANCREATITIS

The most common cause of chronic pancreatitis is ethanolism, which accounts for approximately 70% to 75% of cases. Such patients are predominantly males. The pain of chronic pancreatitis has several characteristic features. It is usually epigastric in location and in the LUQ and often radiates to the back. The pain can be aching, sharp, dull and steady, or gnawing, and it is frequently exacerbated by eating and alcohol ingestion. Pain may be relieved, albeit incompletely, by pancreatic enzyme therapy, either with or without anticholinergic drugs. The diagnosis must be considered in chronic alcoholics with persistent abdominal pain. The diagnosis of chronic pancreatitis is usually established on the bases of composite criteria employing: (1) imaging procedures (ultrasound or CT scanning), which may disclose pancreatic calcification; (2) endoscopic retrograde cholangiopancreatography, which usually discloses an abnormal pancreatic ductal system; and (3) tests of pancreatic function (secretin test and bentiromide or chymex test), which reveal impaired exocrine function.

CANCER OF THE PANCREAS

The most common symptoms of pancreatic carcinoma, in descending order of frequency, are weight loss (85%), abdominal pain (75%), anorexia (70%), nausea (40%), weakness and fatigue (40%), diarrhea (20%), indigestion (20%), fullness after eating (18%), and back pain (15%). Physical examination may reveal

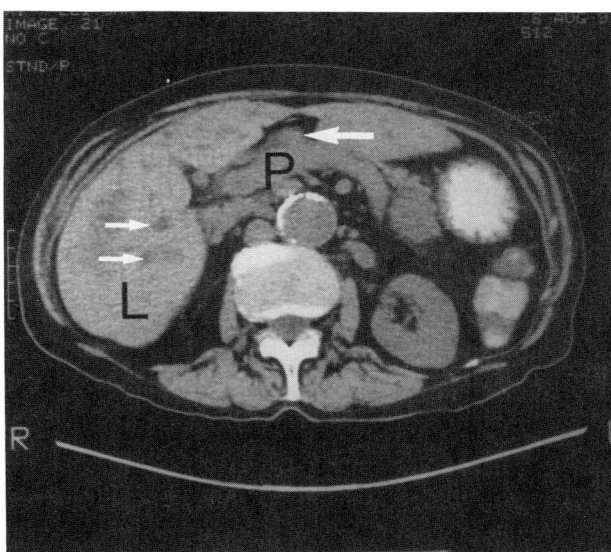

Fig. 5-15 CT scan of the abdomen depicting a lesion in the pancreas consistent with a diagnosis of carcinoma of the pancreas. Note also the lesions in the liver consistent with metastases. *L,* liver; *P,* pancreas; *large arrow,* pancreatic mass; *small arrow,* liver metastases.

evidence of recent weight loss, jaundice, hepatomegaly, epigastric or LUQ mass, a palpable gallbladder, a LUQ bruit, ascites, splenomegaly, edema, and stools positive for fecal occult blood. Painless jaundice, although widely mentioned in textbooks, is infrequent, as most patients do complain of abdominal pain. The pain is variably described as aching, dull, nagging, sharp, steady, or boring and is frequently increased by lying flat, especially at night. Conversely, the pain is often partially ameliorated by sitting in the knee-chest position. These are subtle but important clues. The clinical diagnosis is usually established by imaging procedures (CT scan) (Fig. 5-15), endoscopic retrograde cholangiopancreatography, or percutaneous cholangiography and confirmed by laparotomy or ultrasonically guided needle biopsy of the pancreas.

LACTASE DEFICIENCY

Intolerance of the lactose in milk and milk products because of intestinal lactase deficiency is common, occurring in 60% to 80% of American blacks and Orientals, 30% of Mediterraneans, and 5% to 10% of Caucasians. Ingestion of milk and milk products can cause not only cramping abdominal pain and diarrhea, but also gas, distention, bloating, and nonspecific abdominal discomfort. The clinical diagnosis is usually established by the following criteria: (1) ingestion of milk precipitates symptoms; (2) discontinuation of milk and milk products results in amelioration of symptoms; and (3) ingestion of a lactose load (50 g) results in a rise in breath H_2 excretion. The latter results from the action of colonic bacteria on unhydrolyzed lactose reaching the colon and the resultant H_2 being absorbed and excreted in the breath.

IRRITABLE BOWEL SYNDROME

The irritable bowel syndrome is a common cause of abdominal pain and is characterized by abdominal discomfort, alterations of bowel habit, and no demonstrated organic cause. Abdominal pain occurs with diarrhea or alternating diarrhea and constipation (see Table 5-1). A tentative diagnosis of the irritable

Regional Enteritis (Crohn's Disease)

I. History (especially important if greater than 4 weeks' duration)
   A. Diarrhea
   B. Abdominal pain
   C. Back pain
   D. Weight loss > 10 lbs
   E. Fever
   F. Positive family history of inflammatory bowel disease
   G. History of renal colic
   H. History of gallstone disease or biliary colic
   I. History of perirectal disease
II. Physical examination
   A. Palpable tender mass in RLQ (thickened, inflamed bowel, usually ileum and/or right colon)
   B. Perirectal disease (fistula, fissures, abscess)
   C. Skin lesions (erythema nodosum, erythematous plaques)
   D. Uveitis
   E. Oral ulcerations
   F. Clubbing
   G. Arthritis
   H. Fecal occult blood test is positive
III. Laboratory studies
   A. Anemia, leukocytosis, thromocytosis, ↑ sedimentation rate
   B. Blood in the stool
   C. Decreased serum albumin, cholesterol
   D. Abnormal Schilling test for vitamin B_{12} absorption
IV. Radiologic studies
   A. Characteristic changes in small bowel and/or colon (ileal disease or obstruction, ileocolic disease, fistula, string sign, segmental involvement)
V. Endoscopic studies
   A. Upper GI endoscopy (stomach and/or duodenal abnormalities)
   B. Colonoscopy (linear ulceration, segmental disease, may see ileal abnormalities as well)

bowel syndrome can be made on the basis of the history and physical examination alone if the following are found:

1. The patient complains of recurrent abdominal pain, often with loose bowel movements
2. The patient does not experience discomfort at night after retiring for sleep
3. Defecation relieves lower abdominal pain
4. One to four bowel movements occur daily, the last few being loose, and they usually occur in the morning after breakfast
5. Passage of bowel movements is accompanied by a feeling of incomplete evacuation
6. No systemic symptoms are present (i.e., no history of anorexia, weight loss, or fever)
7. No history of melena or hematochezia is present, and tests for fecal occult blood are negative

Perforated Peptic Ulcer

I. General considerations
   A. Formerly, incidence of 5% to 10% of peptic ulcer patients, but incidence has ↓ 30% in the past 10 years
   B. Much more frequent in males than in females
   C. Most perforations preceded by ↑ in ulcer symptoms
   D. <10% patients deny previous ulcer symptoms
   E. Site of perforation usually anterior wall of first part of the duodenum
II. History and physical examination
   A. Previous history of proven peptic ulcer disease is helpful
   B. In most patients, it is clear that an intrabdominal catastrophic event has occurred
   C. Pain of perforation begins suddenly and is severe, excruciating, agonizing. Pain initially is epigastric and RUQ, later spreads
   D. Abdominal tenderness is marked, abdomen is rigid and boardlike, rebound tenderness is usual, and bowel sounds are diminished or absent
   E. Classic "lull" may supervene, followed by ↑ signs of peritonitis, ↓ bowel sounds and ↑ abdominal distention, hypovolemia, ↑ pulse, and ↓ BP
III. Laboratory findings
   A. ↑ WBC count
   B. ↑ Serum amylase (15% to 20% of cases)
   C. Plain film abdomen, chest film show pneumoperitoneum (75% of cases)
IV. Atypical features in elderly patients

Mechanical Intestinal Obstruction

I. Causes of mechanical intestinal obstruction
   A. Small bowel obstruction
      1. Adhesive bands (usually after previous laparotomy)
      2. Hernias (inguinal, femoral, internal)
      3. Intussusception
      4. Gallstone obstruction
      5. Regional enteritis (stenosis)
   B. Large bowel obstruction
      1. Diverticulitis
      2. Colonic carcinoma
      3. Regional enteritis (stenosis)
      4. Cecal or sigmoid volvulus
II. History and physical examination
   A. Symptoms
      1. Abdominal pain, frequently colicky
      2. Vomiting
      3. Constipation
   B. Physical findings
      1. Abdominal distention
      2. Borborygmi
      3. Palpable abdominal mass (usually implies closed-loop obstruction)
      4. Succussion splash (pyloric outlet obstruction)
III. Laboratory findings
   A. Abnormal plain film (air fluid levels, "stepladder" pattern)
   B. Abnormal contrast studies

> **Renal Colic: History, Physical Examination, and Investigations**
>
>   I. Loin or abdominal pain, colic type, radiating to abdomen, genitalia, inner thigh
> II. Costovertebral-angle tenderness
> III. Dysuria
> IV. Hematuria
>   V. Recovery of calculi in strained urine
> VI. Abnormal imaging procedure showing renal/ureteral calculi
>   A. Plain films
>   B. Intravenous urogram
>   C. Sonogram

8. Female preponderance
9. Long history: no new onset after age 50 (if the latter occurs, suspect structural causes such as carcinoma of the pancreas or inflammatory bowel disease)
10. No anemia is present

Usually, in this setting, additional studies such as a flexible sigmoidoscopy and barium enema will be carried out to exclude a colonic cause for diarrhea.

This discussion has focused on only one form of the irritable bowel syndrome, abdominal pain. Other forms include constipation (see the section on constipation and upper abdominal pain and distention, pp. 211 to 213) and upper abdominal pain (see the section on delayed gastric emptying, pp. 206 and 227 to 228). Both these subsets can be associated with recurrent abdominal pain.

ANTERIOR ABDOMINAL WALL PAIN

Several conditions can cause anterior wall abdominal pain, including the following:

- Scar pain following a surgical procedure, frequently caused by a neuroma
- Hernias (incisional, spigelian)
- Hematomas in abdominal wall musculature (trauma, heparin injection)
- Rectus abdominis nerve entrapment syndrome
- Herpes zoster

As discussed previously, a useful maneuver here is to note whether the patient's flexion of the neck *increases* or *aggravates* abdominal pain and/or tenderness to the pressure of the palpating hand. If so, abdominal pain is most likely localized to the anterior abdominal wall. If the pain is judged to be scar pain because of an entrapment syndrome, a series of local injections with lidocaine and corticosteroids often results in striking relief of abdominal pain.

Gynecologic Causes of Acute Abdominal Pain

I. Pelvic inflammatory disease
   A. History, physical examination, and investigations
      1. Diagnosis of PID must always be considered in young women with *lower abdominal pain* and tenderness
      2. About 50% of acute PID caused by *N. gonorrhea;* nongonococcal PID is caused by several organisms, including *B. fragilis, C. trachomatis,* and anaerobic gram-positive cocci
      3. Risk of PID increased 2- to 9-fold in women wearing an IUD
      4. Abnormal vaginal discharge, abnormal menstrual bleeding, or onset of unusual pain during menstruation
      5. Systemic findings (fever, chills or leukocytosis often present)
      6. Abnormal pelvic exam
         a. Cervical motion causes pain
         b. Adnexal tenderness
      7. Cervical bacterial culture frequently positive
   B. Differential diagnosis
      1. Gonococcal perihepatitis may mimic acute cholecystitis
      2. Perihepatitis also occurs in nongonococcal PID
      3. Differential diagnosis should include
         a. Ectopic pregnancy
         b. Acute appendicitis
         c. Pelvic endometriosis
         d. Tuboovarian abscess
         e. Ovarian tumor
         f. Corpus luteum hematoma
         g. Ovarian cyst
II. Ruptured ectopic pregnancy
   A. History, physical examination, and investigations
      1. Missed menstrual period
      2. Lower quadrant abdominal pain
         a. Without rupture—rhythmic
         b. With rupture—lancinating, severe
      3. Hypotension (BP < 100) or tachycardia (p > 100) in 33% of patients
      4. Abnormal pelvic exam
         a. Cervical exam especially important
      5. Rectal tenesmus
      6. Pelvic sonogram showing tubal pregnancy
      7. Abnormal culdocentesis (bloody fluid)
   B. Pelvic exam → cervical motion → pain; differential diagnosis includes:
      1. PID
      2. Ruptured graafian follicle
      3. Ruptured ectopic pregnancy
III. Twisted ovarian cyst
   A. History, physical examination, and investigations
      1. Gradual onset of increasing lower abdominal pain
      2. Pelvic examination reveals abnormal adnexa (tenderness, and/or mass)
      3. Abnormal ultrasound examination revealing mass on ovary
      4. Abnormal laparoscopic examination

Miscellaneous Conditions Causing Acute Abdominal Pain

I. Dissecting aneurysm of the aorta
   A. History
      1. Abrupt onset of severe chest pain ("ripping" or "tearing" in quality), often radiating to back and arms. Patients frequently describe it as the worst pain they have ever experienced.
      2. Initial pain may be epigastric.
      3. Predisposing factors include hypertension, Marfan's syndrome, pseudoxanthoma elasticum, myxedema, and pregnancy.
   B. Physical examination
      1. Physical signs are related to site and extent of aortic dissection
      2. Unequal peripheral pulses (radial, femoral, and also carotids) and unequal blood pressures
      3. Aortic diastolic murmur
      4. Neurologic symptoms
         (a) Ischemic neuropathy
         (b) Stroke with hemiparesis
         (c) Impaired circulation to spinal cord resulting in paraparesis or paraplegia
   C. Investigations
      1. PA chest film may disclose widening of superior mediastinum and displacement of aortic shadow
      2. Imaging procedures (sonography, CT scan)
      3. Aortography is diagnostic procedure of choice
II. Acute pyelonephritis
   A. History
      1. Abrupt onset of severe pain, which may be back pain, loin pain, RUQ or LUQ pain; pain may radiate to the groin as in renal colic
      2. Fever and chills; nausea and vomiting do occur and may initially obscure the correct diagnosis
      3. Dysuria, cloudy urine, urine frequency
   B. Physical examination
      1. Costovertebral-angle tenderness to palpation or light pressure
      2. RUQ or LUQ tenderness to palpation may also be present
   C. Investigations
      1. Urinalysis classically reveals pyuria, clumps of white blood cells, and bacteriuria
      2. Suitably obtained specimens for urine culture reveal $>10^5$ microorganism/ml
      3. Blood cultures are positive in ~ 10% of cases
      4. Ultrasound and/or intravenous pyelograms may also disclose abnormalities
III. Splenic rupture/splenic infarction
   A. Splenic rupture/subcapsular hematomas
      1. History
         a. Trauma (automobile accident, blow to abdomen, loin, or back)
         b. May rupture with infectious mononucleosis, infarction, or sepsis, especially if large and soft and palpated too vigorously
         c. Intense pain in LUQ or left loin and radiating to the left shoulder should always raise the question of a ruptured spleen or subcapsular hematoma
      2. Physical examination
         a. Signs of shock (hypotension, tachycardia, pallor)
         b. LUQ tenderness; may feel an enlarged tender spleen or just a LUQ mass
      3. Investigations
         a. Imaging procedures with an ultrasound or CT scan accurately identify subcapsular hematoma and ruptured spleens

The Abdomen 259

Miscellaneous Conditions Causing Acute Abdominal Pain—cont'd

  B. Splenic infarction
  1. History
     a. Predisposing factors include vasculitis, bacterial endocarditis, marantic (nonbacterial) endocarditis, left atrial myxoma, polycythemia vera, myelofibrosis
     b. Abrupt onset of severe LUQ pain
     c. Fever
  2. Physical examination
     a. LUQ tenderness; LUQ mass
     b. Splenic fraction rub may be heard if infarction is subcapsular and/or with extensive perisplenitis
  3. Investigations
     a. Ultrasound and/or CT scan often disclose characteristic abnormalities
     b. Leukocytosis
IV. Acute mesenteric vascular occlusion and variants
  A. History
  1. Abrupt onset of acute abdominal pain may have been preceded by the classic triad of findings indicating a severely compromised mesenteric arterial circulation:
     a. Postprandial abdominal pain
     b. Weight loss (usually caused by decreased food intake, the latter associated with decreased postprandial pain)
     c. Epigastric, LUQ, or periumbilical aortic bruit
  2. Factors predisposing to arterial occlusion include severe atherosclerosis (diabetes, smoking) and emboli (atrial fibrillation, bacterial endocarditis, marantic endocarditis).
  3. Factors further compromising an attenuated gut blood flow include cardiac failure and use of digitalis glycosides. Indeed, acute hemorrhagic necrosis of the small bowel can occur without arterial occlusion of the major vessels (celiac, superior mesenteric) in patients with low cardiac output.
  4. Transient melena or hematochezia can occur.
  B. Physical examination
  1. Bruit(s) may be present
  2. Fever and tachycardia initially followed by hypothermia, acidosis, sepsis, and hypotension
  3. Abdominal distention and tenderness
  4. With frank gut infarction no bowel sound will be appreciated
  C. Investigations
  1. Aortography in patients with the classic triad of findings indicative of gut arterial insufficiency will establish the correct diagnosis and, if done early enough, permit operative intervention
  2. Needle aspiration of abdomen may disclose sanguineous fluid, which denotes gut infarction and "dead bowel"
  D. Special note—While the findings noted above are often dramatic and obvious in patients with acute mesenteric arterial occlusion, the clinical picture is more insidious in patients with mesenteric venous occlusion. Such patients often complain of rather severe abdominal pain that is quite out of proportion to the paucity of physical findings. Thus, this diagnosis must always be considered in patients with severe and persistent abdominal pain *and* a disorder known to predispose to mesenteric venous occlusion. These conditions include polycythemia vera, paroxysmal nocturnal hemoglobinuria, sickle cell anemia, myelofibrosis, and abdominal trauma.

Summary

The accompanying checklist is a summary listing all the items that are important in the physical examination of the abdomen. Obviously, many of the findings and maneuvers listed will not apply to every given patient. Rather, the list is a reminder to the student of the skills and techniques that are utilized in the examination of the abdomen, and that should be mastered.

Summary Checklist for Examination of the Abdomen

Inspection
- Malnutrition
- Dehydration
- Hyperpigmentation
- Scars
- Striae
- Visible pulsations
- Visible peristalsis
- Dilated veins
- Diastasis recti

Protuberant Abdomen
- Obesity
- Organomegaly
- Pregnancy
- Cysts
- Intestinal obstruction
- Increased gas/air in gut lumen
- Increased free air in peritoneal cavity
- Neoplasms
- Ascites

Hernias
- Inguinal
- Femoral
- Obturator
- Richter's
- Umbilical
- Spigelian
- Incisional

Ecchymosis
- Jaundice
- Peripheral stigmata liver disease
- Percussion
- Liver
- Spleen
- Bladder
- Shiftness dullness
- Fluid wave
- Puddle sign

Auscultation
- Peristaltic sounds
- Bruits
- Succussion splash
- Friction rubs

Palpation
- Liver
- Spleen
- Gallbladder
- Kidneys
- Aorta
- Masses
- Stomach
- Bowel loops
- Bladder
- Pelvic/rectal
- Hernias
- Tenderness (reproducibility)
- Rebound tenderness
- Jar tenderness
- Rigidity, guarding
- Abdominal pain

Suggested readings

Sleisenger MH, Fordtran, JS; *Gastrointestinal disease,* ed 4, Philadelphia, 1989, WB Saunders.

Greenberger NJ: *Gastrointestinal diseases. A pathophysiologic approach,* ed 4, Chicago, 1989, Mosby–Year Book.

Cattau EL Jr, et al: The accuracy of the physical examination in the diagnosis of suspected ascites, *JAMA* 247:1146, 1982.

Sherlock S: *Diseases of the liver and biliary system,* ed 8, Boston, London, 1989, Blackwell Scientific.

Barkun AN, Camus M. Guen L: The bedside assessment of splenic enlargement, *Am J Med* 91:512, 1991.

CHAPTER SIX

Male Genitalia

CHAPTER OUTLINE

History Taking
Dysuria
Frequency of urination
Urgency
Nocturia
Polyuria
Urinary incontinence
Hematuria
Oliguria and anuria
Pneumaturia
Changes in voiding pattern and prostatism
Penile pain, ulcers, and discharge

Loss of libido and impotence
Infertility
Scrotal swelling and testicular pain
Additional history of importance

Physical Examination of the Male Genitalia
Penis
Scrotum
Prostate
Inguinal canals and groin
Rectal examination

Summary

This chapter emphasizes the importance of history taking and physical examination in delineating several very common problems that affect men. To illustrate, benign prostatic hypertrophy (BPH) occurs almost universally in aging men and is the most common cause of urinary tract symptoms in such patients. Similarly, prostatic carcinoma occurs frequently in elderly men. It has been demonstrated in autopsy studies that after the eighth decade, over 90% of men have prostatic hyperplasia, and the majority of such patients have carcinoma, which is frequently silent.

Infertility is a vexing problem that requires a detailed evaluation and often is related to abnormal testicular function. Testicular dysfunction can be caused by hypothalamic-pituitary disorders or by testicular defects that are developmental (Klinefelter's syndrome), acquired (viral orchitis), or related to abnormal sperm transport (cystic fibrosis).

Inguinal hernias are a common cause of groin pain and careful evaluation is required, especially in the elderly, if complications such as strangulation or incarceration are to be avoided.

Testicular cancer occurs frequently in men aged 15 to 34, with an average of

6000 new cases diagnosed each year. It is extremely important to exclude this diagnosis in all men with testicular masses, as combined orchectomy and chemotherapy is frequently curative.

Finally, genitourinary infections resulting from venereal diseases are very common. In 1988, it was estimated that over 300 cases of gonorrhea were reported for 100,000 population (men and women), and if nongonococcal urethritis is also considered, over 1,000,000 cases of such diseases occur per year.

History Taking

Dysuria

Dysuria is defined as uncomfortable or painful urination. Such pain usually accompanies micturition but also may persist after voiding. Pain felt during urination is often caused by urethritis, urethral obstruction, inflammation of the meatus, or prostatitis. Pain after urination should suggest cystitis, prostatitis, or a bladder calculus. Inflammation of the urethra and bladder often result in bladder spasms, in turn resulting in frequency and urgency. Indeed, the triad of dysuria, frequency, and urgency are characteristic of acute bacterial infections causing cystitis or prostatitis. Dysuria is also frequent in patients with BPH and prostatic cancer.

Frequency Of Urination

Normal adults urinate every 3 to 6 hours (4 to 6 times/day) and occasionally at night; they generally do not need to awaken from overnight sleep for micturition. Obviously, increased daily fluid intake (> 3000 ml/day) will influence both the volume and frequency of urination. The regular requirement to void urine more than once during sleeping hours is termed *nocturia*. As noted above, frequency of urination is a common symptom in patients with acute infections of the genitourinary (GU) tract and BPH.

Urgency

Urgency, as the term implies, indicates the urge to micturate without the ability to voluntarily postpone voiding. Urgency accompanied by dysuria and frequency indicates cystitis or prostatitis. Urgency alone may reflect BPH or a bladder or urethral problem.

Key Symptoms in the Evaluation of the Male Genitalia

- Dysuria
- Frequency of urination
- Urgency
- Nocturia
- Polyuria
- Urinary incontinence
- Hematuria
- Oliguria and anuria
- Pneumaturia
- Changes in voiding and prostatism
- Penile pain, ulcer, and discharge
- Loss of libido and impotence
- Infertility
- Scrotal swelling and testicular pain

Nocturia

Nocturia, as defined above, is present in several disorders, including the following:

- Habitually large daily fluid intake
- BPH
- Treatment with diuretics
- Uncontrolled diabetes mellitus
- Congestive heart failure
- Chronic renal disease

Polyuria

The normal 24-hour urine volume ranges from 500 to 2000 ml, with the average being 1500 ml. Urine volumes greater than 2500 ml/day may reflect the following:

- Inordinate fluid intake
- Psychogenic polydipsia
- Diuretic treatment
- Diabetes mellitus
- Diabetes insipidus
- Hypokalemia
- Hypercalcemia
- Chronic renal disease

CASE 6-1 Benign Prostatic Hypertrophy

A 67-year-old man has been experiencing increasingly severe lower abdominal (hypogastrium) discomfort of 3 days' duration. Questioning reveals that he has had increasing difficulty initiating urination, a considerable decrease in the force of his urinary stream, occasional midstream stoppage, and postvoiding dribbling. Further, he has nocturia 2 to 4 times per night. Importantly, on an occasion 3 days earlier he had great difficulty initiating urination and developed lower abdominal discomfort followed by urinary incontinence. He subsequently was able to urinate but has noted a decreased output.

Physical examination is unremarkable except for the abdominal and rectal examination. Abdominal examination reveals mild tenderness and increased dullness in the hypogastrium extending 8 cm above the pubic symphysis. A poorly defined mass is appreciated, which is felt to be the bladder. Rectal examination reveals a moderately enlarged, firm, rubbery prostate without nodules or undue hardness. No other masses or organs are palpable.

This patient presented with classic symptoms of BPH. The increasingly severe symptoms culminated in an episode of acute urinary retention characterized by inability to void and lower abdominal pain. The mass identified on physical examination is most likely an enlarged bladder, and this finding, coupled with the history and some overflow incontinence, indicates the presence of high-grade obstruction. The prostate is clearly abnormal; it is only moderately enlarged, but this underscores the fact that the relationship between the degree of prostatic hypertrophy and the severity of obstructive uropathy is not direct. The above constellation of clinical features clearly indicates that a definitive procedure (i.e., a transurethral resection of the prostate) is now necessary.

Urinary Incontinence

Urinary incontinence is defined as the involuntary loss of urine. In children, nocturnal incontinence, or *enuresis* (dysfunctional nocturnal urinary incontinence), is often present without any identifiable organic cause. Similarly, incontinence in the elderly may develop for no apparent reason. However, the new onset of urinary incontinence in an adult should always prompt a detailed evaluation. Common causes of incontinence in males include the following:

- Cerebrovascular accidents
- Neurogenic bladder, as may occur in diabetes mellitus and multiple sclerosis
- Normal pressure hydrocephalus
- Fecal impaction
- Prostatism (BPH)

Hematuria

Hematuria, the passage of red blood cells in the urine, can be either microscopic or gross. The latter results in obvious red or reddish-brown discoloration of the urine. However, such discolored urine may not be caused by blood per se. For example, red-colored urine may indicate hemoglobinuria, myoglobinuria, or porphobilinogenuria (see accompanying box). In addition, orange or orange-brown–colored urine may be found in jaundiced patients or patients taking metronidazole or rifampin. The presence of blood in the urine, either gross or microscopic, always warrants a detailed evaluation. Explore in detail the relationship between hematuria and the phases of micturition. In this

---

Causes of Myoglobinuria and Hemoglobinuria

Causes of Myoglobinuria

I. Trauma, crush injuries
II. Coma or obtundation with muscle compression
III. Rhabdomyolysis
   A. Heat stroke
   B. Severe exercise
   C. Seizures
   D. Hypokalemia
   E. Hypophosphatemia
   F. Enzymatic deficiencies (e.g., McArdle syndrome)
   G. Infectious (e.g., influenza, legionella)
   H. Heroin overdose
   I. Alcohol overdose

Causes of Hemoglobinuria

I. Intravascular hemolysis
   A. Hemolytic transfusion reaction
   B. Hemolysis caused by lysins (snake venom)
   C. Paroxysmal nocturnal hemoglobinuria
   D. Paroxysmal cold hemoglobinuria
   E. Extensive burns

regard, hematuria at the initiation of urination should suggest a urethral or prostatic source, blood throughout micturition suggests a renal source, and terminal hematuria suggest a bladder source. Painless hematuria occurs frequently with bladder neoplasms, renal neoplasms, renal tuberculosis, and acute glomerulonephritis.

Oliguria and Anuria

Oliguria and anuria are harbingers of acute renal failure. *Oliguria* is defined as a 24-hour urine volume less than 400 ml, and *anuria* is defined as a 24-hour output less than 100 ml. The examiner must keep in mind the causes of acute renal failure (see accompanying box) in evaluating any patient with oliguria, and especially in evaluating patients with anuria. Patients do not usually complain of or even note decreases in urine volume. In all patients with oliguria, exclude both postrenal causes (obstruction) and prerenal causes (volume depletion) in addition to parenchymal renal causes.

Pneumaturia

Pneumaturia is the passage of urine or stool mixed with air and occurs in the presence of fistula tracts from either the bowel or the vagina into the bladder. This develops following surgical procedures and pelvic infections and with inflammatory bowel disease.

Changes in Voiding Pattern and Prostatism

Patients with BPH may experience irritative symptoms such as dysuria, frequency, and urgency, which actually reflect bladder hyperreflexia. Obstructive symptoms, however, are more characteristic and more frequent. Thus patients with symptomatic BPH often complain of difficulty initiating urination, diminution in the force of the urinary stream, midstream stoppage, postvoiding dribbling or the sensation of incomplete bladder emptying, and nocturia. With increasing urethral obstruction, these symptoms worsen and urinary retention may supervene, causing overflow urinary incontinence. In this setting, infection, alcohol, and certain medications (nasal vasoconstrictors, anticholinergics, and tranquilizers) can precipitate acute urinary retention. No direct relationship exists between obstructive symptoms and prostate size.

Penile Pain, Ulcers, and Discharge

Penile pain may arise from the urethra shaft of the penis or the meatus. Urethral pain is most commonly caused by urethritis, which is further classified into gonococcal and nongonococcal categories.

The most common cause of nongonococcal urethritis is *Chlamydia trachomatis;* less common causes include herpes simplex virus, *Trichomonas vaginalis*, and *Ureaplasma urealyticum.* Gonococcal and nongonococcal urethritis also cause a urethral discharge that often prompts the patient to seek medical attention.

The urethral discharge from nonspecific urethritis is usually more mucoid than the heavy purulent discharge of gonococcal infection. The patient may also have noted ulcers on the penis. The most common causes of penile ulcers are herpes simplex, herpes genitalis, and syphilis. Chancroid resulting from *Hemophilus ducreyi,* formerly an unusual cause of penile ulcers, appears to be increasing in

Causes of Acute Renal Failure

Parenchymal Renal Diseases
  I. Acute glomerulonephritis
     A. SLE
     B. Poststreptococcal
     C. Bacterial endocarditis
     D. Goodpasture's syndrome
 II. Bilateral renal cortical necrosis
     A. Obstetric accidents
     B. Gram-negative sepsis
     C. Hyperacute allograft rejection
III. Diseases of tubules/interstitium
     A. Drug induced (antibiotics, anesthetics)
     B. Infections (acute pyelonephritis)
     C. Hypercalcemia
     D. Acute uric acid nephropathy
     E. Nephrotoxins (heavy metals, organic solvents, contrast material)
     F. Postischemic renal failure
     G. Pigment induced (hemolysis, rhabdomyolysis, heat stroke)
 IV. Diseases of renal vasculature
     A. Renal artery, renal vein occlusion
     B. Malignant hypertension
     C. Systemic scleroderma
     D. Vasculitis
     E. Thrombotic thrombocytopenic purpura

Extrarenal Obstruction
   I. Urethral obstruction
  II. Benign prostatic hypertrophy
 III. Prostatic cancer
  IV. Bladder/urethral calculi
   V. Retroperitoneal obstruction (neoplasms, fibrosis)
  VI. Blood clots
 VII. Bilateral ureteral calculi

Prerenal Failure
   I. Hypovolemia
      A. Blood loss (GI bleeding)
      B. Renal loss (diuretics)
      C. Skin loss (burns)
      D. Pancreatitis
      E. Peritonitis
  II. Congestive heart failure

CASE 6-2 Urethral Discharge

A 24-year-old male presented to his physician because of a urethral discharge, pain in the penis, and dysuria of 3 days' duration. He had sexual intercourse 8 days earlier with a woman whom he had just recently met. Five days later he noted the onset of a urethral discharge. In addition, he began to experience dysuria both at the initiation and termination of micturition. A detailed inquiry into his sexual history revealed the following: (1) he asserted that he was heterosexual and denied any homosexual practices; (2) he had several different sexual partners in the past 6 years; (3) he had 2 episodes of gonorrhea while serving in the armed forces in the Philippines and an additional episode, also diagnosed as but not proven to be gonorrhea, just 4 months ago; and (4) he generally did not use condoms.

Examination of the genitalia revealed no abnormalities. A small amount of purulent exudate was expressed from the penis. Microscopic examination revealed many polymorphonuclear leukocytes, but no organisms were seen on gram stain, and cultures for gonorrhea were negative. He was treated with antibiotics and made an uneventful recovery.

The abrupt onset of urethral discharge and dysuria following a heterosexual exposure pointed to an infectious urethritis. The most common infectious causes of urethritis in a male are *Niesseria gonorrhea* and *Chlamydia trachomatis*. Promiscuous men not infrequently develop both gonococcal and nongonococcal urethritis; the infections can develop either concurrently or sequentially.

CASE 6-3 Penile Ulcer

A 34-year-old male presented to his physician because of a penile ulcer without other symptoms. Importantly, the ulcer was painless. He had a history of repeated heterosexual exposure during the previous 3 months.

Physical examination confirmed the presence of a single, indurated ulcer of the glans penis. Inguinal lymph nodes were palpated bilaterally. Serologic tests and a dark-fluid examination of a swab of the lesion confirmed the diagnosis of syphilis.

While herpes simplex is probably the most common cause of genital ulceration, a *painless* solitary ulcer is characteristic of syphilis. The examiner must exclude syphilis in all such cases. In addition, the patient's sexual contacts need to be identified and screened for syphilis. The presence of *painful vesicles* along with ulceration(s) would point towards a diagnosis of herpes simplex.

frequency. Rare causes of penile ulcers include lymphogranuloma venereum and Behçet's syndrome.

Pain in the shaft of the penis may be caused by trauma, priapism, sustained erection of the penis, edema, or *phimosis* (constriction of the glans penis in uncircumcised men).

Carcinoma of the penis is a rare condition affecting elderly uncircumcised men. The disease may reach a fairly advanced stage before diagnosis if phimosis is present.

Loss of Libido and Impotence

In the male, sexual performance can be impaired by: (1) lack of desire or a diminished *libido;* (2) inability to have an erection; and (3) failure to achieve orgasm. *Impotence* is defined as inability to perform the sexual act (i.e., attaining or sustaining erection of the penis for sufficient time to obtain satisfactory coitus). This is in contrast to *sterility*, which is defined as inability to reproduce. Decreased libido may occur in several general medical illnesses, neurologic disorders, endocrine diseases, psychiatric disorders, and following drug therapy (see the box on pg. 270). Similarly, erectile difficulty or ejaculatory failure may be caused by neurologic or endocrine disorders, psychiatric problems, or drugs. However, the majority of cases are functional in origin and secondary to psychologic problems or anxiety. In this regard, temporary impotence is quite common.

The sexual history should include questions about sexual disease, sexual practices, social habits, marital attitudes, and drug therapy. Importantly, the presence of early morning erections virtually excludes an endocrinologic, neurologic or vascular cause of impotence and clearly points to a functional problem. The differential diagnosis of impotence is listed in the box on pg. 270. Note the special emphasis placed on drug therapy and alcohol use; in particular, antihypertensive and psychotropic drug treatment are important causes of impaired sexual function. Finally, if any doubt exists as to the cause of impotence, check serum testosterone and prolactin levels and exclude the treatable causes of impotence before undertaking psychosexual counseling.

Infertility

Men with normal libido who are not impotent may still develop infertility. The usual complaint is the inability of a couple to have children. This may be caused by *azoospermia* (absence of sperm), *oligospermia* (decreased number of sperm), or nonmotile or defective sperm. Causes of male infertility are summarized in the box on pg. 271.

Scrotal Swelling and Testicular Pain

The scrotum is a double sac containing the testis, vas deferens, and epididymis on each side. The epididymis is closely attached to the posterolateral surface of the testis. The spermatic cord consists of the vas deferens, arteries, veins, nerves, and lymphatic vessels held together by the spermatic fascia. The testis is contained within the fibrous smooth tunica albuginea and is surrounded by a pouch of peritoneum (see Fig. 6-1). The tunica vaginalis with fluid is termed a *hydrocele*. A cystic dilation of the ducts of the upper part of the epididymis is termed a *spermatocele*. A *varicocele* refers to varicosity of the testicular veins (pampiniform plexus), which can result in swelling of the testis. Failure of the testis to descend into the scrotal sac is termed *cryptorchidism*.

Scrotal swelling can occur for several reasons:

- Hydrocele (see Fig. 6-5, C)
- Hematocele
- Spermatocele
- Varicocele
- Massive edema (anasarca) associated with congestive heart failure and nephrotic syndromes
- After paracentesis of ascitic fluid

Organic Causes of Impotence in Men

Neurologic Diseases

  I. Anterotemporal lobe lesions
 II. Diseases of the spinal cord
III. Loss of sensory imput
   A. Diabetes mellitus* and various polyneuropathies
   B. Tabes dorsalis
   C. Diseases of dorsal root ganglia
 IV. Diseases of nervi erigentes
   A. Complete prostatectomy*
   B. Rectosigmoid operations
   C. Aortic bypass surgery

Endocrine Causes

  I. Testicular failure* (primary and secondary)
 II. Hyperprolactinemia

Vascular Disease

  I. Leriche's syndrome

Penile Diseases

  I. Previous priapism
 II. Penile trauma
III. Peyronie's disease

Drugs*

  I. Antihypertensives*
   A. Methyldopa
   B. Guanethidine
   C. Reserpine
   D. Spironolactone
   E. Clonidine
   F. Propranolol
   G. Thiazide diuretics
 II. Tranquilizers, antidepressants, and psychotropic drugs*
   A. Phenothiazines
   B. Thioridazine
   C. Imipramine
   D. Amitriptyline
   E. Doxapin
   F. Benzodiazepines
   G. Haloperidol
III. Drugs of habituation or addiction
   A. Alcohol*
   B. Heroin
   C. Methadone
   D. Cannabis*
 IV. Miscellaneous
   A. Histamine H_2-receptor antagonists (i.e., cimetidine)
   B. Estrogens
   C. Metoclopramide

* = Most common
From Wilson JD, Walsh P: Impotence. In Braunwald E, et al, editors: *Harrison's principles of internal medicine,* ed 11, New York, 1987, McGraw-Hill.

Causes of Male Infertility
Defective Spermatogenesis • Abnormalities in testosterone synthesis • Klinefelter's syndrome • Obstruction in seminiferous tubules (gonorrhea, tuberculosis, nonspecific infections) • Absense/atresia of vas deferens (cystic fibrosis) • Rudimentary epididymis (cystic fibrosis) • Kartagener's syndrome (nonmotile sperm) • Orchitis (mumps, gonorrhea, brucellosis) • Following chemotherapy **Variococele** **Cryptorchidism** **Decreased Testicular Synthesis of Testosterone** • Chronic alcoholism • Starvation/inanition • Estrogen administration **Decreased Secretion of Gonadotropins** • Pituitary/hypothalamic disorders (neoplastic, inflammatory, traumatic, vascular, and degenerative lesions) • Isolated defects (hypogonadotropic hypogonadism)

- Epididymitis
- Torsion of the spermatic cord
- Thrombosis of the inferior vena cava or pelvic veins

If the above conditions develop abruptly, they are quite likely to cause the acute onset of testicular pain. Other causes of acute testicular pain include the following:

- Orchitis (mumps)
- Calculus (bladder, urethra) with referred pain
- Appendicitis with referred pain and incarcerated inguinal hernia

On the other hand, testicular neoplasms infrequently present as acute pain. Rather, they come to attention because of testicular swelling or the patient's perception of a mass in the testis.

Additional History of Importance

In addition to inquiring about sexual desires, sexual practices, and attitudes, ask in detail about previous venereal diseases such as gonorrhea, syphilis, nongonococcal urethritis, and chancroid. Further, in male homosexuals practicing anal-receptive intercourse, inquire about other infections such as salmonella, shigella, amebiasis, giardiasis, herpes genitalis, campylobacter, and chlamydia. In

CASE 6-4 Inguinal Pain and a Testicular Mass

A 25-year-old male law student, while playing tennis, sustained a right groin injury from an errant tennis ball. The initial sharp right inguinal pain was followed by a dull aching discomfort that prompted him to seek medical attention. The patient's past medical history was entirely unremarkable.

The physical examination was normal except for examination of the right inguinal area and testes. Direct palpation just above the inguinal ligament elicited mild-to-moderate pain. No lymph nodes or masses were palpated. However, examination of the testes revealed that the right testis was very firm, irregular, nontender, and 1½ to 2 times the size of the left testis. The apparent right testicular mass did not transilluminate. After additional studies, the patient underwent a right orchiectomy. Examination of the resected specimen revealed a primary testicular tumor that was classified as a seminoma.

This patient had an asymptomatic malignant testicular tumor that came to clinical recognition because of an incidental injury in an area contiguous to the tumor. Most testicular tumors do not cause pain, especially early in their development, and are often discovered quite by accident, as occurred in this case. This case illustrates the need for careful examination of the testes in young men aged 25 to 35, as primary testicular tumors are one of the most common tumors in this age group.

---

patients who are known to be HIV positive, the list expands to include candida, cytomegalovirus, cryptosporidiosis, and *Mycobacterium avium-intracellulare* infections. Finally, ask about previous stone disease (kidneys, bladder) and urologic surgery.

Physical Examination of the Male Genitalia

Penis

The male genitalia are best examined with the patient standing. First, inspect the penis (Fig. 6-1). If it is uncircumcised, retract the foreskin and examine the urethral orifice and glans penis. The terms *epispadias* and *hypospadias* refer to congenital abnormalities in which the urethral meatus opens on the dorsum of the penis or the ventral surface, respectively (Fig. 6-2). Check the glans penis for scars, ulcers, nodules, or a urethral discharge. A single, indurated, painless ulcer is most likely syphilitic in origin. Less common causes include herpes genitalis, chancroid, lymphogranuloma venereum, and Behçet's syndrome. *Balanitis* refers to inflammation of the glans penis and can be caused by diabetes mellitus, candida infection, *Trichomonas* infections, drug reactions, and Reiter's syndrome.

Palpate the shaft of the penis for masses, tenderness, and deviation, either downward or laterally (Fig. 6-3). The latter condition is termed *Peyronie's disease* (see Fig. 6-2) and is caused by inflammation of the corpora cavernosa of the penile shaft. Penile edema is usually obvious and is most apt to occur with anasarca and after paracentesis in cirrhotics with ascites.

Anogenital warts (condylomata acuminata) occur on the skin and mucosal surfaces of external genitalia and perianal areas.

Fig. 6-1 Anatomic relationships depicting penis, scrotum, testicle, prostate, urethra, seminal vesicles, vas deferens, and epididymides.

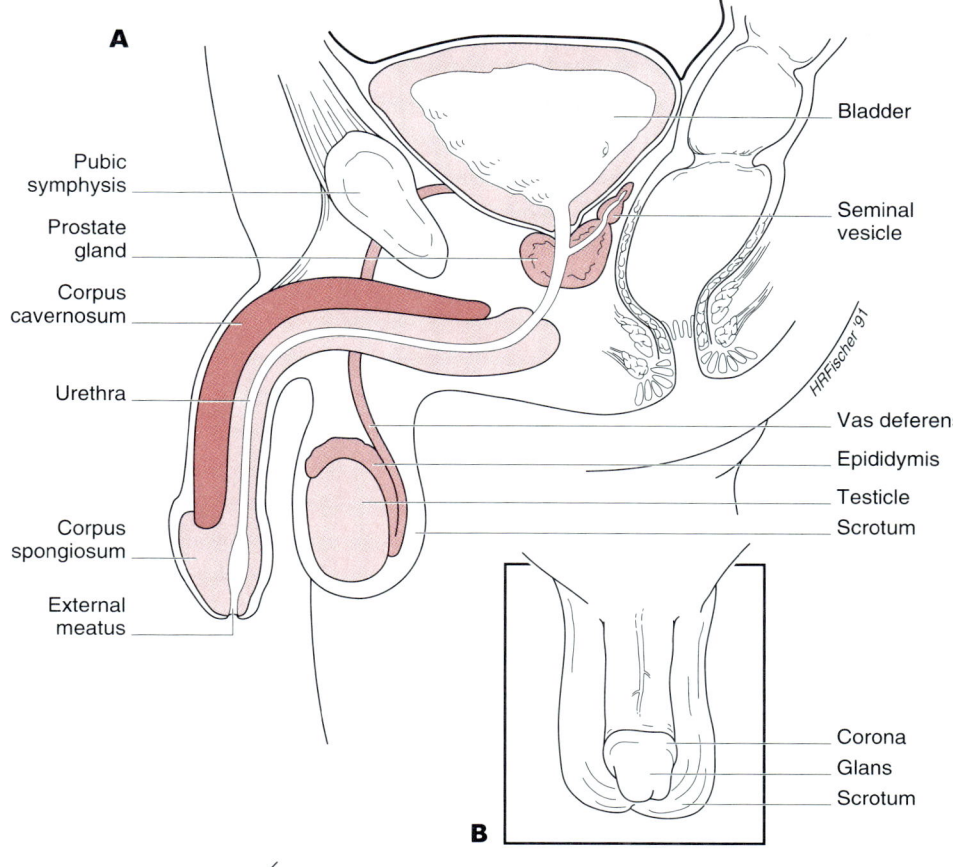

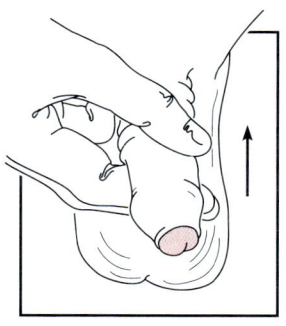

A Phimosis

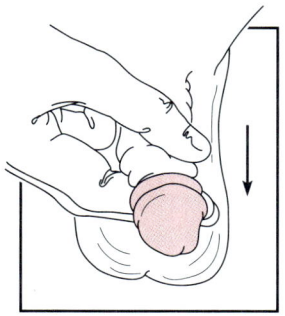

B Paraphimosis

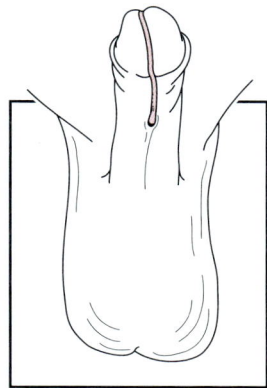

C Hypospadia

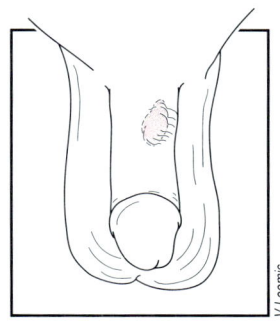

D Peyronie's disease

Fig. 6-2 Scheme depicting congenital abnormality in which the urethral meatus opens on the ventral surface of the penis (hypospadias) and other abnormalities of the penis. For details, see text.

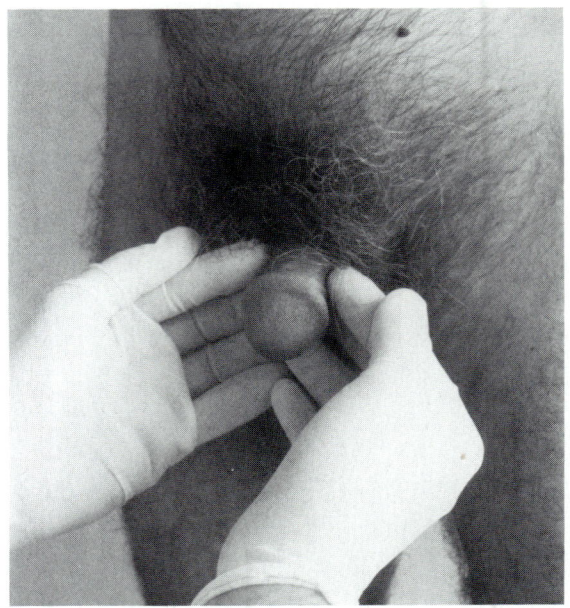

Fig. 6-3 Technique for examining the shaft of the penis and the meatus.

Scrotum

Examine the scrotal contents by palpating the testes, epididymides, and spermatic cords (Fig. 6-4). A normal testis is approximately 4.0 to 4.5 cm by 2.5 cm. A testis measuring less than 3.0 cm in length is atrophic. In normal males, the left testis hangs lower than the right. A reversal of this arrangement may be a subtle clue to the presence of a left renal hypernephroma with occlusion of the spermatic vein and upward retraction of the left testis. Atrophic testes most commonly result from orchitis, trauma, chronic alcoholism, and cirrhosis of the liver. If both testes are quite small, suspect primary or secondary pituitary

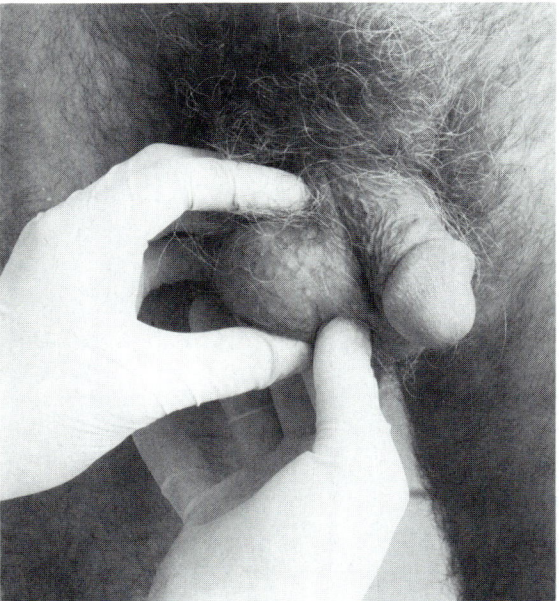

Fig. 6-4 Techniques for examining the scrotum and palpation of the testicle.

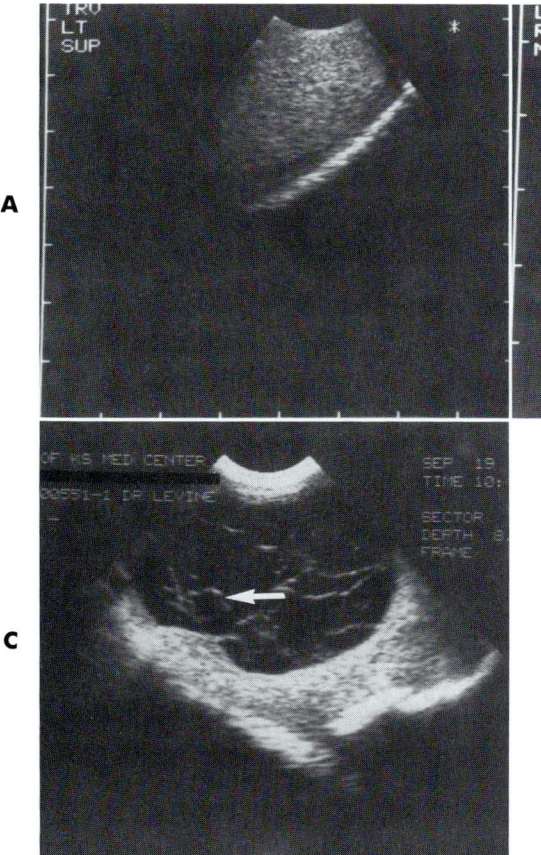
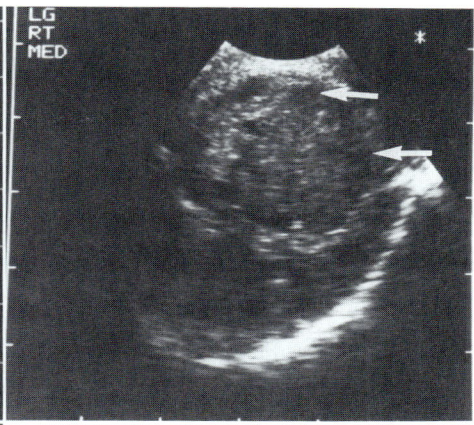

Fig. 6-5 **A**, Ultrasound examination showing a normal testicle. Note homogeneous appearance. **B**, Ultrasound examination showing a testicular mass, with dark, irregular areas highlighted by the arrow. **C**, Ultrasound examination showing a complex fluid collection (hydrocele), which is septated.

gonadotropic failure. The most common cause of primary testicular failure is Klinefelter's syndrome.

Palpate each testis carefully for masses, then palpate the epididymis and spermatic cord. Any marked disparity in testicular size or consistency should raise the question of a testicular lesion. If scrotal swelling or a mass is present, apply transillumination, as hydroceles will transilluminate. Check the inguinal canal, and if hernia is suspected, attempt gentle reduction after auscultating for bowel sounds (see Chapter 5). Epididymal cysts and varicoceles can also be identified by palpation. An empty scrotal sac should raise the question of undescended testes *(cryptorchidism)*.

Neoplasms of the testes are one of the most common tumors in men 25 to 35 years of age. The diagnosis is made by palpating a mass usually firm, smooth, and painless. Neoplasms can usually be distinguished from various cysts by transillumination. Ultrasound is a convenient means of confirming the presence of a testicular mass (Fig. 6-5).

Prostate

The normal prostate is relatively firm and nontender, with the two lateral lobes separated by a median furrow. Because the index finger measures 6.0 to 9.0 cm, the examiner should be able to carefully size up both lateral lobes and the anteroposterior margins of a normal prostate. Any of the following findings are abnormal, especially if these findings are accompanied by pain or urethral discharge:

- Increased size of the prostate
- Asymmetric enlargement of one lateral lobe
- Nodules
- Excessive hardness (prostate carcinomas often result in a prostate feeling rock hard)
- Bogginess or fluctuance

The above constellation of findings is characteristic of acute prostatitis. An enlarged, firm, rubbery prostate is characteristic of BPH. As noted above, no clear relationship exists between the size of the prostate and symptoms of prostatism.

Inguinal Canals and Groin

Examine the inguinal canals with the patient standing (Fig. 6-6). Carefully insert the index finger into the external inguinal ring and ask the patient to cough. Palpation of bowel impulses or a frankly dilated ring with bowel present indicates

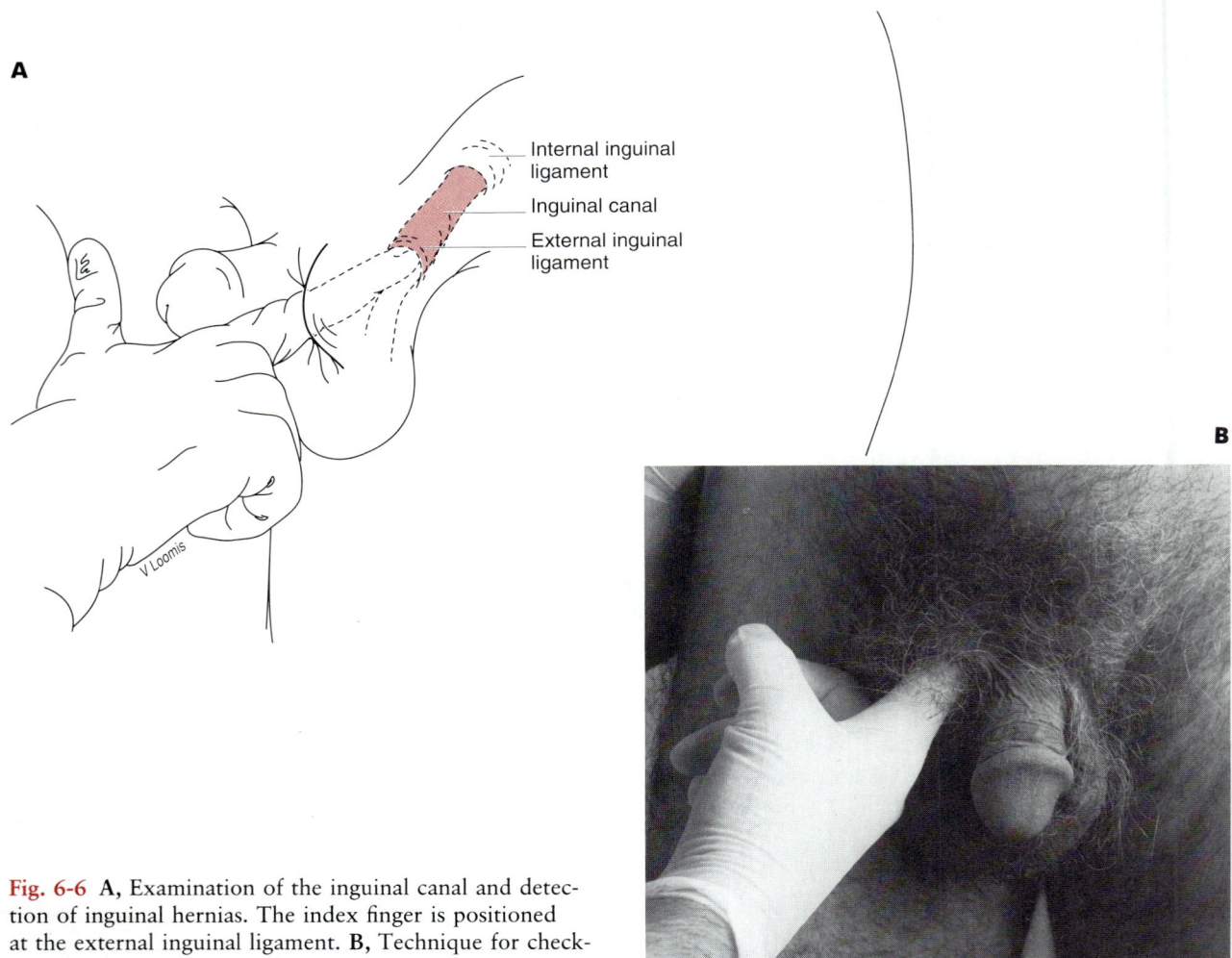

Fig. 6-6 A, Examination of the inguinal canal and detection of inguinal hernias. The index finger is positioned at the external inguinal ligament. **B,** Technique for checking for hernias.

the presence of an inguinal hernia. Carefully palpate both inguinal areas for lymph nodes (Fig. 6-7). Bilateral and enlarged (> 1.0 cm) nodes are found in several disorders, including anorectal infections, venereal diseases, fungi infections of the feet, and neoplastic disorders.

Rectal Examination

See Fig. 6-8 and the discussion on rectal examination in Chapter 5.

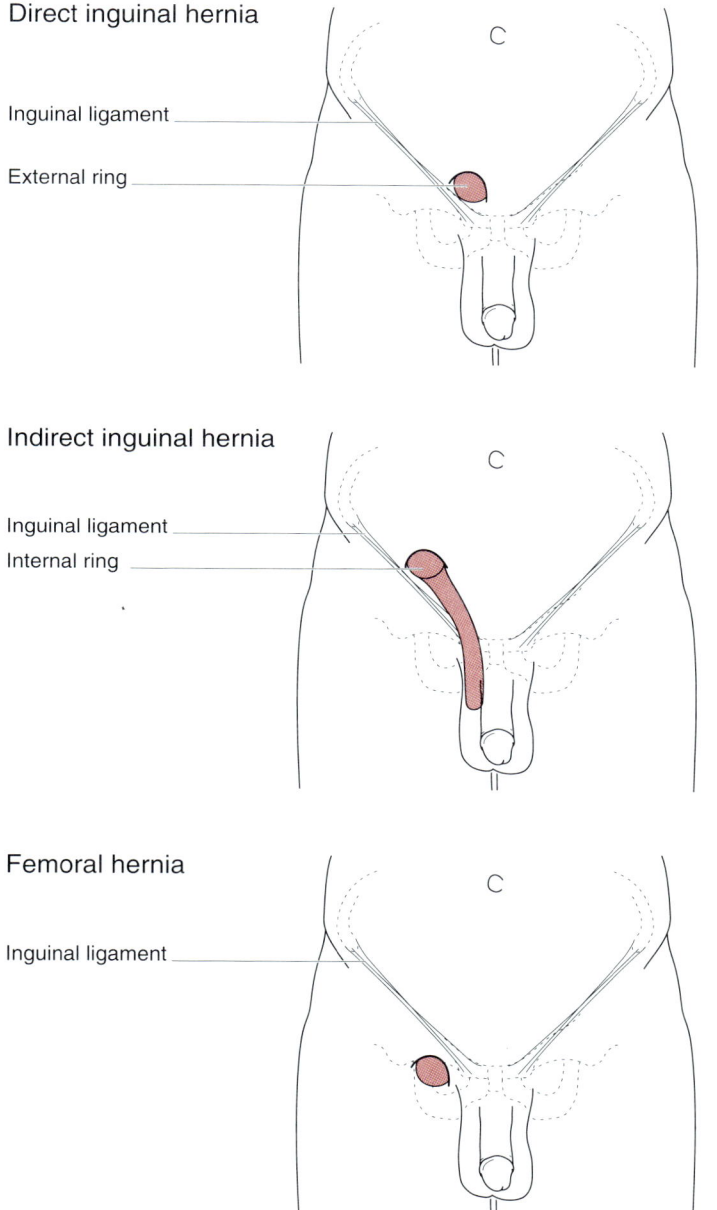

Fig. 6-7 Scheme depicting location of direct and indirect inguinal and femoral hernias.

Fig. 6-8 Technique for examining the rectum. For further details, see discussion on rectal examination in Chapter 5.

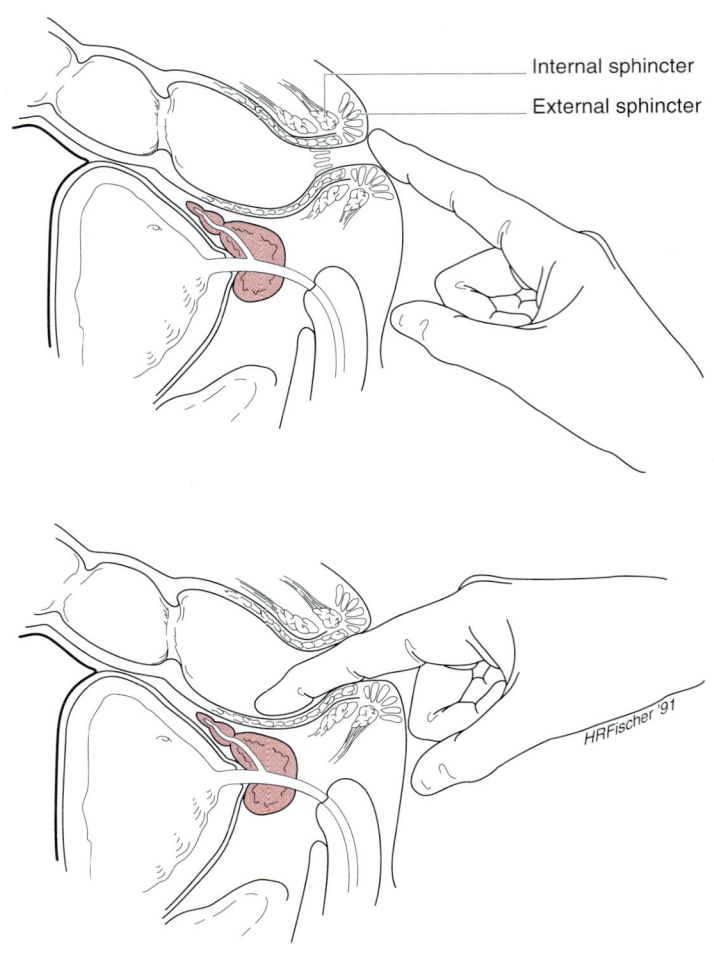

Suggested readings

Garnick MB: Contemporary issues on urologic cancer, *Semin Urol* vol 4, August 1988. *A helpful summary.*

Griffen JE, Wilson JD: Diseases of the testis. In Wilson JD, et al, editors: *Harrison's principles of internal medicine*, ed 12, New York, 1991 McGraw-Hill. *A concise treatise on the pathophysiology and manifestation of testicular disease.*

Klein LA: Prostatic carcinoma, *New Engl J Med* 300:824-833, 1979. *A vintage article on prostatic carcinoma.*

Walsh PC, et al, editors: *Campbell's urology*, Philadelphia, 1986, WB Saunders. *A useful, comprehensive urology textbook.*

Summary

The summary checklist for the examination of the male genitalia is presented below.

Checklist for Examination of Male Genitalia

Symptoms
- Dysuria
- Frequency
- Urgency
- Nocturia
- Polyuria
- Urinary incontinence
- Hematuria
- Oliguria and anuria
- Pneumaturia
- Penile pain, discharge
- Loss of libido and impotence
- Infertility
- Scrotal swelling and testicular pain

Physical Findings

Penis
- Epispadias
- Hypospadias
- Ulcers
- Nodules
- Urethral discharge
- Balanitis
- Peyronie's disease
- Edema

Scrotum

Testes

Mass

Atrophy

Epididymis

Spermatic cord

Empty scrotum (undescended testes)

Inguinal canals and groin
- Hernia
- Lymph nodes

Prostate
- Enlargement
- Nodules
- Consistency (note especially if rock hard)

CHAPTER SEVEN

Female Genitalia

CHAPTER OUTLINE

History Taking
Sensitivity to a woman's concerns during history
Pertinent past history
Abnormalities in menstruation
Nonmenstrual vaginal bleeding
Pelvic pain
Urinary tract infection
Pregnancy and infertility
Abnormalities in sexual function
Rape

Vaginal discharge and itching
Pelvic relaxation
Hirsutism

Physical Examination of the Female Genitalia
Preparation
Examination techniques
Abnormal findings

Summary

Women seek medical care for gynecologic or obstetric problems in 20% of office visits. For adolescent females these problems comprise 40% of office visits. A broad range of problems constitute initial complaints for which treatment is sought.

- Nearly 50% of couples experience some form of sexual dysfunction, though much fewer seek medical help.
- Most women are aware that screening for cervical cancer needs to be done routinely with a pelvic examination and a Papanicolaou smear. This has reduced the mortality from cervical cancer by one-half since the 1950s.
- Relatively few know that cancer of the uterus is now more common than cancer of the cervix, and cancer of the ovary results in nearly one-half of cancer deaths among women.
- Some 10% to 15% of women are affected by endometriosis.
- Infertility affects 15% of women of childbearing age who desire children.
- At present, more than 50% of conceptions are aborted, 15% of which occur spontaneously.

Women may find it difficult to consult a (male or female) physician for gynecologic or obstetric problems because of modesty, social background, religion, or morality. Yet the complete history and physical examination mandates attention to the menstrual history, sexual activity, pregnancies, abortions, pelvic pain, and the pelvic examination.

History Taking

Sensitivity to a Woman's Concerns During History

Although the introductory chapter discussed special techniques in the good bedside manner, a few merit special review. Just as the physician greets a male patient by shaking hands, likewise shaking hands with female patients is appropriate. Greet the patient by name, but not the first name alone unless you expect the patient to call you by your first name too, and you make that clear. Finally, don't make the mistake of saying "Mrs." or "Miss" until you know marital status. Using "Ms." or first and last names together is less offensive. Examples of the initial greeting would be these:

- *Tami Jones, I'm Joe Brown. I'm a second-year medical student. May I talk with you and ask you a few questions?* Notice the use of both first and last names for the patient and for you. Also, you are not trying to pass yourself off as something you are not yet.
- *Ms. Jones, I'm a second-year medical student, Joe Brown.*

Neither women nor men appreciate being called by their first names inappropriately. Another peeve of women would not usually apply to students learning physical diagnosis: women do not appreciate meeting with their physician for the first time when they have already been asked to change to an examining gown and to place their legs in stirrups for a pelvic examination.

Pertinent Past History

When the history does not reveal spontaneous gynecologic complaints, the complete history must include specific questions about possible key complaints and past gynecologic and obstetric history. Ask about the number of pregnancies *(gravida)*, number of deliveries *(para)*, number of terminations (include miscarriages and induced abortions), and the number of living children. Record the date of the most recent pelvic examination and Papanicolaou smear. Any history of radiation therapy for acne, mastitis, or an enlarged thymus may be important in

---

Key Symptoms in the Evaluation of the Female Genital and Reproductive Functions

- Abnormalities in menstruation
- Vaginal bleeding (nonmenstrual)
- Pelvic pain
- Pregnancy
- Abnormalities in sexual function
- Rape
- Vaginal discharge and itching
- Pelvic relaxation (especially urinary incontinence)
- Hirsutism
- Pelvic mass
- Genital ulcers

later development of neoplasms. Use of diethylstilbestrol (DES) by the patient's mother if she was pregnant with the patient between 1947 and 1971 to prevent spontaneous abortion may be a risk factor now. Such a woman has an increased risk of carcinoma of the vagina.

Abnormalities in Menstruation

Menarche is the first menstrual period of a female's life. It usually occurs between 11 and 14 years of age, with age 12.5 as the mean. Cessation of menses, *menopause,* most often occurs between ages 45 and 55. Premature menopause may be caused by surgery or radiation therapy.

Initial menstrual cycles in young girls are typically irregular, occasionally heavy, and usually not associated with ovulation. For women, 24 to 34 days elapse between menses (Table 7-1). The duration of bleeding lasts 3 to 7 days. *Amenorrhea* is the absence of menstruation for 3 months or more. When the interval between menses is more than 35 days but less that 3 months, and if the menstrual flow is normal, *oligomenorrhea* is present. *Hypomenorrhea* refers to a decrease in the volume of flow.

Excessive uterine bleeding is called *menorrhagia* (or *hypermenorrhea*). These terms indicate longer duration of flow than usual. The average woman looses 40 ml (nearly 3 tablespoons) of blood during each menstrual cycle. Menorrhagia refers to loss of 80 ml or more per cycle. Duration of bleeding longer than 7 days is usually associated with loss of greater than 80 ml.

Typical questions to ask about menses would include these:

- *Tell me about your menstrual periods. Are they regular? How far apart are they? How many days do they last? Do you bleed heavily? Pass clots? How many pads do you use? External or internal napkins?*

TABLE 7-1: The Menstrual Cycle

Phase of Cycle	Pituitary	Ovary	Uterus	Exam
Follicular Phase				
From day 1 of menses to surge in LH before ovulation; lasts about 14 days (duration is more variable than in luteal phase)	• FSH production increases after menses and surges before ovulation • LH production increases during phase and surges before ovulation	• FSH stimulates graafian follicle to produce estrogen during second half of phase • Granulosa cells of follicle begin to produce progesterone later in the phase	• Estrogen stimulates proliferation of uterine glands • Progesterone stimulates endometrium to prepare for fertilized ovum	• Vaginal bleeding for 3 to 7 days
Luteal phase				
From preovulatory surge in level of LH to day 1 of menses; lasts 13 to 14 days (more constant part of cycle)	• Levels of FSH and LH decrease in response to hormones from corpus luteum	• Graafian follicle is changed into a corpus luteum; this secretes progesterone and estradiol	• At menses superficial uterine glands slough, leaving basal endothelium	• Progesterone induces an increase in basal body temperature noted at ovulation

AMENORRHEA

For normal menstruation, the hypothalamus, pituitary, ovaries, and uterus must function in concert (see Table 7-1).

Amenorrhea may be primary or secondary. Women with primary amenorrhea are further divided into those who do or do not have secondary sexual development (see the accompanying box). Primary amenorrhea is the absence of menses in (1) a female age 14 or over who has no secondary sexual characteristics (axillary and pubic hair growth, breast development, or change in body habitus), or in (2) a female age 16 years or more who has secondary sex characteristics but no menses. Secondary amenorrhea describes cessation of menses for at least 6 months at some time after the onset of menstrual bleeding.

When a patient complains that she does not have menstrual periods, questions to ask include the following:

- *Have you ever had any vaginal bleeding?* This helps to differentiate primary and secondary amenorrhea.
- *Do you have hair under your arms? Pubic hair? Have your breasts begun to enlarge?* These are better evaluated by examination than by history.
- If the patient has had menses previously, ask, *Could you be pregnant? Have you had any sexual partners during the past few months?*
- *How regular have your periods been in the past? Have you ever experienced a long duration between periods before at anytime?*

Primary Amenorrhea

Most disorders associated with primary amenorrhea (menarche has never occurred) are uncommon. An isolated gonadotropin deficiency could initally appear with primary amenorrhea. Other features include lack of breast development and lack of pubic and axillary hair. One syndrome of sexual infantilism, Kallmann's syndrome, consists of a deficiency of gonadotropin-releasing hormone (follicle-stimulating hormone [FSH] and luteinizing hormone [LH]) with anosmia (inability to smell).

Turner's syndrome Chromosomally incompetent ovaries fail to develop because of an absence of one X chromosome (45,XO). Even at birth, the patient may exhibit characteristic features that suggest the diagnosis: a webbed neck, shield-shaped chest, low-set ears, and coarctation of the aorta. Later there is short

Female Developmental Markers	
Developmental Marker	Average Age (Year)*
Breast bud	11
Pubic hair and axillary hair	12
Menarche	13
Adult distribution of pubic hair	14
Adult development of breasts	15
Menopause	52

*Range is approximately +/− 2 years.

stature for age, no breast development, scanty axillary and pubic hair, and amenorrhea.

Androgen insensitivity syndrome This is called testicular feminization syndrome and is caused by a lack of androgen receptors. These patients are males who look like well-developed females. They have an XY karyotype but absence of virilization. The following are key historical complaints that such patients may exhibit: a female who has had bilateral inguinal hernias (undescended testicles), and amenorrhea. Examination shows a lack of axillary or pubic hair, underdeveloped labia, a blind vaginal canal without a uterus, large breasts, small nipples, and pale areolae.

Uterine and vaginal causes of amenorrhea Congenital abnormalities of the uterus or vagina may result in amenorrhea, such as imperforate hymen, or developmental abnormality of the uterus (agenesis) or the vagina (either a transverse septum or atresia).

An imperforate hymen prevents menstrual flow from exiting. The vagina above the hymen becomes distended with blood and may appear to be bulging. The uterus and tubes may fill with menstrual blood.

Secondary Amenorrhea

Pregnancy, because it requires special management, is the most important consideration. Menopause is a second common cause of secondary amenorrhea.

Psychogenic amenorrhea, or stress-induced absence of menses, occurs in healthy young women. The patient typically develops amenorrhea because of stress of leaving home, going to college, or some exciting event.

Weight-reduction amenorrhea Weight-reduction amenorrhea caused by dieting or illness is associated with decreased gonadotropins and inhibition of ovulation. Decreasing weight by 10% to 15%, or decreasing body fat by one-third, may induce amenorrhea.

The extreme weight loss of anorexia nervosa is important to recognize because of a 5% to 15% mortality rate. *Anorexia nervosa* is most common between age 13 and 25 years. Despite weight losses of up to 25%, the patient's self-image is that she is too heavy. Most such people are otherwise normal psychiatrically. Typically, they have excellent grades in school and are physically active outside of school. Besides amenorrhea, examination shows soft, downy body hair and bradycardia.

Bulimia, self-induced vomiting, may be suggested by callouses on the backs of the fingers (from rubbing teeth when fingers are inserted into the throat) and erosion of teeth by gastric acid. Other features include constipation, cold intolerance, a yellow hue to the skin, or peripheral edema.

Exercise-induced amenorrhea As more women participate in vigorous exercise, exercise-induced amenorrhea has become more common. Such inducing activities include ballet dancing, running, swimming, and gymnastics. The common factor is not the type of activity nor weight loss, but the intensity of exercise. However, usually this involves young women who weigh less than 115 pounds and lose more than 10 pounds. Some who exercise vigorously have irregular menses instead of amenorrhea.

Postpill amenorrhea This has been attributed to the persistent suppressive effects of oral contraceptives. Presumed postpill amenorrhea should be investigated so that another, more serious etiologic cause will not be overlooked.

Pituitary disease as a cause of amenorrhea Sheehan's syndrome is pituitary infarction caused by hypotension resulting from peripartum hemorrhage. Failure to lactate may be the first manifestation. Other symptoms include loss of energy, fatigue, hypotension, loss of axillary and pubic hair, and weight loss.

Premature ovarian failure Ovarian failure is a common cause of secondary amenorrhea. This occurs when a deficit of ovarian follicles is present. Normally ovarian follicles cease to develop at menopause. Premature ovarian failure results in amenorrhea before age 35. Usually no pathology is associated, but viral oophoritis (mumps), radiation therapy to ovaries, or chemotherapy for cancer may be causes.

Uterine causes of amenorrhea Asherman's syndrome is amenorrhea caused by intrauterine synechiae (adhesions) that obliterate part of the uterine cavity. Vigorous dilation and curettage (D and C) that removes the basal layer of endometrium can expose the underlying myometrium. When this occurs in opposing areas of the uterine cavity, adhesions can form, obstructing outflow of menstrual blood.

ABNORMAL MENSTRUAL BLEEDING

Menorrhagia typically occurs in one of the following conditions:

- Uterine fibroids
- Pelvic inflammatory disease (PID)
- Endometriosis
- Polyp in the uterine cavity
- Intrauterine contraceptive device (IUD)

Women with menorrhagia pass clots, fill multiple pads or tampons, or have other historical clues showing excessive volume.

Dysfunctional uterine bleeding (DUB) is abnormal uterine bleeding in which no etiologic cause can be found on pelvic examination and routine studies. *Metrorrhagia* is bleeding at midcycle between menses, and it is caused by the decrease in estrogen secretion following ovulation.

MENOPAUSE

Menopause refers to cessation of menses caused by aging, surgical removal of the ovaries or uterus, or other reasons. The *climacteric* refers to the phase of life in which a women passes from the reproductive years. *Perimenopause* includes the few years before and after menopause.

The average age for menopause, ~52 years, has remained fairly constant for centuries. In contrast, menarche has decreased 2.5 years since 1900.

Clinical symptoms in menopause at first are caused by acute estrogen deprivation. Later the manifestations of prolonged estrogen deprivation occur. Acutely, patients may complain of hot flashes, flushes, and sweats (vasomotor symptoms). Later, dyspareunia (painful intercourse) or pruritus caused by atrophic vaginitis and osteoporosis-induced vertebral fractures occur. Atherosclerotic vascular disease is partly caused by estrogen deficiency. Other symptoms can include skin aging, headaches, irritability, insomnia, anxiety, and depression.

Vasomotor instability occurs in 80% of women with natural menopause but in only 40% following surgical oophorectomy. A hot flush begins as a sudden rush of heat in the face or neck and spreads to the chest. Occasionally a chill, perspiration, dizziness, headache, or nausea supervenes. The subjective warmth may last for 2 minutes, but objective skin changes can last for 30 minutes or longer. Most women have these symptoms only for 1 to 2 years. One-third may have vasomotor symptoms for up to 5 years. These symptoms may be stopped by replacement hormone.

Similarly, symptoms caused by reduced estrogen activity is characteristic of amenorrhea resulting from nutritional deficiency, anorexia nervosa, use of clomiphene citrate (an antiestrogen), during therapy with danazol (decreases estrogen production), and in men who have been treated with estrogens for prostatic carcinoma but who have had the therapy discontinued.

PREMENSTRUAL SYNDROME

Premenstrual syndrome (PMS) is the recurrent constellation of symptoms before the monthly menses that completely subsides during menses. A symptom-free interval follows. PMS includes cyclical emotional, physical, and behavioral changes. Unfortunately, a single etiology for this syndrome has not been found. Symptoms of PMS can be divided into nine categories: affective, cognitive, pain, neurovegetative, autonomic, CNS, fluid and electrolyte, dermatologic, and behavioral (Table 7-2).

DYSMENORRHEA

Dysmenorrhea is the term used for pain associated with menstruation. An estimated 5% of women suffer from severe dysmenorrhea at some time.

Primary dysmenorrhea refers to pain that accompanies menstruation without associated pelvic pathologic condition. It begins a few hours before menstrual flow and lasts for 1 or 2 days. Dysmenorrhea often begins when ovulatory menstrual cycles begin. Lower abdominal colicky pain radiates to the lower back and upper thighs. Other symptoms include nausea, vomiting, headache, nervousness, fatigue, diarrhea, or syncope. Primary dysmenorrhea is believed to be caused by excessive myometrial levels of prostaglandin F_{2a}. Uterine tone, frequency, and strength of contractions are increased.

Secondary dysmenorrhea is pain with menses caused by organic disease of the pelvis (endometriosis, chronic PID), uterus (IUD, polyp, adhesions), or lower genital tract (imperforate hymen). It may begin at any age. Typically pain begins a few days before menses and persists throughout the menstrual cycle. The timing of symptoms may help to separate primary from secondary dysmenorrhea.

Nonmenstrual Vaginal Bleeding

When a female complains of vaginal bleeding, determine whether the source of bleeding is menstrual with a variation in flow or is nonmenstrual bleeding from urethra, anus, or vagina.

Genital (vaginal) bleeding before puberty is always abnormal. Typical causes include trauma, neoplasm, and foreign body, or it may be hormonally related.

When vaginal bleeding not related to menses occurs between ages 12 and 50, consider a possible pregnancy first. Uterine bleeding may be caused by intrauterine pregnancy with various abnormalities or be caused by a tubal or ectopic pregnancy. Neoplasms or polyps of the cervix or endometrium are also possible causes. Infections with resulting erosions or ulcers may bleed. Tampons left in place too long can cause vaginal ulcers. Finally, birth control methods such as the IUD or oral contraceptives with breakthrough bleeding may be responsible.

Bleeding beginning longer than 6 months after menopause is termed *postmenopausal bleeding*. Carcinoma of the cervix and uterus are more common after menopause and may cause bleeding. Atrophic vaginitis was an important

TABLE 7-2: Symptoms Associated with Premenstrual Syndrome

Category	Symptom
Affective	• Sadness
	• Anxiety
	• Anger
	• Irritability
	• Labile mood
Cognitive	• Decreased ability to concentrate
	• Indecisiveness
	• Paranoid ideation
	• Suicidal thoughts
Pain	• Headache
	• Breast tenderness
	• Joint pain
	• Muscle pain
Neurovegetative	• Insomnia or hypersomnia
	• Craving for salt or sugar
	• Anorexia
	• Excessive fatigue and lethargy
	• Agitation
	• Changes in libido
Autonomic	• Nausea
	• Vomiting
	• Palpitations
	• Sweating
CNS	• Clumsiness
	• Seizures
	• Dizziness or vertigo
	• Paresthesia
	• Tremors
Fluid and electrolyte	• Bloating
	• Weight gain
	• Oliguria
	• Peripheral edema
Dermatologic	• Oily skin
	• Greasy or dry hair
	• Hirsutism
Behavioral	• Decreased motivation
	• Decreased efficiency
	• Poor control over impulses
	• Social isolation

cause, but the use of estrogen supplementation has reduced its incidence. Atrophic vaginitis allows trauma from coitus to cause bleeding. Cancers, polyps, infection, trauma, unopposed estrogen use (no progesterone cycling) can be other reasons for bleeding.

Pelvic Pain

Pelvic pain may originate from the ovaries, uterus, fallopian tubes, or pelvic peritoneum. Extragenital pelvic pain sources include the kidneys, bladder, or bowel, and appendicitis, diverticulitis, colitis, or orthopedic problems.

Typical questions to ask women who seek treatment for pelvic pain include the following:

- *Where do you feel pain and what does it feel like?* Determine the quality of the pain, such as constant or cramping.
- *Is it related to menstrual periods? How?* Use timing to consider primary amenorrhea and imperforate hymen, or another cause such as PID.
- *Do you have pain with intercourse?*
- *Have you had any change in bowel habits, such as diarrhea or constipation?*
- *Have you had any urinary tract symptoms? Do you leak urine when you laugh or strain?* Urinary incontinence may be a sign of pelvic relaxation or cystocele.
- *Do you have burning when you pass urine?* This may be caused by vaginitis or by a urinary tract infection.

ACUTE PELVIC PAIN

Mittelschmerz (middle pain) is pain at midcycle, related to ovulation. Ovulation ordinarily occurs 12 to 14 days before the menstrual period. The ovarian follicle ruptures, releasing the ovum and 5 ml of follicular fluid into the peritoneal cavity. In some women a small amount of ovarian bleeding may accompany rupture of the follicle. This causes acute pain. Mittelschmerz tends to be recurrent at menses.

Twisting (torsion) of the ovary occurs more often when the ovary is enlarged with an ovarian cyst. Torsion impairs the blood flow, resulting in ischemia, with the potential for necrosis. This causes acute pelvic pain. Bleeding into an ovarian cyst may also cause acute pain.

A fertilized ovum may implant in a fallopian tube, in the peritoneal cavity, or in the endometrium. In the tube, initial growth occurs slowly so that the tube stretches without pain. However, in early rupture of a tubal pregnancy, a small amount of bleeding produces peritoneal irritation and abdominal pain. When a tubal pregnancy suddenly ruptures, massive bleeding, hypotension, and severe pain result. The history usually reveals symptoms of pregnancy such as breast enlargement or tenderness or a skipped period. These point the clinician to a ruptured tubal pregnancy as the cause of severe pelvic pain with hypotension.

Spontaneous abortion (miscarriage) or induced abortion (therapeutic or otherwise) may be associated with central cramping pain.

CHRONIC PELVIC PAIN

Islands of mucosa (glands and stoma) from the endometrium may implant outside of the uterine mucosa in the peritoneal or pelvic cavity. Cyclic hormonal stimulation causes these ectopic islands to function similar to the endometrium with periodic bleeding. This is termed *endometriosis,* which is associated with the triad of dysmenorrhea, dyspareunia, and infertility. The pain is roughly equivalent to the site of the ectopic endometrial tissue. The distinction between endometriosis and dysmenorrhea tends to be (1) onset at age 25 to 40 for endometriosis (under age 20 for dysmenorrhea), and (2) the pain of endometriosis tends to be referred to the sacrum, rectum, or coccyx (lower abdomen, back, and thighs for dysmenorrhea). The dyspareunia is deep and constant in endometriosis. Infertility is also typical in endometriosis.

Pelvic or lower abdominal pain that is most pronounced during or shortly after menses may result from infection of the vagina, uterus, and fallopian tubes. PID is usually a polymicrobial disease caused by a combination of *Neisseria gonorrheae, Chlamydia trachomatis,* anaerobic streptococci, or *Bacteroides* species, including *B. bivius (Prevotella bivia).* The tube wall becomes edematous and distended (salpingitis). As purulent exudate exudes into the peritoneal cavity, pain and rebound tenderness result.

Typical findings in PID include a history of several sexual partners, nausea, vomiting, fever, and pelvic pain worse during or after menstruation. On pelvic examination, pain increases when the cervix is moved. The adnexa seem tender and enlarged as tubes and ovaries become involved in abscesses.

Urinary Tract Infection

On the basis of symptoms and findings on examination, urinary tract infections (UTIs) are termed *lower tract* or *upper tract* infections. Certain symptoms are found in both upper and lower tract infections; that is, dysuria (painful urination) and frequency (needing to void).

The typical history of lower tract infection is found in young women who have recently become sexually active (formerly called honeymoon cystitis). However, school girls and older women may also be affected.

Lower tract symptoms depend on anatomic sites affected; they can include urethritis (burning while voiding), trigonitis (frequency), and cystitis (suprapubic pain or discomfort). Urine may be dark, have a foul order, or be turbid.

Upper tract symptoms (pyelonephritis) include costovertebral angle pain and tenderness to percussion, abdominal pain, and systemic symptoms including headache, vomiting, fever with chills, and malaise. In some people, neither symptoms nor physical examination findings differentiate pyelonephritis from simple cystitis.

Urinalysis shows pyuria (white blood cells in urine), whether the UTI is caused by *Escherichia coli, Proteus mirabilis,* or vaginitis/urethritis resulting from microbes such as *Chlamydia trachomatis.* Bacterial cultures typically have greater than 10^5 bacteria/ml, but fewer bacteria may sometimes be found.

Chronic or recurrent UTIs may be in either upper or lower tracts. The lower tract chronic/recurrent infections may be caused by sexual activities, hygiene, diabetes, or structural abnormalities of the urinary tract. Examples of the latter include cystocele and failure to completely empty the bladder when voiding. Upper tract chronic/recurrent infections are typical in pyelonephritis because it may not respond to the usual brief courses of antibiotic therapy.

Pregnancy and Infertility

The physician whose practice includes women of child-bearing age needs to be able to diagnose pregnancy. Because of possible teratogenicity during pregnancy, some radiographs, radionuclide scans, and several medications should be avoided.

NORMAL PREGNANCY

Recognizing early pregnancy may be difficult if the patient has missed only one period or has had reduced menstrual flow. Manifestations that suggest *early pregnancy* include the following:

- *Amenorrhea.* The patient may have missed a period or had slight vaginal bleeding at the usual time for her period.
- *Nausea* and *vomiting.* In pregnancy, morning nausea and vomiting is called

morning sickness. These symptoms may range from mild to severe vomiting (*hyperemesis gravidarum*). Nausea may be precipitated by odors, aromas, or thoughts of food. Often morning sickness subsides by 8 weeks into the pregnancy.
- *Breast tenderness.* Mastodynia ranges from slight breast tingling to breast pain.
- *Urinary frequency.* Bladder irritability and frequency may be related to pressure from an enlarged uterus or be caused by hormonal effects.
- *Constipation.* Because progesterone is a smooth muscle relaxant, many women experience constipation early and throughout pregnancy.
- *Weight change.* Weight loss is common early in pregnancy, related to anorexia, vomiting, and nausea. Weight gain begins later.

Later manifestations of pregnancy include several skin changes, including the following:

- Chloasma (the mask of pregnancy) refers to pigmentary darkening of the skin around the eyes, bridge of the nose, and cheeks. It begins after the fourth month and intensifies with sun exposure.
- The nipples, areola, and skin in the midline between pubis and umbilicus often darken.
- *Striae gravidarum* (stretch marks of pregnancy) often develop on the lower abdomen and breasts.
- Vascular spider angiomas may occur in the skin because of the high estrogen levels.
- An increase in acne, oily skin, and facial or body hair is common.

Other changes commonly occur during pregnancy. Breast enlargement continues throughout much of pregnancy. Colostrum secretion may begin after the fourth month. Abdominal enlargement becomes evident after the fourteenth week of pregnancy. Changes in pelvic organs occur, as listed below:

- *Chadwick's sign* is a blue or purple discoloration of the vagina.
- *Leukorrhea,* a clear or white vaginal discharge with a faint musty odor, may occur during pregnancy.
- *Goodell's sign* is a bluish discoloration of the cervix that occurs in conjunction with softening of the cervix.
- *Braxton Hicks* contractions are painless uterine contractions that the patient may begin to notice after the twenty-eighth week.
- *Quickening* is the first fetal movement of which the patient is aware. Quickening is noted at approximately 18 weeks in the primigravida (woman in first pregnancy) and 16 weeks in the multigravida. Adding 22 or 24 weeks respectively gives the approximate delivery date, called the *expected date of confinement* (EDC).

HIGH-RISK PREGNANCY

Pregnancy is deemed to be at high risk if the mother, the fetus, or the newborn is likely to sustain serious health problems or die. A number of conditions may increase the risk to the mother or fetus:

- Maternal age under 16 or over 35 years.
- Previous high-risk pregnancies that have ended in fetal death or serious problems.

- Medical diseases, including hypertension, renal failure, diabetes mellitus, cancer, sickle cell disease, alcoholism, drug addiction, or heavy smoking.
- Exposure to infections that can be transmitted to the fetus, including *to*xoplasmosis, *r*ubella, *c*ytomegalovirus, *h*erpes simplex, and *s*yphilis (TORCHS).

When a pregnancy has the potential for high risk, special attention is needed to preserve the life and health of the mother and fetus.

ECLAMPSIA

Preeclampsia occurs when the pregnant woman develops hypertension, albuminuria, and edema during the last half of pregnancy, between the twentieth and fortieth weeks. If the patient develops coma or seizures, *eclampsia* is said to be present. *Preeclampsia* develops in 1 of 20 primigravidas and, if left untreated, may progress to fatal eclampsia. A potential complication for the fetus is fetal death.

ABORTION

Abortion is termination of pregnancy before 20 weeks' gestation or before the fetus has achieved weight of 500 g. Patients call a spontaneous abortion a miscarriage. The woman about to miscarry observes vaginal spotting or mild bleeding. Pain may be present.

When abortion (miscarriage) is deemed inevitable, the patient experiences cramping low abdominal pain and extensive vaginal bleeding and has a dilated cervix. Both incomplete and complete abortion signify that products of conception have been passed. When all the products of gestation are passed, abortion is complete.

Septic abortion refers to infection involving products of conception either after spontaneous abortion or after induced abortions. These women may become acutely, severely ill.

HYDATIDIFORM MOLE

The hydatidiform mole is an intrauterine or ectopic neoplasm of trophoblastic origin now termed *gestational trophoblastic neoplasia*. This is the end stage of a degenerating pregnancy with proliferating villi. The majority of hydatidiform moles are benign. Findings suggesting a hydatidiform mole include the following:

- The uterus may rapidly increase in size shortly after implantation of the fertilized ovum (in half the cases).
- There is persistent vaginal bleeding, no fetal movement, and no fetal heart tones by 12 weeks.
- Nausea and vomiting can be more intense than is usual for pregnancy.
- Grapelike clusters of tissue may be passed through the vagina.

CONTRACEPTION

One important cause of women not becoming pregnant is their use of contraceptives. The history taken from women between menarche and menopause should include the question, *Do you use any type of contraception?*

Contraception may include male techniques, such as the following:
- Absence of sexual intercourse
- Condom use

- Vasectomy
- Sexual activity that does not include penile insertion into the vagina
- Withdrawal of penis before ejaculation (a risky contraceptive technique)

Female contraceptive techniques include the following:

- Use of diaphragm
- Female condoms
- IUD
- Oral estrogen-progesterone preparations
- Tubal ligation
- Hysterectomy or oophorectomy
- Contraceptive foams or jellys (may be a risky contraceptive technique)

Because the relative contraceptive effectiveness differs between the various techniques, ask about the method used and be prepared to give advice on other possible methods. At the same time, it is appropriate to discuss the use of latex condoms for safer sex to reduce the risk of transmitting sexually transmitted diseases (STDs), including HIV.

Medication questions should include the type of oral contraceptives (sequential versus combination tablets) or other estrogen preparations, the number of years used, and problems associated with their use, such as swelling, phlebitis, headaches, changes in acne, or other problems.

Abnormalities in Sexual Function

The patient may not mention the sexual history unless you inquire. When you come to this area, the patient may relax and cooperate better if you begin questioning by asking the patient's permission.

A typical beginning question is, *I would like to ask you a few questions of a personal nature regarding your sexual history if that would be okay. This is part of our usual complete evaluation.* Sometimes it is better not to take notes at the time so the patient will feel that what she says is confidential.

As the sexual history is obtained, inquire and respond with an open-minded, nonjudgmental, noncritical attitude, especially as the patient discusses the number of sexual partners, abortions, and sexual practices. Some studies suggest that nearly one-half of women are dissatisfied with their sex lives in some way. The caring clinician needs the entire gynecologic history to be able to help.

Examples of questions to begin the sexual history include the following:

- *Are you currently having a sexual relationship? Is this satisfactory?* Such an open-ended question does not exclude the possibility of celibacy, homosexuality, or a heterosexual relationship.
- *How often do you have sex? Is this enough? Too frequent?* This gives you a feeling for the patient's adjustment to her social situation.
- *What percent of the time would you say you have an orgasm during sex?* Lack of orgasm may be an unexpressed concern unless you give permission to discuss it by asking.
- *What types of contraception have you used, and what are you currently using? Have your sexual methods changed recently?* Patients do not always understand "risky" contraceptive practices in terms of pregnancy and disease prevention.

- *What has been the source of your sexual education? Do you need additional information now? Are you adequately protected from exposure to the AIDS (HIV) virus?*
- *What kinds of sexual experiences have you had in the past for which you feel guilty? Have you ever been traumatized sexually, or raped? Have you been able to resolve your feelings about this? Do you have worries or fears you would like help in coping with?* Rape, incest, and other forms of molestation are difficult for patients to remember and discuss until they establish a bond of respect and trust.
- After these questions it is permissible to ask, *Have you ever been married? Number of times? Duration of each marriage? Have you had any problems of this nature that you would like to discuss?*

VAGINISMUS

Vaginismus is reflex involuntary spasm of the muscles around the lower vaginal opening. Vaginismus makes penetration into the vagina by the penis difficult or impossible. In contrast, *dyspareunia* refers to pain during coitus but not necessarily during penetration. Vaginismus may actually result from a physical problem (rigid or intact hymen), or from an unconscious desire to prevent penetration. Take a careful history because rape, incest, or other molestation may be unconscious factors in vaginismus.

DYSPAREUNIA

Dyspareunia refers to painful intercourse. It may appear during the initial attempts at coitus in young women or develop later in life. Dyspareunia may be caused by actual perineal injury, trauma to the hymen, local lacerations, or pressure against the urethra, or it may be psychogenic. Inadequate lubrication, improper direction of intromission, or an infection may contribute. Improper episiotomy repairs, PID, or estrogen deficiency after menopause with vaginal dryness and thin mucosa may also produce dyspareunia.

INHIBITION OF ORGASM

Inhibition of orgasm *(anorgasmia)* is the absence of orgasm despite sexual activity that ordinarily would result in orgasm. Approximately 10% of women do not attain orgasm. More than half of women do not have an orgasm during coitus, but most do with direct clitoral stimulation. Reasons women list as difficulties in attaining orgasm include the inability to relax, too little foreplay, disinterest, a turned-off feeling, and a lack of tenderness or affection after coitus.

INFERTILITY

Infertility is the failure of a couple to conceive despite 12 months of unprotected intercourse occurring at least once per week. When women have unprotected intercourse, ordinarily 25% become pregnant during the first month, 60% within 6 months, and 85% in 12 months. Infertility problems result from male factors in 40%, tubal abnormalities in 20%, peritoneal abnormalities in 20%, ovulatory dysfunction in 10%, and cervical or endometrial disorders in 5% each.

To assess the male for adequate potential to impregnate, consider the spermatozoa count (> 20 million/ml), volume (2 to 5 ml), alkaline pH, motility (> 60% forward moving), and morphology (> 60% normal forms).

CASE 7-1 Infertility, amenorrhea

A 26-year-old woman presented with the complaint that she and her husband were unable to have a child.

She had been married previously and had had a child when she was 23 years old. Subsequently, she had divorced and remarried.

When questioned about menstrual periods, she volunteered that these had stopped after the birth of her first child. Although she did not breastfeed, she noticed some milklike discharge from the nipples occasionally.

Examination revealed a slender white woman. The general examination was normal, with the exception of only a sparse amount of axillary and pubic hair. The breasts were atrophic, but a small amount of milky discharge could be expressed from the nipples.

This case illustrated the problems that may occur in Sheehan's syndrome (amenorrhea, galactorrhea) resulting from pituitary hemorrhage intrapartum.

To assess the female for infertility, consider tubal patency, ovulation, endometrium, and antisperm antibodies. Tubal patency may be interrupted by STDs such as gonorrhea, chlamydia, or ureaplasma. A history of STDs or PID suggests possible obstructed fallopian tubes.

A peritoneum inconducive to pregnancy is present when a patient has a history of endometriosis or has peritubal or ovarian adhesions.

Ovulation usually occurs 2 weeks before the onset of the menstrual bleeding. A simple technique for determining time of ovulation is the basal body temperature graph. To check this, take the oral temperature immediately after awakening each morning. On the day of ovulation the temperature increases by 0.5° F and continues at that level for 14 days, as compared with the temperature taken during the 10 to 14 days previously. This sustained increase in temperature is caused by the effect of progesterone.

Endometrial factors that promote infertility include the previous use of IUDs or the presence of fibroid tumors or uterine synechiae. The IUD can cause inflammatory changes that prevent implantation. Evidence is mounting that uterine fibroid tumors may be associated with infertility. These may be found on examination, whereas uterine synechiae would not be found without a special scope (hysteroscope). Another factor concerns the mucus the cervix normally contains with which the sperm must interact in transit to the fallopian tubes. If antisperm antibodies are present, pregnancy may be prevented.

Rape

Rape is a legal and a moral term instead of a medical term. Rape is defined as the sexual penetration of any body orifice against the will of another, either woman or man. Statutory rape is coitus with a female below the age of consent (age 18) even if she has consented.

A typical rapist is a disturbed, compulsive, violent person who derives sexual excitement from the fear of his victim. Rape is usually planned and not the result of sudden impulse. It is motivated by a desire to terrorize and humiliate; rarely (except possibly date rape) is it caused by frustrated seduction. Rape is usually by someone the patient knows. Most rapes involve a weapon, frequently a knife, and on examination, 50% of female rape victims show signs of physical trauma. All suffer psychologic trauma.

It is extremely important to be empathetic with such a patient during the history and examination. Statements such as, *This is a terrible thing. I want to help you,* begin to show appropriate concern. In the written medical record, use such statements as suspected rape or alleged rape because the occurrence of rape (whether consent was given) is a legal finding.

Vaginal Discharge and Itching

Vaginitis may be accompanied by discharge, vulvar itching, dyspareunia, or dysuria. Vaginal discharge as a manifestation of vaginitis is fairly common and accounts for more patient visits to physicians among women than any other single entity. Table 7-3 discusses how to differentiate between the causes of vaginitis.

Physiologic vaginal discharge occurs at midcycle. A small amount of white vaginal discharge results from cervical mucus. Should this dry on the perineum, it may cause itching or irritation.

Vaginal or vulvar itching or discharge may be caused by several substances or objects:

- Feminine hygiene sprays
- Suppositories
- Spermicidal preparations
- Pinworms
- Clothing
- Soaps
- Items used in masturbation or sexual activity
- A forgotten tampon in the vagina

TABLE 7-3: Vaginitis and Vaginal Discharge

	Etiology	Discharge	Mucosa	Confirmation
Physiologic discharge	Normal at midcycle	Clear or white	Normal	History, timing
Trichomonad	*Trichomonas vaginalis*	Gray, foamy, bad odor	Red, strawberry cervix	Saline suspension microscopy
Gonococcal	*Neisseria gonorrhoeae*	Profuse mucopus, bad odor	Red, tender	Culture
Nonspecific	*Gardnerella vaginalis* with anaerobes	Gray or white, fishy odor	Normal	Clue cells, alkaline pH
Chlamydial	*Chlamydia trachomatis*	Little, yellow mucopus in endocervical canal	Cervical erosion	FA stain of smear shows elementary bodies
Candidal	*Candida albicans*	White, cottage-cheese–like	White patches stuck to a red base	KOH preparation, microscopy for pseudohyphae
Atrophic	Relative estrogen deficiency	Scanty, may be blood tinged	Atrophic, pale or red	History, age, empiric use of estrogen creams

Complaints that suggest a forgotten tampon include dyspareunia, burning pain, tender vagina, an offensive odor not relieved by bathing or douching, and occasionally a bloody discharge.

VAGINITIS IN CHILDHOOD

Vulvovaginitis more accurately defines involvement in childhood because the external vulva and vagina are involved. Contributing factors include constant exposure to feces and urine, the use of plastic pants and diapers, and the use of antibiotics.

Vaginal discharge is unusual in the newborn. However, the influence of maternal estrogen stimulation in utero can cause slight withdrawal bleeding, which subsides in a few days.

Vaginal discharge other than *Candida albicans* in an infant or child should alert you to possible sexual abuse. In children, demonstration of herpes simplex, *Trichomonas vaginalis, Chlamydia trachomatis,* or *Neisseria gonorrhoeae* is evidence for sexual transmission.

CANDIDAL VAGINITIS

Factors that predispose patients to candida vaginitis include therapy with antibiotics, diabetes mellitus, oral contraceptives, pregnancy, AIDS, or cancer chemotherapy. Recurrent candida vaginitis may be ping-ponged back from an uncircumcised sexual partner.

Key symptoms of candida vaginitis include white curdy discharge, pruritus, evidence of scratching (excoriation), dry and red vulva and vaginal mucosa, vulvar pain, dysuria, and dyspareunia.

For microscopic evaluation of vaginal secretions, a solution of potassium hydroxide is added to a drop of vaginal secretions on the microscopic slide. The potassium hydroxide dissolves the vaginal epithelial cells and allows visualization of pseudophyae.

Because candida colonize healthy people, a culture of vaginal secretions may be misleading. When organisms exist in sufficient numbers to be seen on microscopic evaluations of secretions, candida is probably an important pathogen.

TRICHOMONAL VAGINITIS

Vaginitis caused by *T. vaginalis* is common. Most people acquire the organism through sexual contact. Symptoms are absent in many females and nearly all males. Typical symptoms may include a profuse, foamy vaginal discharge, pruritus, a foul genital odor, and dyspareunia.

Trichomonas is confirmed microscopically by observing a drop of vaginal secretion prepared with normal saline. Trichomonads have a characteristic appearance and motility.

A regular sexual partner of an affected patient often harbors *T. vaginalis* and reinfects the patient unless both patient and partner are treated at the same time.

GARDNERELLA VAGINALIS VAGINITIS

G. vaginalis is associated with vaginitis. The actual cause is debated because anaerobic bacteria are also present and may be partly responsible. Characteristic symptoms of nonspecific vaginitis include itching and a gray-white discharge with a fishy odor that is accentuated after intercourse.

Microscopic examination of a gram stain or a wet mount of the discharge

CASE 7-2 *Gardnerella vaginalis* Vaginitis

A 39-year-old married school teacher appeared to have her IUD checked. This had been in place for several years. She had moved two or three times from out of state and so had not received medical follow-up.

Her menstrual periods were regular, occurring every 30 days. Recently she had begun to notice thin, watery, foul-smelling discharge. She also had some discomfort in the pelvic area. She had tried douching but said that did not seem to prevent the foul odor.

On examination she was generally healthy. The abdominal examination was normal.

On vaginal examination, a copious, malodorous, watery discharge was present and was a gray-white color. The vaginal walls appeared slightly erythematous, but there were no ulcers. The cervix appeared normal. The IUD was apparent, with the strings exiting through the cervical os. The uterus was normal in size and anteverted.

The adnexa showed no masses, and there was no pelvic tenderness.

A sample of the discharge was taken for microscopy. Application of 10% potassium hydroxide to a drop produced much foul odor. No fungi or yeast forms were seen. The pH of the discharge was alkaline.

A wet mount of a drop of discharge in normal saline showed many epithelial cells. These were covered with small gram-negative rods (clue cells). A culture was taken for *N. gonorrheae*.

The most likely cause of the problem is *G. vaginalis* vaginitis.

---

shows characteristic clue cells. These are large epithelial cells that have many adherent coccobacilli.

GONOCOCCAL VAGINITIS

The presence of *N. gonorrheae* may be asymptomatic or may cause mild or copious vaginal discharge, rectal discomfort, pharyngitis, dysuria or PID, depending on sites of infection. These sites are related to the type of sexual contact with an infected partner.

Clues to the diagnosis of gonorrhea include purulent vaginal discharge, urinary frequency and dysuria, and pelvic pain.

A gram stain of vaginal secretions showing gram-negative intracellular diplococci is suggestive in women, but not definitive, as in men. Culture is required for confirmation and also to check microbial susceptibility to antibiotics.

CHLAMYDIAL VAGINITIS

C. trachomatis has surpassed gonorrhea in some areas as the most commonly reported sexually transmitted pathogen. It causes vaginitis, cervicitis, urethritis, or tubal infection. The discharge is scanty but may be mucopurulent. Tubal scarring with destruction of epithelium is a common cause of ectopic (tubal) pregnancy.

ATROPHIC VAGINITIS

Atrophic vaginitis is not caused by microbes but by relative estrogen deficiency. It is typically postmenopausal, but it may be caused by low estrogen levels in other situations. A characteristic clinical finding is a dry vagina, which is not well lubricated during sexual activity; this lack of lubrication results in dyspareunia and sometimes bleeding. Atrophic changes may occur in the urethra and bladder, resulting in frequency, dysuria, and urgency.

Pelvic Relaxation

Pelvic relaxation is a loss of pelvic support caused by loss of integrity of muscles and fascia. This tends to occur in some older patients and in patients who have given birth by vaginal delivery. Urethrocele, cystocele, uterine prolapse, or rectocele may occur individually or simultaneously (see Fig. 7-7). Recent studies suggest that the birth process may be less important in pelvic relaxation than the patient's inherent musculofascial tissue strength. Pelvic relaxation tends to be familial.

In *urethrocele,* the urethra herniates and bulges into the vaginal canal. Unless it is large, it is likely to be asymptomatic. A large urethrocele may cause the patient to appear with a complaint of a vaginal mass.

Cystocele is herniation of the bladder into the vagina, which can give symptoms of a mass. Voiding to empty the bladder is difficult because the bladder sags.

Rectocele is herniation of the rectal wall into the vagina. It may produce symptoms of a mass, cause problems with intercourse, or cause difficulty in evacuation of the bowels.

Uterine prolapse is descent of the uterus down into the vagina. Depending on the depth of descent, it is termed first degree (mild), second degree (marked), or third degree (uterus protrudes beyond the vulva). Symptoms include feeling a mass, discomfort during sitting, problems with intercourse, bleeding, and ulceration.

Hirsutism

Hirsutism describes a male pattern of hair in women that is considered to be excessive in the woman's race or culture. Most hirsutism has no apparent medical or hormonal etiology. Male pattern hair distribution involves the sides of the face, chin, chest, and the lower abdomen.

Hirsutism may be ethnic or familial, tending to occur in certain groups of people. Idiopathic hirsutism indicates an unknown etiologic cause after the patient has been completely evaluated and no pathologic condition found.

In contrast to hirsutism, *hypertrichosis* is excessive growth of fine vellus hair and is usually confined to the extremities, head, or back rather than occurring in the male hair pattern distribution.

Causes of hirsutism include (1) androgen excess in an androgen-producing tumor; (2) Cushing's syndrome with excessive corticosteroids; and (3) the Stein-Leventhal syndrome, which is an association of polycystic ovaries, amenorrhea, sometimes obesity, infertility, and hirsutism. Patients with Stein-Leventhal syndrome have inappropriate secretion of pituitary gonadotropins.

Physical Examination of the Female Genitalia

Before performing the examination, don a pair of latex gloves. These will protect from possible bacterial or viral contagion. Gloves are also useful in other areas of the physical examination (see accompanying box) and should be worn for protection of both the examiner and the patient.

Use of Gloves

- Wear gloves when contact with blood can be anticipated.
- Wear gloves before mucous membranes (vagina, mouth, rectum) or nonintact skin (lacerations or abrasions) is touched.
- Wear gloves if potentially infectious (bacterial, viral, fungal, tuberculous) material may be encountered.
- Wear gloves before performing vascular access procedures such as blood drawing or starting intravenous lines.
- Wear gloves when touching contaminated items or surfaces.
- Especially wear gloves when cuts or scratches are present on the skin of the hands if any danger of body fluid contamination (tears, blood, CSF, urine, feces, or saliva) exists.
- Remove contaminated gloves as soon as practical and replace if needed.
- Remove torn or punctured gloves and replace if needed.
- Do not wash gloves and reuse unless the gloves are made for that purpose.

Modified from Occupational Safety and Health Administration: Federal Register, *Code of Federal Regulations* 56:64175-64182, 1991.

Preparation

The environment in which the pelvic examination takes place should inspire the patient's confidence. Be certain the surroundings are private, with adequate protection from visitors. Another female should attend pelvic examinations by male physicians. Provide a private area for the patient to empty her bladder, undress, and put on a gown that opens in the back.

Ask the patient to lie in the dorsal lithotomy position on her back with her feet placed in the foot extensions called stirrups. The end of the exam table should fold down or slide in so the patient can position her perineum at the end of the table. Place a sheet over the patient that extends from the abdomen to the knees to provide modesty. This permits exposure of only the body parts to be examined (Fig. 7-1).

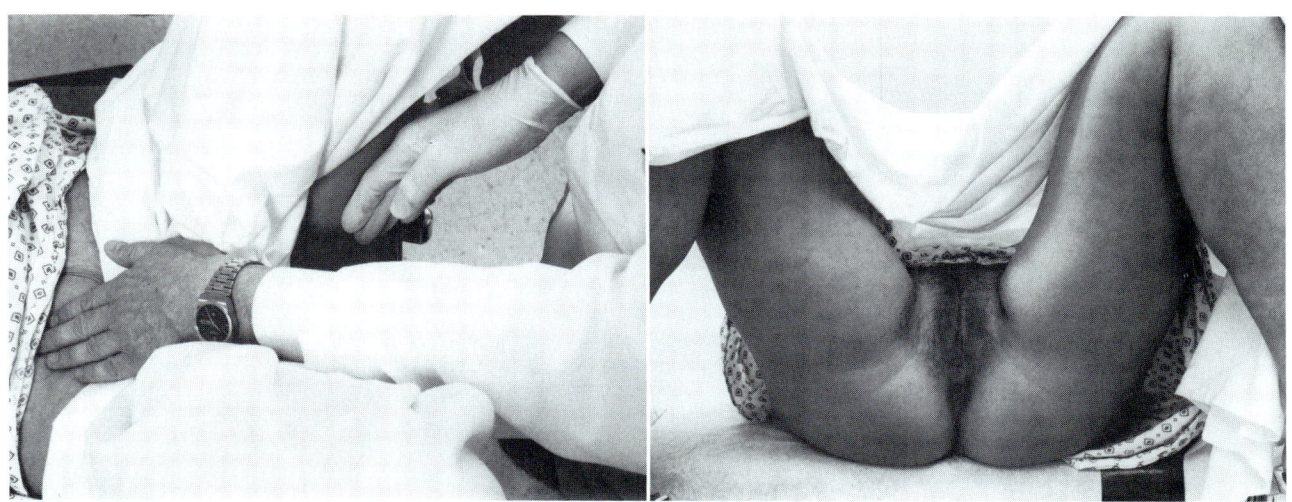

Fig. 7-1 Position for pelvic examination. **A,** Position of examiner. **B,** Position of patient in stirrups.

Examination Techniques

The patient will relax more if you explain what you are going to do and encourage her to ask questions. Ask her to inform you should she sense discomfort so you can evaluate the problem and modify your technique of examination.

In a patient who is debilitated or unconscious, perform the examination with the patient in the left lateral decubitus position with her back near the edge of the examination table. Flex the left thigh slightly and the right hip and knee to 90 degrees. Stand behind and to the side of the patient.

The lower part of the abdominal examination is performed with the pelvic examination. The uterus, tubes, and ovaries may extend up into the abdomen. The four techniques of examination are useful. Inspect for items such as scars, skin or hair changes, discharge, genital ulcers, and evidence of trauma. Palpate for masses, organ enlargement, tenderness, and rebound tenderness of peritonitis. Percussion is not used on examination of the perineum, but it may be used over the lower abdomen. Auscultation is also limited to the abdomen in assessment of the pelvis. Fetal heart tones, hypoactive bowel sounds, or bruits are typical concerns.

Examine the structures of the perineum and pelvis in sequence.

EXTERNAL GENITALIA

The extent of pubic hair growth is assessed according to Tanner's stages of female maturation (Fig. 7-2). In most adult women, hair extends from the perianal region to above the mons pubis. It does not extend up the abdomen to the umbilicus, as for males. Hair does extend toward or onto the medial thighs.

Examine the hair for nits of lice and for infected hair follicles. Before touching the external genitalia, inform the patient that you will now touch her. Then begin by touching the inner thigh with the back of your gloved hand. This avoids startling the patient. Inspect and palpate the labia majora, the lateral external genital folds. Locate Bartholin's glands deep in each of the labia majora at the 4 to 5 and 7 to 8 o'clock positions. These cannot be felt or seen unless they are abnormal. Visualize the labia minora by spreading the labia majora to demonstrate them. The labia minora form a funnel-shaped or boat-shaped entrance to the vagina termed the *vestibule* (Fig. 7-3).

Next inspect the clitoris by gently retracting the skin folds of the clitoral hood, or prepuce, at the apex of the labia minora (Fig. 7-4). The clitoris is usually 1.5

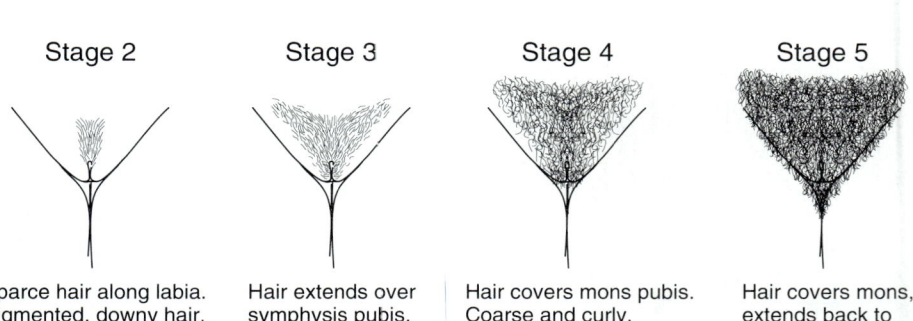

Fig. 7-2 Changes in pubic hair as females mature.

Stage 2: Sparce hair along labia. Pigmented, downy hair, little or no curl.

Stage 3: Hair extends over symphysis pubis. Darker, coarser and more curl.

Stage 4: Hair covers mons pubis. Coarse and curly.

Stage 5: Hair covers mons, extends back to anus, and onto medial legs. Configuration is delta shaped. Curly.

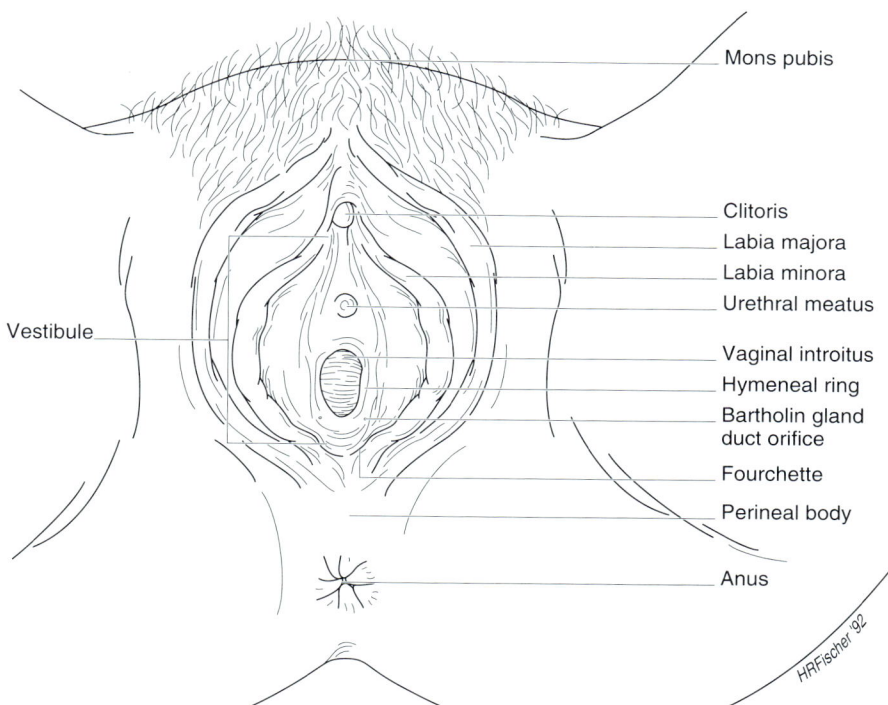

Fig. 7-3 The external female genitalia.

to 2.5 cm long. The urethra is in the midline below the clitoris. Skene's (paraurethral) glands are lateral to the urethra on each side. Inspect and palpate these for tenderness, enlargement, or infection.

The hymen or hymeneal ring is directly below the urethra. At the posterior of the ring are Bartholin's glands (Fig. 7-5). Palpate each for swelling or tenderness. An episiotomy scar may extend from the lower portion of the labia minora, posteriorly toward the fourchette. Usually the episiotomy is lateral to the perineal body and leaves a scar to one side (usually the right) of the fourchette. Place a

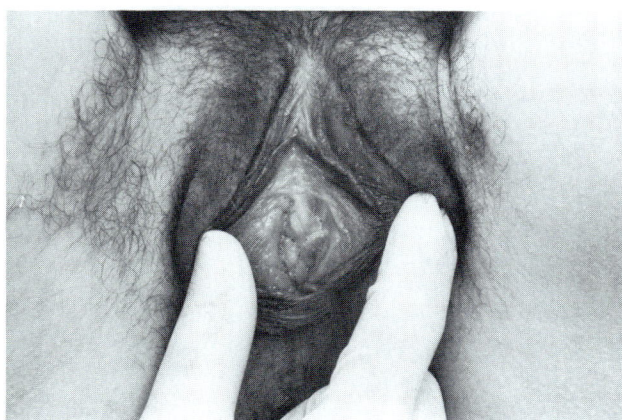

Fig. 7-4 Technique for spreading the labia.

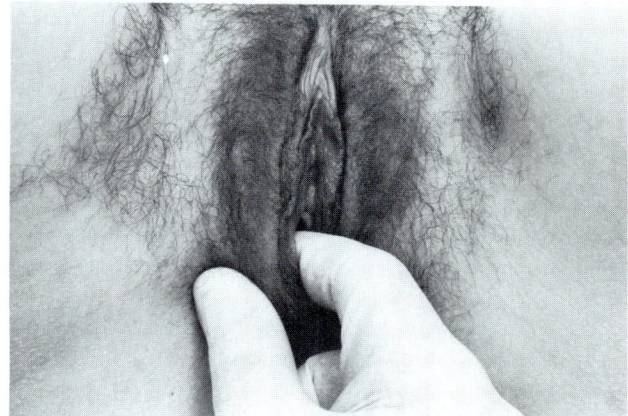

Fig. 7-5 Technique for palpating Bartholin's glands.

Fig. 7-6 Technique for palpating the urethra.

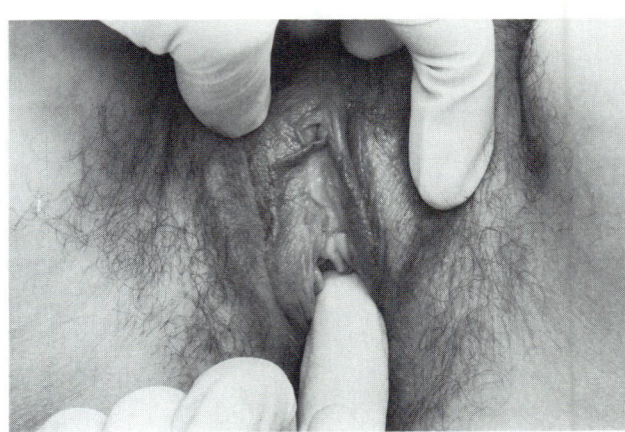

gloved finger inside the hymeneal ring and palpate the lower 3 or 4 cm of the urethra and milk it to look for any urethral discharge (Fig. 7-6).

The hymen may be intact with a small hole in children, young women, and some virgins. Should the hymen be imperforate (no hole), it may bulge with menstrual blood behind it and be the cause of amenorrhea.

To determine if pelvic relaxation is present, insert two fingers along the posterior vaginal wall to see the vaginal contents. Instruct the patient to perform Valsalva's maneuver. This may demonstrate a urethrocele, cystocele, rectocele, or even prolapse of the uterus (Fig 7-7).

Fig. 7-7 Pelvic floor relaxation.

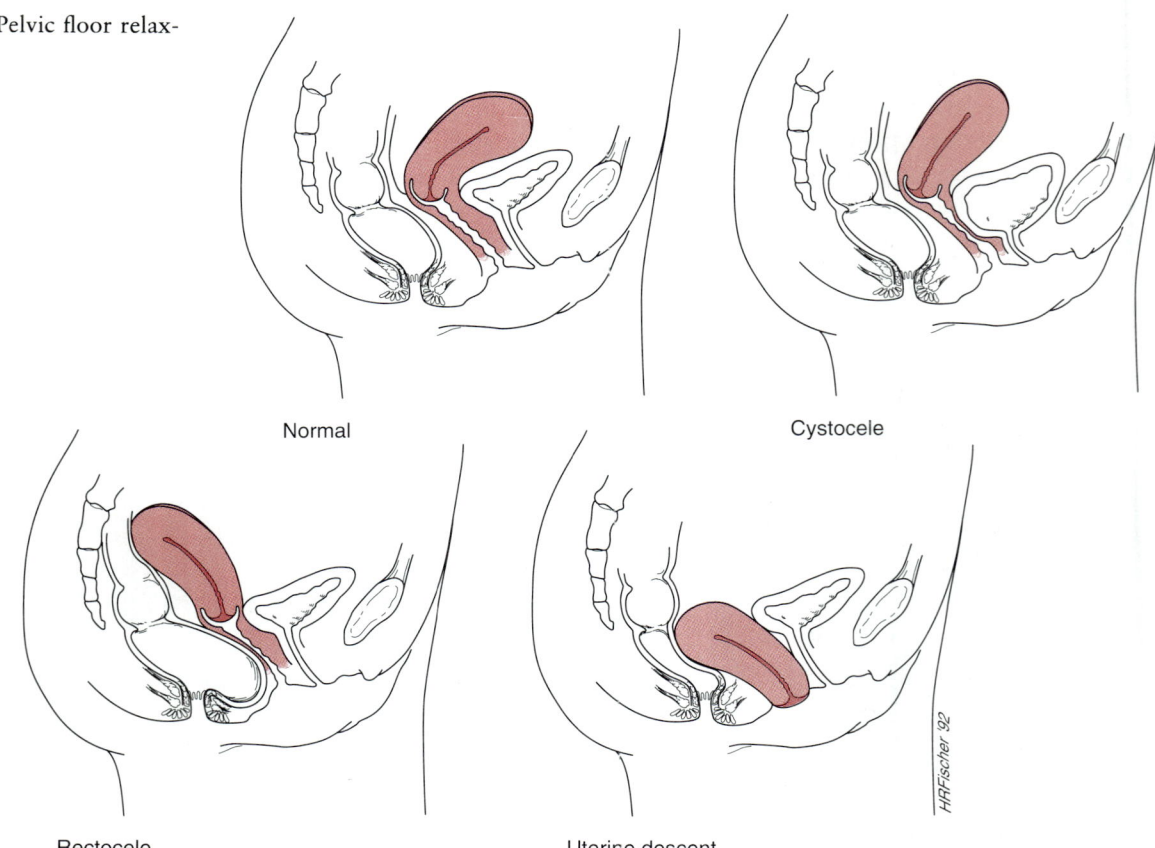

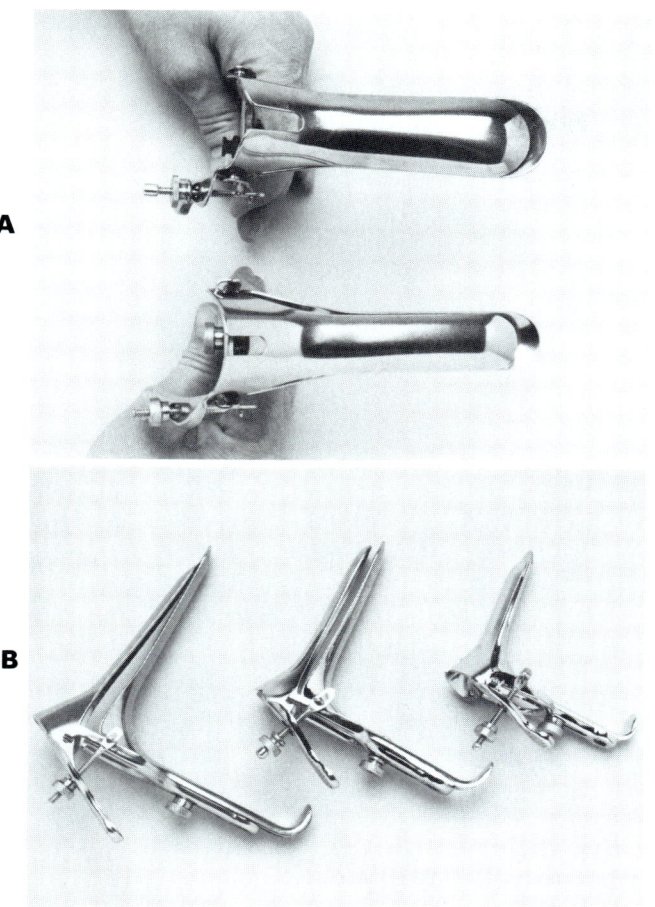

Fig. 7-8 **A**, Graves (top) and Pedersen (bottom) speculums. **B**, Side views.

VAGINAL SPECULUM EXAMINATION

Two types of vaginal speculums are available. The Graves has wider speculum blades, and the Pedersen, narrow blades (Fig. 7-8). The Graves speculum is used for routine examination of multigravida patients. The narrow-blade Pedersen speculum is used for teenagers, virgins, and sometimes for geriatric patients. Each type of speculum is made in several sizes.

To perform the speculum examination, first rinse the speculum with warm water. Avoid lubricating jelly, as it is bactericidal and reduces growth on cultures. To insert the speculum, rotate the blades at a 45-degree angle to enter the hymeneal ring so as to avoid trauma to the urethra. Place one or two fingers of the other hand inside the introitus and press the fourchette down. Insert the speculum and then carefully rotate it to the horizontal while introducing the speculum deeper into the vagina (Fig 7-9). Point the tip of the speculum posteriorly towards the sacrum.

After the speculum is fully inserted, separate the blades so that the cervix comes into view (Fig. 7-10). The nulliparous cervix has a circular entrance, whereas the multiparous cervix has a horizontal linear entrance (Fig. 7-11). The cervix is ordinarily pink, but it may have pale cysts, erythematous eversions, or erosions (Fig. 7-12).

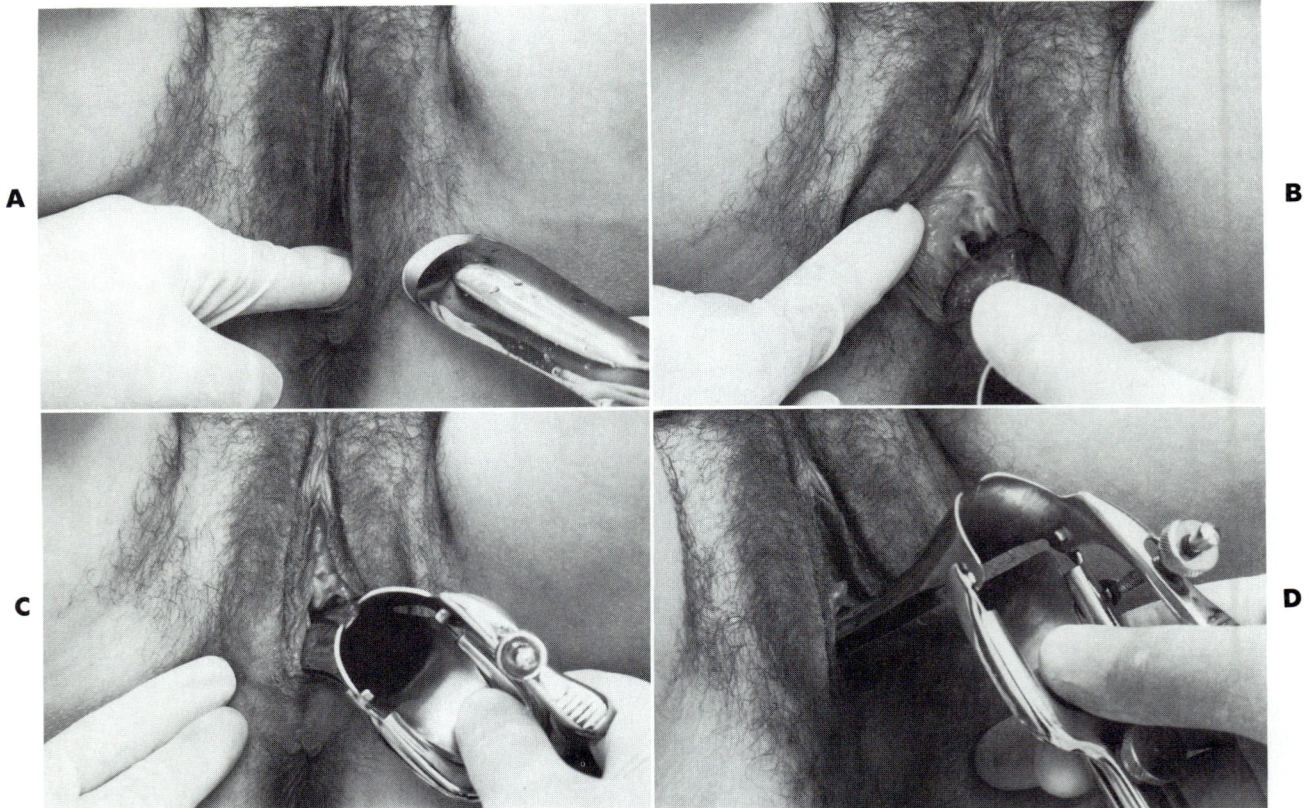

Fig. 7-9 Angles of insertion of the speculum. Locate the vagina **(A)**, then retract the labia to insert the speculum **(B)**. Note the angle during insertion **(C)**. When inserted, turn the speculum to the correct angle **(D)**.

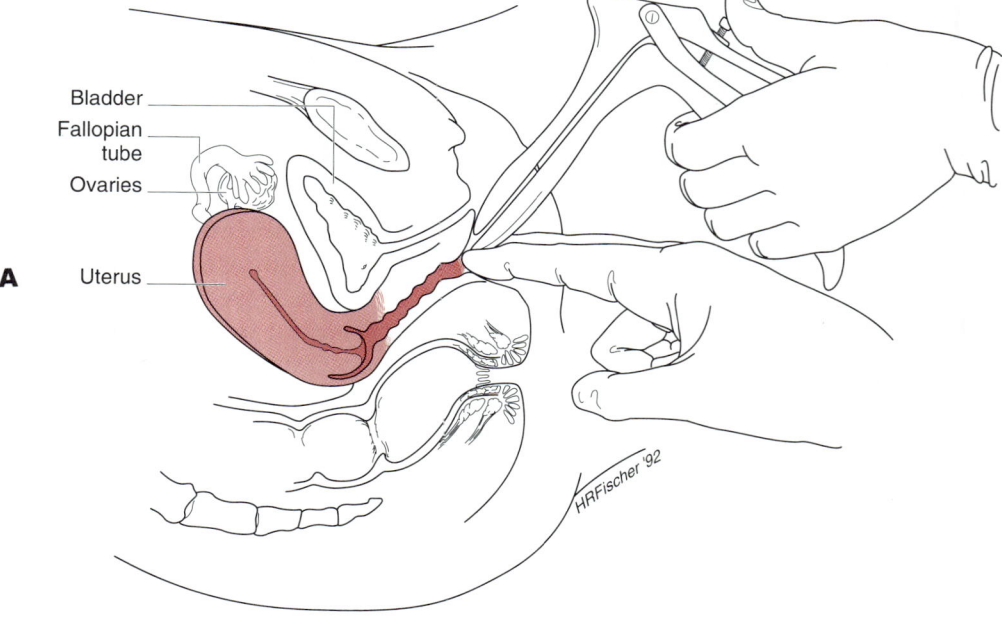

Fig. 7-10 Position of the speculum in vagina. **A,** Approach to vagina. **B,** Insertion. **C,** Opening of blades.

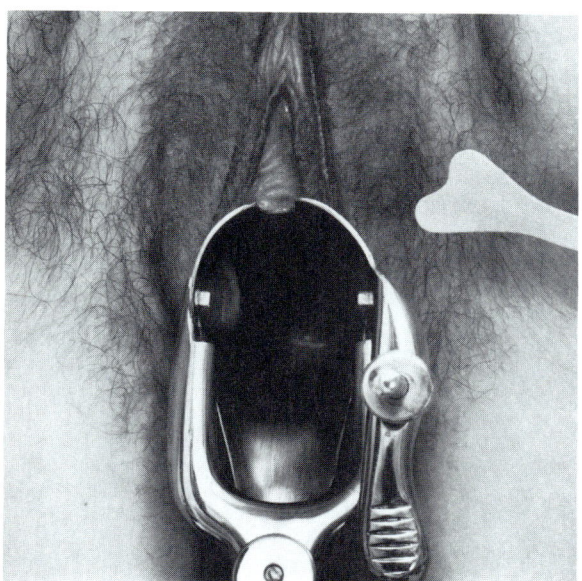

Fig. 7-11 Appearance of the normal multiparous cervix.

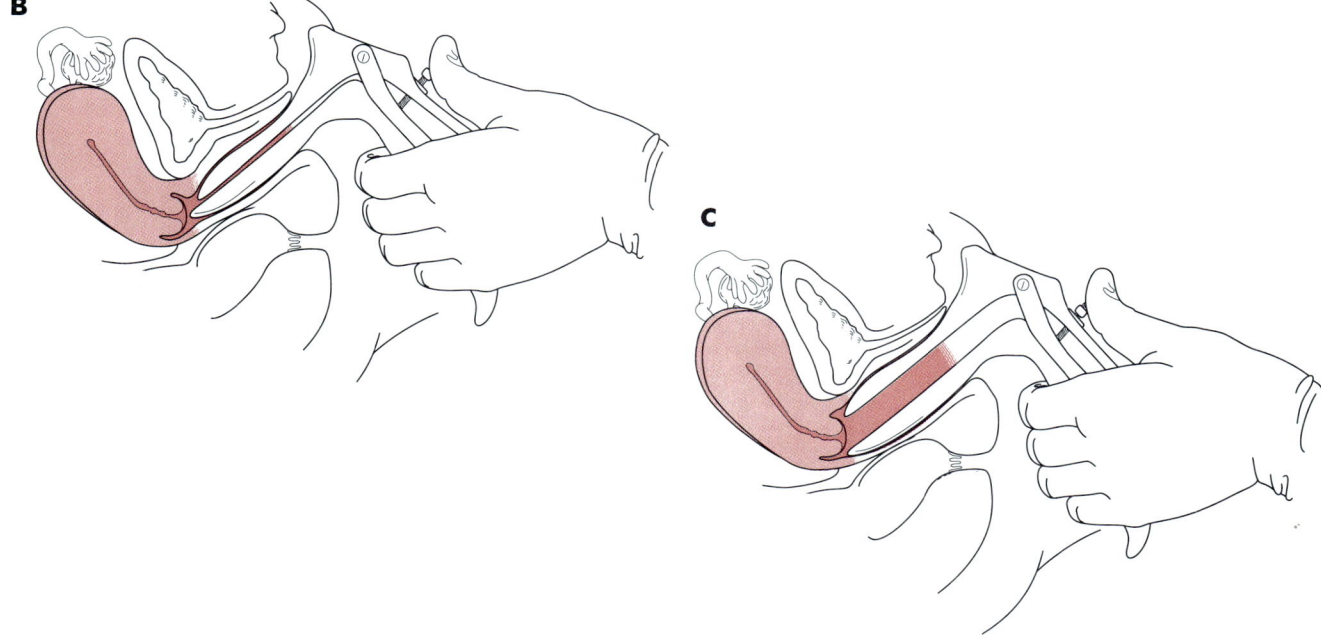

Fig. 7-12 Appearance of the cervix. **A**, Nulliparous. **B**, Multiparous. **C**, Erosion or eversion. **D**, Nabothian cyst of cervix.

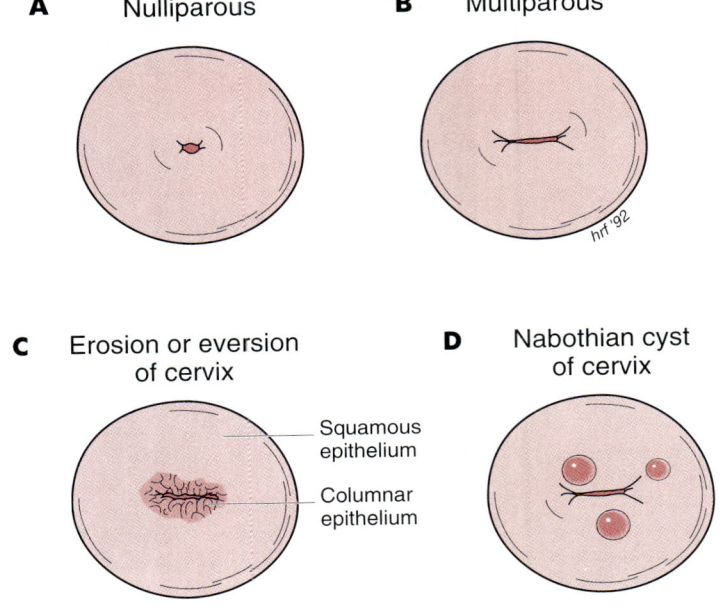

PAPANICOLAOU SMEAR

To take the Papanicolaou (Pap) smear to screen for neoplastic cells, use a wooden spatula to scrape the os cervix in a circular motion. Cells from the transition zone of squamous to columnar epithelium are most important. The specially shaped spatula (Fig. 7-13) allows one end to be inserted into the os. Sweep in a 360-degree motion to ensure adequate sampling of cells. Place the secretions on a microscope slide and fix with aerosol spray. Next, use the other

Fig. 7-13 Obtaining cells for the Pap smear. Place the end of the wooden (Ayers) spatula in the cervical os and twist it to scrape the cervix.

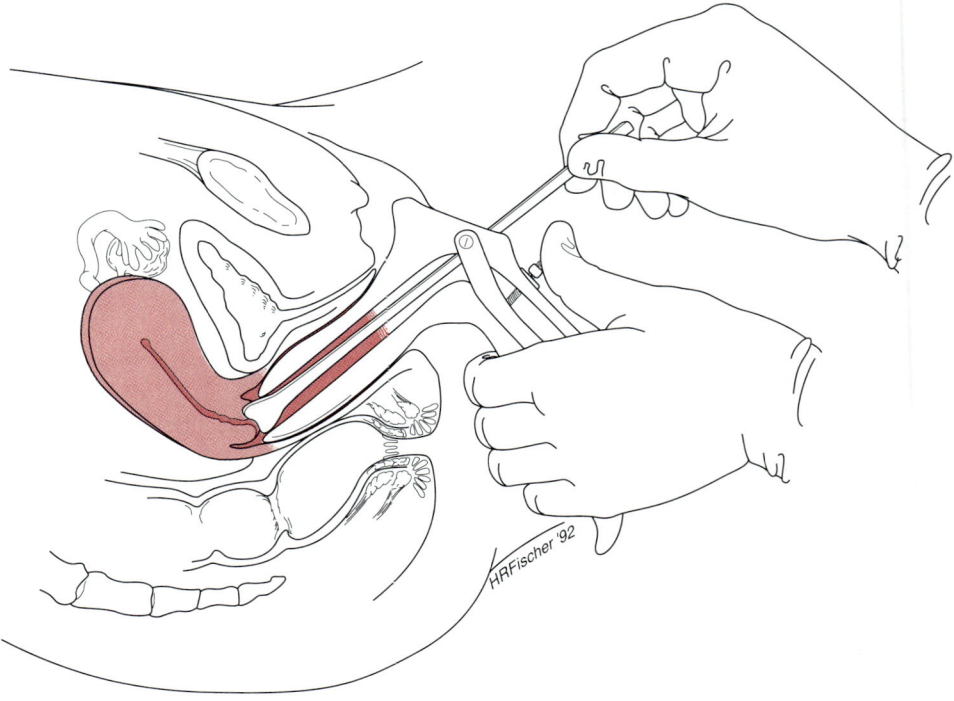

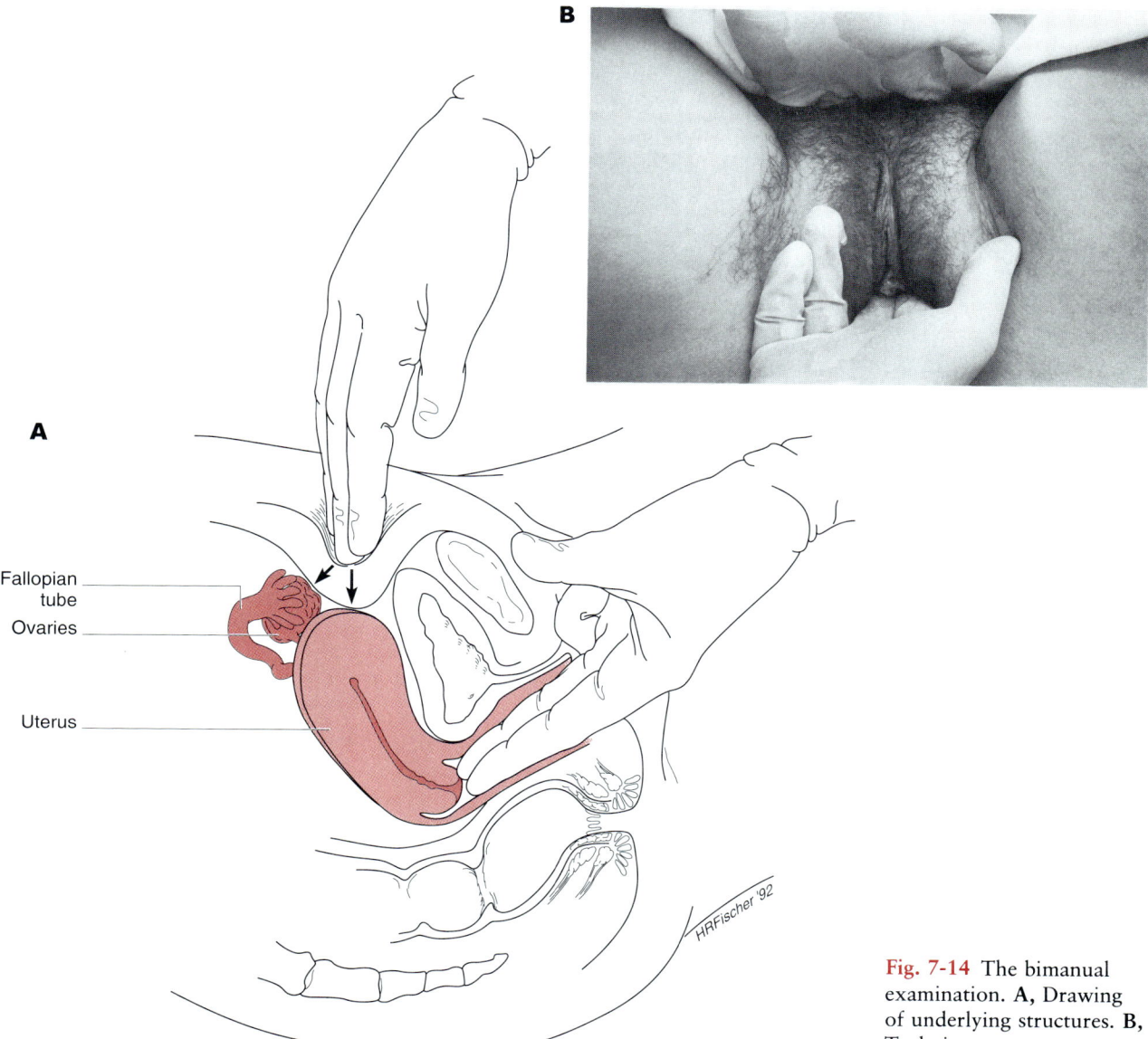

Fig. 7-14 The bimanual examination. **A,** Drawing of underlying structures. **B,** Technique.

end of the spatula to remove cells from the vaginal walls, place on another slide, and apply fixative. Slowly remove the speculum while inspecting the vaginal walls continuously. Should any visible abnormalities be present, the Pap smear is not adequate. Call visible abnormalities to the attention of the clinician for biopsy. Evaluate discharge as shown in Table 7-3.

BIMANUAL EXAMINATION

Place a lubricant (such as KY Jelly™) on the gloved fingers. Insert the index and middle finger of the right hand into the vagina (Fig. 7-14). Palpate the vaginal walls when inserting and later while withdrawing the fingers. The cervix is a circular structure, 3 to 4 cm in diameter. Its consistency feels similar to the tip of the nose or the male prostate gland. While palpating the cervix, place the left examining hand on the patient's lower abdominal wall so that the body of the uterus can be palpated between the two hands (called bimanual exam). The size of the uterus can be determined, whether it is normal, flexed, or turned anteriorly or posteriorly (Fig 7-15).

Next, move the two fingers of the hand in the vagina to each side of the uterus to palpate the adnexa, the ovary, and tube on that side (see Fig. 7-14, *A*). Move the intravaginal fingers and the hand palpating the lower abdominal wall to the same side. Use the intravaginal fingers to elevate the tube and ovary and the abdominal hand to push down so these can be palpated between the two. The ovary, approximately 3 cm long, can be felt. The tube is normally not palpable unless it is enlarged, as in tuboovarian abscess.

After removing your hand from the vagina, change the glove before proceeding to the rectovaginal examination. This practice prevents transmission of pathogens from the vagina to the rectum. Insert the lubricated middle finger into the rectum while placing the forefinger in the vagina (Fig. 7-16). The posterior cervix and uterus are palpated better with this technique. Masses and other irregularities may be easier to feel. Palpate the wall of the rectum for masses, polyps, or fecal material. After removing the gloved finger from the anus, test adherent feces for occult blood.

Fig. 7-15 Common positions of uterus on bimanual examination.

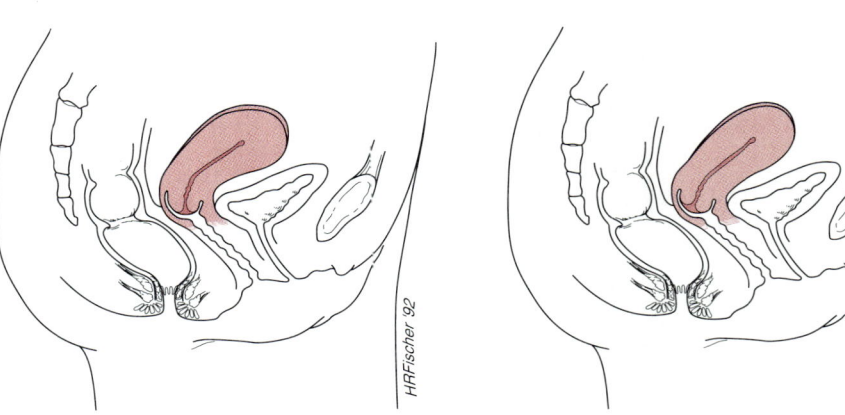

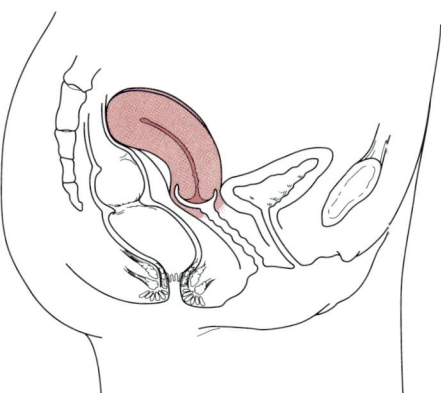

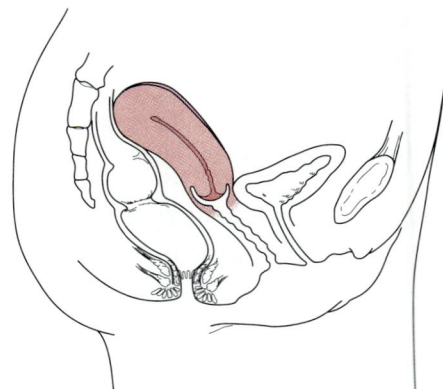

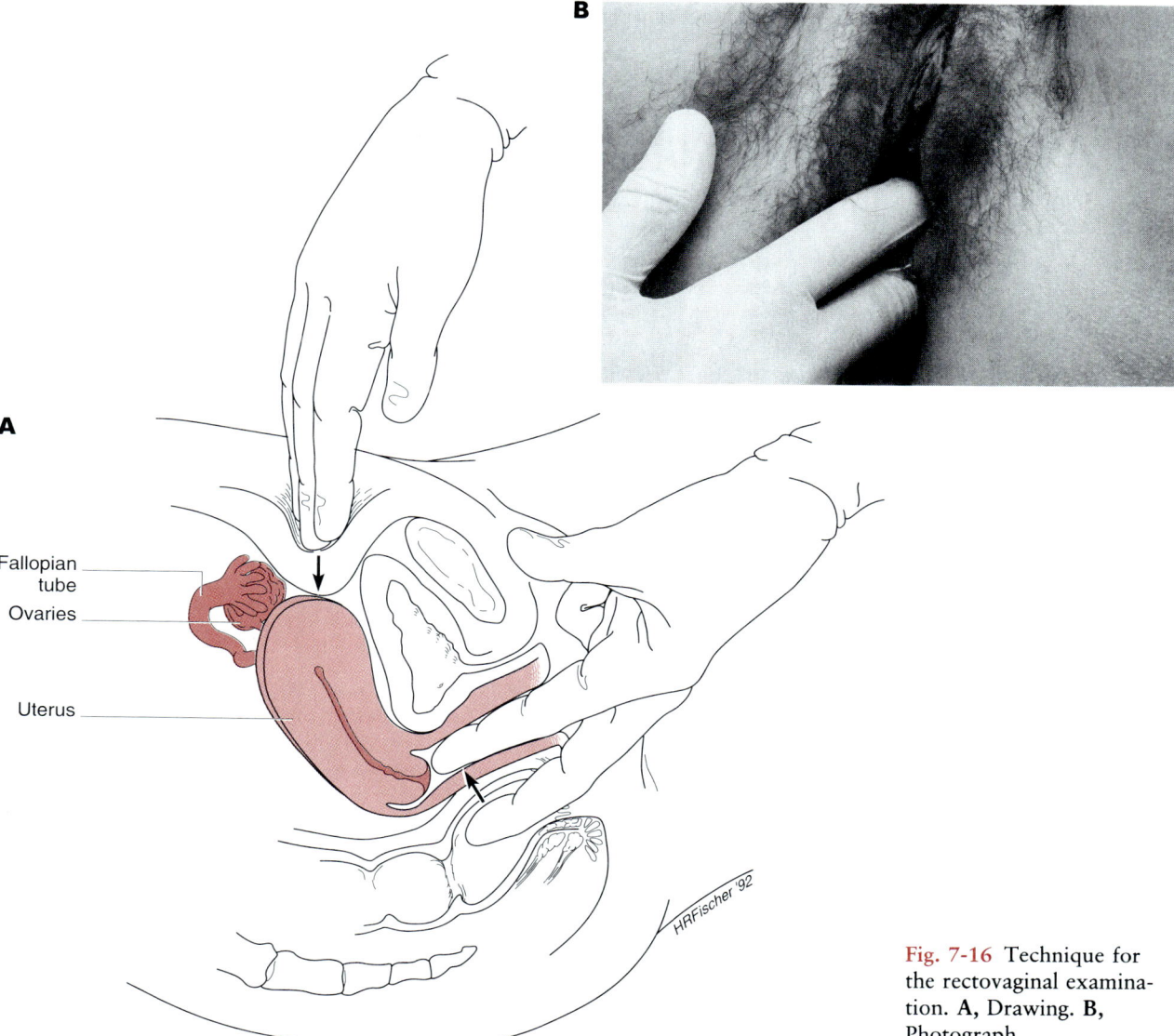

Fig. 7-16 Technique for the rectovaginal examination. **A**, Drawing. **B**, Photograph.

VULVA

Examples of abnormalities that may be present on the vulva are varied (Table 7-4). Vulvar lesions are often associated with symptoms of pruritus. A useful clue to consider is the color of the lesion. Findings in genital ulcers are described in Table 7-5.

The nits of lice may be found on the pubic hair. These are fine, white, tiny, elongated balls no larger than ½ mm in diameter, attached near the base of the hair shaft.

Condyloma lata are flat warty lesions of secondary syphilis, highly contagious. *Condyloma acuminata* are heaped-up irregular warts caused by the human papilloma virus. Although typically seen on the genitalia, these may be found on other parts of the body.

TABLE 7-4: Common Abnormalities of the Vulva

Appearance	Possible Causes
Erythematous Lesions	
Red, dry base, satellite papules	• *Candida albicans*
Folliculitis	• *Staphylococcus aureus*
	• Hidradenitis suppurativa
Symmetric hyperemia	• Reactive vulvitis caused by chemical or mechanical irritants
Dull red with scales, border is sharp	• Psoriasis
Pruritic, greasy looking; symmetric eruption	• Seborrheic dermatitis
Verrucous (warty appearance, elevated)	• Veneral warts caused by (condyloma acuminatum)
	• Vulvar intraepithelial neoplasm (VIN), may be smooth
Fiery red, pruritic, tender	• Paget's disease of vulva
Red and pruritic	• Carcinoma
	• VIN
	• Candidiasis
	• Seborrhea
Pale or White Lesions	
White, pruritic, thickened skin caused by scratching	• Lichen sclerosis
	• VIN
Depigmented skin	• Vitiligo
White debris, cells, odor, pruritus, chafing under skin folds; often has an underlying red base	• Intertrigo
Red, raised, hard with central umbilication	• Molluscum contagiosum
Dark-Colored Lesions	
Flat, well demarcated; no other symptoms	• Lentigo (no malignant potential)
Mole (nevus) with change in appearance or symptoms	• Mole (nevus), could undergo malignant change

VAGINA

In vaginitis, the state of the diffusely erythematous vagina may be caused by infection, trauma, douches, foreign bodies, tampons, or allergic reactions (see Table 7-3).

Gonococcal vaginitis typically causes purulent discharge from the cervix, vagina, urethra, and sometimes Skene's and Bartholin's glands. The vagina becomes red, and the cervix becomes red and eroded.

Trichomonal vaginitis is associated with the reddened mucosa studded with hemorrhagic spots that results in a strawberry appearance. The discharge is typically watery, foamy, and pruritic. *G. vaginalis* vaginitis has a foul (musty, fishlike) odor to the discharge. Atrophic vaginitis caused by relative estrogen deficiency produces a thin mucosa that bleeds easily with trauma.

TABLE 7-5: Symptom: Genital Ulcers

	History	Ulcer Appearance	Other Findings	Diagnostic Test
Chancre (primary syphilis) (uncommon)	• Usually more than one partner • Painless ulcer; single lesion most often	• About 1 cm diameter • Margins are indurated	• Regional node enlarged	• Darkfield microscopy for *Treponema pallidum* • VDRL nonreactive this early
Chancroid (rare)	• Multiple small ulcers; tender	• About 3 to 5 mm diameter • Multiple ulcers	• Regional nodes large	• Culture for *Hemophilus ducreyi*
Herpes simplex (very common)	• Vesicles, itching, burning • History of recurrences at same site (if not primary infection)	• Small, 1 to 3 mm in diameter unless several coalesce	• May leave small scars, often healing	• Virus culture grows the virus
Malignancy	• Prolonged ulcer, nonhealing for weeks, enlarging • Itching and bleeding	• May be red, gray, or white background with an ulcer	• Enlarged inguinal nodes	• Biopsy and histopathology • Squamous carcinoma most common
Behçet's syndrome	• Relapsing oral and genital ulcers	• Shallow or deep, tender (external), destructive ulcers, 2 to 10 mm	• Iritis, uveitis common • May cause blindness	• Nonspecific inflammation • Antibodies to human oral mucosa
Crohn's disease	• Genital and oral ulcers are part of bowel inflammatory disease	• Similar to that in Behçet's	• Very high ESR • Characteristic terminal ileum on radiologic exam	• X-ray pattern and biopsy of bowel
Pemphigus	• Oral and vulvar ulcers	• Similar to that in Behçet's and Crohn's	• May be fatal without therapy (steroids)	• Intracellular IgG pattern is characteristic
Pemphigoid	• Elderly women • Less severe than pemphigus	• Bullous lesions that rupture	• Responds to steroids or Dapsone	• Biopsy shows IgG along basement membrane

CERVIX

The cervix may show healed laceration from trauma, especially from childbirth. The lips of the cervix may be everted because of the growth of columnar epithelium on the ectocervix (Table 7-6). The cervix may appear eroded when the endocervix is infected with chlamydia, herpes, or gonorrhea or when cancer is present. The cervix may appear normal yet be infected with chlamydia, the only manifestation being a small amount of yellow mucopus on a cotton applicator withdrawn from the cervix.

UTERUS

A pelvic mass discovered on the bimanual examination may be caused by the presence of urinary tract, GI, or gynecologic abnormality (Table 7-7).

Leiomyofibromas, a term for fibroid tumors, are hard, painless muscular

TABLE 7-6: Symptom: Abnormalities of the Cervix

Appearance	Possible Cause
Cysts under squamous tissue of cervix	• Nabothian cysts (retention cysts)
Columnar epithelium extending out from cervical os onto cervix	• Ectopy of columnar epithelium over the ectocervix
Cervical erosion early; later may be warty appearance	• Ectropion describes similar appearance (to ectopy) caused by eversion of distal cervical canal, usually after childbirth
	• Cancer of the cervix may resemble this
Bright red polyp in os	• Cervical polyp
Mucopus draining from the cervical os	• N. gonorrheae
	• C. trachomatis
Columnar epithelium covering much of cervix, granular (bumpy) columnar tissue on vaginal wall	• Exposure to DES while in utero
	• Vaginal adenosis or vaginal carcinoma from DES exposure in utero
Clear-cell adenocarcinoma	• DES exposure in utero

nodules, single or multiple, of variable size attached to or in the wall of the uterus. These may become large and cause uterine bleeding, heavy menses, or pressure symptoms.

Endometrial carcinoma is the most common of the gynecologic malignancies, affecting larger numbers than do ovarian and cervical cancer together. Obesity is a significant risk factor. Asymptomatic cancer may be suspected because of

---

CASE 7-3 Cervical Carcinoma In Situ

A 41-year-old cocktail lounge waitress was seen for her annual checkup for oral contraceptives. She had no complaints.

Her menses had started at age 12 and were regular. She had never been pregnant. Her only medications were oral contraceptives and occasional ibuprofen for headache.

She had become sexually active at age 15 and had had numerous partners thereafter. She had been married and divorced three times, and she was currently living with her partner.

On examination, she appeared well generally. The chest, heart, abdomen, and breast examinations were normal. The vulva and vagina appeared normal. Bimanual examination was also normal.

Staining of the vaginal walls and cervix with acetic acid and examining with the colposcope (10× magnification) showed a small area of punctate white epithelium. A biopsy was performed.

Dysplastic abnormal epithelium appears white or opaque, reflecting increased cellular chromatic content. Human papilloma virus types 16 and 18 are now believed to be etiologically significant. Risk factors for this virus include early age at beginning coitus and an increased number of sexual partners, both of which were part of this patient's history. This tissue required biopsy and histologic examination looking for carcimona.

TABLE 7-7: Causes of Pelvic Masses

Masses	Characteristics/Maneuvers
Centrally Positioned	
Urinary tract	
• Full bladder	Have patient void before exam
GI tract	
• Feces in sigmoid or rectum	Usually indents with pressure
• Colonic carcinoma	Rectal or bimanual examination or sigmoidoscopy to show
Gynecologic	
• Pregnancy	Uterus softer than nonpregnant
• Fibroids	Uterus feels irregular, firm
• Uterine enlargement caused by tumor, trapped pus, or blood	Definition may require ultrasound or dilation and curettage (D and C)
Laterally Positioned	
Urinary tract	
• Ptotic kidney	Variable descent; usually not down into pelvis, but may occur
GI tract	
• Feces, flatus, tumor	Feces more often felt on left
	Bowel movement or enema helps to distinguish
• Neoplasm or Crohn's disease	Uncommonly felt in pelvis, but can be if adherent to pelvic organs
Gynecologic	
• Ovarian cyst, tumor	Maximum normal size of ovary is 6 cm
	After menopause, size decreases to 1.5 cm
• Fallopian tube	Normally not felt unless enlarged
Ectopic pregnancy	Measure beta HCG and do ultrasound
Tuboovarian abscess	Patient has other symptoms of PID
• Uterine developmental defects	Two halves of uterus may fail to fuse during embryonic development

glandular atypia in a Pap smear or on endometrial biopsy. Advanced disease may first appear as a pelvic mass. Even later disease may demonstrate ascites and lymphadenopathy.

ADNEXA

In many women, normally sized adnexa may not be palpated. Abnormal adnexa are described by size, shape, consistency, mobility, and structures not normally present (tuboovarian abscesses, ovarian tumors). Examination findings of pelvic pain are variable (Table 7-8).

TABLE 7-8: Examination Findings in Pelvic Pain

Finding	Possible Diagnosis
Tender, enlarged ovarian cysts	• Torsion of ovary • Bleeding into a cyst
Enlarged tube or adnexa; patient hypotensive	• Ectopic pregnancy with rupture
Nodularity of uterosacral ligaments	• Endometriosis • Cancer
Fixed, retroverted uterus	• Endometriosis • Cancer
Motion of cervix is tender; enlarged adnexa	• PID
Enlarged, nodular uterus	• Fibroids (usually not painful), keep looking for another cause

Summary

A summary checklist for the examination of the female genitalia is provided in the box on the opposite page.

Suggested readings

Cowan BD, Morrison JC: Management of abnormal genital bleeding in girls and women, *N Engl J Med* 324:1710-1714, 1991. *A current concepts' review of abnormal bleeding.*

Kahn JG, et al: Diagnosing pelvic inflammatory disease, *J Am Med Assoc* 266:2594-2604, 1991. *This reviews the medical literature from 1969 to 1990.*

Martin CA, Warfield MC, Braen GR: Physicians' management of the psychological aspects of rape, *J Am Med Assoc* 249: 501-503, 1983. *This paper shows how patients initially seek treatment, how the examination should be conducted, and how the victim can be prepared for dealing with friends and possible sequelae.*

Melnick S, et al: Rates and risks of diethylstilbestrol-related clear-cell adenocarcinoma of the vagina and cervix, *N Engl J Med* 316:514-516, 1987. *This report reviews 519 cases of this rare tumor.*

Summary Checklist for Examination of Female Genitalia

External Genitalia
- Mons pubis
- Labia
- Vulva
- Clitoris
- Urethra
- Skene's glands
- Bartholin's glands
- Vestibule
- Fourchette
- Hymeneal ring
- Genital ulcers
- Vaginal discharge
- Condyloma acuminata
- Molluscum contagiosum
- Nevi
- Candidiasis
- Nits
- Puruitus

Speculum Examination
- Vaginal walls
- Cervix
- Cervical erosion
- Cervical polyp
- Cervical mucopus
- Atrophic vaginitis
- Cervical carcinoma
- Vaginal adenosis
- Dysplastic epithelium

Bimanual Examination
- Pelvic mass
- Retroflexed, retroverted uterus
- Soft cervix
- Fibroid tumors
- Full bladder
- Adnexa
- Fallopian tube
- Tuboovarian abscess (PID)
- Ovarian cancer
- Ovarian cyst

Rectovaginal examination
- Uterine positions
- Posterior pelvis
- Rectal examination
- Stool for occult blood

CHAPTER EIGHT

The Breast

CHAPTER OUTLINE

History taking
The breast lump or mass
Multiple lumps
Pain or tenderness
Changes in size or shape

Abnormalities of the nipples
Importance of the past medical history in breast disease

Physical Examination of the Breasts
Inspection
Palpation

Special Concerns in the Breast Examination
After mastectomy
The male breast

Summary

Although many other diseases may affect the breast, cancer is the most common concern of patients who seek treatment for breast complaints. Overall, 1 in 11 women in America develop cancer of the breast. The ratio is higher in white (1 in 10) than in black (1 in 14) women.

In 1983, 34,000 American women died of breast cancer, which represents 18% of all female deaths caused by cancer. In men, breast cancer is 100-fold less common than in women. It is usually recognized late and carries a poor prognosis.

Because 90% of breast lumps are discovered by women, we discuss breast self-examination each time we do a breast exam. However, most lumps are not cancer. Of 676 women who went to a breast clinic for periodic examination or evaluation of a problem, only 5.5% had cancer (Table 8-1). Most complaints by women to physicians about their breasts are not cancer related.

History Taking

The Lump or Mass

Studies of over 1200 women established that more than 75% of women who had the diagnosis of breast cancer sought medical care with the complaint of a breast lump (Table 8-2 and Fig. 8-1). Thus most cases of breast cancer first manifest as a breast lump. Alternatively, 95% (or more) breast complaints evaluated in a breast clinic during a physical examination are not caused by malignancy.

TABLE 8-1: Diagnosis in Women Presenting to a Breast Clinic

	Number	Percent
Fibrocystic disease	197	29.1
Normal examination	195	28.8
Fibroadenoma	72	10.7
Unexplained breast pain	50	7.4
Infections	41	6.1
Carcinoma	37	5.5
Nipple discharge	23	3.4
Gynecomastia	16	2.4
Mass	15	2.2
Lipoma	6	.9
Fat necrosis	5	.7
Enlarged axillary node	4	.6
Duct ectasia	3	.4
Inappropriate lactation	3	.4
Fibrous disease	2	.3
Intraductal papilloma	2	.3
Superficial thrombophlebitis (Mondor's disease)	2	.3
Amastia	2	.3
Polymastia	1	.1
TOTAL	676	

Modified from Donegan WL: Diagnosis. In Donegan WL, Spratt JS, editors: *Cancer of the Breast*, ed 3, Philadelphia, 1988, WB Saunders.

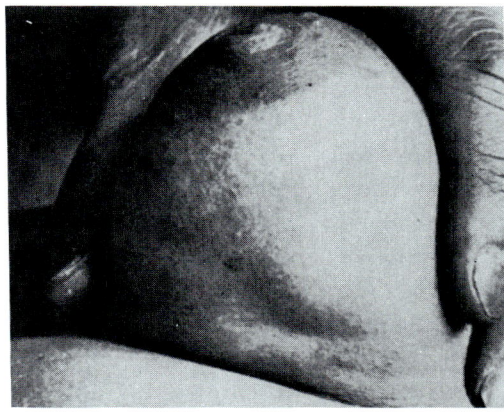

Fig. 8-1 A breast lump of cancer.
From Haagensen CD: *Carcinoma of the breast,* New York, 1950, American Cancer Society.

TABLE 8-2: Presenting Symptoms In Patients with Breast Cancer (N = 1205)

Symptoms	Percent
Discrete lump	76
Swelling	8
Pain	5
Nipple retraction	4
Nipple bleeding, discharge, or crusting	2
Others	5

Data from Donegan WL, Spratt JS, editors: *Cancer of the breast,* ed 3, Philadelphia, 1988, WB Saunders; and Donegan WL: *Br J Surg* 70:350, 1983.

Key Symptoms in the Evaluation of the Breast
• A lump or mass • Change in size or shape of breast • Multiple lumps • Abnormalities of the nipples • Pain or tenderness • Discharge from the nipple

Some patients refer to a thickening rather than a lump. Some just say that an area of the breast feels different. Women who practice self-examination become aware of their own breast thickenings. Whenever a new thickening or a change in the breast occurs, a patient often detects it first during her own examination.

The three most common types of breast masses have age-related distributions (Table 8-3). Fibroadenomas are common from age 15 to the mid-forties, with smaller numbers of cases before and after these age groups. Fibrocystic breast disease begins increasing during the mid-twenties and achieves maximal frequency between the ages of 35 and 50. Carcinoma begins during the twenties, rapidly increases in incidence in the forties, and continues into old age.

Cancer metastasis may also be present in the lymph nodes. The breast tissue is well-drained with lymphatics (Fig. 8-2). Lymph nodes important to the breast

CASE 8-1 Breast Lump in a Young Woman

A 22-year-old woman presented with the chief complaint of a lump in the right breast.

She said that after jogging 3 days ago, she noticed a different sensation in the upper part of the right breast while taking a shower. At first she didn't want to admit anything might be wrong, but by the next day she had felt it again.

She denied any family history of breast cancer. She didn't smoke. She was not married and was not taking oral contraceptives.

On examination, she was a thin, worried, white woman. Vital signs were normal. The examination was normal except for the breast examination. The contours of the breast were normal in all positions, sitting, arms up and down, leaning forward.

In the upper outer quadrant of the right breast, she had a 1 cm nodule, firm and nontender. There was no attachment to skin or underlying fascia.

No discharge from either nipple was evident. No nodes were felt in the axillae, supraclavicular, or infraclavicular regions.

Because she was due for a menstrual period in a few days, the patient was asked to return in 2 weeks for reexamination. If the nodule remained palpable, she would have ultrasonography to determine whether this is a cystic or solid mass.

The concern was whether this lump would resolve rapidly when not under the influence of hormonal stimulation. If not, and if cystic, it would be aspirated. If solid, mammography would be performed with plans to do an excisional biopsy for definitive histopathologic diagnosis. The most likely diagnosis in this patient would be fibroadenoma.

TABLE 8-3: Benign and Malignant Breast Lumps

Parameter	Fibroadenoma	Fibrocystic Change	Cancer
Median age (years)	20	30	60
Range (years)	15 to 40	20 to 60	40 and over
Relative frequency found on biopsy for breast lumps (%)	20	35	30
Palpable mass	More so in older patients	Maybe; may feel "lumpy"	Yes, usually
Characteristics of lesions	Multiple and bilateral, solid, rubbery, painless	Multiple and bilateral, tenderness, fullness	Solitary, hard, irregular, painless; other lesions may be present
Moveable	Mobile	Yes	May be fixed to skin or other tissues
Skin or nipple changes	No	No	Dimpling, retraction
Radiologic Studies	In younger patients with more dense breasts, contrast with ultrasound or mammography may be lacking	Ultrasound may detect cysts >7 mm	Mammography is better to show cancer; normal mammogram does not exclude cancer

include the internal mammary (not palpable), axillary nodes (central, interior or pectoral, lateral along the arm, and posterior toward the scapula), infraclavicular, and supraclavicular. These may enlarge because of local or systemic infections, develop metastases in cancer, or be enlarged for other reasons.

Multiple Lumps

Multiple lumps may be found on examination in as many as 25% of women. These may be diffuse or localized, especially in the upper outer quadrant (the axillary tail).

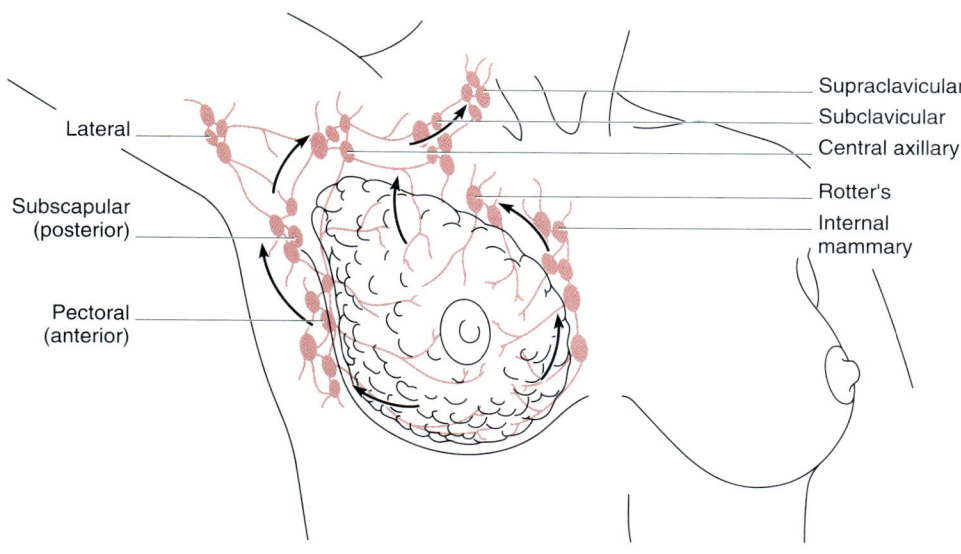

Fig. 8-2 Lymphatic network draining the breast.

Typical questions to ask a patient who comes in with a breast lump, or other breast complaint, include the following:

- *What have you noticed about your breasts?* An open-ended question allows the patient to pace the history and give her own words for any abnormality.
- *Would you call this a nodule, lump, a thickening, or something else?* Help the patient become more specific.
- *When did you first notice it?* Determine its onset.
- *When have you noticed it since?* This allows assessment of a lesion that comes and goes or of inconsistency in the patient's own evaluation.
- *Have you ever had this or anything like it before?* The past history of similar lesions is important in breast lumps.
- *Is it tender?* Cancer is usually not tender, but it may be sometimes.
- *Have you seen any change in the skin or the size of your breasts?* Look for a clue regarding dimpling or contour change caused by cancer.
- *Have you had any discharge from the nipple or any other changes in the nipple?* Discharge does not necessarily mean cancer, but patients often think otherwise.

Pain or Tenderness

Breast discomfort may be localized or diffuse, involving one breast or both. Generalized breast tenderness commonly parallels the menstrual cycle. Tenderness occurs a few days before and stops with the onset of menses. Discomfort is noted most often in the axillary tail of the breast (Fig. 8-3). Generalized tenderness with breast swelling are common in early pregnancy. Physiologic breast tenderness may occur at puberty (11 years, ± 2 years), when hormonal changes promote rapid breast development (Fig. 8-4).

Breast tenderness may be caused by trauma to the breast from blunt injury, vigorous sexual activity, friction, or pressure from clothing. Fat necrosis from trauma may result in a localized tender mass.

Other causes of breast pain include acute localized pain resulting from bleeding into a cyst, diffuse pain caused by postpartum mastitis, or a postpartum abscess. If breast pain is severe, consider inflammation or infection as possibilities.

Most breast pain does not mean cancer. However, pain has been reported in

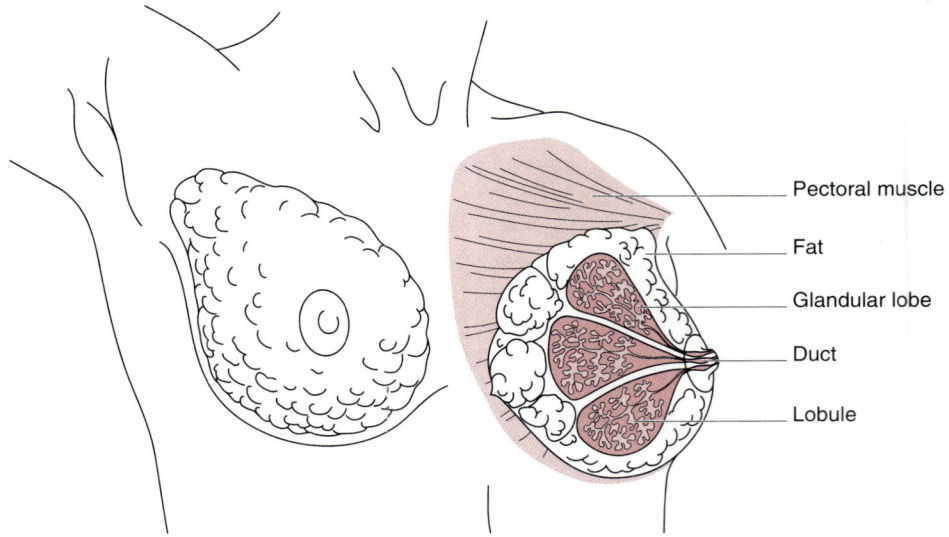

Fig. 8-3 Anatomy of the breast.

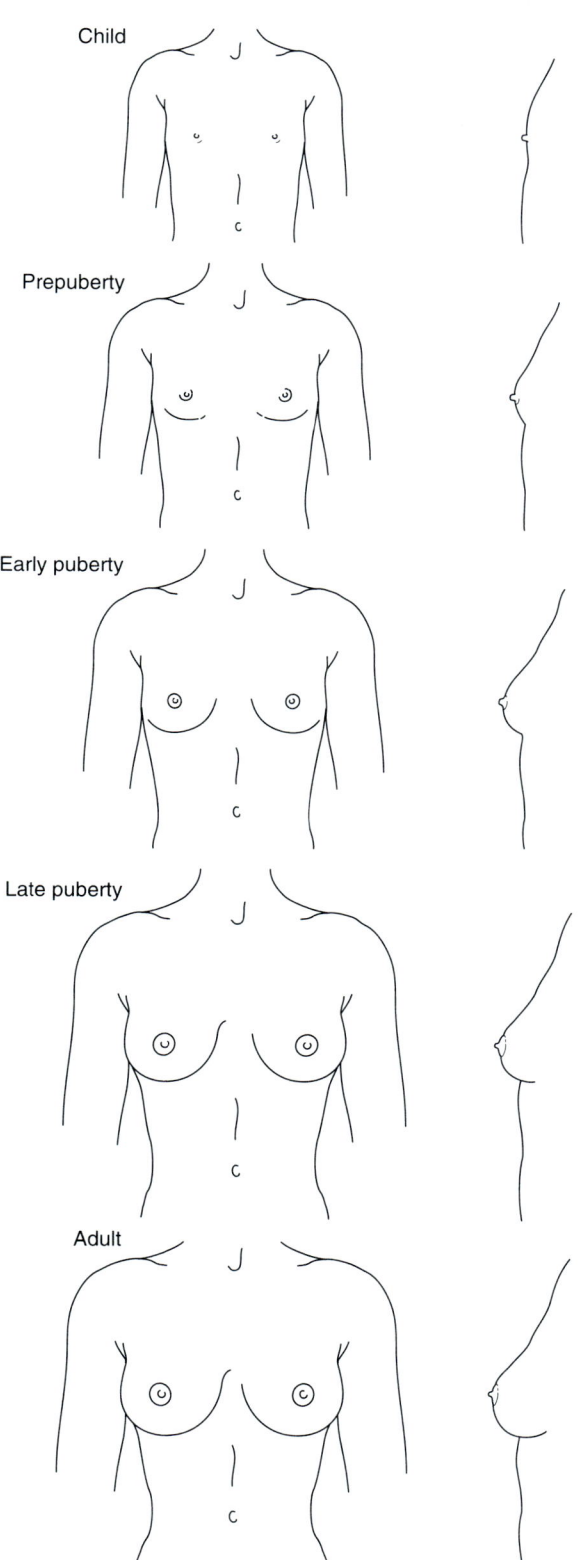

Fig. 8-4 Stages of maturity of breasts. *Stage 1,* Nipple is elevated (preadolescent). *Stage 2,* small mound of areola with nipple (breast bud). *Stage 3,* Beginning of enlarging breast around areola and nipple without separate contours. *Stage 4,* Areola projects beyond breast. *Stage 5,* Nipple only projects, whereas areola has no separate contour from breast.
Modified from Tanner JM: *Growth at adolescence,* Oxford, 1961, Blackwell Scientific Publications.

20% of patients with breast cancer. Clearly a painful site cannot be ignored or called benign without complete evaluation.

Questions to consider in patients who complain of breast pain include the following:

- *Where is the pain?* Determine whether the pain is localized, generalized, or involves one or both breasts.
- *When did it begin? Have you had it before?* Check for duration and recurrences.
- *Do you notice any changes with your menstrual cycle?* Some pain does increase shortly before menses.
- *Do you have any idea why you may be having pain?* Causes include trauma, medications, and clothing.
- *Have you noticed any other changes in your breasts? The way they look, or the way they feel?* This may point to skin or nipple contour changes.
- *Have your breast been enlarging? Has your weight changed? Could you be pregnant?* Breasts usually increase in size with weight gain and increase in size and become tender during pregnancy.

Changes in Size or Shape

Changes in breast size may be accompanied by tenderness. Enlarging breasts are more likely to be tender than are breasts undergoing atrophy. Early in pregnancy, breast enlargement and fullness are often prominent. The areola grows darker. Striae (stretch marks) may result when breast size increases markedly.

As breasts atrophy following pregnancy or during hormonal decreases in menopause, they become ptotic (hang down). This reduction in size remains symmetric if the breasts were previously symmetric. However, at any age it is common for one breast to be slightly larger than the other.

After menopause, the breasts begin to involute. The glandular tissue reduces in size as hormonal stimuli decrease. Fat tissues usually increase, and connective tissue becomes less resilient.

When a patient observes a change in appearance, usually she is looking down on top of the breasts, or looking at her reflection. A complete examination of the patient's complaint of change in appearance needs to consider what she saw and how she became aware of the changes. Abnormal surface contours may be apparent in one view but not from other angles.

An important change is dimpling of the skin. Tumors cause dimpling by retracting a fibrous strand of *Cooper's ligament* (see Fig. 8-2), the suspensory connective tissues supporting the breast. This retraction results in skin indentation. Other diseases that may be associated with dimpling include fat necrosis, plasma cell mastitis, and Mondor's disease (superficial thrombophlebitis).

Abnormalities of the Nipples

Glandular tissue is composed of 15 to 20 lobes that empty into ducts, which come together so that only a few empty onto the skin of the areola (Fig. 8-5). These terminal ducts have short milk sinuses that are useful during nursing. During development, the areola usually begins to darken, more so in women with dark complexions. Sebaceous glands around the areola *(Montgomery's glands)* often become prominent as small 1 to 2 mm superficial nodules.

Along the milk line from the axillary area to the groins, supernumerary nipples may appear (Fig. 8-6). Patients usually do not mention supranumerary nipples as a complaint; usually they consider these to be a mole or a birthmark. Three nipple

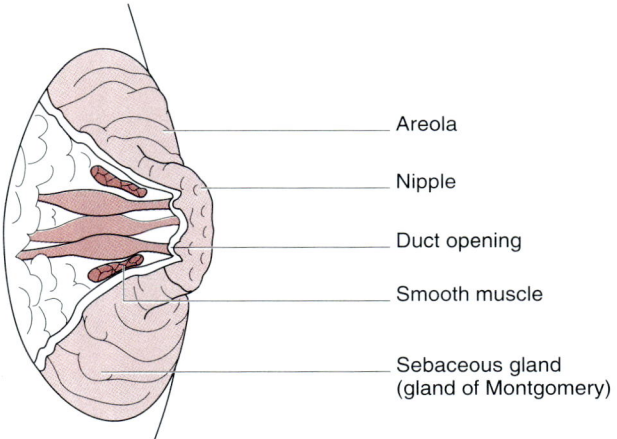

Fig. 8-5 The areola and nipple.

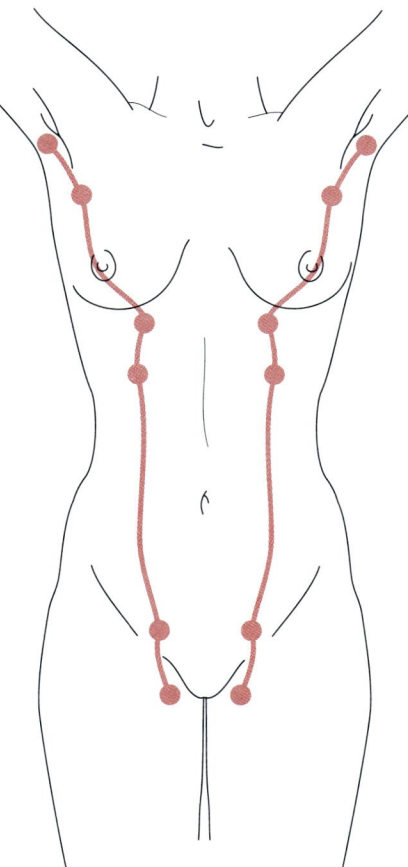

Fig. 8-6 The milk line and supernumerary nipples.

abnormalities of which patients may complain are retraction, ulceration, and discharge.

RETRACTION

Nipple retraction is a drawing back or drawing to one side of the nipple. Such a change in appearance is potentially significant. Usually retraction directly inward of a nipple is abnormal, but it may be normal in some women (Fig. 8-7).

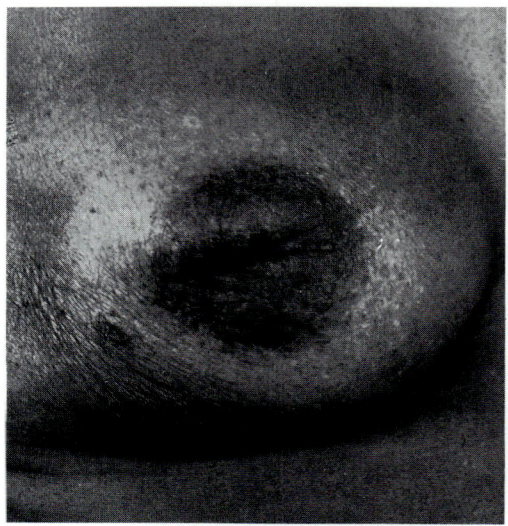

Fig. 8-7 Retraction of the nipple.
From del Regato JA, Spjut HJ, Cox JD: *Ackerman and del Regato's cancer: diagnosis, treatment, and prognosis*, ed 2, St Louis, 1985, Mosby–Year Book.

If palpated or squeezed during examination, usually a normal nipple protrudes straight out. If it does not protrude normally, or if it continues to retract to the side instead of centrally, evaluate the breast for an underlying neoplasm or inflammatory process.

ULCERATION

Ulceration or fissures may appear in the nipple. Ulceration may be caused by trauma, such as by friction of clothing against the nipple while jogging when not wearing a bra.

Paget disease of the breast gives an appearance of eczema of the areola and nipple. Malignant ductal cells from inside the nipple grow externally and involve the areola. Serous drainage crusts around the nipple, and initially the patient usually attributes this to trauma. Patients often call the lesion eczema and are comforted by the cyclic appearance of healing. Ulceration of the nipple or areola occurs late.

DISCHARGE

Women who have never been pregnant usually have little or no secretion from the nipples. As many as 25% of previously pregnant women have nipple secretions at some time. Nipple secretions may be milky, serous, or bloody.

Galactorrhea, defined as inappropriate (not following pregnancy) milky discharge, has several potential causes, listed below:

- Prolactin secretion (chromophobe tumor)
- Increased prolactin-releasing factor (hypothyroidism)
- Failure to inhibit prolactin release (antidepressants, methyldopa, opiates, or encephalitis)
- Pituitary necrosis caused by hemorrhage at childbirth (Sheehan's syndrome, amenorrhea with galactorrhea)

Other types of spontaneous nipple discharge include serous, watery, serosanguinous, and bloody secretions. These may occur in 1% to 8% of patients with breast cancer. Spontaneous discharge from one or two ducts of one nipple is more suspicious for cancer than if all ducts from both breasts have discharge. Benign intraductal papillomas may also result in serous or bloody discharge. Oral contraceptives have been associated with bilateral serous drainage.

In males, bloody or serous discharge from the nipples must raise a strong suspicion of cancer.

Importance of the Past Medical History in Breast Disease

The past history of the patient with breast disease may reveal pertinent information regarding the influence of menses, the use of hormones, and previous breast diseases.

Breast complaints are evaluated considering any potential relationship to hormones of the menstrual cycle. Pain, lumps, or discharge may be cyclic. Women who have had a hysterectomy but not an oophorectomy may continue to have cyclic breast changes.

Oral contraceptives do not increase the risk of breast cancer according to most current studies. The use of unopposed estrogen (no progesterone) may stimulate growth of an existing breast tumor. Usually oral contraceptives do reduce breast tenderness and nodularity. Breast size may increase or decrease. Use of medication with a higher estrogen content tends to increase nodularity. When progesterone alone is used to treat PMS, breast tenderness and nodule size also may be decreased. The use of estrogen replacement therapy is increasing in menopausal women in an attempt to reduce or delay osteoporosis. This usage may also have a beneficial effect on coronary artery disease.

Previous breast disease may provide a clue to the patient's present diagnosis. A previous biopsy showing fibroadenoma suggests, but does not prove, that a newly discovered lump may be the same. However, if a previous biopsy showed a lesion with malignant potential (e.g., epithelial hyperplasia or intraductal papillomatosis), be alert to an increased chance of malignancy in any new lump.

The personal history and family history may be important in suggesting potential for breast cancer (see the box on pg. 326).

CASE 8-2 Breast Cancer

A 62-year-old woman who worked as a nurses' aide in a nursing home sought treatment because of a breast lump. The patient said she had first felt a lump in the left breast over 2 years before. She was afraid it might be cancer because her mother and an older sister both had mastectomies for cancer.

The patient said she was not able to work because of tiredness, and she had lost some weight recently (she was not certain how much). She denied smoking. She had never had children. Menopause had occurred at age 52.

On examination, she was an obese black woman. Vital signs were normal. The general examination otherwise was not remarkable.

The breasts were not symmetric. The left breast showed dimpling of the lateral surface at the level of the areola. Palpation showed a 3 × 5 cm hard mass extending up toward the axilla. Two 1 cm lymph nodes were found on the medial axillary wall. There was no nipple discharge.

The patient had a presumptive diagnosis of breast cancer and was scheduled for admission to the hospital in 2 days.

Risk Factors for Breast Cancer
Personal History 　Age over 40 years 　Previous breast cancer 　Nulliparous, or first child born after age 30 　Exposure to irradiation 　Obese woman, high-fat diet 　Menarche before age 11 or menopause after age 50 **Family History** 　Mother had bilateral breast cancer before menopause 　First-degree relative had breast cancer

Physical Examination of the Breasts

The examination of the breasts begins with the patient unclothed to the waist, facing the examiner. Because this may be embarrassing for women, the attitude of the examiner can help ease tension. Discussing techniques of the breast self-examination while performing the exam on the patient and encouraging her to do these herself often helps her relax. The optimum time to perform the examination is 1 week after a menstrual period because there will be less engorgement and less breast tissue stimulation by hormones, and real masses become more apparent.

The breasts are examined with the patient in the following positions:

- Sitting with arms at the sides
- Sitting with arms over the head
- Sitting with the hands pressed firmly against the waist
- Sitting and leaning toward the examiner
- Supine with a folded towel or small pillow under the back on the side being examined

Inspect the breasts for size, symmetry, shape, contour, skin changes, and color or venous abnormalities. Inspect the nipples for shape, discharge, retraction, deviation to the side, and symmetry. Palpate the breasts for lumps, masses, tender areas, skin thickening, or adenopathy.

Inspection

The rationale for examining the breasts with the arms down and then overhead and with the hands pressing against the waist (Fig. 8-8) is to enhance one's ability to recognize subtle changes in shape, contour, or symmetry caused by bulging or retraction of the skin over a lump. A lesion may be attached to the skin or underlying fascia, or the nipple may be deviated because of a mass. When the arms are down, changes in the superior half of the breast are more prominent, but with the arms up, abnormalities of the lower half of the breasts and the inframammary folds are more apparent.

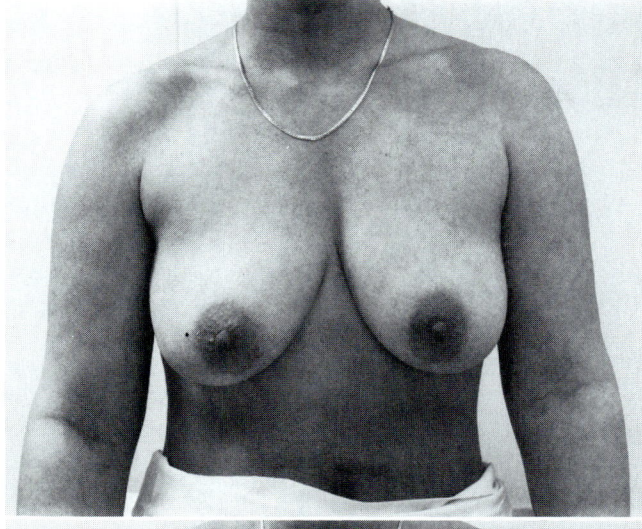
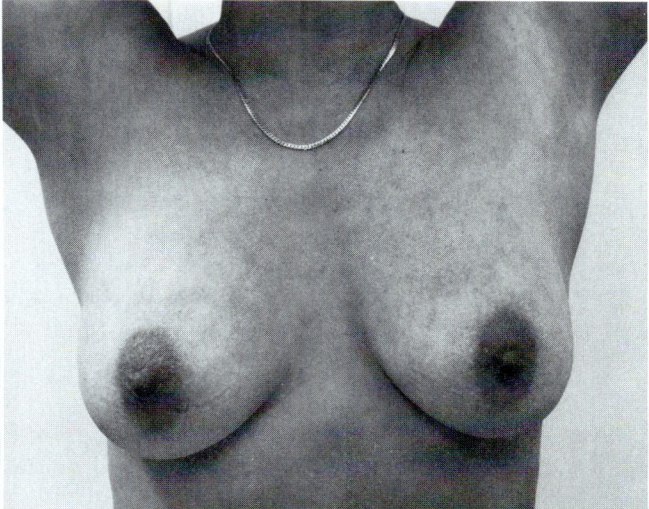
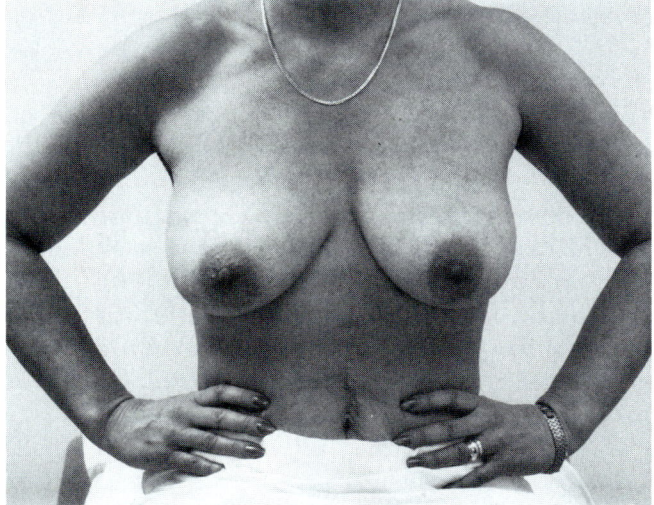

Fig. 8-8 Inspection of the breasts with the patient's arms at the sides (**A**), overhead (**B**), and hands on the waist (**C**). Note how various positions reveal anatomy to different advantages.

Pressing the hands against the waist or hips contracts the pectoralis major muscle, which sometimes demonstrates a skin retraction that would otherwise remain inapparent. Similarly, when the patient leans forward toward the examiner, some types of asymmetry may be observed more readily (Fig. 8-9). When any abnormality is observed, that breast requires special attention during palpation.

Compare the size and shape of the breasts. For some women, cyclic changes in size are the rule. Often one breast is slightly larger. If the asymmetry is recent, a serious disorder may be responsible. Otherwise, unequal size of breasts are of cosmetic importance only.

Skin changes that signify the need for closer attention include the following:

- Swelling
- Dimpling
- Retractions
- A groove
- Ulceration
- Edema
- Venous prominence

Fig. 8-9 Inspection of the breasts with the patient leaning forward.

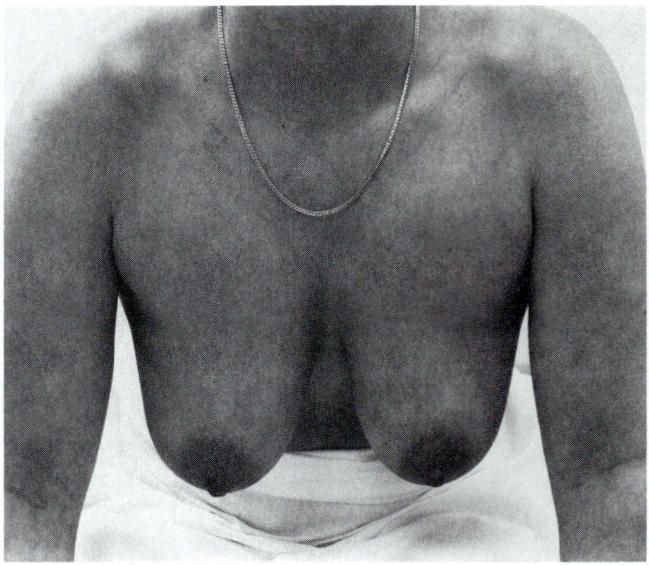

Nipple ulceration or erythema may extend to the areola in Paget disease.

Stretch marks, or *striae*, are irregular purple, red, or white lines that occur with pregnancy, weight gain, Cushing's syndrome, and other causes of breast enlargement. Recent striae are reddish or purple, whereas older striae are pale or white. Prominent bilateral veins over the breasts are less likely to indicate a pathologic condition than are veins prominent on only one side.

Mondor's disease refers to thrombosis of the thoracoepigastric vein of the breast and chest wall. Originally, Mondor's disease was believed to be found only in the presence of malignancy, but the two are not necessarily related. Healing of a thrombosed vein may leave a superficial groove.

Edema of the breast is more common on the lower, rather than the upper, half. The skin may become thickened and edematous because of obstruction of lymphatic drainage. This *peau d'orange* appearance in breast cancer refers to the marked skin edema with tiny dimples that resembles an orange peel.

Palpation

Palpate the breasts while the patient is sitting and then again when she is supine. Concentrate on each area of abnormality noted during inspection as the entire breast is examined. Palpate for nodes in the supraclavicular, infraclavicular, pectoral, and axillary areas with the patient sitting.

Palpation is performed in two ways. First, use the flat of the hand to compress the breast against the chest wall. Press the flat surface of the fingers as a unit (Fig. 8-10). This functions better than using the tips of the fingers, because the fingertips may suggest masses when none are present. Because young women may have tender breasts during parts of the menstrual cycle, begin with gentle pressure. Next, use the fingers and thumb to compress the breast tissue. Take special care not to mistake breast tissue for a mass. Experience is needed for the examiner to be able to differentiate the feeling of normal breast variations from masses or lumps.

To be sure to evaluate each area of every breast, develop a plan. This could follow one of three patterns:

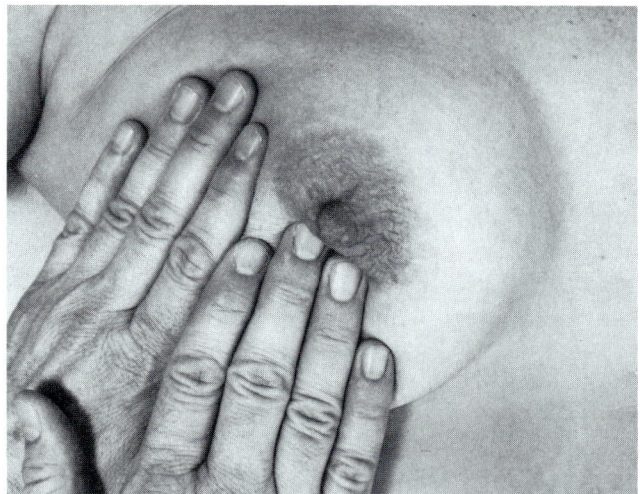

Fig. 8-10 Palpation of the breast, first with the flat of the fingers (as shown), then between the examiner's fingers and thumbs.

- Palpate each of the four quadrants (Fig. 8-11, *A*)
- Palpate along the imaginary spokes on a wheel (Fig. 8-11, *B*)
- Palpate in each of the imaginary concentric circles around the nipple and outward (Fig. 8-11, *C*)

Use care to assess the entirety of both breasts. To complete the examination, palpate the nipple, areola, and deeper ductal tissues (Fig. 8-12).

Examine the axillae by using the right hand to examine the patient's left axilla and left hand for the right axilla. Flex the patient's arm at the elbow and lay the patient's forearm across your arm. Begin palpation of the axillae for nodes or masses at the axillary tail of the breast, compressing it against the chest wall (Fig. 8-13). Slightly cup the fingers of the examining hand and insert them high into the axilla. Press the finger tips against the chest wall, and gradually move them downward. Enlarged nodes can be felt "popping" out from under the fingers. Similarly, palpate the anterior, posterior, and lateral areas of the axillae for nodes, masses, or tenderness.

Count the palpable nodes, estimate the size of each, and record the site and

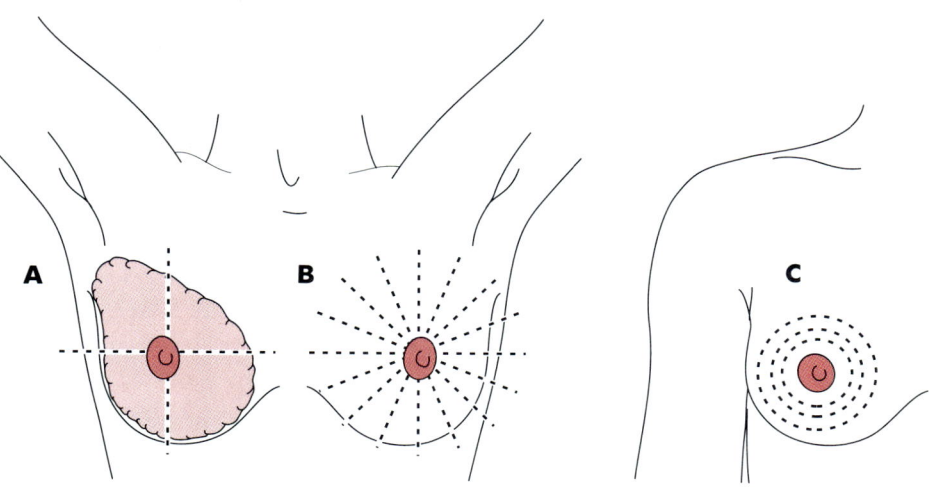

Fig. 8-11 Methods of breast palpation. **A,** The four quadrants. **B,** The "spokes-on-a-wheel" approach. **C,** The "concentric circles" approach.

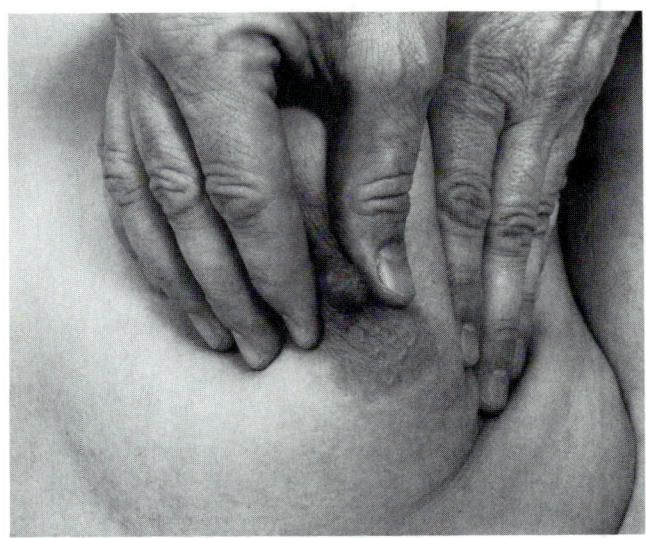

Fig. 8-12 Palpation of the nipples.

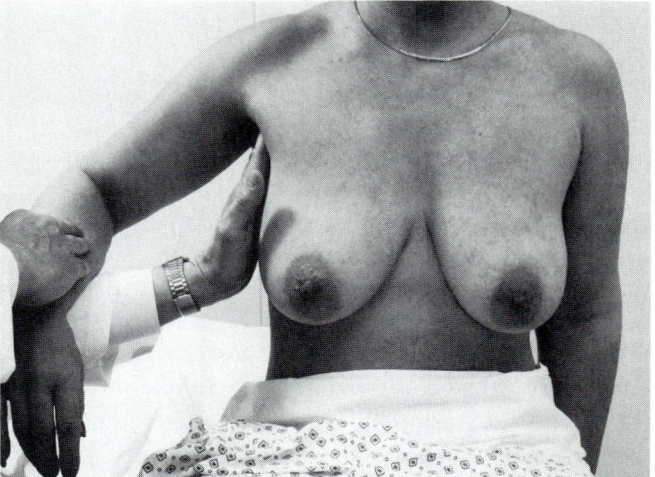

Fig. 8-13 Palpation of the axilla.

whether each is fixed or mobile and soft or firm. Axillary nodes may be enlarged because of lymphatic drainage from the breast or arm or because of systemic diseases. Infections of the fingers or hands, systemic syphilis, or Hodgkin's disease are a few examples of the many diseases besides breast cancer that may result in axillary adenopathy. A common error is to misinterpret the axillary fat pad as a single large lymph node. Differentiate this by trying to palpate it between the forefinger and thumb. The margins of nodes are discrete; those of the fat pad are indiscrete.

The breast is best examined when it is spread over the chest wall, with the least thickness of breast present between the skin and the chest wall. When the patient is lying with the arm above the head, and a pillow is under the shoulder on the side to be examined, the examiner can perform the most accurate evaluation.

At times a lump with a diameter of 1 cm may be palpable. Large breasts may harbor larger lumps that are not palpable. When lumps are found shortly before the menstrual period, the examination should be repeated 1 or 2 weeks after

TABLE 8-4: Comparison of Adjunctive Studies for Breast Abnormalities

Mammography	Ultrasonography	Thermography
• Detects cancer earlier than any other means noninvasively • 12% to 16% of palpable tumors not demonstrated by this tool • Less valuable in young women with dense breast tissue • Good for cancer screening after age 30 years	• 12% to 16% of palpable tumors not demonstrated by this tool • Cystic disease well visualized • Use when woman has had mammary implant	• Less valuable in young women with dense breast tissue • Several benign lesions produce more heat than surrounding tissues • False positives are higher than for physical exam, and false negatives may be found in 25% of cancers

menses to determine whether these have resolved (see Case 8-1). When a lump is found, record the site, size, shape, consistency, mobility, attachments, and whether regional lymph nodes are palpable.

Benign fibroadenomas and cysts are usually smooth and mobile. Fibroadenomas often measure about 1 cm in diameter and are freely movable. They are the most common nodules in young women. Radiologic studies or biopsy may be required to distinguish these from other tumors (Table 8-4).

Cysts are fluid-filled rounded masses. Their consistency is related to the pressure of the fluid. Cysts may appear at once or be present for years, and they may be single or multiple. Ultrasound may distinguish fluid-filled from solid nodules. Many clinicians confirm cysts by needle aspiration and cytologic examination of any aspirated cells.

Bloody fluid obtained at aspiration may be found in either benign cysts or in cystic carcinomas. Bloody fluid from a needle aspirate mandates surgical biopsy for possible cystic cancer.

Malignant breast tumors are typically firm and irregular. The amount of fibrous tissue present determines the firmness of the tumor. Immobility of a mass does not necessarily indicate malignancy. However, a lump or mass that is not freely moveable is characteristic of cancer. It may be adherent to the overlying skin or to the underlying fascia, muscle, or bone.

Special Concerns in the Breast Examination

After Mastectomy

The postmastectomy patient requires special attention to both sides of the chest when looking for metastatic masses. On the involved side, cancer nodules are commonly found along the incisional scar. Axillary or supraclavicular node enlargement may appear soon or many years after the original operation. The remaining breast is also at greater risk of developing cancer.

The Male Breast

Male breasts should also be inspected and palpated. *Gynecomastia* (excessive breast development in men) is typical of cirrhosis, Klinefelter's syndrome, and eunuchs. Men taking medications such as diethylstilbestrol, spironolactone, or digitalis may also develop gynecomastia. This condition is distinguished from simple deposition of fatty tissue caused by aging by the firmer breast tissue, which also has glandular proliferation.

Cancer of the breast is uncommon in men as compared with women. Only 1% of breast cancer occurs in men. A breast lump may become apparent early in men because of the smaller thickness of breast tissue. In men, breast cancers grow quite rapidly and are highly malignant.

Summary

A summary checklist for evaluating the breast is shown in the box below.

Summary Checklist for Breast Examination

Inspection
- Standard positions
- Breast size, symmetry, contour
- Retraction, dimpling
- Nipple discharge
- Ulceration
- Striae
- Mondor's disease
- Peau d'orange

Palpation
- Breast lumps
- Breast cysts
- Fibroadenoma
- Malignant tumor
- Axillary nodes
- Tenderness
- Galactorrhea

Suggested readings

Fletcher SW, et al: How best to teach women breast self-examination, *Ann Intern Med* 112:772-779, 1990. *Comparison of methods for teaching breast self-examination. Use of a silicon model for practice identifying lumps with instruction by a nurse and some physician input enhanced patients' findings of lumps.*

Kinne DW, Kopans DB: Physical examination and mammography in the diagnosis of breast disease. In Harris JR, et al, editors: *Breast diseases*, New York, 1987, JB Lippincott. *This is a thorough chapter in an excellent book covering most aspects of breast diseases, especially breast cancers.*

McKinna JA: Clinical features of breast disease. In Parsons CA, editor: *Diagnosis of breast disease*, Baltimore, Md, 1983, University Park Press. *This chapter discusses the symptoms of breast diseases for which patients commonly seek treatment, and shows pictures of abnormalities seen on physical examination.*

CHAPTER NINE

The Musculoskeletal System

CHAPTER OUTLINE

History Taking
Pain
Stiffness
Weakness
Fatigue

Physical Examination of the Musculoskeletal System
Principles of examination
Regional approach to the examination

Diagnosis of Arthritis

Summary

Musculoskeletal symptoms are important reasons patients seek medical attention. Ten percent of out-patients have musculoskeletal complaints. With aging, bone and joint disorders account for an increasing amount of morbidity. Young people, enjoying physical fitness activities, sustain acute injuries and chronic trauma, resulting in the need for medical care. The elderly often have acute musculoskeletal problems, especially from falls and chronic degenerative diseases.

When evaluating musculoskeletal complaints, establish whether the problem is acute or chronic. The history, examination, and additional studies will be modified thereby. Usually the history and physical examination will be important in assessing musculoskeletal conditions.

History Taking

Initial questions in the history are not unique to the musculoskeletal system, and concern the following areas:

- Age
- Sex

- Race
- Family history of musculoskeletal diseases
- Events surrounding onset
- Tempo of change in symptoms
- Events that seem to initiate onset of symptoms
- Structures that are involved and how this changes with time
- Symptoms that have also occurred but do not seem musculoskeletal

Skillful use of these questions can be helpful in diagnosis.
The patient's age may favor certain diagnoses:

- Childhood—juvenile rheumatoid arthritis (RA) or rheumatic fever
- Young adults—Reiter's syndrome or systemic lupus erythematosis (SLE)
- Middle age—fibrositis
- Old age—osteoarthritis

The patient's sex may favor certain diagnoses:

- Males—gout
- Females—SLE or RA

The patient's race may be important:

- Black—SLE or sarcoidosis
- White—polymyalgia rheumatica

The patient's family history may be a useful clue if gout, RA, or Heberden's nodes are recalled.

The tempo (time course) of the illness may be characteristic. The acutely swollen joint at the base of the great toe *(podagra)* typically begins during the night and becomes very painful. Pain moving from joint to joint *(migratory pain)* is characteristic of rheumatic fever, or of disseminated gonococcal disease.

The associated findings besides musculoskeletal complaints are numerous. Disseminated gonococcal disease may exhibit skin rash, tenosynovitis, and urethritis. *Reiter's syndrome* is characterized by a rash on the palms and soles (keratoderma blenorrhagia) and on the penis (circinate balanitis) in addition to joint manifestations.

Activities or medications that exacerbate or relieve symptoms may yield important clues. Rheumatoid joints tend to loosen up as the day progresses. Changes in atmospheric conditions occasionally tend to make musculoskeletal pain worse.

When a patient seems to have an illness or injury more trivial than expected, search for a deeper reason for the patient's seeking medical care. Is he concerned about possible cancer, a potential deformity, a prolonged recuperation time, inability to work to earn a living, or pending legal action? Is he exhibiting drug-seeking behavior? Sometimes patients "just put up with it" for as long as possible before seeking care. At times, an x-ray film showing no fracture is enough to get a patient moving again.

The clinician usually focuses on the cardinal symptoms for analysis when working toward a differential diagnosis. In the analysis of musculoskeletal diseases, key symptoms and key signs are considered together (see accompanying box).

Each of the key signs in the box may be symptoms, brought to the attention

> **Symptoms and Signs of Joint Disease**
>
> **Key Symptoms**
> - Pain
> - Stiffness
> - Weakness
> - Fatigue
>
> **Key Signs**
> - Swelling
> - Deformity
> - Erythema or warmth
> - Limitation of motion
> - Tenderness
> - Joint noises or locking

of the clinician by the patient, but pain, stiffness, fatigue, or tenderness are commonly presenting complaints.

Generally the history of the present illness begins with the complaint and focuses on its location, time course, and the nature of how it has changed. Initiating events such as trauma are considered because the later physical examination is modified if injury may be involved (i.e., avoid flexing the neck of an injured patient with neck pain until a radiograph shows no fracture).

After the cardinal manifestations of musculoskeletal disease are reviewed and sometimes even during the review, questions regarding past medical history, family history, or social history may become appropriate to ask. A logical time to do this would be when a patient makes a statement such as the following:

- "I think my symptoms are just like my dad's." Pursue the family history at this time.
- "I had something like this before, but it was a little different." Pertinent past history can be reviewed.
- "I have a new boyfriend and he wanted me to come to see you." Questions about social history and sexual history would be appropriate at this time.

The past medical history may suggest a diagnosis. The skin rash of psoriasis raises the possibility of psoriatic arthritis. Rheumatic fever after streptococcal infection characteristically is associated with joint pain, which may recur. In a patient in whom previous medical investigations have failed to reveal the cause of arthritis, the examiner must consider the possibility of joint manifestations of other processes, such as endocarditis or immune complex disease, and the need for more extensive evaluation.

Stress and psychologic factors may be related to episodes of increased joint pain in several diseases. The effect of the illness on the patient's lifestyle and activities of daily living help in defining the extent of the patient's disability.

The family history is particularly important because certain musculoskeletal disorders, such as osteoarthritis, gout, or RA, may have a familial component (see first box on pg. 336). Finally, medications and other therapy may give clues to future requirements for the patient.

Pain

Whether pain is from tendons, muscles, bursa, ligaments, or joints, it is often described as joint pain. Articular cartilage and compact bone lack sensory

Arthritis In Which Other Family Members May be Affected
• Akylosing spondylitis • Gout • Heberden's nodes (osteoarthritis) • Hemophilia (with bleeding into joints) • Hemoglobinopathies (e.g., sickle cell disease)

innervation. Thus other structures that have innervation are responsible for pain.

Pain originating in muscles is often a continuous deep ache, but may be called tender or cramping.

Pain arising from bone is often deep or boring pain. Although bone pain commonly interferes with sleeping at night, ordinarily bone pain is not increased with movement unless a fracture or dislocation coexists. Joint pain or pain from tenosynovitis may also be produced by movement.

Pain from the periosteum is usually localized. In general, pain arising from a musculoskeletal structure feels either local or diffuse because of relation to the depth of the site of origin and to the size of the area involved more than the tissue involved: the deeper the structure, the more diffuse the pain.

Often pain in a muscle of an extremity is perceived in *(referred to)* the joint that the muscle moves. An example of referred pain occurs when pain originating in the quadriceps femoris muscle is felt in the knee. Pain from the anterior tibial muscle may be felt in the ankle joint. The box below shows examples of problems that may cause joint pain either because of referred pain or because of direct joint involvement. Bone tumors and osteomyelitis may result in either joint pain or bone pain. Trauma to periarticular soft tissues or bursa may result in soft-tissue or joint discomfort. Inflammation of a tendon *(tendinitis)* or tendon sheath may mimic joint pain. Pressure over the tendon or movement of the tendon in the

Some Causes of Joint Pain	
Bone Disease • Tumors • Osteomyelitis **Soft Tissue** • Bursitis • Tenosynovitis • Trauma **Referred Pain** • To shoulder from diaphragm • To knee from hip	**Systemic Infections** • Viral diseases • Gonococcemia • Rheumatic fever **Joint Diseases** • RA • Osteoarthritis • Septic joint • Joint trauma

tendon sheath may reproduce the pain even if joint motion is minimal.

Arthralgia may be defined as joint pain without objective signs of inflammation. Patients typically complain that "My joints ache" or "My ankle hurts," or "I have the rheumatism." Arthralgia is a fairly common manifestation of diseases, including immune diseases or systemic infections caused by bacteria, viruses, or rickettsia. Possible examples include influenza, rubella, typhus, or endocarditis. Arthralgia or arthritis may be confined to a single joint *(monarticular)*, involve several joints *(polyarticular)*, involve one joint and later other joints simultaneously *(additive)*, or involve several joints successively *(migratory)* and be symmetric or asymmetric.

In contrast to arthralgia, arthritis has objective changes of inflammation in one or more joints (Table 9-1). Patients often complain that "My rheumatism is acting up," "I have arthritis," or "My knee is swollen." Thus the patient's spontaneous

TABLE 9-1: Symptom: The Painful Joint

Diagnosis	Cause/History	Usual Joint Involved	Examination Findings
Trauma	• Injury of a joint, bone, or supporting structures	• Any	• Mechanical problems • Joints lock or give way • Crepitus or popping • Tenderness may localize to one side of joint
Degenerative	• Single or multiple joints involved	• Fingers, hip, knees	• Pain, tenderness, deformity
Septic joint	• Gonococcal: migratory arthralgia, skin pustules, tenosynovitis • Staphylococcal: intravenous drug abusers, infected intravascular lines	• Knees, ankles, hands	• Hot, red, tender joint that is painful with movement
	• Rheumatoid with secondary *S. aureus* infection, preexisting joint abnormality; now acutely inflamed		• Red, warm, swollen, painful
	• Tuberculosis: adjacent bone may be infected; slow progression, mild pain		• Joint is "cool," unlike in bacterial infections
Rheumatoid	• Usually multiple joints, but may be single; attacks are more brief (1 to 4 days) than gouty attacks	• Fingers, hands, many others	• Joint red, hot, tender; hurts to move it • Exam shows evidence of deformities • Loss of grip strength is common
Gout	• First MTP joint—unable to tolerate weight of bedsheet on it; untreated lasts 10 to 14 nights.	• Great toe, knees, ankles	• Red, hot, tender joint
Neuropathic joint disease	• Painless or only slight pain for the marked swelling and hypermobility of the joint; consider diabetes, syphilis	• Knee, ankle	• Loss of pain sensation allows joint damage with grinding sounds, loose bone bodies, and eventually unstable joint
Bursitis	• Swelling and fluid distention of bursa must be differentiated from joint pain		• Tender, swollen, red bursa with increased fluid

Cardinal Signs of Inflammation
• Calor (heat) • Rubor (redness) • Tumor (swelling) • Dolor (pain) • Functio laesa (loss of function)

history may not distinguish between arthralgia or arthritis unless specific questions are asked about signs of inflammation (see the accompanying box).

Examples of questions to ask about joint pain and the rationales for these questions are as follows:

- *Describe your joint discomfort.* This allows the patient to tell his own story.
- *When did the joint pain begin? When did it start this time?* Duration helps to differentiate acute from chronic processes.
- *How did the pain start?* Sudden onset of pain is more in keeping with an infectious etiologic cause, trauma, or gout. Gradual onset is characteristic of degenerative arthritis.
- *What do you think brought on the joint pain?* Trauma or excessive activity often give clues to the cause.
- *What do you do that makes the pain worse? What relieves it?* This gives a clue to diagnosis, disability, and ability to manage the problem.
- *Which joints have been involved? What joint was first affected? For how long? How have subsequent joints been affected?* Sometimes only one joint may be involved (Table 9-2). At other times many joints may be painful (Table 9-3). Migratory arthralgia is characteristic of acute rheumatic fever (Table 9-4), gonococcal arthritis, and early rheumatoid disease. Finally, determine the most severely affected joints so these can be given special attention during the examination.
- *What times during the day is your discomfort worse?* RA is worse in the morning. Osteoarthritis becomes uncomfortable later in the day.

The pattern of symptoms in relation to the time of day or night is important. Rheumatoid disease typically begins with morning stiffness that subsides as the patient becomes mobile during the day. Untreated, the average patient with rheumatoid disease has some stiffness that may last as long as 3 or 4 hours. On the other hand, degenerative disease tends to become more painful with use during the course of the day. Night pain and interference with sleep is typical for the painful great toe proximal interphalangeal joint (the *podagra* of gouty arthritis). Pain from bone tumors is often worse at night. Questions asked to determine patterns include the following:

- *Do you have pain every day?* Tendinitis, bursitis, and fibromyalgia wax and wane depending on weather, exercise, or other factors.
- *What gives you relief?* Activity in the morning tends to relieve rheumatoid disease. Inactivity or immobility associated with a catnap during the day may

TABLE 9-2: Diseases that may Cause Arthritis in a Single Joint

Disease	Clinical Features	Additional Studies
Gout	• Males • First MTP joint • Onset at night • Recurrent attacks	• Serum uric acid high • Urate crystals in joint fluid • WBC in joint fluid; 10 to 50,000 cells/mm^3 or more — mostly polys
Pseudogout	• Elderly • Knee or large joint • Previous attack • Flexion contracture	• Radiograph may show calcification in joint • Calcium pyrophosphate crystal in joint fluid • WBC count as for gout
Calcific tendinitis	• Tendon or capsule of large joint • Previous attack	• Calcification on radiograph • WBCs have ovoid bodies phagocytosed
Septic joint	• History depends on microbe • May be a primary septic focus • Duration: hours to days	• Joint fluid has WBC count of 50,000 to 200,000 cells/mm^3, nearly all polys
Fungal or tubercular arthritis	• Duration: weeks or longer • May be infected focus elsewhere	• Joint fluid may yield positive smear or culture • WBC with polymorphs predominately

CASE 9-1 Rheumatoid Arthritis

A 44-year-old woman secretary came to the general medicine clinic for fatigue, joint pain, and morning stiffness.

During the past few weeks the patient had an unusual sense of fatigue so that by midafternoon she did not feel like staying at her job. She would go home early and go to bed before getting up later to fix dinner for the family.

She volunteered that after the fatigue had begun, she also began to notice a stiffness in the mornings when she got out of bed. After she took a warm shower and had breakfast she usually felt a little better. Several mornings she had to take a few aspirins to "help get going."

On examination she had several tender joints, including the wrists, the metacarpophalangeal joints, and both knees. Several proximal interphalangeal joints were swollen, giving a fusiform appearance to the fingers. There was discomfort when either forefinger was moved passively.

The patient did not have any signs of advanced disease: no ulnar deviation of fingers, swan neck, boutonniere deformities of the fingers, rheumatoid nodules of the elbows, or Baker's cysts at the knees. In short, she seemed to have early disease.

Her laboratory studies showed a normochromic, normocytic anemia. The erythrocyte sedimentation rate was elevated to 78 mm/hour. The ANA and VDRL were negative. The rheumatoid factor was positive at 1:640.

This case shows the extreme fatigue that patients with RA often suffer in the course of the disease. Morning stiffness persisting for several hours is typical unless the patient receives antiinflammatory medications. Criteria needed to make a diagnosis of RA are shown in Table 9-5.

TABLE 9-3: Diseases that may Cause Arthritis in Several Joints at Once

Disease	Clinical Features	Additional Studies
Rheumatoid arthritis (RA), seropositive	• Seropositive • Females more often • Symmetric • Synovial thickening, nodules	• Rheumatoid factor positive • Joint fluid 5000 to 30,000 WBC majority polys • CH50 decreased in joint fluid • Radiography shows bone erosions
RA, seronegative	• Seronegative • Sex — either men or women • Symmetric involvement but may be asymmetric	• Rheumatoid factor absent • Joint fluid up to 20,000 WBC, 20% to 60% polys • CH50 not reduced in joint fluid • Radiograph shows no bone erosions
Systemic lupus erythematosus	• Females • Symmetric joints as in RA • Rash, hair loss, per criteria	• Joint fluid 1000 to 2000 WBC • Radiograph shows no erosions • Serum CH50 reduced • ANA titer elevated Anti-DNA titer increased
Scleroderma	• Raynaud's phenomenon • Tight skin, visceral involvement • Symmetric tendon contractures • Not much synovial thickening	• Positive ANA; pattern is speckled or nuclear
Dermatomyositis	• Proximal muscle weakness of pelvic and pectoral girdles • Tender muscles • Erythema of knuckle pad • Symmetric joint involvement	• EMG abnormal: myopathy and denervation • Increased serum creatinine and phosphokinase • Abnormal muscle biopsy
Mixed connective-tissue disease	• Symmetric joint involvement • Raynaud's phenomenon • Swollen hands, skin is tight	• Positive ANA (speckled) • Anti-RNP increased • Radiograph joint erosions
Juvenile rheumatoid arthritis	• Symmetric joint involvement • Rash, fever • Iridocyclitis if ANA positive	• Rheumatoid factor negative • Radiograph periostitis early, and later erosions • HLA B-27 may be positive
Psoriatic arthritis	• Often single joint, may be multiple • Asymmetric joint involvement • Skin and nail lesions may follow arthritis or be minimal • DIP especially involved	• Rheumatoid factor negative • CH50 normal in joint fluid • Radiograph periostitis or erosions
Rheumatic fever	• Young person, age 2 to 30 years • Migratory arthritis • Recent streptococcal sore throat (group A, *Streptococcus pyogenes*) • Jones criteria for diagnosis (see end of chapter)	• Systemic potential • Elevated ASO titers or streptozyme titer • Dramatic response to aspirin
Reiter's syndrome	• Males • Sexually active • Asymmetric joints • Urethritis, iritis, conjunctivitis	• May follow yersinia, chlamydia infection • Joint fluid 5000 to 30,000 WBC • Serum CH50 is increased

TABLE 9-3: Diseases that may Cause Arthritis in Several Joints at Once—cont'd

Disease	Clinical Features	Additional Studies
Reiter's syndrome—cont'd	• Sacroiliac and lower extremity joints • Keratoderma blennorrhagica on palms and soles • Circinate balanitis on glans penis	• Macrophages in joint fluid with phagocytosed polys (Reiter's cell)
Gonococcal arthritis	• Either sex • Migratory arthritis • Tenosynovitis • Skin lesions, often pustules	• Pustules often have gram-negative diplococci that do not grow on culture • Culture positive from urethra, rectum, pharynx, or cervix
Gout	• Usually single joint initially • Symmetric arthritis • Previous attacks • Tophi; may have flexion contractures	• Urate crystals in joint fluid
Pseudogout	• Usually single joint initially • Symmetric arthritis • Previous attacks • May have flexion contractures • MCP, shoulders, hips, or knees involved	• Pyrophosphate crystals in joint fluid

TABLE 9-4: Revised Jones Criteria for Rheumatic Fever

Criteria	Manifestations

Two major or one major and two minor criteria required. Patients must have evidence for recent streptococcal infection.

Major

1. Carditis		
	a. Myocarditis	• Gallop rhythm, congestive heart failure, arrhythmias, ST-T changes on ECG, nodal tachycardia
	b. Pericarditis	• Precordial chest pain, pericardial friction rub, pericardial effusion, ECG findings of pericarditis
2. Polyarthritis		• Arthritis involving several large joints at once; begins with migratory arthralgia; responds so promptly to salicylate therapy that this is a therapeutic test
3. Chorea		• Purposeless movements of various muscle groups; these disappear during sleep
4. Erythema marginatum		• Pink circular rash on trunk and proximal arms (erythema annulare, erythema circinata)
5. Subcutaneous nodules		• 1 to 5 cm granulomas on the joint extensor surfaces, wrist, nodules elbows, occiput, and palms; tender, moveable, not attached to skin; cardiac involvement commonly discovered when these are found

Continued.

TABLE 9-4: Revised Jones Criteria for Rheumatic Fever—cont'd

Criteria	Manifestations
Minor	
1. Clinical criteria	
a. Previous rheumatic fever or rheumatic heart disease	
b. Arthralgia	• Joint pain without findings on examination except tenderness
c. Fever	• Usually afternoon, rarely over 39.5° C, responds rapidly to aspirin therapy
2. Laboratory criteria	
a. Acute phase reactants	• Increases in erythrocyte sedimentation rate (this is so commonly elevated in other disorders that a normal ESR is useful against the diagnosis), C-reactive protein, leukocytosis
b. ECG	• Prolonged PR interval without other manifestations of cardiac abnormalities
c. Recent streptococcal infection	• Throat culture, recent scarlet fever, antibodies suggesting streptococcal infection (ASO titer or streptozyme titer high)

cause midday stiffness. Rest relieves pain from degenerative arthritis. Heat often relieves pain of musculoskeletal origin. Aspirin may relieve pain of arthritis, but if used in modest doses aspirin may exacerbate attacks of gouty arthritis by reducing urinary excretion of uric acid.

- *What types of activities are you able to do yourself, and what do you need help with?* Pain or other symptoms may force the patient to seek help with tasks of daily living, such as cooking, dressing, performing usual work, shopping, or driving a car. Note how disabled the patient says he is so that appropriate insurance and disability forms can be filled out later if needed.

TABLE 9-5: Diagnostic Criteria for Rheumatoid Arthritis

Criterion	Definition
1. Morning stiffness	Morning joint stiffness lasting at least 1 hour
2. Arthritis of 3 or more joint areas	At least 3 joints simultaneously have soft tissue swelling or effusion (not just bony overgrowth) observed by a physician. The joints include right or left PIP, MCP, wrist, elbow, MTP, ankle, knees.
3. Arthritis of hand joints	At least 1 swollen wrist, MCP, or PIP joint.
4. Symmetric arthritis	Simultaneous involvement of the same joints on both sides of the body. (Involvement of small joints of both hands or both feet need not be absolutely symmetrical to qualify).
5. Rheumatoid nodules	Subcutaneous nodules over joints or extensor surfaces (observed by a physician).
6. Serum rheumatoid factor	Serum rheumatoid factor positive (using a method with < 5% positive controls).
7. Radiographic changes	Typical radiographic changes on hand and wrist radiographs, including erosions or bony decalcification in or adjacent to the involved joints.

Adapted from Arnett FC, et al: Revised criteria for the classification of rheumatoid arthritis, Arthr Rheum 31(3):315-324, 1988.
A patient has rheumatoid arthritis if 4 of these 7 criteria are satisfied. Criteria 1 through 4 must have been present for at least 6 weeks. Designation as classic, definite, or probable rheumatoid arthritis is no longer made.

TABLE 9-6: Symptoms in Selected Types of Arthritis

Manifestation	Rheumatoid Arthritis	Osteoarthritis	Gouty Arthritis	Traumatic Arthritis	Septic Arthritis
Pain tempo	Gradual	Gradual	Abrupt	Abrupt	Abrupt
Pain	During activity	Follows activity	During the night	May have constant pain	Constant pain
Stiffness	Morning, for several hours, generalized	Morning for several minutes	Of involved joint	Present	Of involved joint
Weakness	Present, often severe	Some	No	Marked	Of involved joint
Fatigue	Severe, onset in afternoon	Not usually	No	No	Maybe

- *What other symptoms do you experience?* Associated symptoms may give clues to etiologic cause (Table 9-6). For example, general malaise is typical of inflammatory arthritis. Rash may be present with juvenile RA, SLE, and other conditions.

Stiffness

Patients with joint diseases may have the complaint of stiffness of the joints. Some patients may not distinguish joint pain from morning stiffness until asked to do so. Stiffness of RA occurs in the morning or during the day after periods

---

CASE 9-2   Gout

A 56-year-old obese man had been in reasonably good health. The evening in question, he had gone to bed after the evening news. About 2 AM he was awakened by severe pain in the right great toe. At first the pain was of moderate intensity, but it became more intense during the next hour.

The patient felt chilly but had no shaking chills. He found it difficult to get comfortable, and kept changing position and moving the foot for relief. The base of the great toe was too tender for even a bedsheet to touch.

Near morning he broke into a light sweat and got back to sleep. When he awakened the proximal joint of the great toe was swollen but less painful.

He did not seek medical help at that time. The toe continued to swell and be painful each evening, relenting towards morning. Skin over the persistently red, swollen joint began to exfoliate. After the left great toe became affected, he saw his physician.

Blood studies showed the serum uric acid was elevated to 9.1 mg/dl and the urinary excretion of uric acid was above normal. The pain of acute attacks was controlled with colchicine. The serum uric acid was reduced to normal, using allopurinol.

This case shows the acute onset of nocturnal pain in acute gout. The painful toe may continue to give nightly episodes of pain if the patient remains untreated. Some untreated patients can expect additional joints to become involved.

of joint disuse. The duration of morning stiffness is an indicator of severity of inflammation, and it is believed to be caused by the supporting structures of the joint. Effective therapy tends to reduce duration of morning stiffness. To determine the duration of morning stiffness, ask the patient, *What time do you get out of bed in the morning?* and then *What time do your joints feel as limbered up as they are going to feel?* If the patient is asked the single question, *How long are your joints stiff after you get up in the morning?* the response may be shorter than the actual duration of morning stiffness.

Degenerative arthritis may also be associated with stiffness but it usually lasts only a few minutes. After getting out of a chair, someone who is stiff from

---

CASE 9-3 Systemic Lupus Erythematosus

An 18-year-old black woman was seen for pain in both knees. She had recently changed insurance carriers and had brought a packet of old medical records with her.

She stated that she had had lupus for 2 years. The diagnosis was first made when she had a low-grade fever of 100.5, became fatigued easily, and had a weight loss of 15 pounds. She said there were also sores in her mouth and several areas where hair fell out of her scalp.

She denied ever having had a rash across the bridge of her nose or cheeks, even though she had been in sunlight some on her job at an outdoor restaurant. She tried to avoid sunlight because the joint pain seemed to get worse after she had been in the sun a lot.

Her records showed that she had had urinary tract infections, but at other times she had had hematuria and proteinuria. Red blood cell casts had been noted on one occasion.

The ANA was positive at 1:1280. The VDRL was weakly reactive, but the FTA-ABS and the rheumatoid factor were both negative.

Thus this patient had more than 4 of the 11 criteria needed for diagnosis of SLE:

1. Malar rash (over bridge of nose and on cheeks)
2. Discoid rash (red patches healing with atrophic scars)
3. Photosensitivity (rash caused by sunlight)
4. Oral ulcers (usually painless)
5. Arthritis (tenderness, swelling, or fluid in two or more joints)
6. Serositis (pleuritis, pericarditis)
7. Renal disorder (proteinuria or cellular casts)
8. Neurologic disorder (seizures or psychosis)
9. Hematologic disorder (hemolytic anemia, leukopenia, or lymphopenia, or thrombocytopenia)
10. Immunologic disorder (positive LE preparation, anti-DNA or anti-Sm nuclear antigen, or biologic false-positive test for syphilis)
11. Antinuclear antibody (in the absence of drugs to cause drug-induced lupus)

These criteria are used to identify patients for clinical studies. A patient is said to have SLE if 4 or more of these 11 criteria are present during any time interval. Rodman GP, Schumacher HR: *Primer on the rheumatic diseases,* ed 8, Atlanta, 1983, Arthritis Foundation.

osteoarthritis may find the initial step or two difficult, but subsequent steps feel normal. In contrast, the patient with RA is typically stiff for 3 or 4 hours.

Weakness

Weakness may be a symptom the patient complains of or a sign that can be quantitated during the examination. Patients may confuse weakness and fatigue. *Weakness* refers to strength, whereas *fatigue* refers to endurance. Weakness of the proximal muscles (upper arm or upper leg) may occur in myopathies and in polymyalgia rheumatica. Proximal muscle weakness may be caused by the remote effects of tumors (Eaton-Lambert syndrome) or by nerve root impingement. Weakness of distal muscles (lower arm or leg) is more likely to be related to arthritis, tendinitis, or peripheral neuropathy.

Fatigue

Fatigue (tired weariness, or decreased endurance) in healthy people has many causes, including stress, work, and loss of sleep. In normal people it begins late in the day.

Fatigue caused by rheumatic diseases often begins in the morning. Fatigue is a subjective phenomenon not specific for disease. In RA, the time elapsing after a patient has arisen from bed before the onset of fatigue is an indicator of severity of inflammation. A patient with severe untreated RA may be out of bed only 3 or 4 hours before becoming fatigued.

Patients with chronic fatigue syndrome may experience fatigue all day or beginning in midday. Patients with insomnia or sleep apnea may have excessive daytime sleepiness, whereas patients with anemia or metabolic diseases may have fatigue. In this setting, try to differentiate between sleepiness and fatigue.

Patients who have RA often have sleep disturbances, which may contribute to fatigue and depression. Taking effective antiinflammatory medication reduces symptoms.

Depression is a common symptom in patients with RA. It often begins about the time severe fatigue begins. Manifestations may be crying spells, temper tantrums, or withdrawal.

Physical Examination of the Musculoskeletal System

The examination of bones and joints must be an active process to search for specific information to help generate a differential diagnosis and a specific diagnosis. Questions for the examiner to ask himself include the following:

- What structures am I examining?
- What techniques should I use to assess this structure?
- What am I looking for to guide my diagnostic thinking?
- How does the structure and function of this joint differ from normal?

Because the hands and feet are so often involved with rheumatic diseases, the examination may begin with the hands. Some clinicians prefer to start at the head and proceed down. The examiner should be systematic so that no joints or muscle groups are overlooked. As a systematic regional approach is developed, head and neck, the upper extremities, the back and sacroiliac joints, and the lower extremities are examined. The patient is usually sitting for the upper extremities

Definitions of Terms Applying to Musculoskeletal Disorders	
Term	Definition
Abduction	To move from the midline of the body
Adduction	To move towards the middle
Eversion	To turn outward from the midline
Extension	To straighten at joint
External rotation	To rotate laterally at a joint
Flexion	To bend at the joint so the distal part moves toward the body
Internal rotation	To rotate a limb medially at the joint
Inversion	To turn inward
Kyphosis	Rounded curvature of the spine, normally found in the thoracic area, characterized by extensive flexion.
Kyphoscoliosis	Combination of kyphosis and scoliosis.
Lordosis	The concave curvature of the spine similar to that usually found in the lumbar and cervical areas.
Pronation	Applied to the foot, combination of eversion and abduction, when the medial edge is lowered. Applied to the palm, the hand faces backward or downward.
Scoliosis	Lateral curvature of the spine in a **C** shape or **S** shape.
Supination	Applied to the foot, combination of inversion and abduction, the medial edge is elevated. Applied to the forearm, the palm faces forward or upward.
Varus	Deviation of the distal portion of a joint toward the midline (genu varum—bowleg)
Valgus	Deviation of the distal portion of a joint from the midline (genu valgum—knock-knee)

and head-and-neck examinations. He may need to stand and bend over for more complete examination of mobility of the back and sacroiliac joints. The patient then may be supine or sitting for examination of the lower extremities. Finally, weight bearing and gait are evaluated.

Principles of Examination

In the examination of muscles, bones, and joints, adequate body exposure and good light are important. Compare the unaffected side and affected sides. Inspection and palpation are used together routinely, whereas auscultation or percussion are needed only occasionally.

Joint assessment begins with general observation and inspection of range of motion, followed by palpation, and must occasionally be followed by percussion (ballottement) or auscultation for joint noises (see accompanying box).

Inspect skin, soft tissues, and scars overlying bones, joints, and muscles. Red, shiny skin may reflect an underlying bone or soft tissue abnormality. Observe the bones and joints for alignment, deformity, shortening, or asymmetry, comparing sides. Soft tissues may show asymmetry caused by swelling, inflammation, or muscle wasting.

The type of movement expected from each joint depends on the anatomic structures (Fig. 9-1) forming the joint.

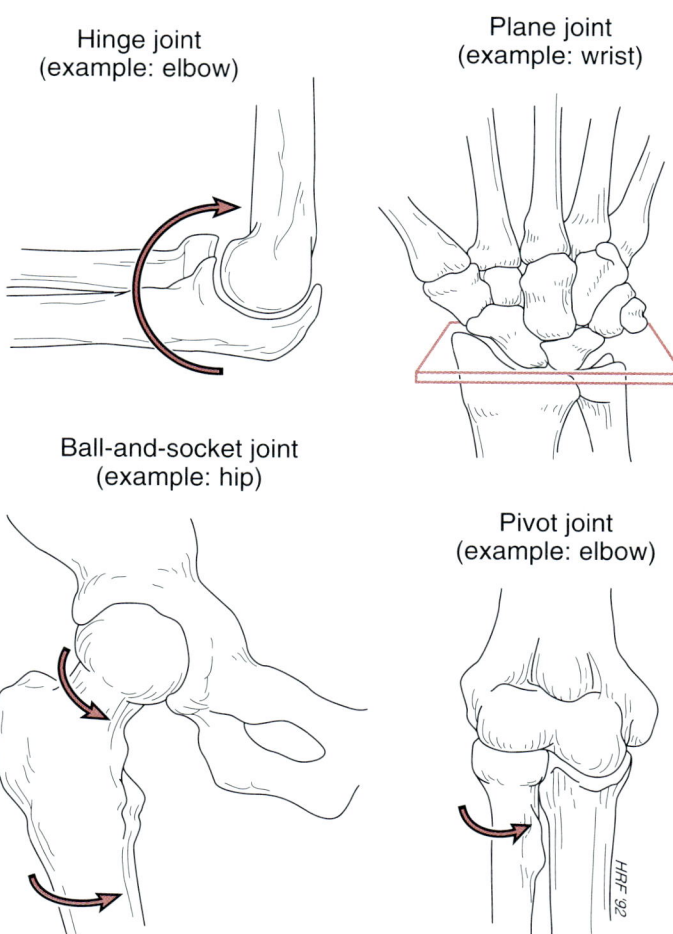

Fig. 9-1 Types of joints: hinge, plane, ball and socket, and pivot.

INSPECTION

Stability of joints depends on the articular surfaces and the supporting structures. A joint may be unstable, showing excessive range of motion, motion in an abnormal plane for the joint, or dislocation. When evaluating a joint that may be unstable or show abnormal range of motion, ask the patient to relax to prevent obscuring the instability. Some unstable joints may show instability better with stresses (such as weight bearing). Instability is more important in evaluating a patient's disability than in arriving at a diagnosis because instability is often a late finding.

PALPATION

Palpation is often done simultaneously with inspection for musculoskeletal disorders. This gives more complete information on swelling, increased temperature, range of motion, and tender sites. To fully assess information offered by palpation, the examiner must know which anatomic structures are being pressed by the examining hand. A corollary is that some instruction is required on the location of the more important sites to allow palpation of each joint. These sites are discussed and shown in a later section.

Pressure of palpation depends on the patient's symptoms at each joint. For joints that are tender, begin with a light touch. Firm pressure, even enough to

TABLE 9-7: Signs in Selected Types of Arthritis

Manifestation	Rheumatoid Arthritis	Osteoarthritis	Gouty Arthritis	Traumatic Arthritis	Septic Arthritis
Swelling					
Synovium thickened	Marked	No	No	No	No
Effusion	Common	May occur	Yes	May occur	Yes
Deformity	Common	Common	Late in course	Can occur if untreated	Can occur if untreated
Erythema and warmth	Transient early, common	Absent Absent	Common Common early	Absent Absent	Common Common
Limitation of motion	Common	Not usually severe	Mild	May be marked acutely	Marked acutely
Tenderness	Usual, indicator of inflammation	Usual	Usual	May be localized	Usual

blanch the nailbed of the examining finger, is applied only to joints or structures that do not seem tender, and the intent is to rule out tenderness. Whether tenderness is caused by a low pain threshold in the patient or by an abnormal structure must be determined.

Abnormalities to inspect and palpate on examination of joints include the following (Table 9-7):

- Swelling
- Deformity
- Erythema and warmth
- Limitation of the range of motion
- Tenderness
- Joint noises or locking (they may be palpated or heard by auscultation)

Swelling

Joint swelling is usually caused by synovial swelling, or effusion. Swelling or deformity may be caused by dislocation, fracture, periarticular swelling, or bony enlargement.

In normal patients, the synovium is thin and not palpable. When the synovium is thickened, the joint appears variably swollen depending on severity. The synovium becomes palpable around the entire circumference of the joint, taking on a doughy feeling as it gets thicker. This is easier to show in joints that are close to the skin surface, such as the finger joints, metacarpophalangeal joints, wrists, elbows, knees, ankles, feet, and toes. Synovial thickening is characteristic of RA.

Synovial thickening may occur in a tendon sheath to produce the sausage-shaped digit. Examples of conditions causing this include Reiter's syndrome and psoriatic arthritis.

Effusions collecting in the joint space distend the capsule. Fluid may appear more prominently on one side of the joint than the other, so that pressure applied over the fluid can cause the fluid to shift to the opposite side. The sensation is somewhat like that of poking a water-filled balloon. Fluid results from many causes, including excessive exercise and other trauma, rheumatoid disease, bleeding, and infections.

Examination of Joints
Cardinal signs of inflammation (heat, redness, swelling, pain, function loss) Deformity of joint Crepitus Stability of joint Muscle strength Circulation Sensory perception (position, vibratory sense)

Fluid is more commonly found in the knee than in most other joints. Ballottement of the patella often helps to demonstrate knee effusion (see Fig. 9-26). Use the left hand to grasp the thigh above the knee and compress it above the patella, applying pressure to collapse the suprapatellar bursa. While holding the leg, use the fingertips of the right hand to gently touch the patella. Then give the fingers a swift push, pushing the patella directly back against the femur. The sensation of the patella moving through the fluid-filled layer, striking the underlying bone, confirms the presence of fluid.

To quantitate swelling for later comparison, measure the circumference of each side. Use a bone landmark such as the tibial tuberosity. At the same distance above it bilaterally, check the circumference. Record each of the measurements (distance above tuberosity, and circumference), because it is easy to forget precisely where the knee was measured previously.

Deformity

Dislocations and fractures often result in deformities because of the distorted alignment, soft-tissue edema, and bleeding into the tissues.

Enlargement of bones in osteoarthritis may be caused by hypertrophic bone formation or spurs (see accompanying box). Typical sites of enlargement include distal and proximal interphalangeal joints, the knees, and the feet.

Periarticular swellings include ganglia, rheumatoid nodules, gouty tophi, and bursitis. *Ganglia* are typically found at the wrist. These are fluid-filled cysts that are found along joint capsules, often attached to a tendon sheath. Rheumatoid nodules are firm nodules often found on extensor surfaces or bony prominences. These have mononuclear cell infiltrates and fibrosis. *Tophi* are nodules occasionally found near joints that contain urate deposits. Typical sites include the elbow, where they may be confused with rheumatoid nodules; the achilles tendon; the extensor surface of the forearm; or the feet. *Bursitis* is inflammation of a *bursa*, a synovial fluid-filled sac located over areas subject to friction, such as where a tendon passes over a bone (knee) or a bone is near the skin (elbow).

The fingers deviate laterally at the distal interphalangeal joints in some patients with osteoarthritis (see Fig. 9-18). Lateral or ulnar deviation of the entire finger at the metacarpophalangeal joints is characteristic of RA. Nodules appear on the dorsum of the fingers above the distal interphalangeal joints in osteoarthritis (Heberden's nodes). Swan neck and boutonniere deformities of the fingers are characteristic of RA.

Erythema and Warmth

Usually erythema and warmth of the skin may be found over an inflamed joint. An acute septic joint or acute rheumatic fever produces an erythematous joint. The typical color of the first metarsophalangeal joint in acute gout is a violaceous red. Distinctly red joints are infrequently found in RA.

To assess temperature, use the back of the fingers to palpate each side comparatively. Sometimes, comparing skin temperature by moving toward and away from the site in question is helpful.

Temperature changes are important in inflammation, but may be a less sensitive indicator than is tenderness. Small variations from normal in skin temperatures may be difficult to assess because of temperature variation distally down an extremity. Also temperatures depend on how the site was covered before the examination, and whether one side was lying against the other. In contrast, most normal structures are normally nontender, so mild tenderness may be easier to assess.

Tenderness

Tenderness is the subjective sensation of pain felt by the patient as the clinician applies pressure with the examining fingers. Tenderness is a less reliable indicator of inflammation than are the more objective swelling and erythema. Nonetheless, tenderness can be useful diagnostically. A septic joint or a joint with RA may be tender all around. A small, localized, tender site may be found with a torn meniscus of the knee. In "tennis elbow," the lateral epicondyle is tender.

Tender sites are analyzed as to the anatomic structures involved for diagnostic clues. A grading scale is used in an attempt to quantitate tenderness, as shown below:

Grade	Definition
0	No tenderness
1+	Patient says it is tender
2+	Patient complains of pain and winces
3+	Patient complains of pain, winces, and pulls back
4+	Patient will not allow palpation

Certain patients have an unusual amount of tenderness. For example, those with fibromyalgia have multiple trigger points which produce pain when palpated, or they may complain of pain when touched nearly anywhere (see box opposite). Patients with the "touch-me-not" reaction are psychoneurotic individuals who grab the examiner's hand even before he palpates, thus not allowing palpation. Of course, this would not receive a 4+ designation.

AUSCULTATION

Joint noises and locking include crepitus and clicking. *Crepitus* is a grating or grinding sensation felt by the patient, or a sound palpated or heard by the examiner. Destruction of articular cartilage allows bones to rub when a joint is flexed and extended. Apply the stethoscope over the joint to hear fine or coarse crepitus. Abnormal rubbing of tendons may also produce crepitus.

> **Criteria for Diagnosis of Fibromyalgia**
>
> 1. History of widespread pain.
>   Definition—all of the following should be present: pain on the left and right sides of the body and above and below the waist. Skeletal pain involving cervical spine, anterior chest, thoracic spine, or low back must be present.
> 2. Pain is present on palpation of 11 of 18 points.
>   Definition—Pain is produced by palpation, must be present in 11 of the following 18 sites (each side of the body counts as 1):
>   Occiput: at the suboccipital muscle insertions
>   Low cervical: at the anterior aspects of the intertransverse spaces at C5-C7
>   Trapezius: at the midpoint of the upper border
>   Supraspinatus: at origins, above the scapula spine, near the medial border
>   Second rib: at the second costochondral junctions, just lateral to the junctions on upper surfaces
>   Lateral epicondyle: 2 cm distal to the epicondyles
>   Gluteal: in upper outer quadrants of buttocks in anterior fold of muscle
>   Greater trochanter: posterior to the trochanteric prominence
>   Knee: at the medial fat pad proximal to the joint line
>   Palpation should be performed with a force of about 4 kg by the palpating fingers. For a tender point to be considered "positive," the subject must state that the palpation was painful. "Tender" is not to be considered "painful."

Adapted from Wolfe F, et al: Criteria for the classification of fibromyalgia, Arthr Rheum 33(2): 160-172, 1990.

Joints of most people make an occasional *crackling* or *snapping* sound that does not necessarily indicate a joint pathologic condition. Joint clicking repeatedly can indicate joint abnormality. *Clicking* may be caused by a damaged meniscus of the knee or an abnormality of the temporomandibular joint (TMJ). A loose foreign body may be present in such a joint. At times, such a foreign body may cause locking, preventing flexion or extension of the joint.

MUSCLE STRENGTH

Muscle strength may be decreased because of muscle disease, nerve diseases, other systemic disease, or when bone or joint abnormalities are present. Weakness may be caused by disuse, muscle atrophy, or pain associated with movement. Atrophy occurs with disuse in bone, joint, and neuromuscular diseases, with an attendant decrease in muscle mass circumference, mass, and strength.

Muscle strength or power is compared by having the patient move against resistance exerted by the examiner. Muscle strength is graded according to the following:

Grade	Definition
5	Normal muscle strength
4	Strength to move against gravity and added resistance
3	Strength to move against gravity without additional resistance
2	Muscle contracts but strength is insufficient to move against gravity (can move side-to-side)
1	Muscle contracts with little or no movement
0	No muscle contraction

The most comfortable position for an inflamed or injured joint is usually slightly flexed.

RANGE OF MOTION

The range of motion shows how far the patient can comfortably move a joint himself *(active range)* and how far the examiner can move it *(passive range)*. These results are compared with normal ranges. To perform this part of the examination, have the patient undress enough to observe joint range but remain discreetly covered for modesty.

Not every patient needs to have range of motion checked routinely on every joint. Check range of motion in patients who have symptoms such as those which:

- Suggest a specific joint abnormality. ("My knee hurts." Check both knees).
- Suggest joint manifestations of a systemic disease that might involve joints. ("I have psoriasis." Check the distal interphalangeal joints.)
- Indicate a pattern of disease that typically involves certain joint groups beside the joints the patient has mentioned. ("I have the gout in my toe." Check also joints such as the knees, ankles, and elbow.)

The range of motion is occasionally estimated as the number of degrees of flexion or extension. However, because estimates of degrees are imprecise, use of the goniometer is preferred. The *goniometer* is a device use to measure the angles at joints. It consists of two arms attached at one end to a protractor. Place the point of attachment over the joint and open the arms of the goniometer to correspond with the joint range. Read the degrees of movement from the protractor (Fig. 9-2).

The normal range of motion for joints commonly evaluated is shown in Fig. 9-3. When the range of motion is abnormal, special attention is given to that joint in evaluating stability of the joint and its extension, flexion, adduction, abduction, and internal and external rotation. Occasionally an examiner can move a joint over a greater range passively than the patient can actively. Pain on active motion but no pain on passive motion excludes several abnormalities. Palpate painful sites to delineate tender anatomic structures.

Loss of normal range has many causes. A joint may be dislocated, a joint capsule fibrosed and contracted, an effusion present, or synovium thickened. A loose foreign body in the joint; tendons inflamed, shortened, or ruptured; a fracture; or a muscle spasm may cause limitation of motion.

In arthritis, joint restriction is typically evident in all directions. Mechanical

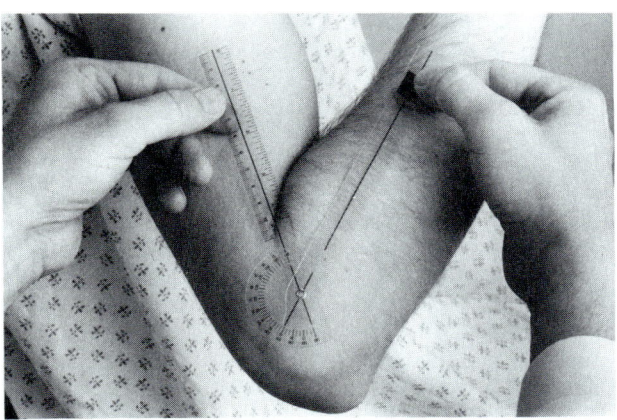

Fig. 9-2 Use of a goniometer to measure range of motion.

A.1

Shoulder

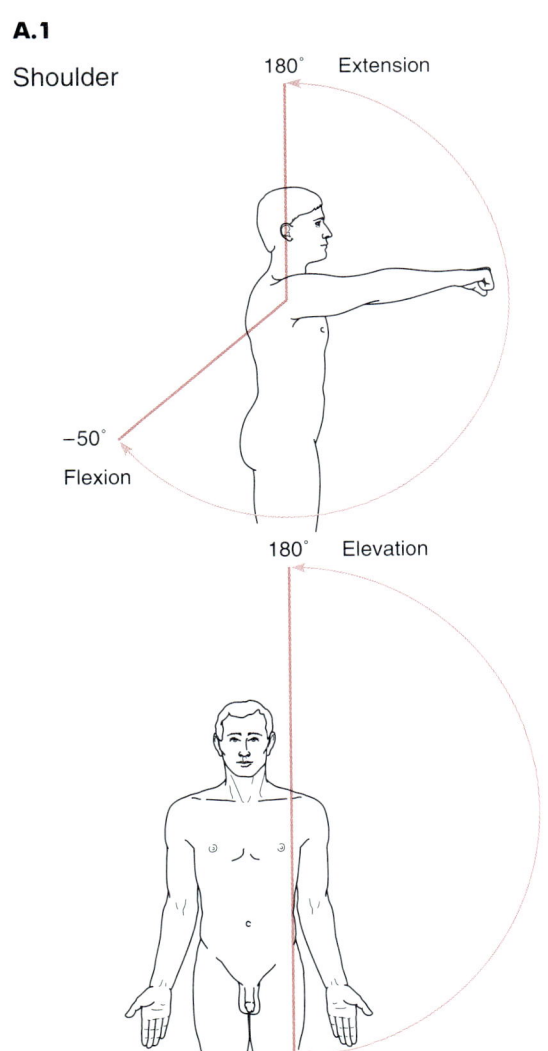

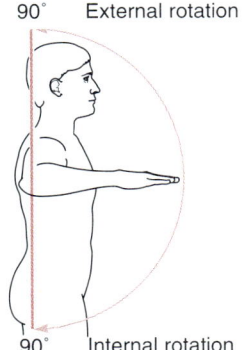

Fig. 9-3 Range of motion of selected joints. **A**, Upper limb.

Continued.

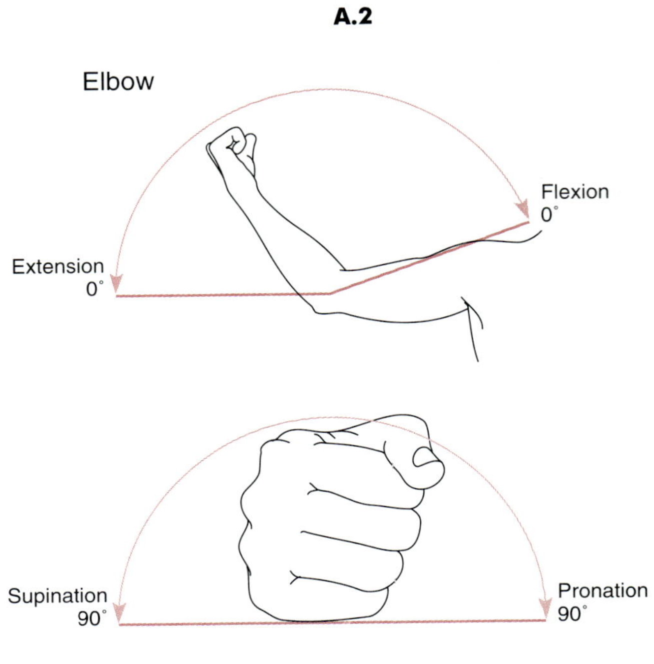

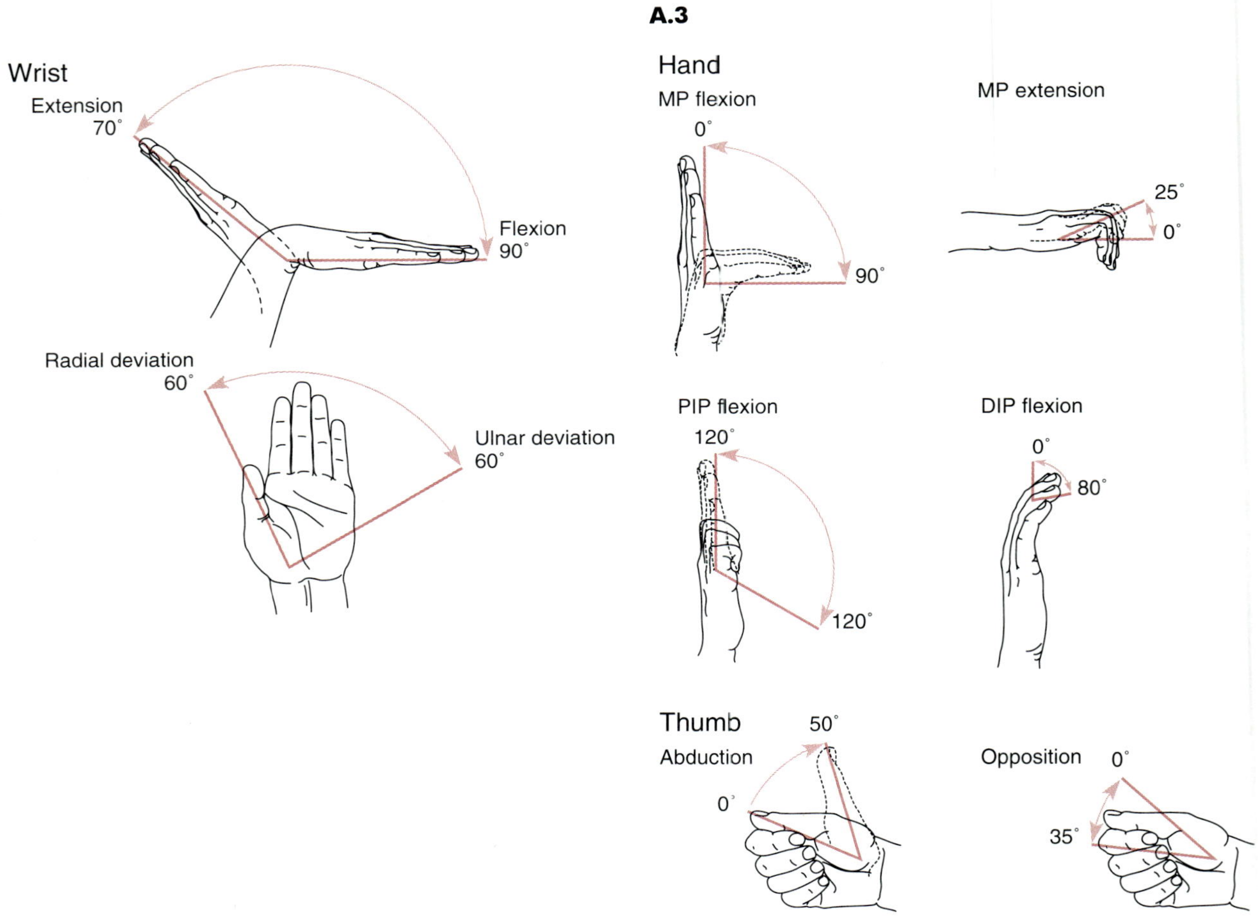

354 History Taking and Physical Examination

Fig. 9-3, cont'd Range of motion of selected joints. **A,** Upper limb.

A.2

Elbow
- Flexion 0°
- Extension 0°
- Supination 90°
- Pronation 90°

A.3

Hand
- MP flexion 0° / 90°
- MP extension 25° / 0°
- PIP flexion 120° / 120°
- DIP flexion 0° / 80°

Wrist
- Extension 70°
- Flexion 90°
- Radial deviation 60°
- Ulnar deviation 60°

Thumb
- Abduction 0° / 50°
- Opposition 0° / 35°

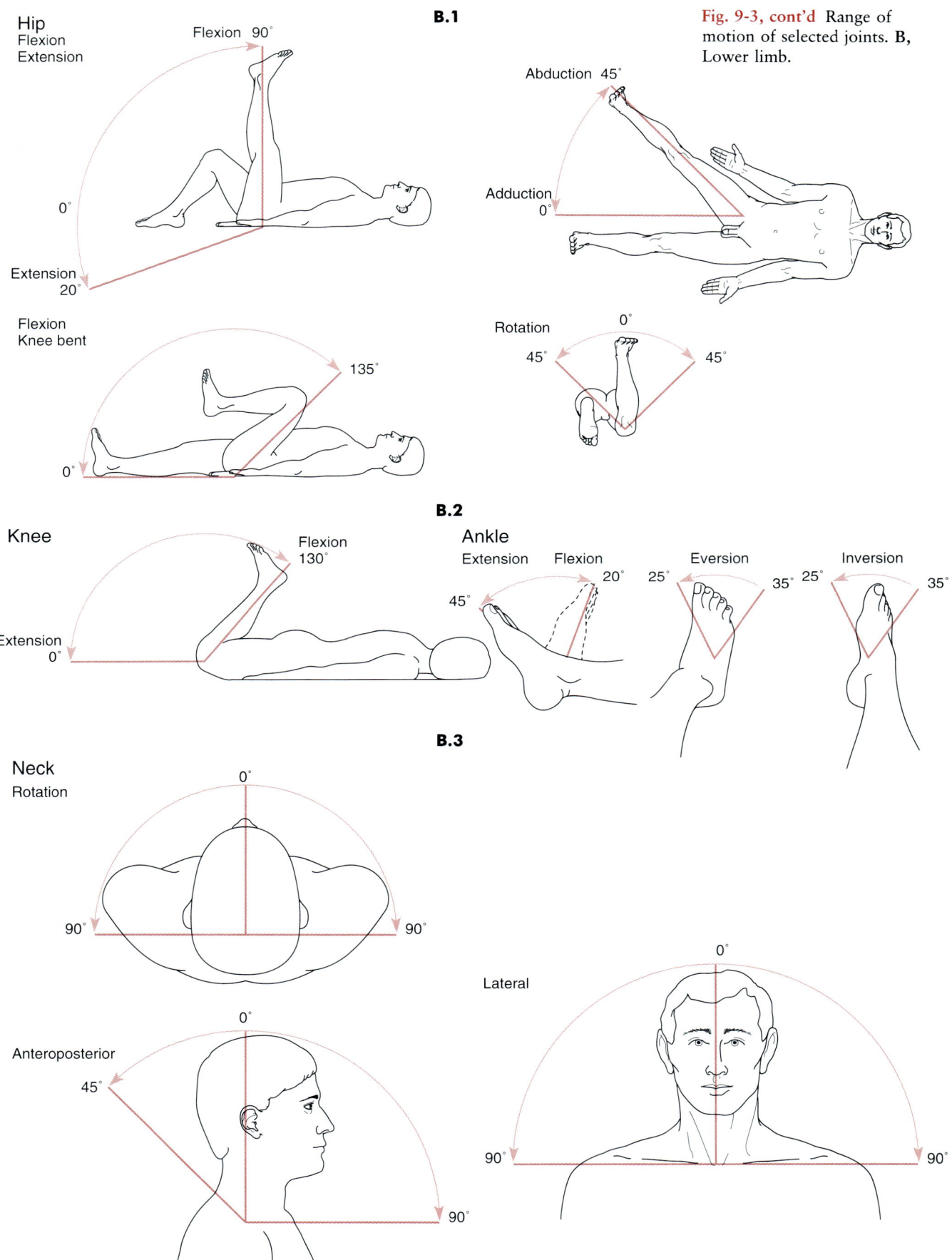

Fig. 9-3, cont'd Range of motion of selected joints. B, Lower limb.

problems limit joint motion in a single direction. Passive range of motion exceeds active range when muscles responsible for motion are paralyzed or when tendons are torn.

Alternatively, some joints may develop excessive joint motion. The unstable knee of osteoarthritis may be hypermobile, with excessive motion either in extension or laterally.

OVERALL FUNCTION

After testing muscle strength in individual muscle groups, overall function is observed. Although this part of the examination is similar to that performed during the neurologic examination, the examiner performing the musculoskeletal analysis checks for functional disabilities in activities of daily living. Observe the patient buttoning his shirt, tying shoes, combing hair, walking, standing on tiptoes, and standing after having been squatting or climbing stairs. Functional impairment may be quite severe in certain diseases, especially RA.

Regional Approach to the Examination

We begin the description of the musculoskeletal examination at the head and proceed down, although others begin with the hands.

THE HEAD

Begin with the TMJ just in front of the external auditory canal, below the zygomatic arch (Fig. 9-4). Use the fingers to palpate over the joint for tenderness or swelling. Ask the patient to open his mouth so that the examining finger drops into the joint space (Fig. 9-5). Then insert the examining fingers into the external auditory canal while you palpate the joint space anteriorly. Observe the range of jaw motion, joint tenderness, clicking, or locking of the jaw. Normally, the front teeth can be opened two or three finger-breadths wide.

Examples of TMJ Abnormalities

TMJ abnormalities may be caused by dental malocclusion, trauma to the jaw, or RA.

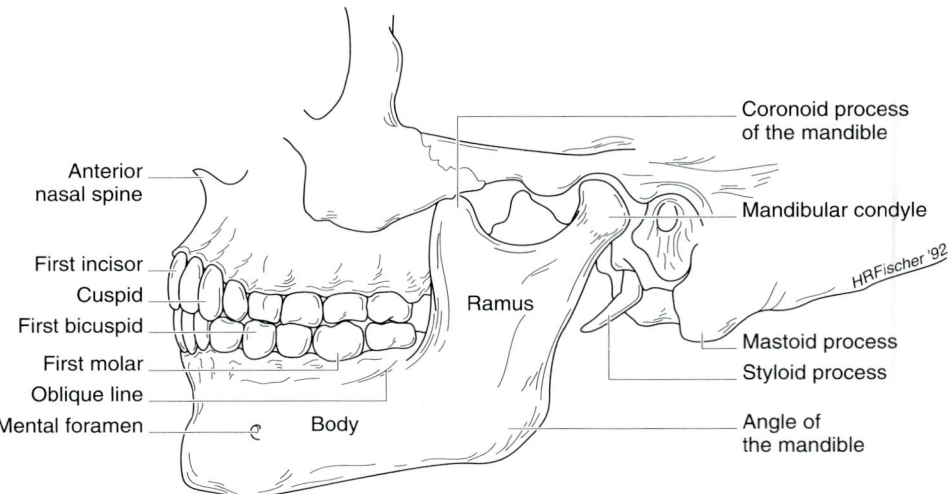

Fig. 9-4 Anatomy of the TMJ and jaw.

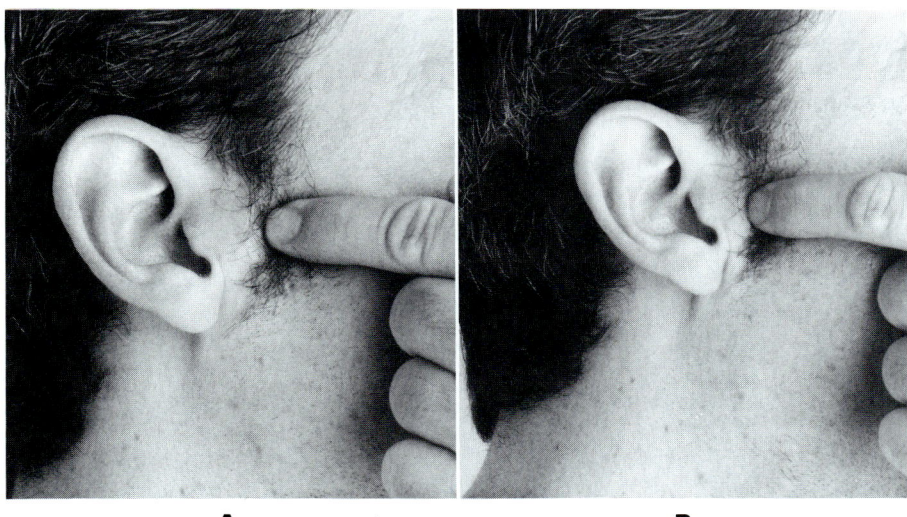

Fig. 9-5 Palpation of the TMJ. **A,** Jaw closed. **B,** Jaw open.

THE CERVICAL SPINE

Next check the cervical spine. The cervical spine should have a slight lordosis when the patient sits at rest. Assess neck flexion by asking the patient to bend the neck and touch the chin to the chest. Assess neck rotation by asking him to touch the chin to each shoulder. Next have the patient touch each shoulder with the respective ear to assess lateral flexion. Finally test neck extension as the patient tilts the head as far back as possible. Normal people move the occiput to three finger-breadths from the spinous process of C7 (see Fig. 9-3).

Examples of Cervical Spine Abnormalities

Arthritis may limit rotation or lateral flexion before limiting flexion and extension. When cervical flexion becomes acutely painful in any patient without joint disease, consider meningeal irritation caused by meningitis, cervical fracture, or dislocation. Palpate the base of the neck for the painful trigger points of fibromyalgia.

THE SHOULDER

Next examine the shoulder. Movement occurs at several joints in the shoulder (Fig. 9-6), including the acromioclavicular (AC) joint, the glenohumeral (GH) joint, and the sternoclavicular (SC) joint.

Inspect the shoulders for symmetry, deformities, or atrophy. Don't forget to inspect the scapulas posteriorly for symmetry and movement. Apply pressure over the joints for tenderness and palpate for deformity of the AC and SC joints. Palpate along the bicipital groove for tenderness (Fig. 9-7). Ask the patient to move the shoulder through a complete range of motion (see Fig. 9-3). If restriction is evident, actively move the shoulder by holding the patient's wrist or elbow.

Test for muscle strength and function of the shoulder by asking the patient to lift his arms in front of and out from his body while you hold them against his chest. Then ask him to lift both hands over his head with the elbows straight and place palms together (external rotation), and then to lower his hands palms down

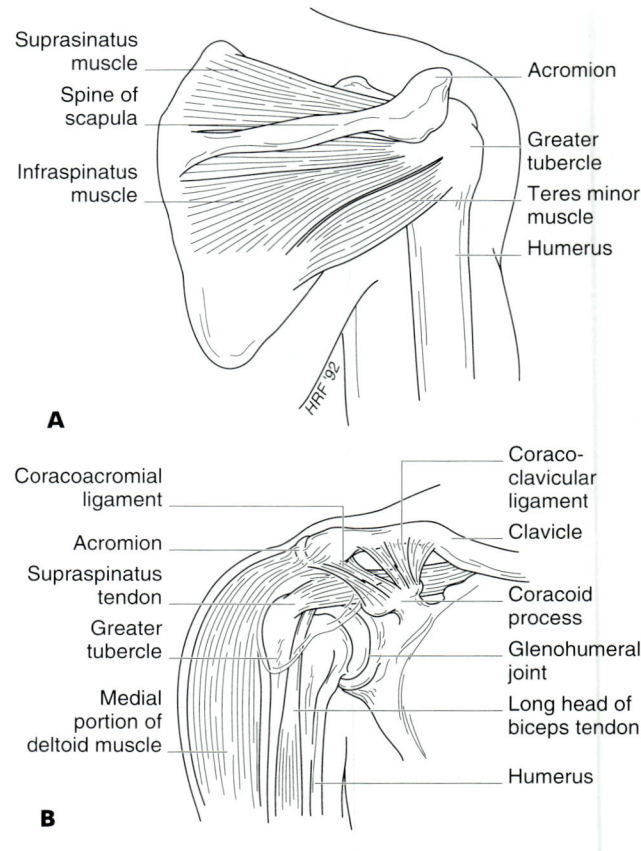

Fig. 9-6 Anatomy of the shoulder. **A,** Muscle attachments. **B,** Bones, ligaments, and tendons.

on his upper back with the elbows held up alongside the head (internal rotation). Finally, have him hold each arm straight out at the side and lift above his head.

Examples of Shoulder Abnormalities

Important causes of a painful shoulder that should not be forgotten include referred pain such as that caused by coronary artery disease or diaphragmatic irritation. Musculoskeletal causes of shoulder pain include the following:

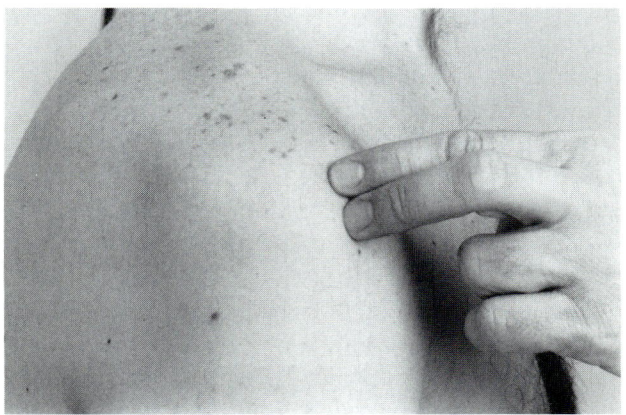

Fig. 9-7 Palpation along the bicipital groove.

- Adhesive capsulitis (frozen shoulder)
- AC arthritis
- Bicipital tendinitis
- Acute bursitis
- Calcific tendinitis
- Rotator cuff tendinitis (impingement syndrome)
- Rotator cuff tears (Table 9-8)

To understand shoulder disorders, some review of the complex anatomy of the rotator cuff is required. The rotator cuff has four muscles that hold the humerus in the glenoid cavity at the GH joint and stabilize the shoulder. The tendons of these four muscles are fused to the capsule of the joint (see Fig. 9-6).

When the humerus is abducted, the tendon of the supraspinatus muscle is exposed to friction midway by the acromial process. Normally the subacromial bursa protects it. Degenerative changes in the bursa allow damage of the supraspinatus tendon. This may extend to the other three tendons of the rotator cuff. Pain and spasm begin near the midrange of abduction.

The tendon may rupture or may calcify, giving similar types of symptoms.

Adhesive capsulitis is referred to as a frozen shoulder. A diffuse, dull, aching pain occurs unilaterally. Fibrosis of the GH capsule increases, and range of motion decreases. On examination, tenderness is diffuse rather than at one point. Later, pain decreases but movement remains restricted.

AC degenerative arthritis may result from trauma. Movement is painful when

TABLE 9-8: Symptom: Painful Shoulder Joint

	History	Range of Motion	Pain	Examination Technique
Adhesive capsulitis	Generalized dull shoulder pain	All movements decreased; frozen shoulder	Tender around GH joint but no point tenderness	Decreased range of motion
Acromioclavicular arthritis (AC joint)	Initially injured, later degeneration	Normal so long as scapula not moved	Tender over acromioclavicular joints; scapular movements tender	Scapular movements tender, but GH movement is not
Bicipital tendinitis (tendon of long head of biceps)	Pain as arm is elevated laterally	Unable to abduct humerus above horizontal	Tender over tendon in bicipital groove	Pain in bicipital groove area when patient tries to supinate forearm against resistance
Calcific tendinitis (calcification in supraspinatus tendon)	Arm held at side	Usually painful		Calcification on radiograph in supraspinatus tendon
Rotator cuff tendinitis (supraspinatus tendon)	Sports injury or trauma	Restricted	Pain when attempting to reach overhead	Resisting forced abduction increases pain
Rotator cuff tears (supraspinatus tendon)	Trauma, falls	Normal with external rotation of humerus	Tender over greater tuberosity of humerus	Abduct the humerus; patient lifts shoulder to prevent GH joint movement

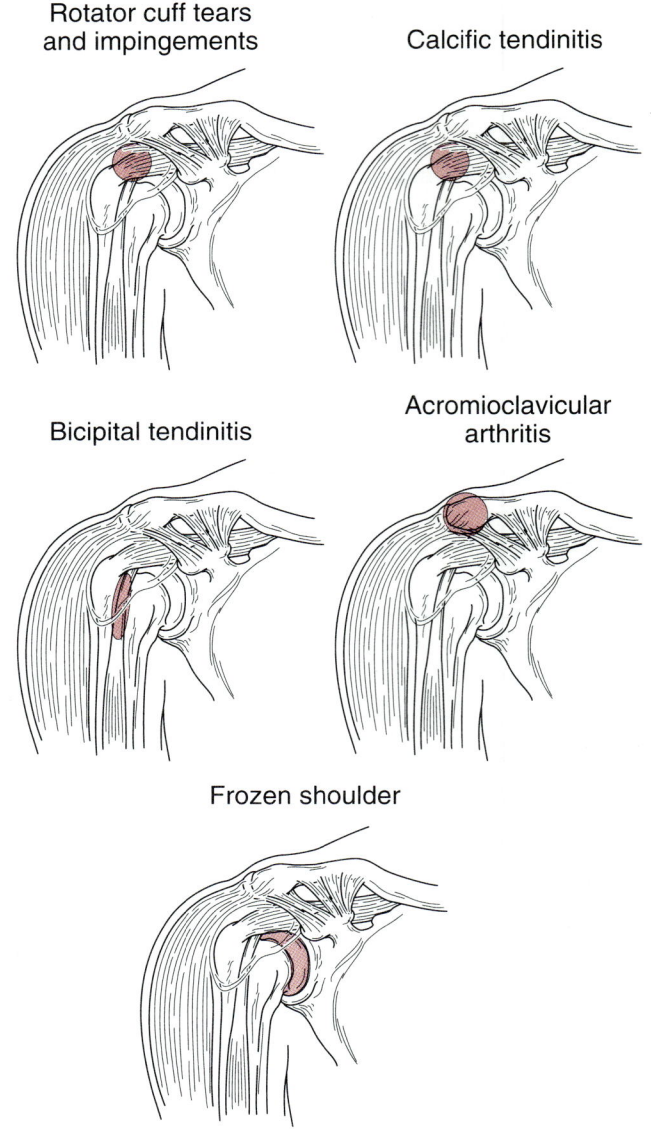

Fig. 9-8 Abnormalities of the shoulder: rotator cuff tears and impingement, calcific tendonitis, bicipital tendonitis, acromioclavicular arthritis, frozen shoulder.

the scapula is moved (at the AC joint). Point tenderness is present over the AC joint.

Bicipital tendinitis is inflammation of the biceps tendon along the bicipital groove of the humerus. Palpation over the tendon in the bicipital groove shows tenderness. With the patient's elbow flexed to 90 degrees and at the side, ask him to supinate the hand and forearm while you hold it still. This increases pain along the bicipital groove.

Rotator cuff tendinitis, or *impingement syndrome,* is caused by inflammation of the tendon of the supraspinatus muscle (Fig. 9-8). Later, other muscles and tendons of the rotator cuff may become involved. As the arm is raised, the rotator cuff impinges against the underside of the AC ligament and is painful.

Calcific tendinitis refers to prolonged supraspinatus tendon inflammation with resulting calcification. Both calcific tendinitis and rotator cuff tendinitis usually involve the supraspinatus tendon.

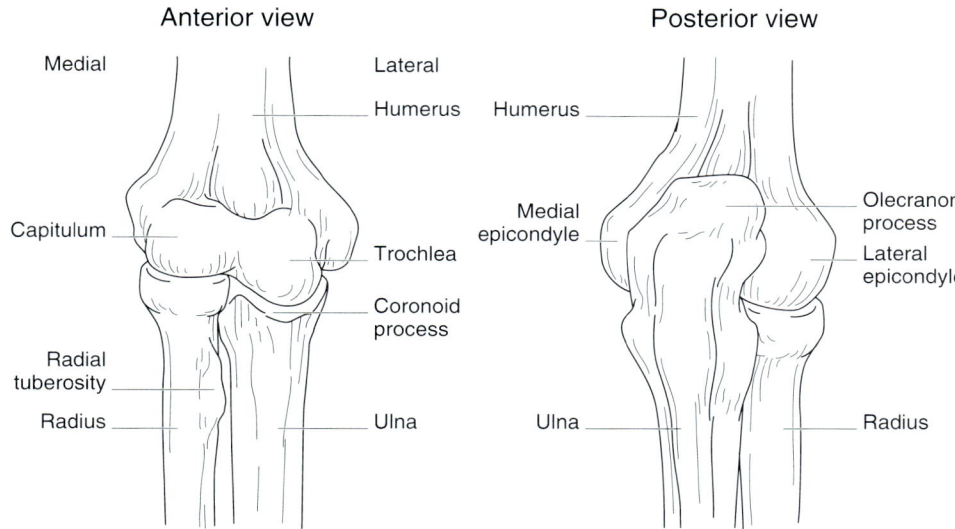

Fig. 9-9 Anatomy of the elbow.

Rotator cuff tears result in limitation of abduction so that the arm extended out to the side cannot be elevated beyond about 90 degrees, the extent to which the deltoid muscle can abduct. As disuse continues, muscles atrophy.

THE ELBOW

The elbow is a complicated joint because of its anatomic structures and functions. At the humerus, it operates with the ulna as a hinge joint, allowing flexion and extension. Because the radial head is attached to the ulna by an annular ligament and is not attached to the humerus, it is free to rotate, allowing pronation and supination of the forearm (Fig. 9-9; see also Figs. 9-1 and 9-3).

Muscle strength of each of these functions is assessed by asking the patient to move against resistance.

Inspection and palpation of the elbow proceeds with the medial and lateral epicondyles of the humerus (Fig. 9-10). A tender and inflamed lateral epicondyle caused by repeated pulling of the extensor muscles of the forearm on the lateral epicondyle occurs in *tennis elbow.*

Ask the patient to extend the elbow while you hold it firm. This dramatically increases the pain at the epicondyle. Ask the patient to lift a heavy object with the

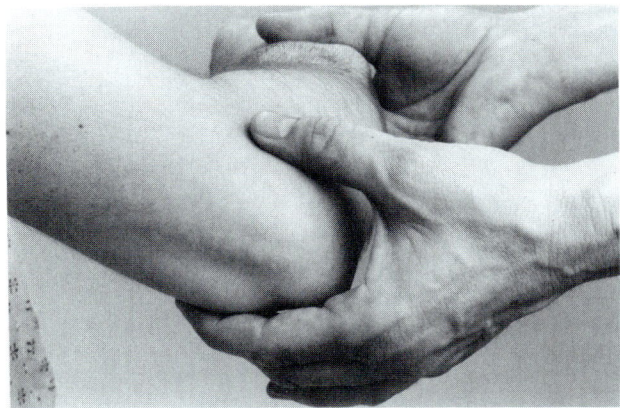

Fig. 9-10 Palpation of the elbow, medial and lateral epicondyles.

Fig. 9-11 Abnormalities of the elbow: epicondylitis and olecranon bursitis.

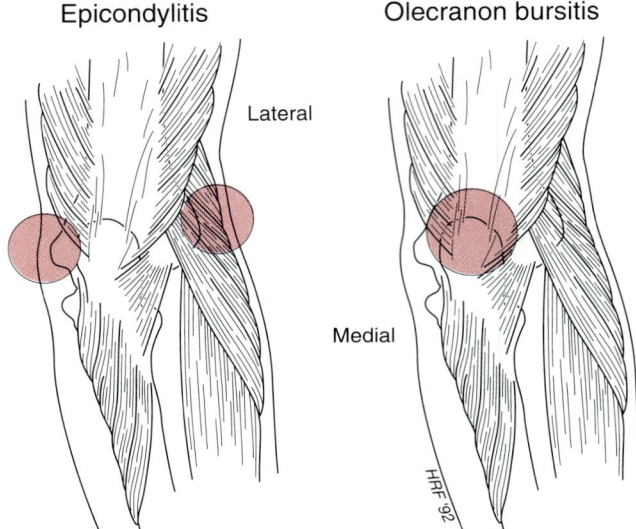

palm downward. This also increases pain. With the palm up, pain is not so severe. *Golf elbow* caused by medial epicondylitis typically shows pain when lifting with the palm up.

The olecranon bursa is located over the olecranon. Palpate for swelling, tenderness, or effusion. The elbow joint space is palpated in the antecubital fossa and between the epicondyles and olecranon for synovial thickening, effusion, and tenderness.

Examples of Elbow Abnormalities

One example of an abnormality at the elbows is olecranon bursitis (Fig. 9-11). Also, either rheumatoid nodules or gouty tophi may overlay the extensor surface of the ulna.

THE WRIST

Its large number of joints gives the wrist the potential for numerous disorders (Fig. 9-12).

Ask the patient to flex and extend the wrist and to move it medially and laterally while the forearm is held stable (see Fig. 9-3). Palpate each of the small joints in the wrist by placing your fingers under the wrist and thumb on top of the wrist joints (Fig. 9-13). Look for thickened synovium, joint effusions, and tenderness. Also palpate the extensor and flexor tendons, and look for ganglions.

Examples of Wrist Abnormalities

DeQuervain's tenosynovitis involves the extensor tendon of the thumb. Pain occurs near the junction of the lower third and middle third of the forearm; this is where the tendon crosses over the radius. To reproduce pain, ask the patient to apply pressure with the thumb against the forefinger (Fig. 9-14). Palpation shows tenderness over the tendon.

A *ganglion* is a cyst caused by herniated synovium into soft tissues. It is filled with synovial fluid but is a closed sac separate from the original joint space. It does not move with tendons.

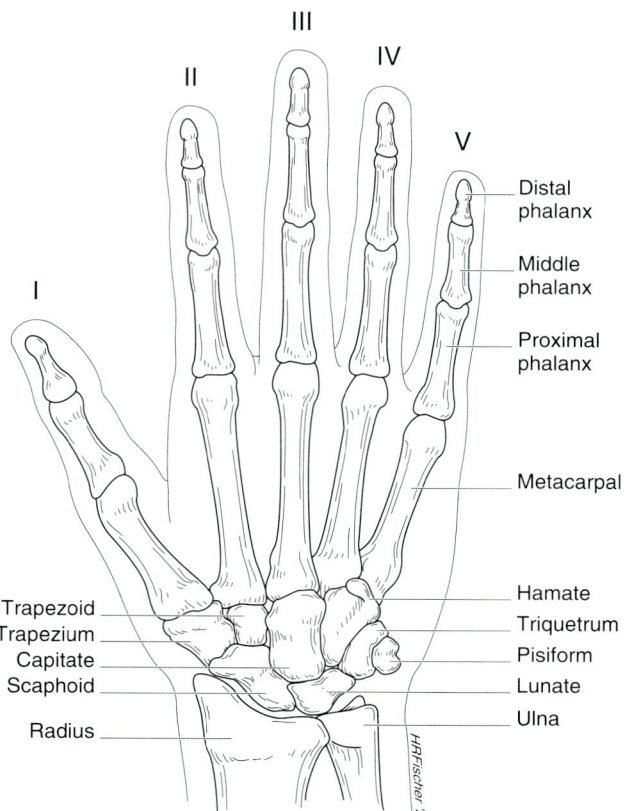

Fig. 9-12 Anatomy of the hand and wrist.

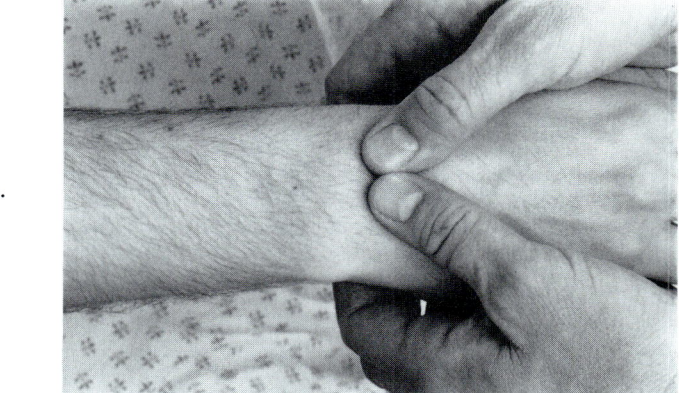

Fig. 9-13 Palpation of the wrist.

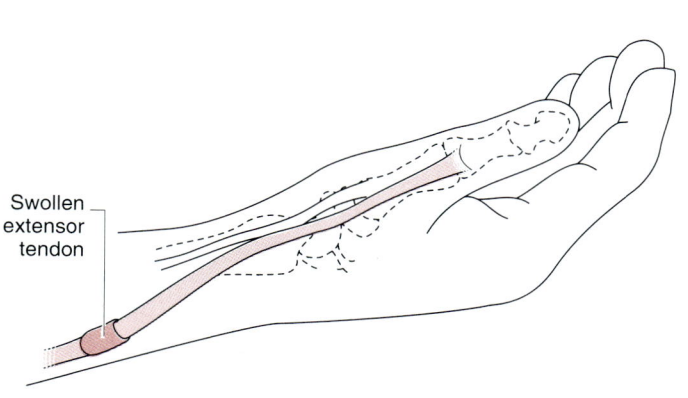

Fig. 9-14 Abnormalities of the wrist: DeQuervain's tendinitis and ganglion.

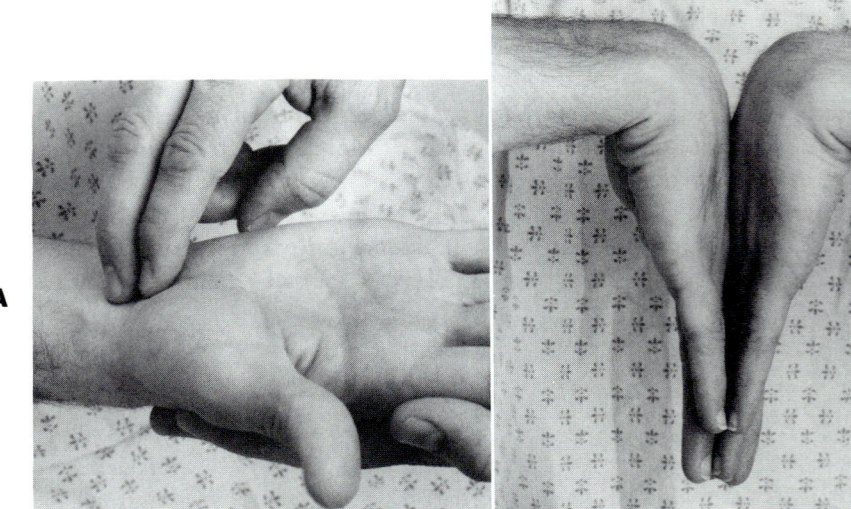

Fig. 9-15 Tests for carpal tunnel syndrome. **A,** Tinel's sign. **B,** Phalen's test.

Carpal tunnel syndrome is caused by compression of the median nerve by the carpal ligament. Patients complain of numbness and tingling. Pain or paresthesias may be felt in the fingers. Two physical examination signs are linked with this diagnosis: Phalen's test and Tinel's sign (Fig. 9-15). *Phalen's test* is performed by asking the patient to flex each wrist in a 90-degree angle for 1 minute. A positive test occurs if the patient develops numbness and tingling over the distribution of the median nerve: the thumb, forefinger, middle finger, and part of the ring finger. *Tinel's sign* consists of tingling shots of pain in the distribution of the median nerve when the nerve is lightly percussed at the wrist.

THE HAND AND FINGERS

Inspect and palpate the hands and fingers. Ask the patient to flex and extend each (see Fig. 9-3) and to make a tight fist. Do the fingertips tuck into the palm with no space between?

Evaluate grip strength by placing your forefinger in the patient's palm and asking him to squeeze tightly. If two fingers are used, some patients squeeze so tightly as to make this painful for the examiner. The grip strength is recorded as normal or weak.

Next, ask the patient to pinch a piece of paper with a thumb and forefinger while you tug. Abnormal pinch ability may be caused by either weakness or limited motion.

The metacarpophalangeal (MCP) joints are positioned 1 cm distal to the knuckles (see Fig. 9-12). Press these together as a unit. If these are tender, palpate each joint individually, medially and laterally, for synovial hypertrophy, effusion, and tenderness (Fig. 9-16).

Joint swelling of MCPs may be identified visually. Ask the patient to clench the fist. Examine the grooves between the MCP joints. Loss of grooves occurs with small amounts of swelling.

In the finger exam, assess each proximal interphalangeal (PIP) and distal interphalangeal (DIP) joint individually (Fig. 9-17). Examine each for swelling,

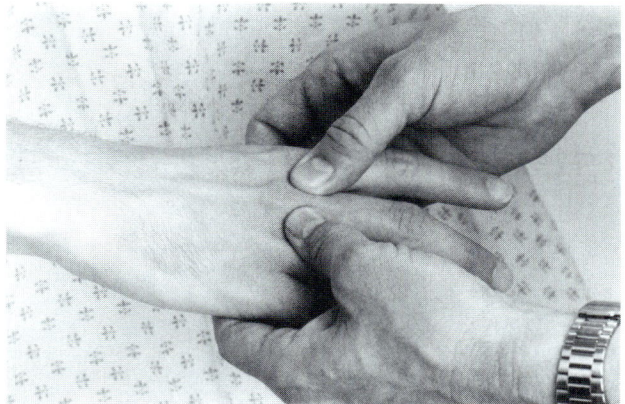

Fig. 9-16 Palpation of the metacarpophalangeal joint.

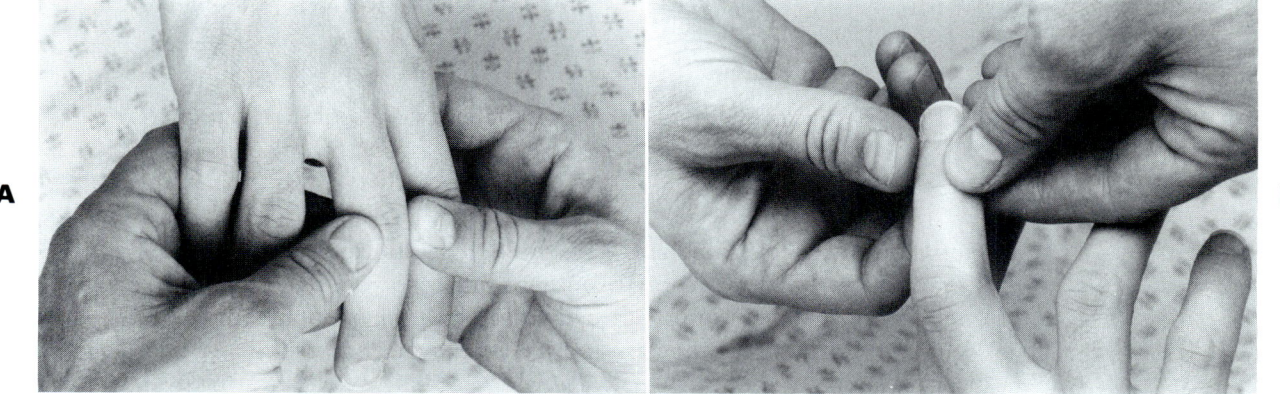

Fig. 9-17 Palpation of the interphalangeal joints. **A,** PIP. **B,** DIP.

tenderness, range of motion, and deformity. These joints are palpated using the thumb and finger on the lateral and medial sides of the joint. Swelling of the PIP joints, *Bouchard's nodes,* may be less common than is DIP swelling.

Examine the DIPs and PIPs individually. Swelling of these joints may show loss of skin wrinkles on the dorsum. A digit may take on a fusiform or sausage shape. A slight flexion contracture occurs in some elderly people who keep the hand closed while performing tasks.

Examples of Hand and Finger Abnormalities

Limited range of MCP motion reduces strength and fist formation. The fingers begin to deviate toward the ulnar side of the hand at the MCP joint in RA (Fig. 9-18). This is called the ulnar drift of the fingers, or *ulnar deviation.* Ulnar deviation is not specific for RA, however.

Examine the palm of the hand for related abnormalities, including loss of muscle mass of the thenar and hypothenar eminences. *Dupuytren's contractures* are fibrous bands stretched across the palm lengthwise from the base of the fingers toward the wrist (see Fig. 9-18). These may be found in rheumatoid disease or alcoholism, or they may be familial.

Heberden's nodes are bony overgrowths on the dorsum of the DIP joints typical of osteoarthritis (see Fig. 9-18). They occur more often in women than in men and, in women, often begin shortly after menopause.

Fig. 9-18 Abnormalities of the fingers: ulnar deviation, Dupuytrens's contractures, Heberden's nodes, boutonniere deformity, swan neck deformity.

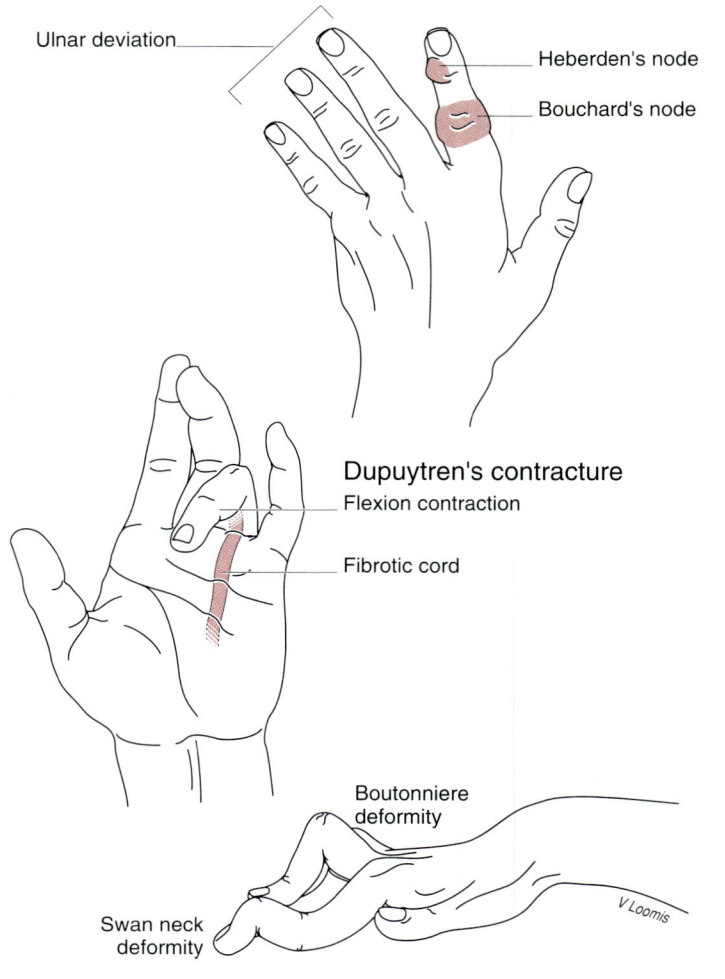

The DIP joints may be inflamed unilaterally in *psoriatic arthritis*. (A clue for the diagnosis may be found by checking the fingernails for tiny pits). Symmetric DIP arthritis is characteristic of RA.

The *boutonniere (button hole) deformity* is a flexion contracture of the PIP joint with a hyperextension at the DIP joint of the same finger (as if one is forcing a button through a buttonhole) (see Fig. 9-18). A single boutonniere deformity may be caused by trauma; multiple deformities are usually caused by RA.

The *swan neck deformity* (see Fig. 9-18) consists of hyperextended PIP joints and flexed DIP joints, just the opposite of the boutonniere deformity. These deformities may accompany RA.

THE SPINE

The examination of the spine and sacroiliac (SI) joints follows (Fig. 9-19). For parts of this exam, the patient will be standing.

Examine the thoracic spine with the patient standing. Ask the patient to bend to each side laterally and to rotate right and left (see Fig. 9-3). The normal thoracic spine has a slight kyphosis.

Ask the patient to bend forward. Compare the paravertebral muscle mass on each side. In *scoliosis,* the muscles are more prominent on one side than on the other (see Fig. 9-21).

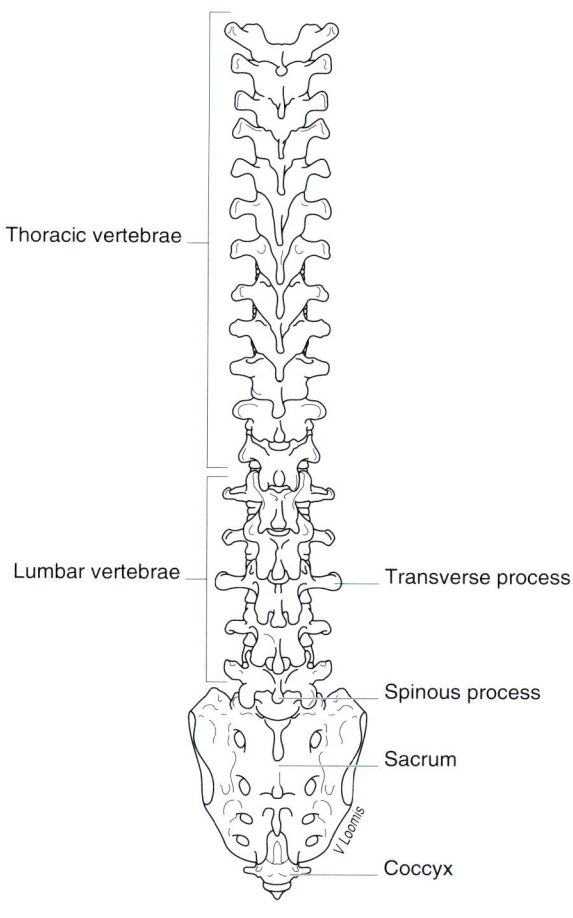

Fig. 9-19 Anatomy of the spine.

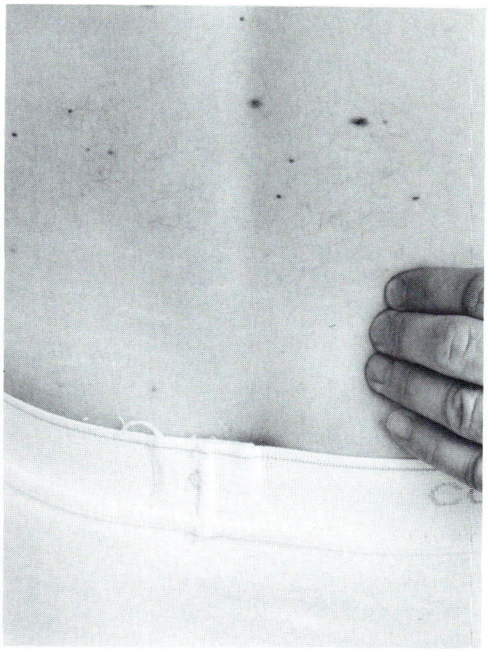

Fig. 9-20 Palpation of the sacroiliac joint.

The lumbar spine normally has a slight lordosis. While the patient leans forward, backward, and laterally and twists the torso in each direction, evaluate mobility and symmetry. Look for lumbar kyphosis, scoliosis, or *gibbus* (an angular deformity caused by a collapsed vertebra; see Fig. 9-20).

Palpate each spinous process from C7 down to the sacrum for tenderness. Palpate the sacroiliac joints for tenderness or swelling. As the patient bends over again, observe and palpate for mobility of the sacroiliac joints (Fig. 9-20).

Examples of Spinal Abnormalities

The straight-back syndrome lacks normal thoracic kyphosis. *Kyphosis* may be accentuated in severe osteoporosis, after vertebral body fractures, or with degenerative disc space disease. Marked kyphosis of dorsal spine (Fig. 9-21), when observed in elderly women, is known as the *Dowager's hump*.

Ankylosing spondylitis usually begins with reduced SI joint mobility and then affects the lumbar spine (Table 9-9).

Reiter's syndrome may be associated with sacroiliitis, along with a rash on the palms and soles called *keratoderma blennorrhagia*, and a penile eruption called *circinate balanitis* (circular red rash).

Lumbosacral strain is a rather common diagnosis applied to back pain. Chronic lumbosacral strain may be characterized by generalized low back discomfort.

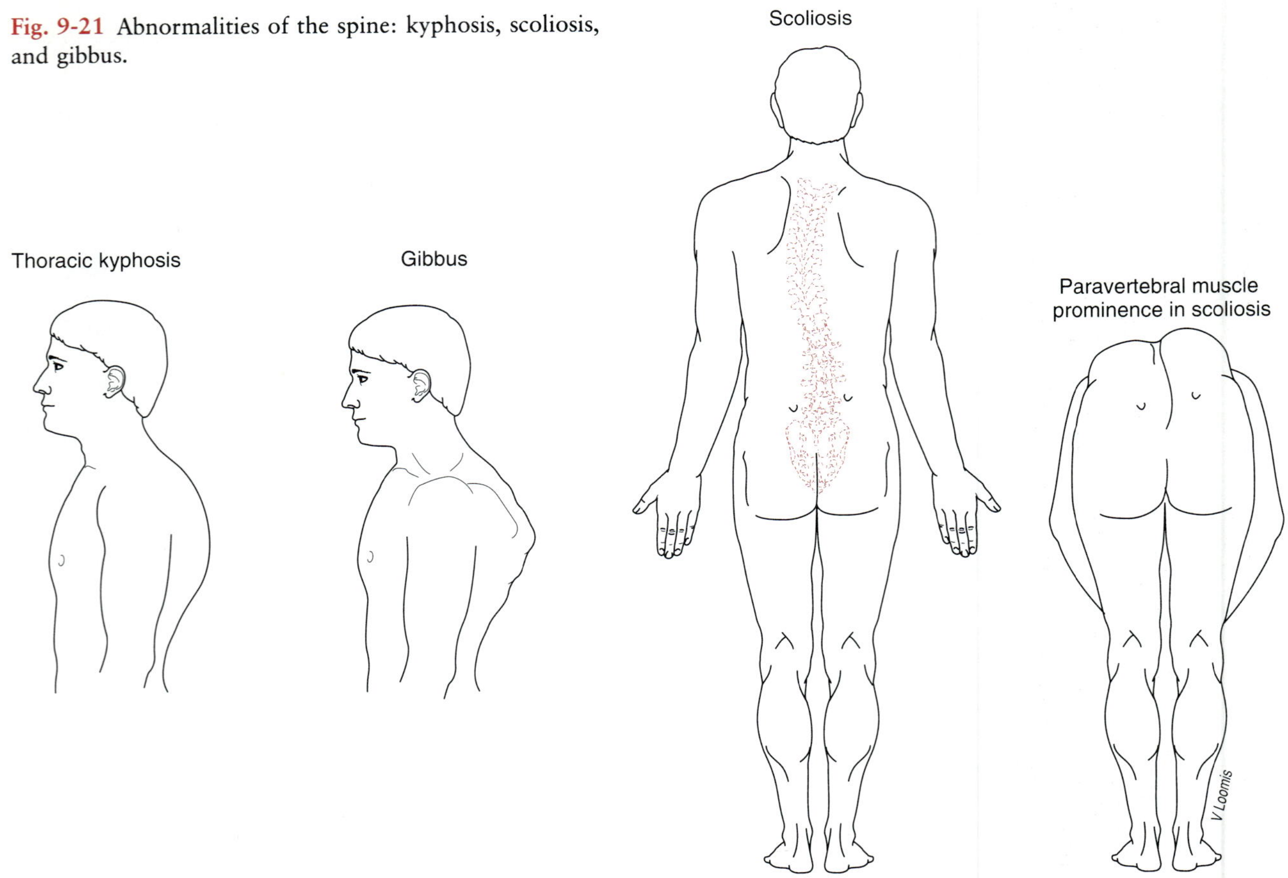

Fig. 9-21 Abnormalities of the spine: kyphosis, scoliosis, and gibbus.

Thoracic kyphosis

Gibbus

Scoliosis

Paravertebral muscle prominence in scoliosis

Fatigue is prominent, but neither fatigue nor back pain are much relieved by rest. Typically, the patient is flabby, has poor posture, and is overweight. Mild paraspinous muscle spasm may be present.

Acute lumbosacral strain usually results from back injury, especially lifting. Muscle spasm occurs, but as the patient tries to work it out, the spasm becomes incapacitating. Examination shows muscle spasm and tenderness.

Herniated nucleus pulposus, or *intervertebral disc*, is associated with pain radiating along the distribution of the irritated nerve. Changing positions may intensify the pain, as does coughing, sneezing, or straining during a bowel movement. Bed rest usually relieves it.

Sciatica, or *sciatic neuritis*, is characterized by pain radiating down the back of the leg in an L5-S1 distribution. This may be caused by a herniated nucleus pulposus. For diagnosis, use the straight leg-raising test. With the patient supine, the examiner flexes the patient's hip. Holding the thigh flexed and the leg straight, the examiner slowly dorsiflexes the ankle (Fig. 9-22). This maneuver produces pain in the thigh of the patient with sciatica.

THE HIP

Because the hip joint is deep within soft tissue and supporting structures (Fig. 9-23), it is more difficult to examine. The hip joint is examined with the patient supine and later with the patient standing.

With the patient supine, the examiner flexes the hip to 90 degrees, then rotates

TABLE 9-9: Diseases that may Cause Sacroiliac Arthritis

Disease	Clinical Features	Additional Studies
Ankylosing spondylitis	• Males • Symmetric involvement of SI joints • Uveitis • Limitation of spinal movement • Complete ankylosis	• Radiographs show SI erosion and calcified spinal ligaments • HLA-B27
Reiter's syndrome	• Males with STDs • Asymmetric SI involvement • Asymmetric involvement of other joints • Urethritis • Keratoderma blennorrhagia, iritis, spurs • Partially ankylosing	• Radiograph shows spur on heel • Skip areas of spinal involvement
Psoriatic spondylitis	• Either sex • Asymmetric SI involvement • Asymmetric arthritis • Skin and nail lesions may be present	• Radiograph • Skip areas of spinal involvement
Inflammatory bowel disease (ulcerative colitis or Crohn's disease)	• Usually symmetric SI involvement • Bowel disease may be in remission • Peripheral arthritis in some patients • Uveitis in some	• HLA-B27 occasionally present

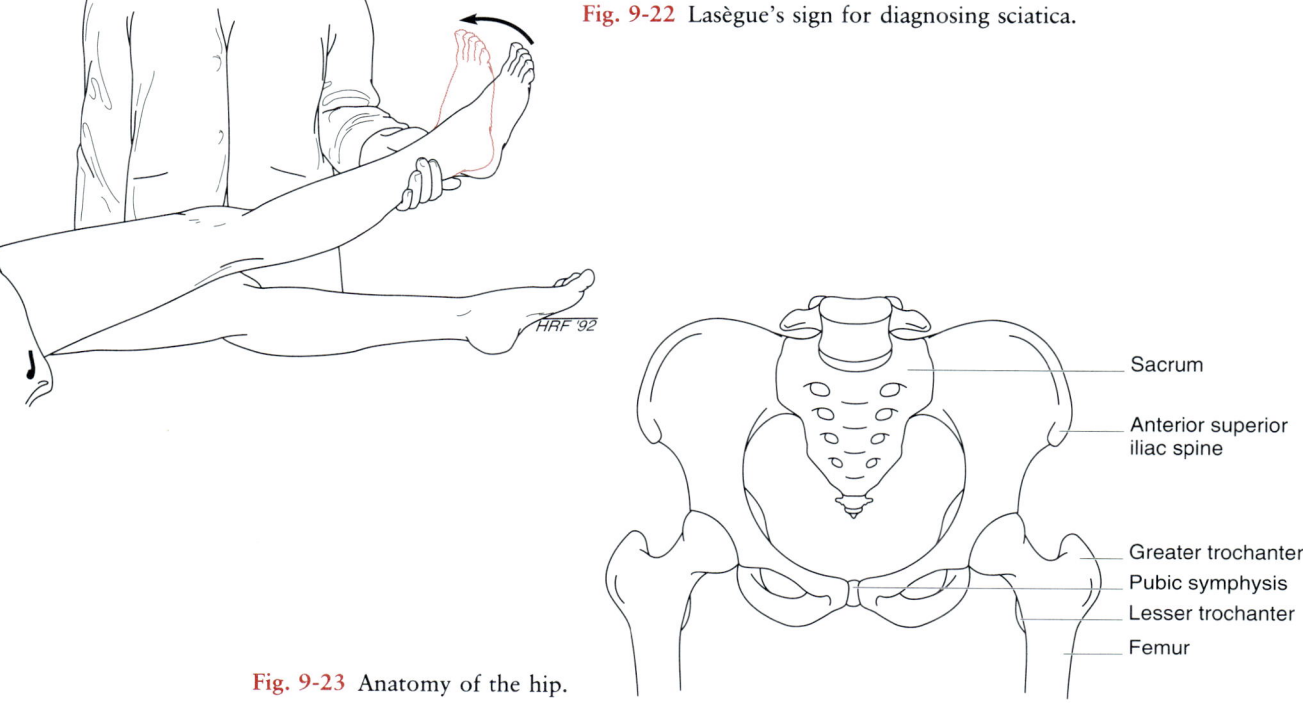

Fig. 9-22 Lasègue's sign for diagnosing sciatica.

Fig. 9-23 Anatomy of the hip.

Fig. 9-24 The Trendelenburg test. **A,** Normally, when standing on left foot, right pelvis rises. **B,** Positive Trendelenburg test indicated by right pelvis falling when standing on left foot (weak abductors).

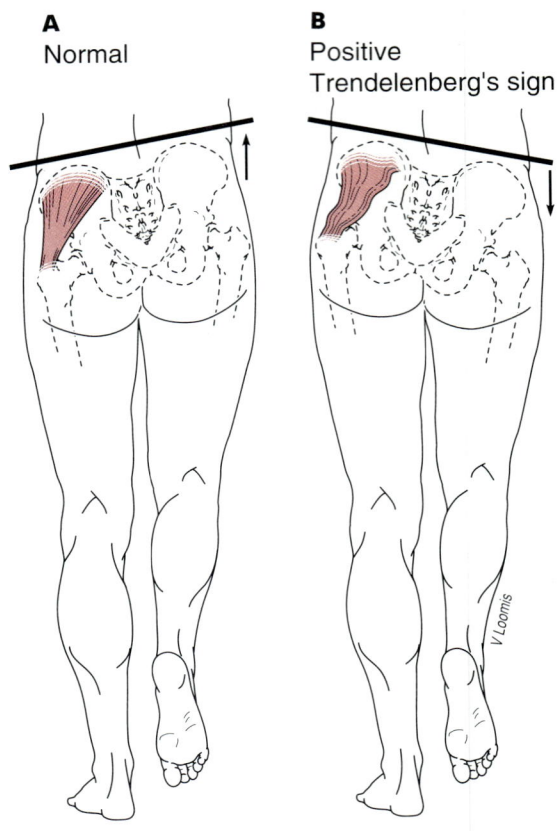

the leg internally and externally (see Fig. 9-3). This is a good test for hip joint disease. If one leg is shorter than the other as measured from the anterosuperior iliac spine to the medial malleolus and the legs are otherwise symmetric, hip disease is likely.

A test for ability of the hip muscles to function is the *Trendelenburg test* (Fig. 9-24). Ask the patient to stand on one leg and then on the other. When the patient has normal muscles, the opposite thigh and hip normally elevate because the pelvic muscles to the greater trochanter are sufficient to elevate the hip not bearing weight. However, if the gluteus medius muscle is too weak to pull the pelvis upward on the opposite side, or if the abductors are tender, the pelvis tilts downward on the side with the leg elevated. This is a positive Trendelenburg test.

With the patient lying on one side, compress the hip joint in the inguinal area from above, and then laterally. This maneuver may demonstrate trochanteric tendinitis or bursitis. Trochanteric bursitis occurs in some patients who regularly sleep on their sides.

Finally, observe the patient walking for clues to disorders. A patient may walk in such a way as to prevent pain (the *antalgic* gait). He may shift weight to the involved side to prevent muscle contraction and spasm.

Examples of Hip Abnormalities

The patient leans away from the abnormal hip in arthritis or dislocation. A waddling gait is used to shift weight from side to side when the abductor muscles are weak or when bilateral hip disease is present.

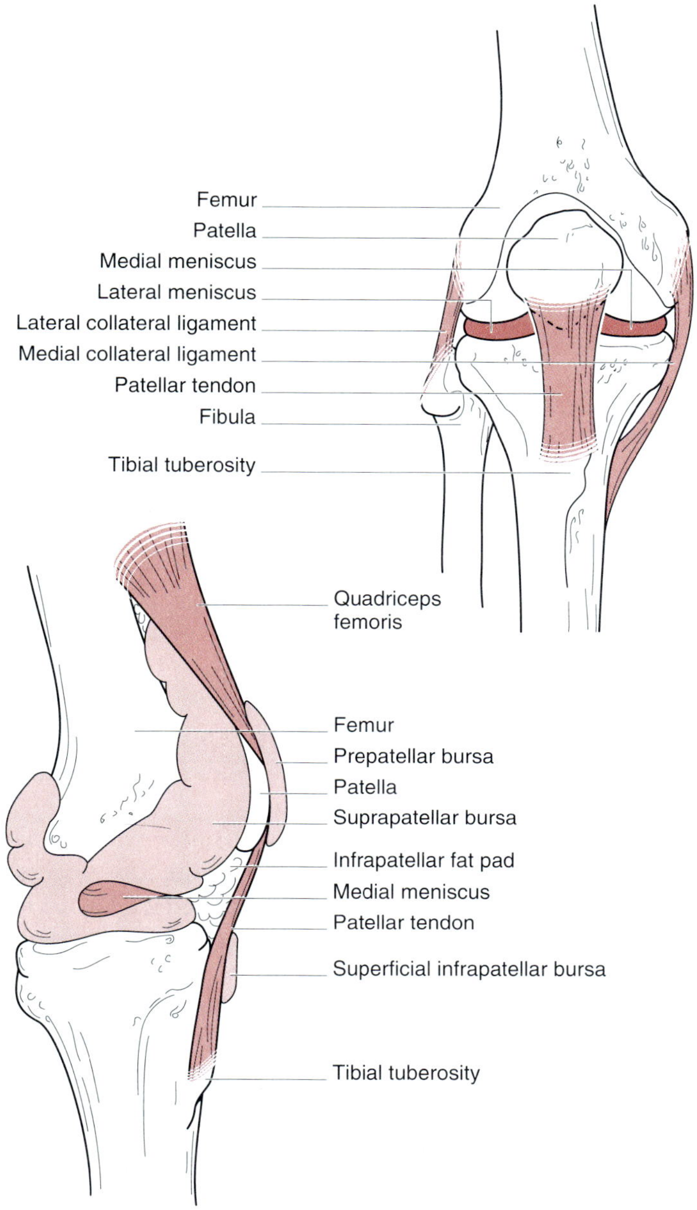

Fig. 9-25 Anatomy of the knee.

Femur
Patella
Medial meniscus
Lateral meniscus
Lateral collateral ligament
Medial collateral ligament
Patellar tendon
Fibula
Tibial tuberosity

Quadriceps femoris
Femur
Prepatellar bursa
Patella
Suprapatellar bursa
Infrapatellar fat pad
Medial meniscus
Patellar tendon
Superficial infrapatellar bursa
Tibial tuberosity

THE KNEE

Pain, usually worse when bearing weight, occurs more often in the knee than in other joints. Pain may radiate into the thigh, calf, or shin. Palpate the quadriceps, the patella, synovium, and the prepatellar bursas (Fig. 9-25). Diffuse swelling of the capsule gives diffuse tenderness. Point tenderness may be found over a torn meniscus. Pain may severely limit range of motion (see Fig. 9-3).

Palpate the posterior knee for a popliteal cyst, called *Baker's cyst,* an extension of the synovium into the popliteal space. Baker's cyst may enlarge further and dissect down into the posterior calf, mimicking thrombophlebitis.

The quadriceps femoris inserts on the tibial tuberosity. In the adolescent, a

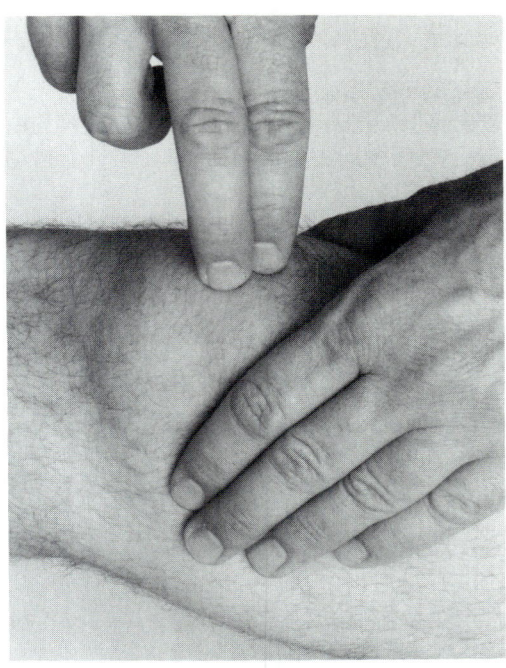

Fig. 9-26 Ballottement of patella to determine joint effusion.

partial separation at the tuberosity may occur in *Osgood-Schlatter disease*. The tibial tuberosity becomes swollen and tender. In later life, the patient may be left with a prominent tibial tubercle.

Using ballottement, examine the knee for joint effusion with the patient supine. With your left hand, grasp the leg in midthigh with the four fingers facing away from you and the thumb towards you (Fig. 9-26). Then slide your hand down to the patella. This collapses the joint space on each side of the leg under the quadriceps tendon. Should joint effusion be present, this action will make it more prominent. Quickly but gently press the patella straight down with the fingers of the right hand, feeling for a click. The click demonstrates excessive joint fluid is holding the patella away from the underlying femur. In the absence of joint effusions, the patella remains in contact with the femur and does not demonstrate the movement and click.

Small amounts of joint effusion may be compressed back and forth from one side of the patellar tendon to the other. This maneuver can produce a visible bulge of small amounts of fluid.

Moving the patella from side to side or flexing the knee may produce crepitus in chronic arthritis.

Check the stability of the knee ligaments. Support comes from the medial and lateral collateral ligaments and the anterior and posterior cruciate ligaments. Test for collateral ligament stability with the patient supine (Fig. 9-27, *A*). Place one hand against the knee joint and use your other hand to grasp the ankle and pull it laterally and then medially while supporting the knee to keep it from moving. Ordinarily, little lateral motion occurs at the knee.

To test the cruciate ligaments, ask the patient to flex the knee to 90 degrees (Fig. 9-27, *B*). Grasp the leg below the knee, then (1) pull the lower leg from the patient (open drawer sign), and (2) push it toward the patient (close drawer sign). Normally this technique will move the proximal tibia very little in relation to the femur.

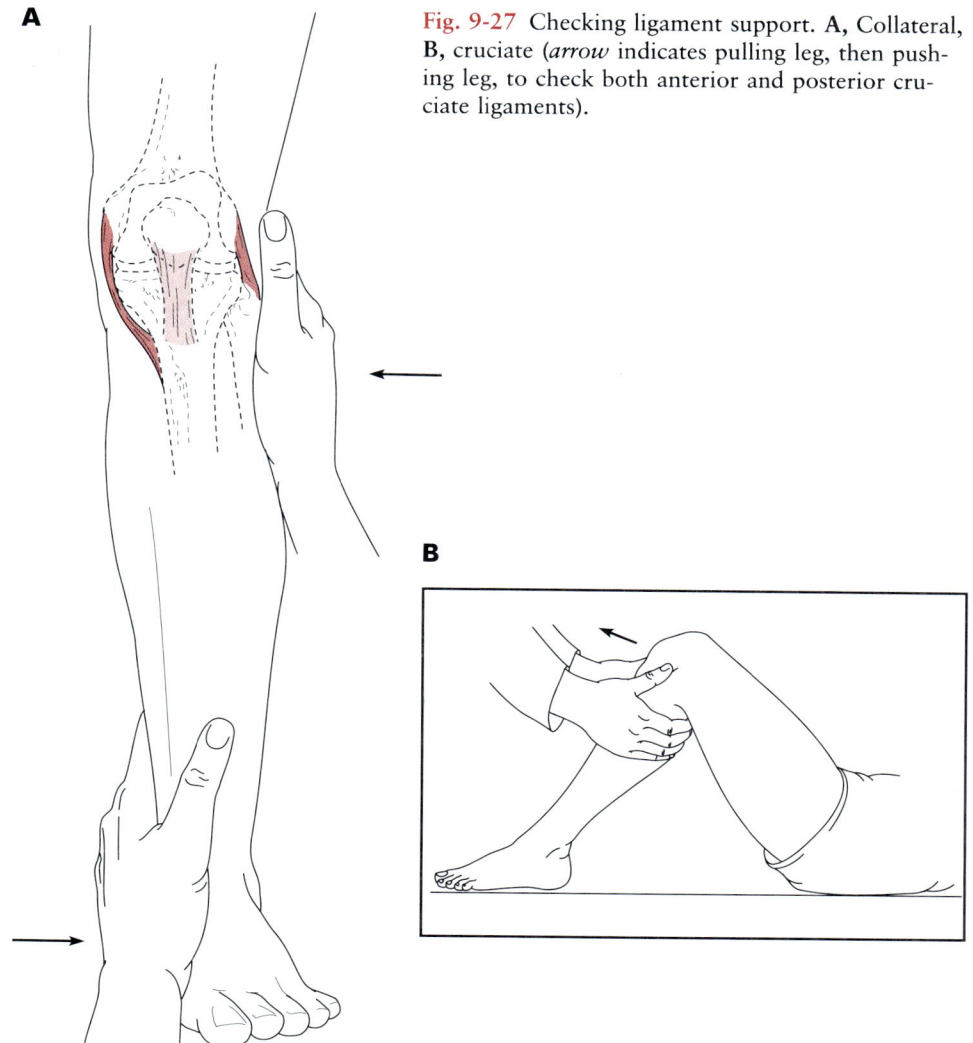

Fig. 9-27 Checking ligament support. **A**, Collateral, **B**, cruciate (*arrow* indicates pulling leg, then pushing leg, to check both anterior and posterior cruciate ligaments).

Examples of Knee Abnormalities

Genu valgus is the knock-kneed deformity (Fig. 9-28). This may be present in childhood or appear later because of arthritis. Genu varus (bowleg) indicates the apex angle at the knee is outward (see Fig. 9-28). *Genu recurvatum* signifies excessive extension of the knee (see Fig. 9-28).

Pain and swelling of both knees is typical of several types of arthritis: rheumatoid, ankylosing spondylitis, Reiter's syndrome, gout, pseudogout, connective tissue diseases, and osteoarthritis. Any of these may show unilateral (asymmetric) involvement.

THE ANKLE AND FEET

First examine the ankle (tibiotarsal) joints, then the subtalar (talonavicular and talocalcaneus) joints (Fig. 9-29; see also Fig. 9-3).

Palpate the ankles and feet for swelling, tenderness, or deformities (Fig. 9-30, *A*). Edema is differentiated from synovial thickening or joint effusion by the characteristic pitting of an edematous ankle after direct pressure of the fingertips.

Compress the tarsal joints and also the metatarsal joints medially to laterally

374 History Taking and Physical Examination

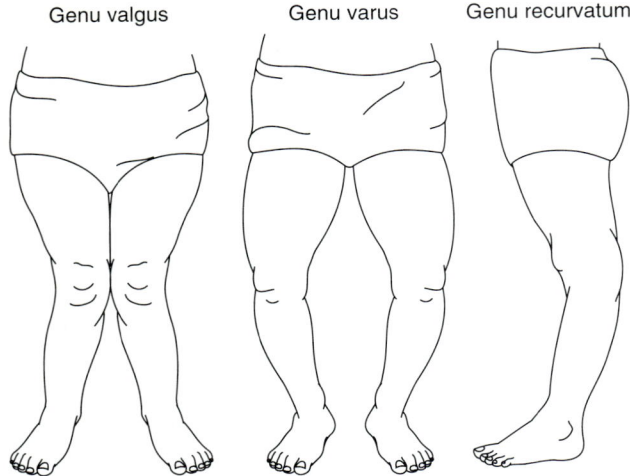

Genu valgus   Genu varus   Genu recurvatum

Fig. 9-28 Abnormalities of the knee: genu valgus, genu varus, and genu recurvatum.

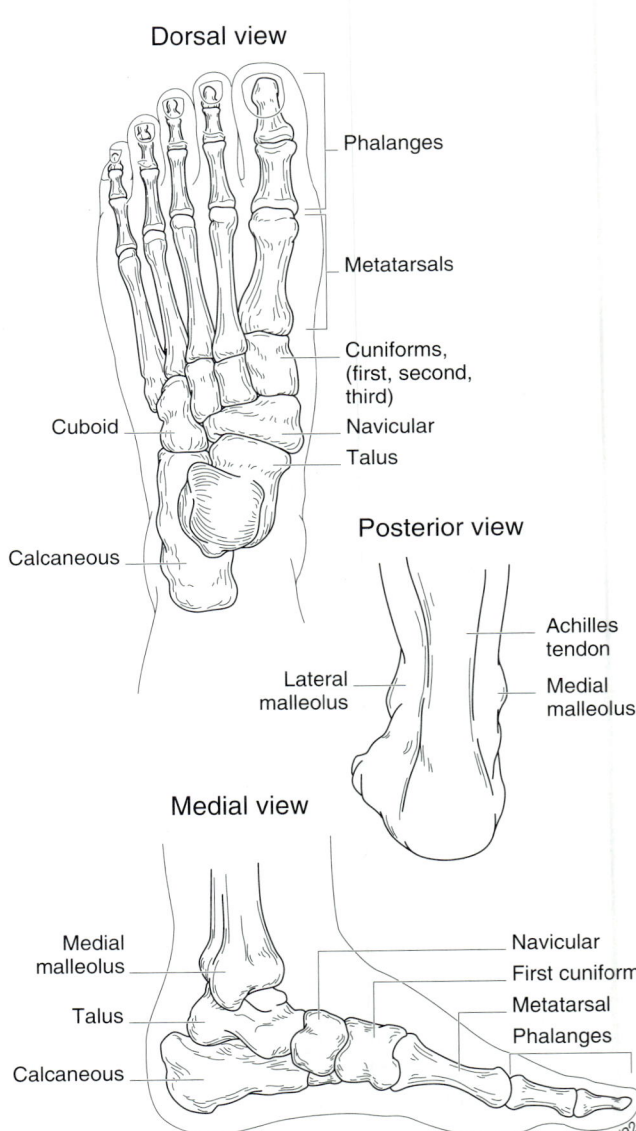

Fig. 9-29 Anatomy of the ankle and foot.

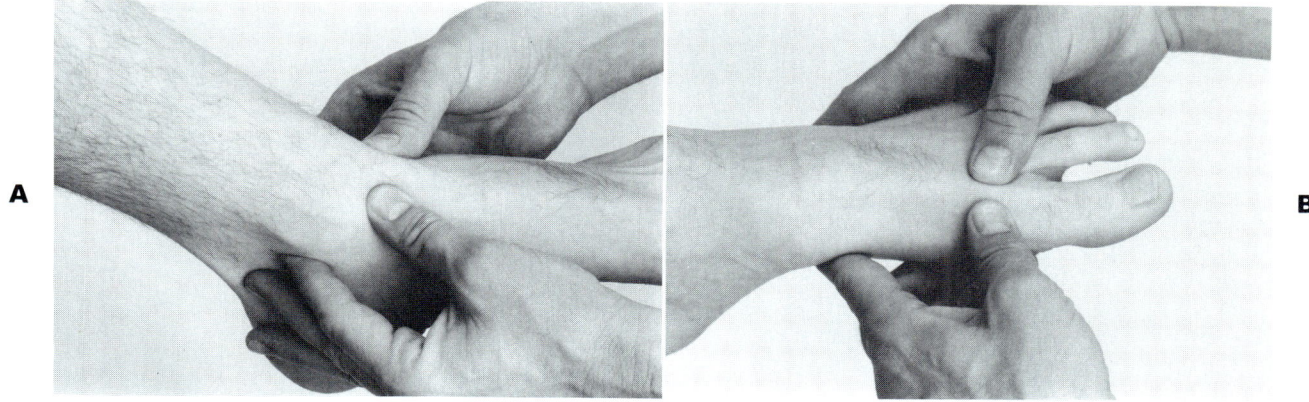

Fig. 9-30 Palpation of the ankle and foot. **A,** Ankle. **B,** Metatarsophalangeal joints.

with the examining hand (Fig. 9-30, *B*). If any is tender, palpate each joint separately. Check each of the toes for erythema, swelling, tenderness, and deformity. Gently separate each toe to inspect the web. An ulcer or a sinus tract may exit there and serve as a clue to soft-tissue infection or osteomyelitis. Observe for corns, nailbed abnormalities, lateral deviation of each toe, and hammer toes.

Examples of Ankle and Foot Abnormalities

The ankle is probably the joint most often subjected to sprains. Pain and tenderness of a sprain is ordinarily over the medial or lateral malleolus. Flexing or extending the ankle joint typically produces little discomfort in sprains, but inversion or eversion is quite uncomfortable.

A *bunion* involves a swelling of the first metatarsophalangeal joint (Fig. 9-31). Typically the distal great toe deviates laterally (hallux valgus). Development of a bunion is common when shoes do not fit well or the patient has osteoarthritis or RA.

Much foot pain results from abnormal longitudinal or transverse arches. When the longitudinal arch relaxes, the middle portion of the foot flattens *(flat foot, pes planus)* (see Fig. 9-31). Patients with flat feet tend to wear down the soles of their shoes on the medial side. Normally people wear the sole fairly evenly, with a little more wear along the lateral margin. Patients who have excessively high arches *(pes cavus)* (see Fig. 9-31) typically have excessive shoe sole wear under the metatarsal heads and the back of the heels.

A *heel spur* (see Fig. 9-31) may result in tenderness at the insertion of the plantar longitudinal tendon of the calcaneus. A spur may occur in otherwise healthy people. Patients with Reiter's syndrome also develop spurs. These may result from plantar tendinitis.

Morton's neuroma can give severe burning pain caused by pinching of a fibrous neuroma between the metatarsal heads.

Calluses on the soles (see Fig. 9-31) may act as foreign bodies in patients who have peripheral neuropathy. Trauma from walking on these or from home surgical techniques may result in foot ulcers. Mal perforans ulcers of the soles may be found in those with diabetes or other peripheral neuropathic conditions.

Tenderness at the first metatarsophalangeal joint is typical of *gouty podagra* (see Fig. 9-31). In the absence of a typical history, other disorders may be the cause of joint abnormality here.

Fig. 9-31 Abnormalities of the ankle and foot: pes planus, pes cavus, heel spur, bunion, calluses, and podagra.

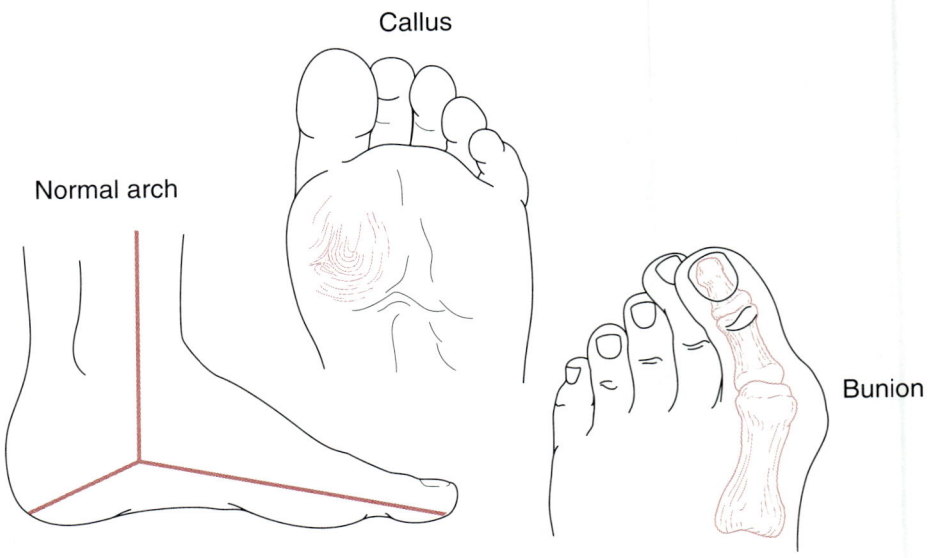
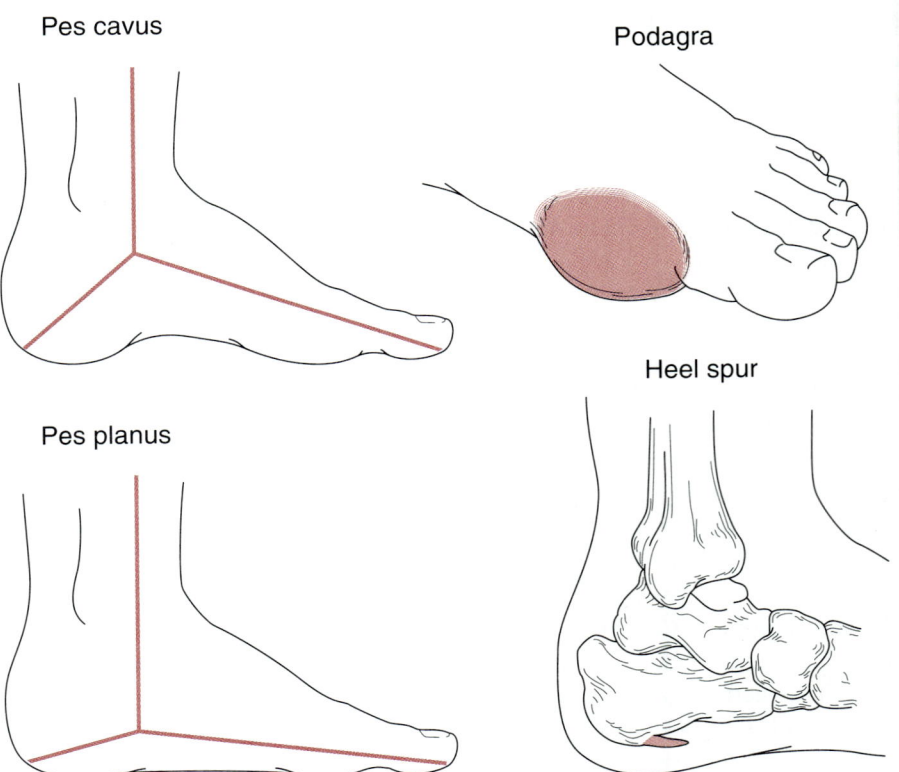

Summary of Deformities in Arthritis

Rheumatoid Arthritis

Proximal interphalangeal (PIP) joints: swollen early to give sausage shape
Metacarpal phalangeal (MCP) joints: fingertips deviated toward ulnar side of arm
Boutonniere deformity: flexion of PIP joint, hyperextension of distal interphalangeal (DIP) joint
Swan neck deformity: flexion of MCP joint, hyperextension of PIP joint, flexion of DIP joint
Wrist: synovial hypertrophy
Elbows: rheumatoid nodules, reduced range of motion
Knees: Baker's cysts, reduced range of motion, synovial hypertrophy, chronic effusion
Feet: lateral deviation of toes, overriding toes, first metatarsal phalangeal (MTP) joint prominent

Osteoarthritis

DIP joints: swollen, prominent bones (Heberden's nodes)
Hip pain, limp
Knee: crepitus, reduced range of motion, Baker's cysts
First MTP joint prominent (bunion)

Gouty Arthritis

First MTP joint, ankle, or knee swollen
Tophi containing urates around joints

Pseudogout

Rarely affects first MTP joint of great toe
Most often affects the knees, wrists, MCP joints

Psoriatic Arthritis

DIP joints: enlargement with nail pitting, fragmenting, discoloration
PIP, MCP joint involvement may mimic rheumatoid arthritis
Fingers may swell to resemble sausages
May precede skin psoriasis

Diagnosis of Arthritis

Differentiating between the types of arthritis can be difficult. The examiner must rely on the medical history, examination findings, and additional laboratory studies to arrive at the correct diagnosis. The major causes of arthritis commonly seen in medical practice are summarized in Table 9-10. Each of these may be distinctive or may be confused with the others, depending on how typical or atypical the manifestations are in each patient.

TABLE 9-10: History and Examination Finding in Selected Disorders of Joints

Disorder	Usual Age at Onset	Sex	Joints Involved	Signs and Symptoms
Gonococcal arthritis	15 to 45; any age	Women 4 : 1	• 1 to 4 joints, knee most common, ankle and wrist common, asymmetric	• Severe pain, swelling • Often arthralgia precedes arthritis; effusion common • Most have migratory arthritis
Rheumatic fever	2 to 30	M = F	• Symmetric joint involvement, but can be monarticular • Migratory, several joints • Knees, ankles, wrists, elbows hips or feet	• Follows streptococcal pharyngitis by about 2 wks • Joints become red, hot, tender, swollen in one day; pain is severe; joint pain may be transient and fleeting
Rheumatoid arthritis	20 to 60	Women 3 : 1	• Initially: hands, feet knee 50% (as single joint) wrist, hip • Ultimate involvement: PIP joints wrists or knees in majority; MCP, ankles, shoulders, MTP, toes	• Joint stiffness in AM • Pain, fatigue, weight loss • Classic signs of inflammation • Joint effusions • Muscle wasting • Elbows, cervical spine, hips, DIP, all common
Osteoarthritis	40 to 65	Women	• Knees • DIP (Heberden's nodes) • PIP, 1st MTP (bunion)	• Usually joint pain evenings • Brief (10 to 30 min) morning stiffness; knees grate, swell • Baker's cysts, Heberden's nodes
Gouty arthritis	30 to 60	Males 20 : 1 (females if postmenopausal)	• Base of great toe 75% (first MTP—podagra) • Ankle, knee, fingers, or other toes	• Red, hot, swollen joint • Onset is sudden, typically during the night; attacks precipitated by salcylates, alcohol, starvation, and other medication, all of which increase uric acid
Pseudogout (pyrophosphate arthropathy)	Usually over 60	M = F	• Knees, hips, ankles, shoulders, toes, fingers • Rarely first MTP joint • Usually monarticular	• Acute, red, hot, swollen and tender; effusion common
Psoriatic arthritis	20 to 50	M = F	• Polyarticular, DIP or PIP may mimic rheumatoid, but negative rheumatic factor • Sacroiliitis may occur	• Acute or chronic, morning stiffness; joints red, hot swollen, termed sausage-shaped digit
Reiter's syndrome	20 to 40	Males 2 : 1	• Asymmetric knee, ankle, feet, shoulder, wrist elbow, hip, spine, sacroiliac joints	• Often follows urethral discharge or diarrhea • Acute joint pain, red, hot, tender; fever, pain in the heel, or SI tenderness

Course	Associated Findings	Radiographs	Laboratory
• Begins 3 to 15 days after infection; untreated chronic synovitis with deformities	• Tenosynovitis—25% to 75% • Maculopapular, pustular or hemorrhagic skin lesions in 70% • Fever in majority	• Early—normal; late—cartilage loss gives narrow joint space • Joint destruction	• Microbe cultured from blood, urethra, cervix, anus, throat, or synovial fluid
• Untreated lasts 2 weeks • Rapid relief with aspirin • No permanent deformities	• Carditis, pericarditis, (rub) myocarditis with tachycardia; subcutaneous nodules, erythema marginatum nodosum (Jones criteria)	• Normal • No joint damage after subsides	• Throat culture positive for group A streptococci in 25% • ESR high in nearly all • ASO titer high in 75%
• Episodic or persistent arthritis • Episodic course is 6-month attacks of arthritis each 2+ years • Persistent course, arthritis waxes and wanes; joints tend to remain involved but may become inactive as develops	• Multisystem involvement of joints, periarticular soft tissues, heart, lungs, nerves, eyes, lymph nodes • Patients are ill other than joints	• Characteristic early and late radiographic changes	• Rheumatoid factors • Elevated ESR is usual • Synovial fluid, characteristic abnormalities
• Slowly additive pattern of joints involved	• Patient may be healthy except for joints in contrast to rheumatoid arthritis • Other diseases may exhibit osteoarthritis (e.g. injuries, obesity, gout)	• Loss of joint space • Osteophyte formation	• Normal ESR • Negative rheumatoid factor
• Fever may be present acutely • Attack lasts 10 to 14 days • Joints normal between attacks; chronic attacks	• Obesity, hypertension, alcoholism, family history	• Punched-out lucent areas around joint	• Serum uric acid elevated • Negative birefringent needle-shaped crystals in synovial fluid
• Attacks last for weeks to months; slowly progresses, leaving osteoarthritis-like deformity. • May be intermittent or progressive; some types are deforming	• Surgery or medical illness provoke attacks in some • Fingernail changes include pitting and onycholysis	• Calcifications in knees and wrists, may have linear calcification of cartilage • Radiographic erosions, sclerosis, cysts, destruction of bone ends	• Brick-shaped crystals positively birefringent in synovial fluid • ESR usually normal • Rheumatoid factor is negative
• Initial attack lasts few months; one-half have repeat attacks without urethritis or diarrhea	• Triad of arthritis, urethritis and conjunctivitis; skin lesions are circinate balanitis, keratoderma blennorrhagica, Achilles tenosynovitis, spurs, and iritis	• Radiographs show bilateral sacroiliitis, ankylosing spondylitis in less than one-half	• HLA-B27 in majority

TABLE 9-10: History and Examination Finding in Selected Disorders of Joints—cont'd

Disorder	Usual Age at Onset	Sex	Joints Involved	Signs and Symptoms
SLE	20 to 40	Women 9 : 1	• Resembles rheumatoid PIP, MCP, wrists, knees, ankles, elbows, spine, TMJ, symmetric	• Pain, stiffness, morning stiffness, fever, slight soft tissue involved
Lyme disease	Any age	M = F	• Asymmetric joint involvement; large joints, knees most often; ankle, wrist, shoulder, TMJ, hip, elbow, hands	• Often begins monarticular with swelling, effusion, tenderness, warmth

Summary

The summary checklist for the examination of the musculoskeletal system is shown in the box opposite.

Suggested readings

Huskisson EC, Hart FB: *Joint disease: all the arthropathies,* Bristol, England, 1987, Wright Publishing. *This is a crisp presentation of the topic and is quite helpful.*

Katz WA: *Diagnosis and management of rheumatic diseases,* ed 2, Philadelphia, 1988, JB Lippincott. *Well-written textbook on musculoskeletal problems.*

McCarty DJ: *Textbook of rheumatology,* ed 10, Philadelphia, 1985, Lea & Febiger. *Comprehensive presentation of joint problems, beginning with history and physical examination and going on to analyze differential diagnosis, laboratory and x-ray studies, therapy, and prognosis.*

Rodman GP, Schumacher HR: *Primer on the rheumatic diseases,* ed 8, Atlanta, 1983, Arthritis Foundation. *Gives important diagnostic information on rheumatic diseases in an authoritative and succinct manner.*

Course	Associated Findings	Radiographs	Laboratory
• Stress or sunlight may precipitate onset or make worse	• Usually little joint deformity; renal involvement may be fatal	• Radiographs erosions bone destruction, necrosis	• All increased ESR, ANA, anti-DNA, ENA
• Caused by *Borrelia sp.* and acquired by tick bite	• Skin lesion, erythema (chronicum) migrans • Neurologic abnormalities include meningitis, Bell's palsy	• Radiographs normal	• Antibodies to *Borrelia sp.* may be present

---

Summary Checklist for the Musculoskeletal System Examination

Inspection
  Symmetry
  Deformity, peripheral and spine
  Distribution of deformity
    Joints and synovium
    Bursa
    Ligaments and tendons
    Bones and muscles
  Limitation of active range of motion, loss of function
  Erythema of joints and surrounding structures
  Instability
  Movement, gait
Palpation
  Deformity
  Synovial effusion
  Ballottement
  Thickened synovium
  Tenderness
  Warmth
  Joint locking
  Range of passive motion
  Use of goniometer
  Muscle strength
  Fracture
Auscultation
  Crepitus
  Joint clicking
Individual joint evaluations
  Temporomandibular joint
  Cervical spine
  Shoulder joint abnormalities
    Adhesive capsulitis
    Acromioclavicular arthritis
    Bicipital tendinitis
    Calcific tendinitis
    Impingement syndrome
    Rotator cuff tears
  Elbow
    Golf elbow
    Tennis elbow
  Wrist
    DeQuervain's tenosynovitis
    Ganglion
    Carpal tunnel syndrome
      Phalen's test
      Tinel's test
  Hands and fingers
    Grip strength
    Heberden's nodes
    Bouchard's nodes
    Boutonniere deformity
    Swan neck deformity
  Spine
    Scoliosis
    Kyphosis
    Kyphoscoliosis
    Gibbus
    Sacroiliitis
  Legs
    Trendelenburg's test
  Knee
    Baker's cyst
    Stability testing
    Genus varus and valgus
  Feet
    Bunion
    Flat feet
    Spur

CHAPTER TEN

The Neurologic Examination

CHAPTER OUTLINE

History Taking
Headache
Syncope and loss of consciousness
Seizures
Changes in vision
Changes in hearing
Changes in speech
Paralysis or weakness
Numbness and paresthesia
Changes in mood and sleep pattern
Alcohol and drug use and sexual practices

Essentials of the Neurologic Examination
Examination of motor functions
Sensory Examination

Cerebellar function and tests of coordination
Reflexes
The cranial nerves
The mental status examination
Recognition of some common neurological problems

Approach to the Comatose Patient

Approach to the Patient with Delirium and Acute Confusional States

Approach to the Patient with a Peripheral Neuropathy

Approach to the Patient with Signs of Meningeal Irritation

Summary

    Symptoms and signs suggestive of a disorder of the nervous system are among the most common clinical problems. The prevalence of cerebrovascular diseases in the United States may be as high as 750 per 100,000 population, and this helps explain the occurrence of over 400,000 hospitalizations for stroke each year. Seizures and convulsive disorders afflict 1% to 2% of the population. Alzheimer's disease is an ever-increasing problem in our aging population and, along with multiinfarct dementia, accounts for the vast majority of elderly patients with dementia. Trauma to the head and spinal cord continues to be a vexing problem affecting several thousand individuals each year. Other important disorders of the nervous system include the following:

- Neoplastic diseases, which cause approximately 100,000 deaths each year
- Infectious diseases, especially bacterial and aseptic meningitis
- Nutritional and metabolic disorders
- Demyelinating diseases such as multiple sclerosis
- Neuromuscular disorders such as myasthenia gravis
- Peripheral neuropathies

Finally, evaluation of the patient in coma as well as the patient with an altered mental status merits special attention.

When patients seek treatment with symptoms or signs suggestive of a disorder of the nervous system, a detailed examination is clearly indicated. On the other hand, if no evidence of disturbed functions is present, an abbreviated examination can be carried out. The latter might well include assessment of gait and station, deep tendon reflexes, strength in the arms and legs, examination of the pupils, ocular assessment and funduscopic examinations, evaluation of the cranial nerves, and a brief mental status exam. If abnormalities in the mental status examination are detected, the examiner must distinguish between a neurologic and psychiatric disorder, a distinction that may be difficult. Evaluation of the patient with dementia, especially of recent onset, is particularly appropriate because a small but significant fraction (approximately 10% to 15%) of such patients have treatable disorders.

This chapter emphasizes the importance of symptoms and signs of neurologic dysfunction, which often point to the site of a lesion as well as to the cause of a lesion. In few areas of medicine is the clinical evaluation so vital.

History Taking

An obviously important element in the diagnosis of neurologic disorders is an accurate and complete history. Several key symptoms merit detailed evaluation (see accompanying box).

Headache (Table 10-1)

Most patients experience occasional mild headaches that are of no consequence. However, a headache that differs from a patient's normal pattern, an unusually severe headache, recurrent severe headaches, or headaches associated with other symptoms warrant more detailed questioning. Be especially concerned if a patient not prone to recurrent headaches suddenly develops a severe headache

---

Key Symptoms in the Neurologic Evaluation

- Headache
- Syncope and loss of consciousness
- Seizures
- Changes in vision
- Changes in hearing (also tinnitus and vertigo)

- Changes in speech
- Paralysis or weakness
- Numbness and paresthesia
- Changes in mood and sleep patterns
- Alcohol, drug use, and sexual practices

TABLE 10-1: Clinical Features of Some Common Headaches

Type	Location	Clinical Characteristics	Associated Symptoms	Precipitating Factors
1. Migraine	• Frontotemporal • Usually bilateral	• Throbbing or dull ache, generalized headache, visual prodrome (scintillating lights)	• Nausea, vomiting, possible transient neurologic defects (numbness, vertigo, confusion)	• Tension, alcohol, noise, caffeine
2. Tension	• Bilateral • Generalized • Occipital	• Pressure, tightness, aching, occurs more frequently in women	• Anxiety, insomnia, nervousness	• Nervous strain • Fatigue
3. Cluster	• Orbital, frontal • Unilateral	• Intense pain, usually nocturnal • May persist for several days	• Unilateral nasal congestion • Unilateral lacrimation	• Alcohol
4. Meningeal				
a. Meningitis	• Generalized	• Variable severity, may be worse in the neck	• Fever, nuchal rigidity, altered consciousness, • Positive Kernig's/Brudzinski's signs	
b. Subarachnoid bleed	• Generalized	• Intense, sudden onset, frequent complaint, "worst headache I have ever had"	• Nuchal rigidity, altered consciousness	
5. Hypertension	• Variable	• Check for hypertensive retinopathy	• May develop stroke, hypertensive encephalopathy	• Discontinue medications
6. Brain tumor	• Variable	• Variable frequency (minutes to hours), and intensity, may awaken at night	• Papilledema, nausea, projectile vomiting, altered mental status	
7. Temporal arteritis	• Unilateral • Temporal or occipital	• Aching or burning discomfort • Check temporal artery pulsations	• May be associated with loss of vision (retinal artery occlusion)	

and spontaneously states something to the effect that, "This is the worst headache I have ever had." Such an event may be the harbinger of a subarachnoid hemorrhage caused by a leaking berry aneurysm or AV malformation. Suspicion of this diagnosis should be heightened if the patient has a history of transient loss of consciousness or evidence of *meningismus* (stiff neck) on physical examination.

A history of recurrent headaches should prompt a detailed inquiry into antecedent events, precipitating factors, associated symptoms, relationship to emotional events if any, and the effect of various therapies. For example, patients with migraine headaches often note an aura that precedes the headache, and associated weakness, numbness, and paresthesia may be present. Tension headaches also tend to be recurrent. They usually occur late in the afternoon, are

CASE 10-1 Sudden Onset of Severe Headache

A 30-year-old woman came to the emergency room complaining of the sudden onset of a severe headache that radiated to the back of the head and neck. She spontaneously volunteered the information that "this is the worst headache I have ever experienced. . . . it is as if something burst in my head." The patient's family history was noteworthy in that an older brother died of a 'stroke' at age 40.

The physical examination revealed normal vital signs and no evidence of ptosis or cranial nerve palsies, but equivocal signs of meningeal irritation (i.e., stiffness of the neck). Because of the unusually severe and persistent headache, the resident physician ordered a noncontrast CT scan of the head, which showed evidence of a subarachnoid hemorrhage. Subsequently a cerebral arteriogram demonstrated a berry aneurysm involving the anterior cerebral artery. The aneurysm was subsequently clipped, and the patient recovered unevenfully. The clue to the correct diagnosis was the unusually severe nature of the headache, along with its abrupt onset.

---

often stress-related and not accompanied by other symptoms, and are usually relieved by conventional analgesics.

Cluster headaches are characterized by male predominance, constant unilateral orbital localization, and onset within 2 to 3 hours after falling asleep. The pain is usually intense, with lacrimation, rhinorrhea, and sometimes flushing, all lasting around 1 hour.

Headaches accompanied by other symptoms are also worrisome. A morning headache associated with vomiting, which may be projectile, should raise the question of a CNS lesion such as neoplasm causing increased ICP (see Figure 10-30). A headache accompanied by an obvious change in personality or daily habits should alert the examiner to the possibility of a frontal lobe lesion; this is often the presentation of a patient with a primary brain tumor such as a glioma or metastasis from an occult bronchogenic carcinoma. A headache associated with fever and a stiff neck should raise the question of meningitis. Headaches accompanied by markedly elevated blood pressure and funduscopic changes should alert the examiner to the likelihood of accelerated hypertension and to the possibility of hypertensive encephalopathy. Finally, a headache accompanied by loss of consciousness, albeit transient, should always raise the question of a cerebrovascular accident (CVA), subarachnoid bleed, or cardiovascular cause of syncope.

Syncope and Loss of Consciousness

Ask all patients whether they have ever lost consciousness or passed out. Avoid the use of nonspecific terms such as "dizziness," "light-headed," or "blackout spells," which may mean different things to a patient. Syncopal episodes are usually caused by a transient decrease in cerebral blood flow, and this in turn has several causes. Syncope is also discussed in Chapter 4, and only key causes are considered here (see accompanying box).

A syncopal episode is often heralded by a prodromal stage characterized by weakness, unsteadiness, visual changes, ringing in the ears, and nausea. The pa-

Etiology of Syncope, Weakness, and Faintness*

I. Circulatory (deficient quantity of blood to the brain)
   A. Inadequate vasoconstrictor mechanisms
      1. Vasovagal (vasodepressor)
      2. Postural hypotension
      3. Primary autonomic insufficiency
      4. Sympathectomy (pharmacologic caused by antihypertensive medications such as methyldopa and hydralazine, or surgical)
      5. Diseases of central and peripheral nervous systems, including autonomic nerves
      6. Carotid sinus syncope (see also bradyarrhythmias, below)
   B. Hypovolemia
   C. Mechanical reduction of venous return
      1. Valsalva's maneuver
      2. Cough (posttussive)
      3. Micturition
      4. Atrial myxoma, ball-valve thrombus
   D. Reduced cardiac output
      1. Obstruction to left ventricular outflow: aortic stenosis, hypertrophic subaortic stenosis
      2. Obstruction to pulmonary flow: pulmonic stenosis, primary pulmonary hypertension, pulmonary embolism
      3. Myocardial: massive myocardial infarction with pump failure
      4. Pericardial: cardiac tamponade
   E. Arrhythmias
      1. Bradyarrhythmias
         a. Atrioventricular (AV) block (2° and 3°), with Stokes-Adams attacks
         b. Ventricular asystole
         c. Sinus bradycardia, sinoatrial block, sinus arrest
         d. Carotid sinus syncope (see also inadequate vasoconstrictor mechanisms, above)
         e. Glossopharyngeal neuralgia (and other painful states)
      2. Tachyarrhythmias
         a. Episodic ventricular fibrillation with or without associated bradyarrhythmias
         b. Ventricular tachycardia
         c. Supraventricular tachycardia without AV block
II. Other causes of weakness and episodic disturbances of consciousness
   A. Altered state of blood to the brain
      1. Hypoxia
      2. Anemia
      3. Diminished carbon dioxide resulting from hyperventilation (faintness common, syncope seldom occurs)
      4. Hypoglycemia (episodic weakness common, faintness occasional, syncope rare)
   B. Cerebral
      1. Cerebrovascular disturbances (e.g., TIAs)
         a. Extracranial vascular insufficiency (vertebrobasilar, carotid)
         b. Diffuse spasm of cerebral arterioles (hypertensive encephalopathy)
      2. Emotional disturbances, anxiety attacks, and hysterical seizures

Modified from Martin JB, Ruskin T: Faintness, syncope, and seizures. In Wilson J, et al, editors: *Harrison's principles of internal medicine,* ed 12, New York, 1991, McGraw-Hill, p 134.
*See also Chapter 4.

tient may appear pale or ashen gray. During the syncopal episode the patient may lose consciousness or may merely be obtunded and confused but be able to respond. The patient often falls to the floor and may remain there from a few seconds to several minutes. A detailed evaluation is indicated in all patients with either a documented syncopal episode or a convincing history suggestive of syncope.

Seizures

When asking patients about seizures, ascertain whether they (1) have a history of seizures or "fits"; (2) have ever had a convulsion; and (3) have ever had epilepsy. In addition, as noted above, also ask whether they have ever lost consciousness. If a history consistent with seizures is elicited, ask the patient about any prodromata such as an aura, which may include nausea, palpitations, vertigo, tinnitus, or headache. Patients may also mention feelings of fear and deja vu, which are common features of complex partial seizures. In addition, ask the patient about frequently associated symptoms such as a bitten tongue, incontinence of urine or stool, transient amnesia, postictal weakness, and whether tonic-clonic movements were noted by anyone who witnessed the seizures.

Grand mal seizures begin with a sudden loss of consciousness, a cry, a fall to the ground, tonic then clonic movement of limbs, sometimes sphincteric incontinence, and other autonomic disorders. Petit mal seizures come without warning and are notable for their brevity (usually last only a few seconds) and minimal motor accompaniment.

Onset of seizures after age 35 without an obvious cause such as head trauma should raise the question of an intracranial mass lesion such as a brain tumor, metabolic disorder, or cerebral vascular disorder. Temporal lobe seizures in adults may be associated only with a transient diminution of consciousness or periods of being unable to speak (i.e., periods of unreality without any abnormal movement or other seizure phenomena). The accompanying box is a detailed list of the causes of seizures.

Changes in Vision

Ask the patient about any recent changes in vision, especially blurred vision, *diplopia* (double vision), or transient loss of vision (see also Chapter 2). A sudden

---

Major Causes of Seizures According to Age

I. Adolescents (12 to 20 years)
   A. Idiopathic
   B. Trauma
   C. Drug and alcohol withdrawal
II. Young adults (20 to 35 years)
   A. Trauma
   B. Alcoholism
   C. Brain tumor

III. Older adults (> 35 years)
   A. Brain tumor
   B. Cerebrovascular disease
   C. Metabolic disorders
     1. Hyponatremia
     2. Hypoglycemia
     3. Hepatic failure
     4. Uremia
   D. Alcoholism

Modified from Dichter MA: The epilepsies and convulsive disorders. In Wilson JD, et al, editors: *Harrison's principles of internal medicine,* ed 12, New York, 1990, McGraw-Hill, p 1971.

CASE 10-2 Sudden Loss of Vision

A 67-year-old man came to the clinic with a chief complaint of sudden transient loss of vision in his right eye. The patient was a heavy smoker and had a long history of hypertension reasonably well controlled with medication. He described a transient (i.e., about 10 minutes) loss of vision and stated, "It was as if a black curtain descended over my right eye and I could not see anything for a few minutes."

Physical examination revealed a blood pressure of 150/90 mm Hg and a loud bruit over the right carotid artery. Doppler ultrasound studies demonstrated high-grade stenosis of the right common carotid artery; this finding was subsequently confirmed by angiography. The clues to the correct diagnosis were the history of transient monocular blindness (amaurosis fugax) and the loud carotid bruit. The patient subsequently underwent a successful carotid endarterectomy.

---

transient loss of vision in one eye *(amaurosis fugax)* should raise the question of internal carotid artery stenosis. This suspicion is heightened if the patient states something to the effect that, "A curtain was pulled down over my eyes and I could not see anything for a few minutes." Not infrequently, other symptoms such as transient weakness and numbness and paresthesia in an upper extremity accompany amaurosis fugax. Transient monocular blindness, lasting a few days to a few weeks, also occurs with retrobulbar neuritis, which may develop in multiple sclerosis. New onset of blurred vision or unexplained change in normal acuity can occur with diabetes mellitus.

Changes in Hearing

A common but often neglected cause of decreased hearing is excess cerumen in the external ear canal. In any patient with a change in hearing, also inquire about tinnitus and vertigo. The presence of the latter two symptoms should raise the question of labyrinthine dysfunction. Recurrent tinnitus and vertigo are found in Ménière's disease.

Changes in Speech

Changes in speech can occur with *dysarthria* (difficulty in articulating words), *dysphonia* (difficulty speaking because of impaired function), and *aphasia* (inability to produce or understand spoken or written words), which are discussed in detail under the neurologic examination (see page 417). Transient dysarthria, especially if accompanied by transient diplopia, should raise the question of vertebral basilar transient ischemic attacks.

Paralysis or Weakness

Explore in detail any history of paralysis or weakness, albeit transient. Note whether the weakness involved a single limb, one side of the body, trunk, head, or neck, and whether it had any associated symptoms such as numbness, *paresthesia* (abnormal sensations), diplopia, and dysarthria. Recurrent transient weakness should cause the examiner to consider myasthenia gravis, periodic paralysis resulting from hypokalemia, and transient ischemic attacks (TIAs); the

> ### Differential Diagnosis of Peripheral Neuropathies
>
> - Drugs (e.g., nitrofurantoin, isonicotine hydrazine, pyridoxine in excess, vincristine, DDI)
> - Alcohol
> - Nutritional (pernicious anemia, thiamine, B_6)
> - Guillain-Barré syndrome
> - Toxins (heavy metals such as arsenic and lead)
> - Hereditary (e.g., Charcot-Marie-Tooth, Refsum disease)
> - Endocrine (diabetes mellitus, hypothyroidism)
> - Renal failure
> - Amyloidosis
> - Porphyria
> - Infections (syphilis, mononucleosis, diphtheria, leprosy, AIDS)
> - Systemic disorders (rheumatoid arthritis, SLE, vasculitis, sarcoidosis)
> - Tumor
>
> NOTE: Mnemonic to remember the classification—DANG THERAPIST

Modifed from Griffin, JW. In Harvey AM, et al, editors: *The principles and practice of medicine,* ed 21, Norwalk, Conn, 1984, Appleton-Century-Crofts, p 1315.

last would be suggested by recurrent transient weakness in an upper extremity accompanied by numbness and paresthesias. Such a history often heralds a full-blown cerebrovascular accident.

Limitations of space preclude a detailed listing of all the causes of continued muscle weakness or paralysis. The most common causes include the following:

- Sequelae of a stroke
- Peripheral neuropathies (see accompanying box)
- Diabetic neuropathy
- Demyelinating diseases such as multiple sclerosis
- Connective tissue disorders such as polymyositis and dermatomyositis
- The muscular dystrophies

Numbness and Paresthesia

The presence of numbness and paresthesia, especially if either persistent or recurrent and accompanied by other symptoms, suggests a number of diagnostic possibilities. A partial listing includes the following:

- Peripheral neuropathies (see box above)
- Nerve root compression caused by cervical spine disease or a cervical disc (especially if confined to the upper extremities) or a lumbar disc (if confined to the lower extremities)
- Metabolic causes (hypocalcemia, hypomagnesemia)
- Hyperventilation syndrome
- Medications (isoniazid, metronidazole)
- Paraneoplastic syndrome, as may occur in bronchogenic carcinoma

Changes in Mood and Sleep Pattern

Changes in mood and sleep pattern may point to a specific diagnosis. For example, the constellation of symptoms and signs that includes anorexia, early morning insomnia, and feelings of helplessness and hopelessness clearly point to a diagnosis of depression. Loud snoring, periods of apnea, mood changes, and inordinate fatigue during the day should suggest sleep apnea syndrome.

Alcohol and Drug Use and Sexual Practices

In any adult patient, and especially if neurologic symptoms are elicited, inquire about alcohol and drug use. Criteria useful in the diagnosis of chronic alcoholism are detailed in the accompanying box. Review any medications used chronically and any illicit drugs used to determine their potential for injury to the nervous system. In younger adults appearing with unexplained alterations in behavior or

---

Diagnosis of Chronic Alcoholism

I. Evidence of alcohol withdrawal syndromes
   A. Tremulousness
   B. Alcoholic hallucinosis
   C. Withdrawal seizures or "rum fits"
   D. Delirium tremens
II. Evidence of tolerance to alcohol
   A. Ingestion of a fifth or more of whiskey per day
   B. No gross evidence of intoxication with blood alcohol level >150 mg/dl
   C. Random blood alcohol level >300 mg/dl
   D. Accelerated clearance of blood alcohol (>25 mg/dl per hour)
III. Psychosociologic factors
   A. Continued ingestion of alcohol despite strong contraindication to do so
      1. Threatened loss of job
      2. Threatened loss of spouse and/or family
      3. Medical contraindication known to patient
   B. Admission of inability to discontinue use of alcohol
IV. Presence of alcohol-associated disorders
   A. Erosive gastritis with upper GI bleeding
   B. Pancreatitis (acute and chronic) in the absence of cholelithiasis
   C. Alcoholic liver disease (fatty liver, alcoholic hepatitis, cirrhosis)
   D. Alcoholic diseases of the nervous system
      1. Peripheral neuropathy
      2. Cerebellar degeneration
      3. Wernicke-Korsakoff syndrome
      4. Beriberi
      5. Alcoholic myopathy
   E. Alcoholic cardiomyopathy
V. "CAGE" criteria
   C = Concerned about drinking and unable to cut back
   A = Annoyed about questions on drinking
   G = Guilty about drinking
   E = Eye opener (i.e., morning drink needed)

From Greenberger NJ, et al: *The medical book of lists: a primer of differential diagnosis in internal medicine,* ed 3, Chicago, 1990, Mosby–Year Book, p 95.

CASE 10-3 Diagnosis of Chronic Alcoholism

A 50-year-old woman with complaints of numbness and paresthesias and evidence of peripheral neuropathy and peripheral stigmata of chronic liver disease appears in the clinic. Chronic alcoholism is suspected, but the patient initially denies a history of use.

- Open-ended questions are asked to begin with—*Tell me more about your use of alcoholic beverages.*
- Because the patient appears reticent to admit to excessive use of alcohol, questions are asked in a permissive manner—*Although you may not be drinking heavily now, was there a time some years ago when you were drinking heavily?*
- If the answer to the above questioon is yes, you can proceed to ask how much alcohol was being drunk. Start with large numbers (i.e., a half fifth of liquor or a half case of beer per day). The patient may amend the numbers downward.
- Ask about retching ("dry heaves") in the morning, as this is a symptom of alcohol withdrawal, especially if the patient needs an alcoholic drink in the morning to "get going."
- Ask questions incorporating the CAGE criteria (see the box on pg. 390).

signs of early dementia, inquire about sexual practices and IV drug use. Distressingly, patients with HIV infection and AIDS may appear initially with just dementia or focal neurologic findings.

Essentials of the Neurologic Examination
Examination of Motor Functions

The motor system is evaluated by assessing muscle strength as well as muscle tone in a systematic fashion, and then noting whether any abnormal motor functions are present (see box on pg. 392).

ASSESSMENT OF MUSCLE STRENGTH

With the patient sitting, ask him to extend and separate the arms and hold them in that position, preferably with the eyes closed (Fig. 10-1). A downward drift with or without pronation suggests upper extremity weakness, which is often the occult residua from a remote CVA.

Evaluate and compare the strength of both upper and lower extremities. Use a five-point scale of strength:

Grade	Definition
0	No contraction
1	Trace of a contraction
2	Moves if gravity is eliminated
3	Moves against gravity
4	Moves against gravity with some resistance
5	Moves against gravity with full resistance

Assessment of Muscle Strength, Muscle Tone, and Abnormal Muscle Functions

Assessment of Muscle Strength
- Upper extremities
- Drift
- Deltoids
- Biceps
- Triceps
- Wrist flexion and extension
- Fingers
- Lower extremities
- Hip flexion, extension, abduction, and adduction
- Leg flexion and extension
- Ankle flexion and extension
- Trunk musculature

Assessment of Muscle Tone
- Spasticity
- Cogwheel rigidity
- Contractures
- Flaccidity
- Atrophy

Abnormal Motor Functions
- Fasciculations
- Tics
- Tetany
- Tremors

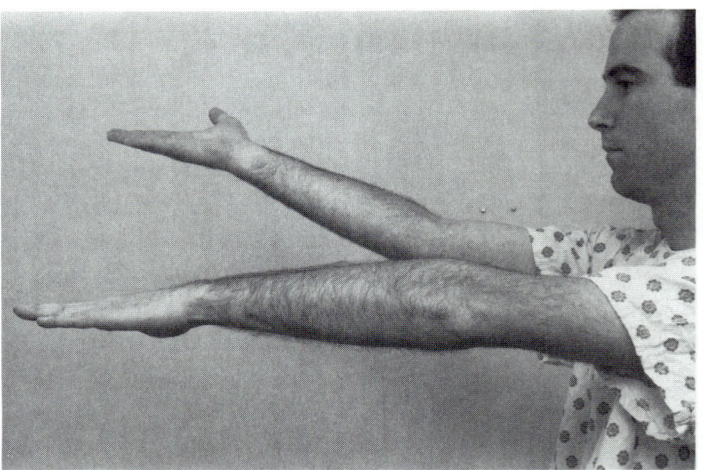

Fig. 10-1 Ask the patient to extend both arms with palms upward. Downward movement as well as pronation of the left arm is evident; such drift usually indicates weakness of the affected extremity.

Begin by having the patient abduct the arms with the forearms flexed and press on his arms to assess deltoid strength (Fig. 10-2). Next, with the patient's forearms flexed, attempt to pull them down to assess biceps strength. Also with the patient's forearm flexed, evaluate the triceps by having the patient press both dorsal surfaces of the wrist downward against your thumbs (Fig. 10-3). Alternatively, the triceps can be tested (with the arm fully extended) by the examiner attempting to flex it against resistance. Evaluate the wrist flexors and extensors by having the patient make a fist and then push upward and downward against your hand (Fig. 10-4). Assess finger strength by having the patient attempt to spread his fingers against resistance of your fingers (Fig. 10-5).

With the patient supine, ask him to extend his leg and raise the thigh. Assess hip extensors by placing your hand over the tibias and asking the patient to push

The Neurologic Examination 393

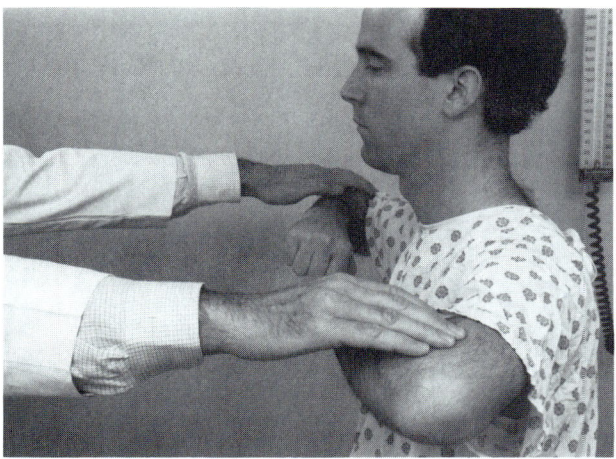

Fig. 10-2 Technique for assessing strength of the deltoid muscles.

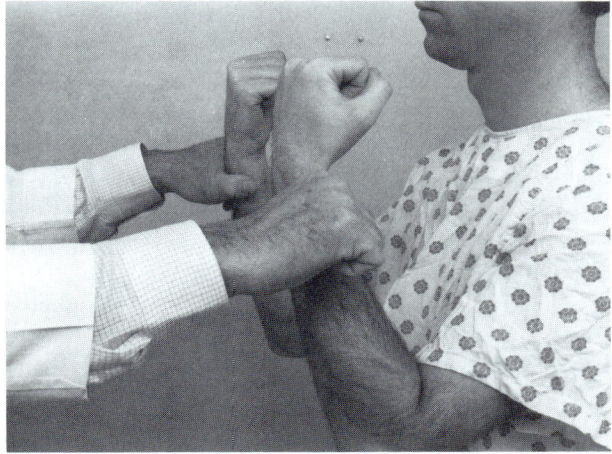

Fig. 10-3 Technique for assessing strength of the triceps muscle. Note the examiner's thumbs placed across the dorsal surface of the lower arm.

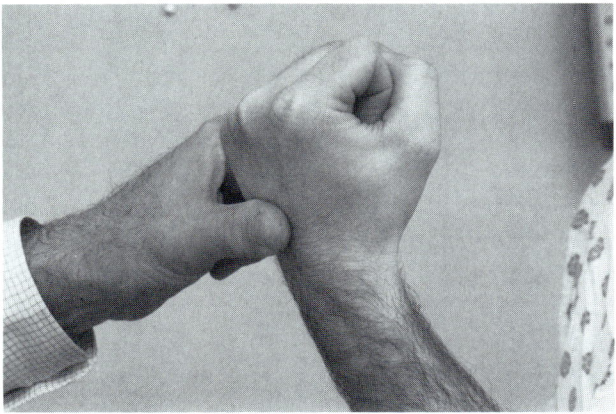

Fig. 10-4 Technique for assessing strength of the wrists. Ask the patient to dorsiflex the wrist against the examiner's thumb.

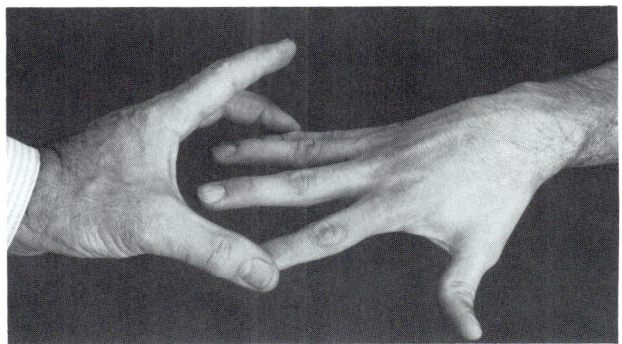

Fig. 10-5 Technique for assessing finger strength.

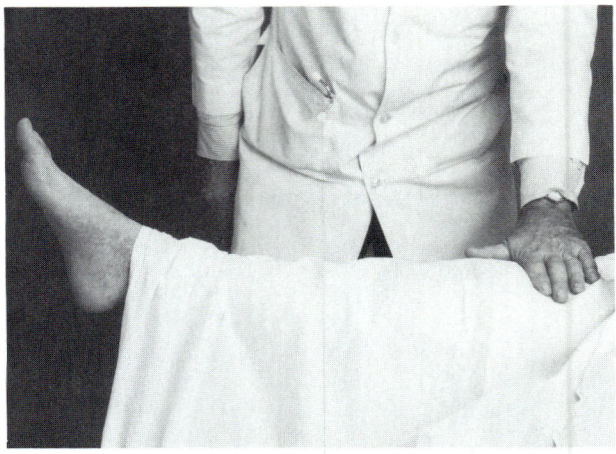

Fig. 10-6 Technique for assessing strength of hip extensors. Ask the patient to lift the thigh against resistance.

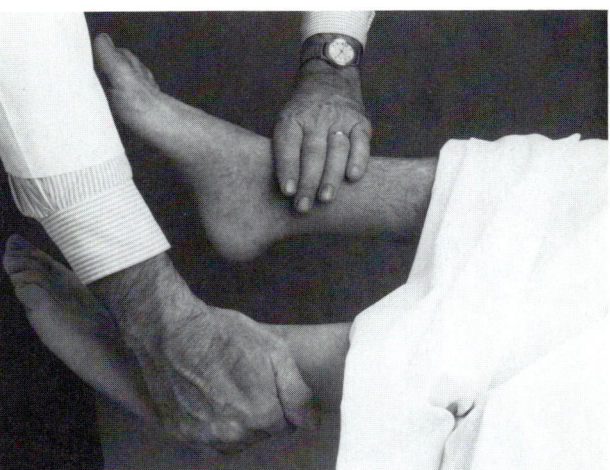

Fig. 10-7 Technique to determine spurious weakness of the lower extremities. Note the position of the examiner's hands. For details, see text.

upward (Fig. 10-6). Check hip flexor strength conversely by placing your hands under the calves or ankles and asking the patient to press downward. Assessment of leg flexion and extension and ankle flexion and extension also involves checking these muscle groups against resistance.

One can detect spurious weakness of the lower extremities, as may occur in hysteria, by a variant of the above maneuvers. With the patient supine, place one hand on the dorsum of the ankle of the affected limb and the other hand under the achilles tendon of the other leg (Fig. 10-7). Instruct the patient to elevate the affected limb. With organic disease, one will perceive a downward movement in the unaffected limb as the patient attempts to compensate for the weakness in the affected limb. By contrast, in hysteria, no movement is noted in the unaffected limb.

Assess the strength of the trunk musculature by noting how the patient arises from a supine to a sitting position. If a patient has to use his arms to prop himself up and/or swings his thighs and legs over the side of the bed to enlist the aid of gravity in lifting the trunk, suspect weakness of the trunk muscles. Such weakness may occur with polymyositis, the muscular dystrophies, and a paraneoplastic syndrome.

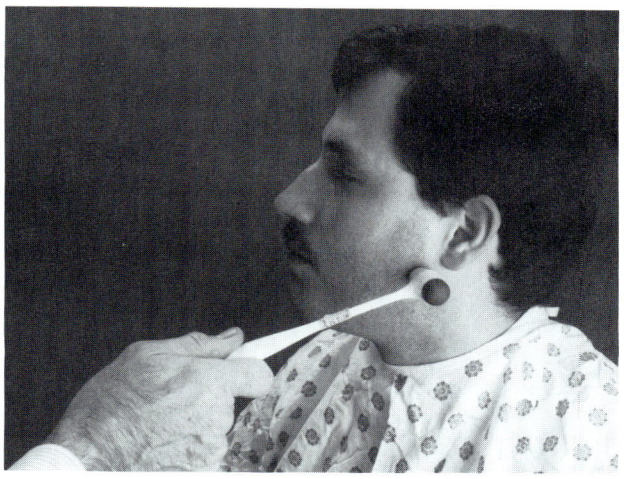

Fig. 10-8 Technique for eliciting Chvostek's sign.

ASSESSMENT OF MUSCLE TONE

Muscle tone is evaluated by passively but rapidly moving a segment of the patient's limb. In a limb weakened because of an upper motor neuron lesion, tonus of the muscle may be increased, causing *spasticity*. When the limb is extended, the resistance may suddenly cease, giving a clasp-knife effect. By contrast, when *cogwheel phenomenon* is present, as in parkinsonism, the limb flexes or extends as if being released by a series of cogs. If paralyzed limbs are neglected and not regularly moved passively, muscle fibrosis and shortening occurs, resulting in contractures. With lower motor neuron lesions, as may occur in poliomyelitis, paralysis is flaccid. Muscle atrophy occurs with both upper and lower motor neuron lesions and with marked weight loss, as in cancer cachexia.

ABNORMAL MOTOR FUNCTIONS

Fasciculations are twitchings observed in resting muscles. Sporadic coarse fasciculations may be observed in fatigued muscles or after cold exposure. Persistent fasciculations, especially in the presence of muscle weakness, may be the harbinger of a serious underlying disorder such as amyotrophic lateral sclerosis.

Tics are normal movements of muscle groups (such as winking or grinning) that occur *involuntarily* and seemingly inappropriately. They can be controlled with beta blockers, and they disappear during sleep.

Tetany is involuntary muscle spasms that may occur with several different disorders, including tetanus, hypocalcemia, hypomagnesemia, and hyperventilation syndrome. Two useful tests to check for latent tetany are Chvostek's sign and Trousseau's phenomenon. Chvostek's sign is elicited by tapping over the facial nerve anterior to the ear and checking for contraction of the facial muscles, especially the orbicularis oculi (Fig. 10-8). Trousseau's phenomenon is elicited by inflating a blood pressure cuff to systolic pressure and maintaining that for 2 to 3 minutes; induction of carpal-pedal spasm indicates latent tetany.

Tremors are oscillating movements caused by involuntary contraction of muscle groups. Fine tremors occur in several disorders but most commonly in alcohol withdrawal syndrome and hyperthyroidism; they may also be familial. A weak resting tremor is characteristic of parkinsonism and is often evident in the

Modalities of Sensation Tested
• Pain (superficial and deep) • Tactile (light touch) • Position sense • Vibration sense • Stereognosis • Two-point discrimination • Sensory extinction • Temperature (should be tested if abnormalities in pain and sensation are detected)

face and hands, the latter classically being a pill-rolling tremor. Interestingly, tremors disappear during sleep.

Sensory Examination

A complete evaluation of sensory function is generally not done in the routine physical examination. However, a history of pain in an extremity or the face and trunk, numbness, tingling, or the finding of motor deficits indicates the need for a detailed sensory evaluation (see accompanying box).

Fig. 10-9 details nerves subserving cutaneous function in the anterior and posterior aspects of the body.

PAIN

Testing for pain is a difficult part of the neurologic examination, and examiners are prone to errors, especially if they "lead" patients to answers. Avoid suggestions such as, "Is this pain sharper on this side?" Cutaneous pain sensation is evaluated by having the patient close his eyes and indicate whenever he feels a pinprick (Fig. 10-10). Ask the patient to compare pinprick sensation between the two sides of the face, trunk, upper extremities, and lower extremities. Pinprick sensation is evaluated on a longitudinal axis and can be related to specific dermatomes (see Fig. 10-9). This is important, for example, in determining a sensory level in patients with spinal cord injury or spinal cord compression by a tumor.

In checking pinprick sensation, ask the patient to indicate if sensation changes, especially below the midforearm as the hands are approached and in each leg as the ankles are approached. As discussed in more detail below, such a change is important in several disorders but especially so in patients with diabetes mellitus or chronic alcoholism with a peripheral neuropathy, in whom diminished sensation to pain and tactile sensation characteristically occurs in a "stocking-and-glove" distribution. The sensation of cutaneous pain may be normal, reduced *(hypalgesia)*, increased *(hyperalgesia)*, or absent *(analgesia)*.

If uncertain about the response to pinprick, mix a sharp sensation (pinprick) and a dull sensation (pin-guard on a safety pin). Deep pain can be tested for by pressure on the sternum, eyeballs, or the achilles tendon. Discard pin after use to prevent spread of disease.

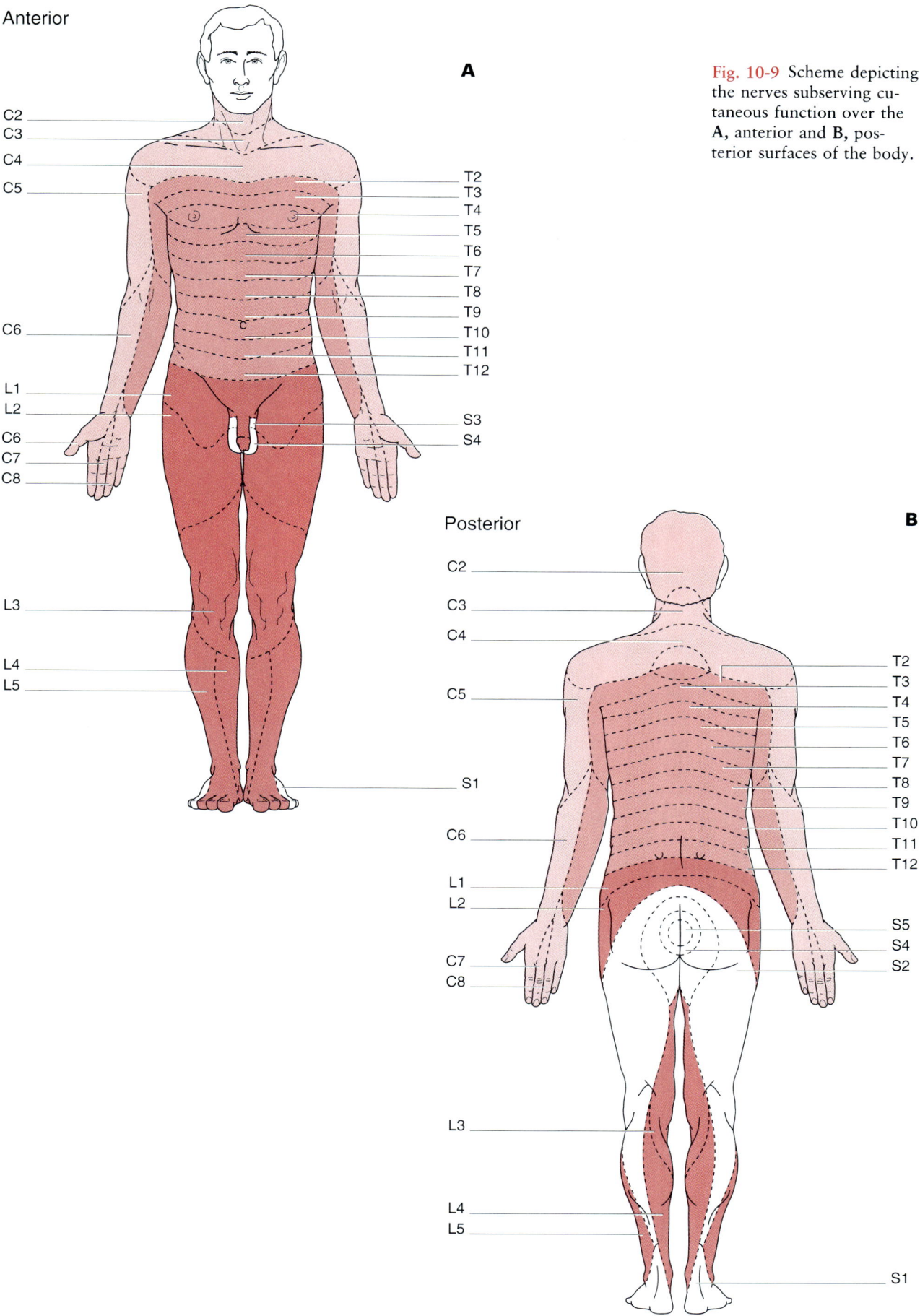

Fig. 10-9 Scheme depicting the nerves subserving cutaneous function over the **A**, anterior and **B**, posterior surfaces of the body.

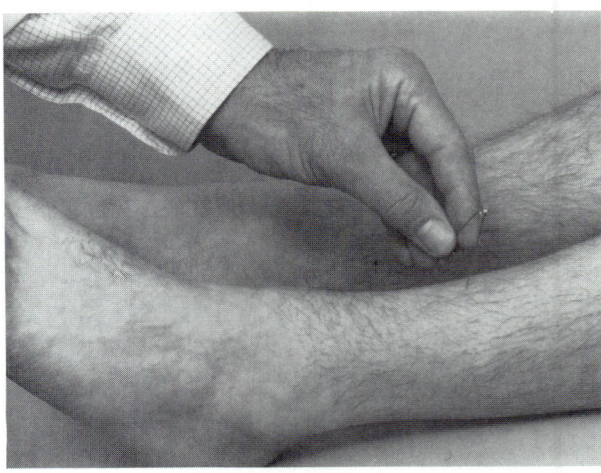

Fig. 10-10 Technique (pinprick) for assessing pain and abnormalities in pain sensation, especially hypalgesia or analgesia.

In the patient with an impaired pain response, also evaluate for temperature sensation (see below).

LIGHT TOUCH

Test for the sensation of light touch by gently stroking the patient's skin with a wisp of cotton and comparing the response at symmetric points (Fig. 10-11). An easy way to do this is to ask the patient to close his eyes and simply say "yes" each time he perceives the cotton touching him. As in testing for pain, test the two sides of the face, trunk, upper extremities, and lower extremities in an organized fashion. To ensure reliability of the findings, insert a few control tests when you do not actually touch the patient but ask him whether he does or does not feel the cotton.

Impaired light-touch sensation is termed *hypesthesia,* loss of light-touch sensation is termed *anesthesia,* and an exaggerated response is termed *hyperesthesia* or *hyperpathia.* Patients with peripheral neuropathy caused by diabetes or chronic alcoholism frequently have a stocking-and-glove hypalgesia and hypes-

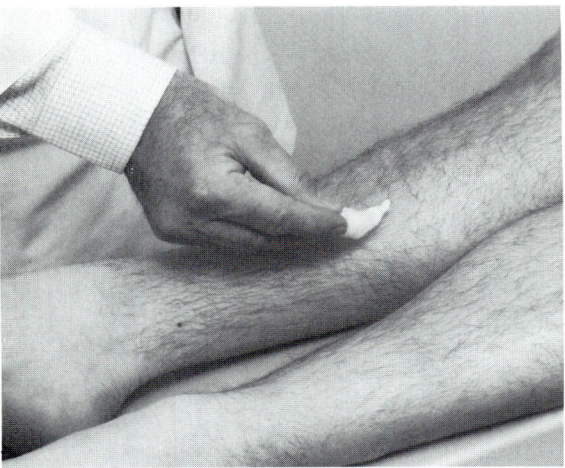

Fig. 10-11 Technique for assessing light touch and altered touch sensation (i.e., hypesthesia or anesthesia). For further details, see text.

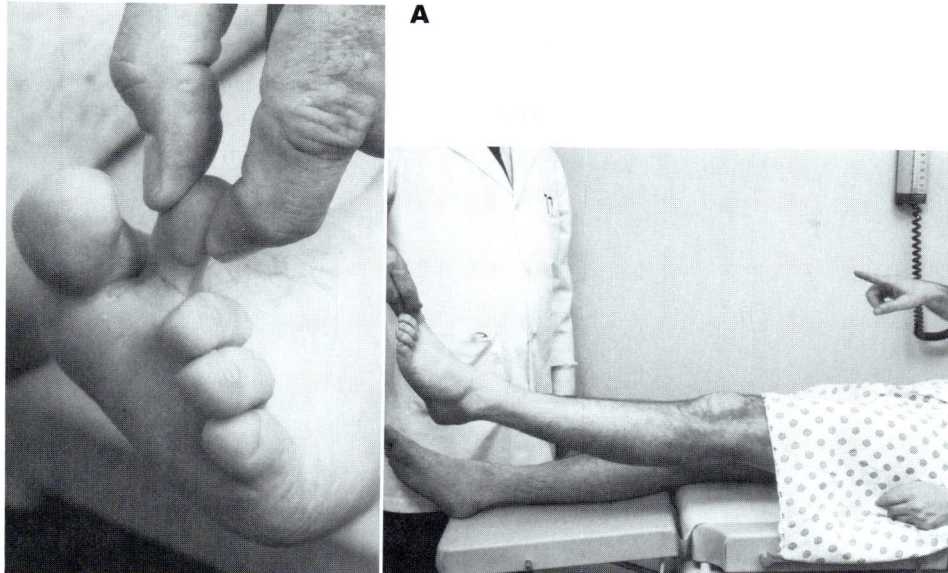

Fig. 10-12 A, Techniques for assessing position sense by moving the toe slowly in either an upward or downward direction. B, Alternative technique for assessing position sense by having the patient point with his right index finger towards the position of his left toe, which is being moved by the examiner. For details, see text.

thesia. Patients with a middle cerebral artery–occlusive lesion characteristically have a contralateral hypesthesia and hypalgesia in addition to the usually more obvious hemiparesis.

POSITION SENSE

Position sense is usually investigated using the toes and fingers by having the patient close his eyes, after which the examiner moves the toe or finger slowly in a vertical direction and asks the patient to identify whether the toe or finger is up, down, or midposition (Fig. 10-12). It is important for the examiner's fingers not to touch adjacent toes or fingers and to move the digit slowly so as not to give additional tactile clues to the direction of movement.

Another maneuver to evaluate position sense involves having the patient close his eyes while the examiner lifts the left foot by its big toe. Then ask the patient to point to the left big toe with his right hand (Fig. 10-12, B). Move the elevated foot and toe in different directions and again ask the patient to point to them. Impaired position sense occurs frequently with diseases involving the posterior columns such as pernicious anemia and tabes dorsalis and with peripheral neuropathies.

VIBRATION SENSE

Vibratory sensation is tested by placing the handle of a vibrating tuning fork with a 128 frequency on a bony prominence such as the malleoli of the ankles, knuckles of the hands, or epicondyles of the femurs (Fig. 10-13). Normally a modest decrease in vibratory sense occurs in the lower extremities in elderly patients. The patient should indicate whether he feels the vibrations and when they cease. Make control tests by getting the tuning fork to vibrate audibly and then unobtrusively stopping it before applying the handle to the patient. Impaired vibration sense occurs with diseases affecting the posterior columns and with peripheral neuropathies.

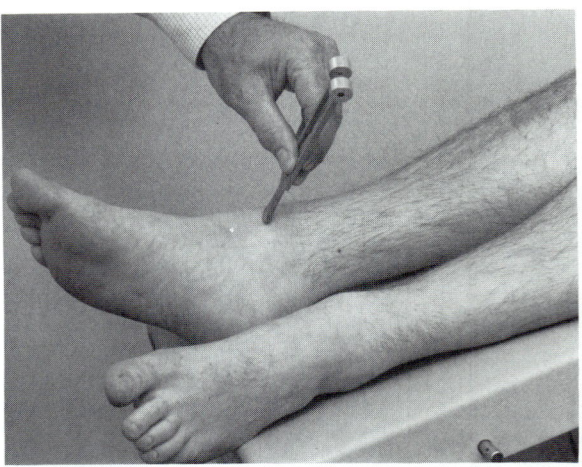

Fig. 10-13 Testing for vibratory sense with a tuning fork placed over a bony prominence such as the medial malleolus.

STEREOGNOSIS

Stereognosis is a higher integrative function wherein patients are able to determine the form, size, texture, and identity of familiar objects. This is tested by having the patient close his eyes and placing in his hand objects such as different coins, a pencil or pen, paper clip, and eyeglasses, all of which should be readily identified. *Astereognosis,* or the inability to define common objects by touch, occurs with cortical diseases, as in dementia, and after CVAs.

TWO-POINT DISCRIMINATION

Two-point discrimination is tested by touching the skin with two pinpoints simultaneously and determining the distance at which a patient can distinguish between one and two points. The distance for two-point distinction varies considerably, from 3 mm on the finger tips to 8 millimeters on the hands, to a few centimeters on the arms and several centimeters on the thighs.

SENSORY EXTINCTION

Sensory extinction is tested by applying the same stimulus (i.e., a pinprick) simultaneously to two sides of the body. If a parietal lobe lesion is present, the patient may correctly perceive the pinpricks if they are applied to the two sides *consecutively.* However, if they are applied *simultaneously,* he does not perceive the pinprick on the affected side; it is masked.

TEMPERATURE

Temperature sensation is not tested for routinely, but it is clearly indicated if the pain sense is impaired. A simple way to do this is to fill small glasses or test tubes with either hot or cold water and place these sequentially in the same position on the patient's skin. Another clue to impaired temperature sensation is burns on the skin that the patient did not appreciate. Lesions in the lateral spinothalamic tract may result in impaired pain and temperature sensation but preserved light-touch sensation, as exemplified by the rare disorder syringomyelia.

Cerebellar Function and Tests of Coordination

Several tests are available and done routinely to evaluate coordination, which in turn largely reflects cerebellar function (see box opposite).

Tests of Cerebellar Function and Coordination

Dysnergia, Dysmetria, Intention Tremor
- Finger-to-nose test
- Finger-to-finger test
- Heel-to-shin test

Dysdiadochokinesia
- Rapid alternating movement
- Hand clapping
- Heel tapping
- Rebound sign

Speech
- Test phrases for scanning speech

Gait and Station
- Normal walking
- Tandem walking
- Walking on heels and then toes
- Romberg's sign
- Titubation
- Specific gait disturbance

DYSERGIA, DYSMETRIA, AND INTENTION TREMOR

Dysergia is defined as improper coordinated function of given muscle groups. *Dysmetria* is defined as the inability to gauge properly the distance between two points or objects. Three tests are used to test for dysergia and dysmetria. In the finger-to-nose test, ask the patient to extend his elbow and rapidly move the tip of the index finger to the tip of the nose (Fig. 10-14). This can be done both with the patient's eyes open and then closed.

The finger-to-finger movement is a variation of this test, in which the patient moves his index finger back and forth between the tip of his nose and your finger (Fig. 10-15). You can then vary the position of your finger. In both tests,

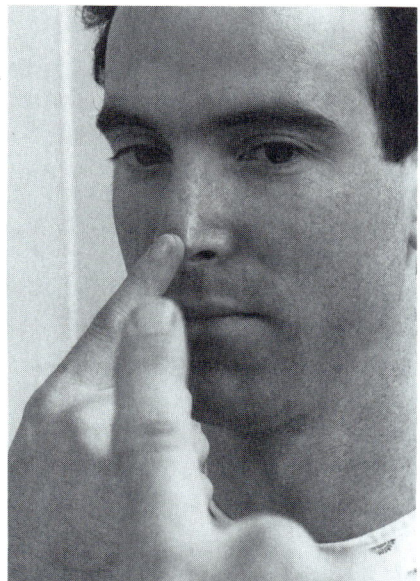

Fig. 10-14 Technique for performing the finger-to-nose test. The examiner's finger indicates how far the patient should extend his finger before touching his nose. For details, see text.

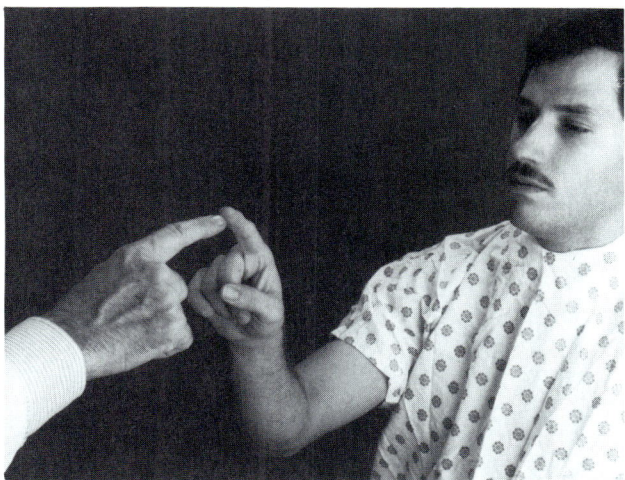

Fig. 10-15 Technique for performing the finger-to-finger test. Ask the patient to repeatedly touch the examiner's index finger as it moves laterally and up and down.

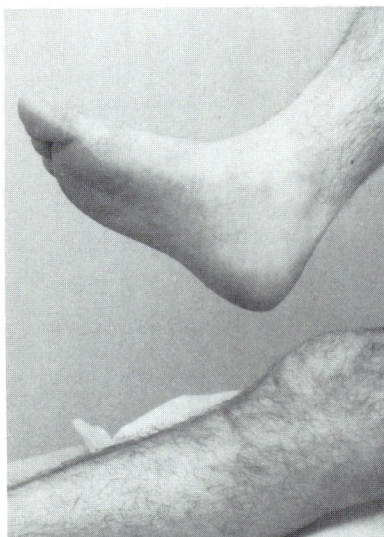
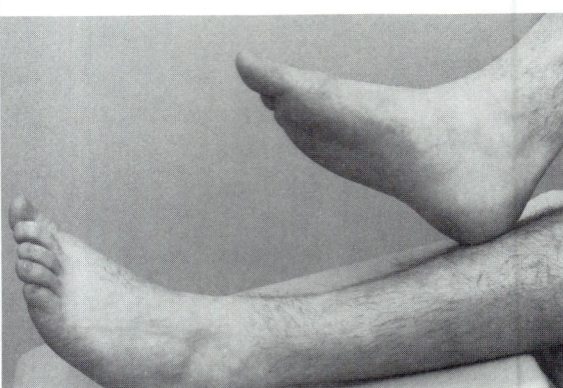

Fig. 10-16 The heel-to-shin test is useful in assessing cerebellar function. Ask the patient to position his heel a few inches above the knee **(A)**, then slide it straight down the shin **(B)**. For details, see text.

specifically look for tremulous or uncoordinated movement and "overshooting" either the nose or your finger.

The heel-to-shin test is done when the patient is supine. Ask the patient to place one heel directly over the opposite knee and hold it there 3 to 6 inches above the knee. Then ask the patient to slide the heel down the shin to the ankle (Fig. 10-16). Again, note any uncoordinated, jerking, or inaccurate movements.

An *intention tremor*, in which initiation of a voluntary movement results in tremor, occurs frequently in cerebellar disease such as multiple sclerosis, alcoholic cerebellar degeneration, and after cerebellar infarction.

DYSDIADOCHOKINESIA

Dysdiadochokinesia is defined as the inability to arrest abruptly one motor impulse and substitute its opposite. To test rapid alternating movements, ask the patient to pronate and supinate his hand on a flat surface such as a table or his thigh (Fig. 10-17). Alternatively, ask the patient to clap his hands in a triplet,

Fig. 10-17 Technique for assessing rapid alternating movements by rapidly **A,** pronating and **B,** supinating the wrists on the anterior thighs.

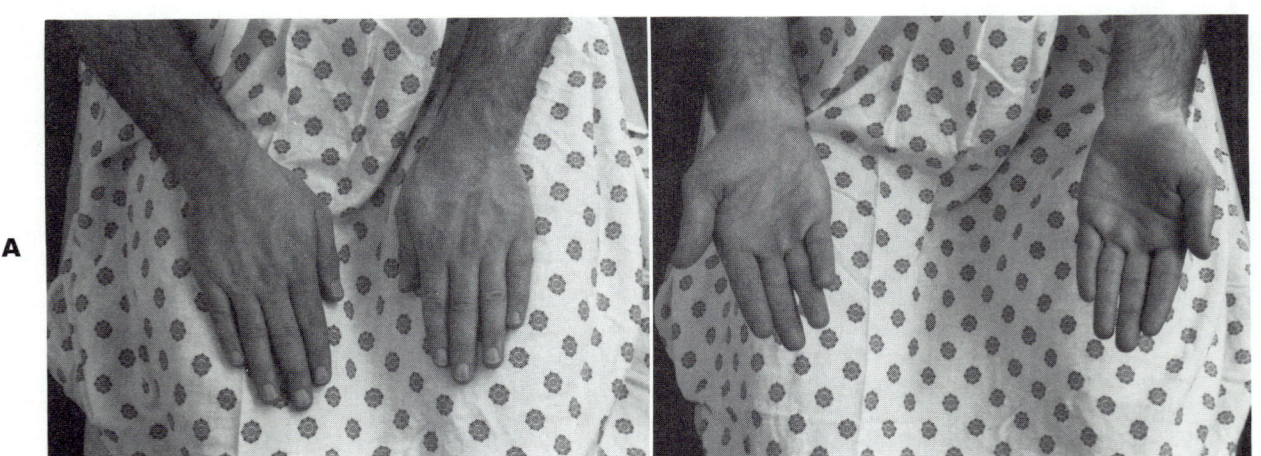

TABLE 10-2: Disturbances of Gait and Station

Condition	Abnormality
1. Hemiplegia–hemiparesis	• Affected area immobile, with elbow, wrist, and fingers flexed. • Difficulty flexing hip and knee and dorsiflexing ankle so that on walking either paretic leg swings outward or patient drags foot, scraping the toe.
2. Parkinsonism	• Characteristic posture of flexion with thoracic spine and head bent forward, arms flexed and immobile, and steps short and shuffling. Steps may become more rapid (festination).
3. Cerebellar ataxia	• Gait is wide based, unsteady, and staggering. Attempting to stand with feet together provokes swaying or falling whether the eyes are open or closed.
4. Sensory ataxia	• Loss of position sense in the feet and legs caused by disease processes in the posterior columns of the spinal cord, dorsal roots, and peripheral nerves results in a characteristic gait disorder. The gait is unsteady with the feet wide apart as the patients watch the ground for guidance. The legs are lifted higher than normal and the feet thrown forward and outward, coming down first on the heels and then on the toes, resulting in a characteristic double tapping sound.
5. Foot drop	• This can result from peripheral neuropathy (lead poisoning, drugs such as isonicotinic acid hydyrazide [INH]) and lower motor neuron disease. Such patients either drag their feet or lift them high, with knees flexed, and bring them down with a slap onto the floor, thus appearing to be walking up stairs. They are unable to walk on their heels.

accentuating the third clap. Similarly, ask the patient to rapidly tap his heel rhythmically on the floor. During all three of these tests, note any uncoordinated movements.

Finally, check the rebound sign. Place downward pressure on the patient's wrist while holding the arm in an extended and lateral position; as you quickly release your hand, the patient's arm "overshoots" in an upward movement; such a reaction is abnormal. The lateral extended position is advised to minimize the likelihood of the patient striking himself with this maneuver.

SPEECH

Scanning speech, in which there is undue separation of syllables while words seem to run together, occurs frequently in cerebellar disease. To check for scanning speech, ask the patient to repeat phrases such as "third riding Massachusetts artillery brigade" or "Methodist Episcopal."

GAIT AND STATION

Some common disturbances of gait and station are highlighted in Table 10-2. The examiner can initially assess a patient's gait when the patient enters the examining room. A further test of gait is having him walk back and forth. In addition, ask the patient to turn quickly and walk in tandem (i.e., heel to toe; walk on the heels and then walk on the toes). Note whether the walk is wavering, lurching, or staggering and whether the gait is wide based.

Abnormalities in gait can be caused by either cerebellar disease or posterior column disease. Patients with *central* cerebellar lesions are unsteady when walking and stagger from one side to the other and have difficulty in turning, but may show none of the so-called conventional cerebellar signs such as dysmetria

Fig. 10-18 Assessing station by having the patient stand with feet close together and eyes closed and gently nudging the patient to see if balance is lost.

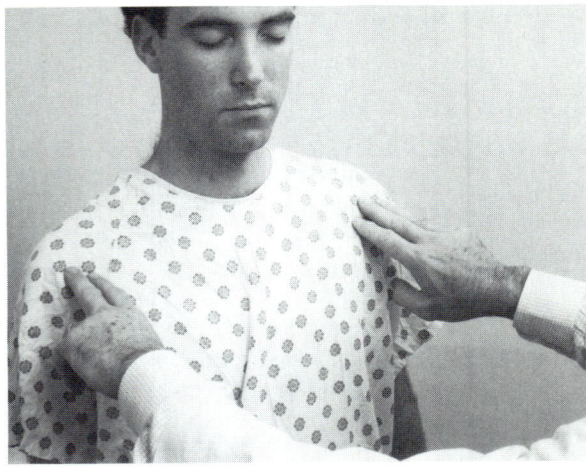

or past pointing, which are associated with *hemisphere* lesions. With diseases of the posterior columns, proprioceptive impulses are impaired and gait disturbance (i.e., ataxia) is much greater with the eyes closed.

To further test equilibratory function, ask the patient to stand with the feet touching each other and assess his ability to maintain his balance. Then nudge the patient gently on the sternum or shoulders to see if balance is maintained—but be sure to safeguard the patient against a fall. Perform these tests with the eyes open and then closed; a loss of balance with the eyes closed is termed a *positive Romberg sign* (Fig. 10-18). *Titubation* refers to a body tremor that is most evident when standing or walking. It is often a sign of cerebellar disease.

Other disorders result in characteristic abnormalities in gait. The gait seen in Parkinson's disease, *festinating gait,* is characterized by rapid, short shuffling steps, absence of swinging arm movement, and trunk and neck flexed in a forward position as if the patient is about to fall. Patients with hemiparesis after a CVA may have an obvious disparity in leg movements while the arm remains in a dependent position. In patients with chorea, walking is accompanied by bizarre, often uncontrollable movements. Finally, in evaluating gait disturbances, one should also be mindful of arthritic, traumatic, or musculoskeletal problems that can result in an abnormal gait (see Chapter 9).

Reflexes

Evaluation of normal reflexes and detection of abnormal reflexes is an integral part of the neurologic examination, as this segment of the examination often provides key findings pointing to a specific diagnosis (see box opposite).

NORMAL REFLEXES

Deep Tendon Reflexes

Evaluation of the deep tendon reflexes of the upper extremities should include the biceps, triceps, and brachioradialis. The *biceps reflex* is elicited by placing your thumb over the biceps tendon with the patient's arm in flexion and relaxation (Fig. 10-19). With the reflex hammer, strike a series of blows against your thumb, which will transmit the blow to the patient. The normal reflex response is elbow flexion. The *triceps reflex* is obtained by having the patient's arm abducted at the

Key Reflexes to Check

Normal Reflexes

- Deep tendon reflexes (DTRs)
- Biceps
- Triceps
- Brachioradialis
- Patellar (quadriceps) and variants
- Ankle (achilles)
- Superficial reflexes
- Abdominal
- Cremasteric
- Brainstem reflexes
- Corneal reflex
- Pupillary reaction to light
- Gag reflex
- Orbicularis oculi
- Jaw jerk

Abnormal Reflexes

- Pyramidal tract disease
- Hyperactive DTRs
- Muscle clonus
- Babinski's sign and variants (Chaddock's, Oppenheim's, and Gordon's signs)
- Hoffmann's sign
- Absense of superficial reflexes
- Primitive reflexes
- Snout/suck
- Grasp
- Palmomental

Application of reflexes in determining death

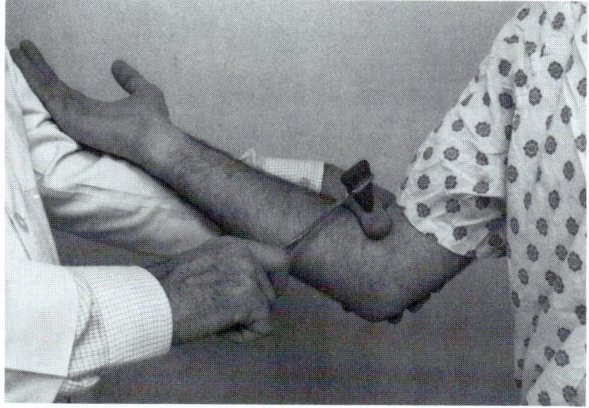

Fig. 10-19 Technique for eliciting biceps reflex.

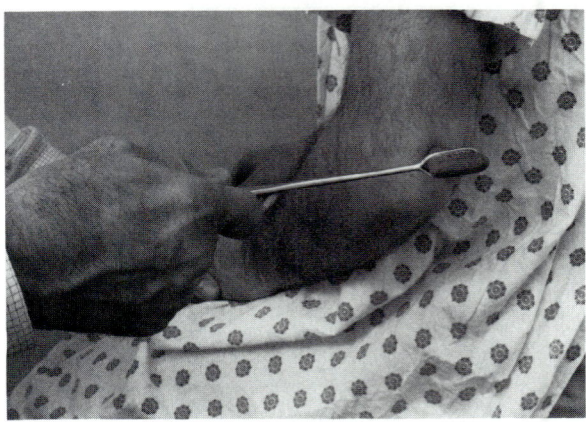

Fig. 10-20 Technique for eliciting triceps reflex.

shoulder, flexed at the elbow, and supported by your hand or resting on the thigh (Fig. 10-20). Tap the triceps tendon part above the olecranon process. The normal response is extension of the forearm. The *brachioradialis reflex* is elicited by placing the patient's arm on his thigh in a relaxed and partially pronated position and tapping the distal radius (Fig. 10-21). A normal response is contraction of the brachioradialis, resulting in flexion and partial supination of the forearm.

Evaluation of the deep tendon reflexes of the lower extremities consists of patellar, suprapatellar, and achilles reflexes. The *patellar reflex* is obtained by direct percussion of the patellar tendon just distal to the patella (Fig. 10-22). The normal response is extension of the leg and contraction of the quadriceps muscles, which may be quite obvious. This reflex can be elicited either with the patient sitting and legs dangling over the side of an examining table, or with the patient supine with the knees slightly bent and supported by your forearm to effect

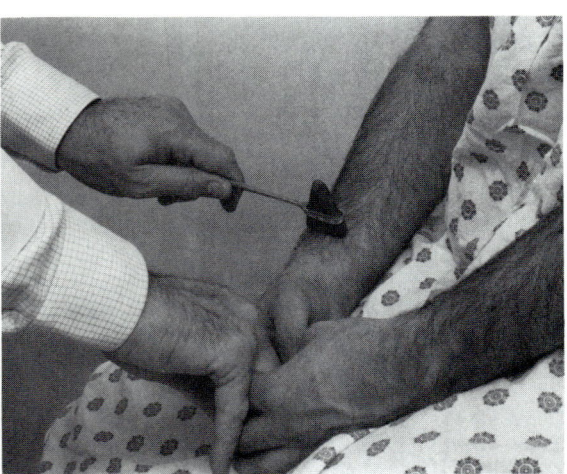

Fig. 10-21 Technique for eliciting brachioradialis reflex.

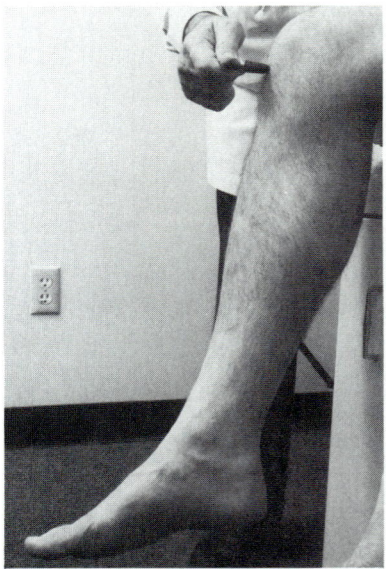

Fig. 10-22 Technique for eliciting patellar reflex (knee jerk).

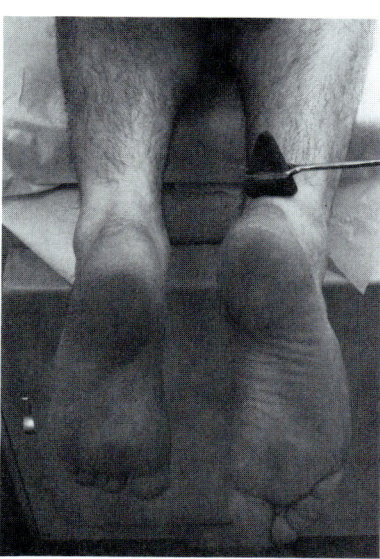

Fig. 10-23 Technique for eliciting achilles reflex (ankle jerk). Note the downward movement of the right foot in response to tapping the achilles tendon.

relaxation. The *suprapatellar reflex* is elicited by tapping above the patella; the response is extension of the leg. This reflex is often hyperactive with upper motor neuron lesions, as discussed below.

The achilles reflex is elicited by tapping the achilles tendon; the normal response is plantar flexion of the foot. The *achilles reflex* can be obtained in several ways, as listed below:

- Have the patient kneel on the examining table with his feet extending over the side (Fig. 10-23)
- Have the patient sit with his legs dangling over the edge of the examining table while you gently support the foot in dorsiflexion
- Have the patient place his leg over the other shin while you dorsiflex the foot

Deep tendon reflexes are conventionally graded on a five-point scale, as follows:

Grade	Definition
0	Complete absence of the reflex
1	Reflex present but diminished
2	Normal reflex
3	Hyperactive reflex
4	Markedly hyperactive reflex, often with *clonus,* a rhythmic contraction of muscles initiated by stretching (see below for more details)

If the grading of a reflex is in question and especially if it appears to be diminished or absent, repeat the testing with reinforcement. This is accomplished by having the patient pull on his interlocked fingers or clinch his fists just before the test (Jendrassik's maneuver).

Fig. 10-24 Technique for eliciting ankle clonus. Note the examiner's right hand dorsiflexing the patient's right foot. For details, see text.

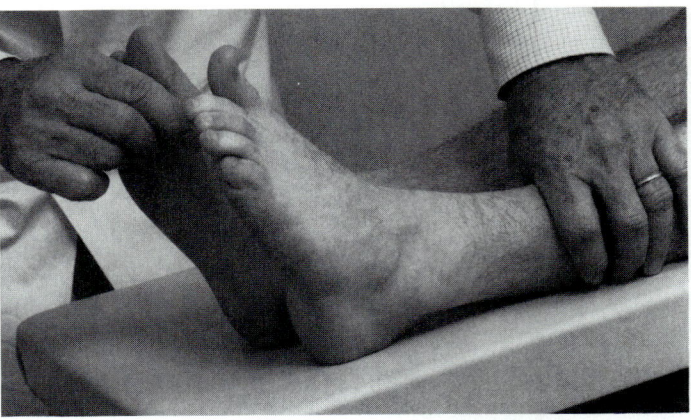

Superficial Reflexes

The superficial reflexes frequently tested are the upper and lower abdominal and the cremasteric reflexes. The *upper abdominal reflexes* are elicited by stroking the skin in the RUQ and LUQ with a split-tongue blade or head of a pin and noting whether ipsilateral contraction of muscles occurs on the stroked side. Similarly, the *lower abdominal reflexes* are obtained by stroking the skin in the RLQ and LLQ. In males, the *cremasteric reflex* is elicited by stroking the inner aspect of the thigh in a distal direction. The normal response is contraction of the cremaster muscle, with elevation of the testis on the ipsilateral side.

Brainstem Reflexes

Brainstem reflexes frequently tested include the corneal reflex, the pupillary reaction to light, and the gag reflex (all discussed in detail below under the cranial nerves), the consensual pupillary response, the orbicularis oculi reflex, and the jaw jerk. If light is shone in one eye, the other pupil constricts *(consensual pupillary response)*. If bright light is shone in the eye, the pupil constricts; the *orbicularis oculi reflex* is the closing of the eyelids when the eye is exposed to bright light. If the lateral margin of the cornea is stroked with a wisp of cotton, the eyelids blink. If the pharynx is gently stroked with a tongue blade, gagging occurs. The *jaw jerk* is the closure of the mouth when the chin is tapped with the mouth partially open.

ABNORMAL REFLEXES

Pyramidal Tract Disease

Lesions in the pyramidal tract (upper motor neuron), which may occur following a CVA, result in several abnormal reflexes. First, the deep tendon reflexes are hyperactive. Second, an additional abnormality of the stretch reflex may be present, such as clonus, the rhythmic contraction of muscles. Clonus can be elicited by dorsiflexing the foot; it may be sustained (Fig. 10-24). Third, pathologic reflexes may be present, the most important of which is Babinski's sign.

Babinski's sign is elicited by applying a firm stimulus to the lateral plantar surface of the foot (Fig. 10-25). The stimulus is usually the blunt end of a key, the pointed end of a reflex hammer, or the split edge of a wooden tongue blade. Importantly, the stimulus should not be painful. Before the stimulus is applied, advise the patient that his foot is about to be scratched and not to jerk his foot.

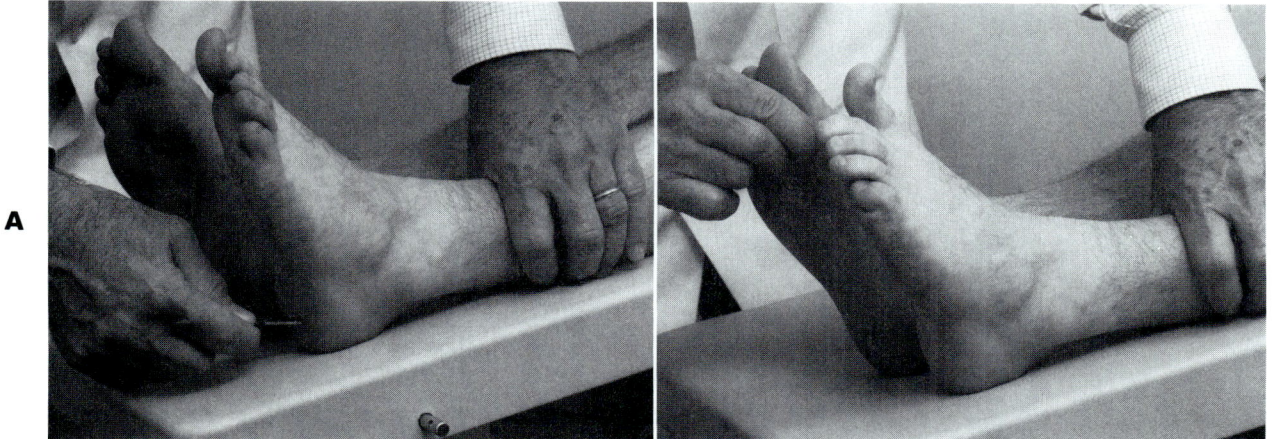

Fig. 10-25 Technique for eliciting Babinski's reflex. **A,** A key is placed over the lateral inferior margin of the heel and **B,** moved upward and medial. Note the positive response of dorsiflexion of the great toe. For further details and use of equivalent tests to assess for pyramidal tract signs, see text.

Hold the heel or ankle in one hand and apply the stimulus laterally on the sole of the foot from the heel to the ball of the foot where the course curves to follow the base of the toes. A normal response consists of all the toes curling down in plantar flexion. A positive Babinski's sign consists of dorsiflexion of the great toe and, usually, fanning of all the other toes. The dorsiflexion of the great toe is a hallmark of pyramidal tract lesions.

Because applying a firm stimuli to the side of the foot is a noxious stimulus, other tests can be employed. A positive response in all of them is dorsiflexion of the great toe, and this has the same significance as a positive Babinski's sign. *Chaddock's reflex* is elicited by using a key or dull point to scratch around the lateral malleolus and then along the lateral aspect of the dorsum of the foot. *Oppenheim's sign* is elicited by applying the knuckles to the skin of the tibia and sliding them downward to the ankle. *Gordon's sign* is elicited by squeezing the calf muscles and noting the response of the great toe.

Hoffmann's sign is elicited by first having the patient extend the middle finger and place it on the index finger of your hand (Fig. 10-26). With the patient's middle finger slightly dorsiflexed, flick the finger of the patient's extended middle finger. A positive response consists of flexion and adduction of the thumb. A unilateral positive Hoffmann's sign suggests pyramidal tract disease, especially if accompanied by the long tract signs discussed above. A bilateral positive Hoffmann's sign is of uncertain significance.

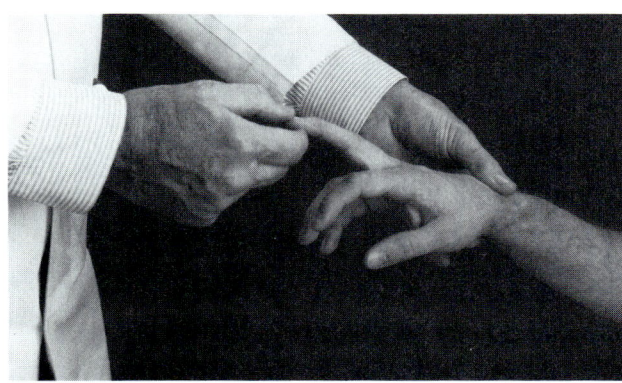

Fig. 10-26 Technique for eliciting Hoffmann's sign. The examiner flicks the nail of the extended middle finger of the dorsiflexed wrist and checks for flexion and adduction of the thumb.

Absence of Superficial Reflexes

The absence of superficial reflexes can be noted in several disorders. Characteristically, lesions of the pyramidal tracts that occur after a CVA result in complete unilateral suppression of superficial reflexes. Another example would be preservation of the upper abdominal reflexes but loss of the lower abdominal reflexes. Because the upper abdominal reflexes are innervated by thoracic nerves TN5 to TN9 and the lower abdominal reflexes by TN11 to TN12, this finding indicates a lesion involving TN10.

Primitive Reflexes

The primitive reflexes frequently reflect frontal lobe disease. The *snout*, or *suck, reflex* is elicited by gently tapping or rubbing the upper lip, which results in a puckering or sucking movement. The *grasp reflex* is obtained by stroking the patient's palm so that he grasps the examiner's finger between his thumb and index finger. A positive response is when the patient cannot release his fingers. The *palmomental sign* is elicited by scratching or rubbing the thenar eminence and noting whether this results in ipsilateral contraction of the muscles of the chin.

APPLICATION OF ABSENT REFLEXES AND OTHER FACTORS IN DETERMINING BRAIN DEATH

The criteria for brain death adopted by the staff at the Massachusetts General Hospital and the Harvard Committee on brain death are as follows:

1. Death occurs when all signs of receptivity and responsivity are absent
2. All brainstem reflexes are absent, including pupillary reactions, ocular movement, blinking, swallowing, and oculocephalic and caloric responses
3. The electroencephalogram (EEG) is isoelectric or flat
4. Spontaneous respiration has ceased

The Cranial Nerves

All of the cranial nerves except CN1 are tested as part of the routine physical examination and routine neurologic examination. Table 10-3 summarizes pertinent information on (1) tests to evaluate the cranial nerves, (2) interpretation of the findings, and (3) key disorders affecting cranial nerve function. (For a detailed discussion of the facial nerves, see Chapter 2.)

TABLE 10-3: The Cranial Nerves

Number of Nerve	Function	Tests to Evaluate	Interpretation of Findings and Disorders Affecting Function
I — Olfactory	Smell	• With the eyes closed, have the patient identify familiar aromatic substances such as coffee, peppermint, tobacco, or vanilla; only complete absence or some obvious perversion of smell is significant	• Causes of *neural* olfactory loss include head trauma with and without fracture of cribriform plate, neoplasm of anterior cranial fossa (meningioma, glioma, pituitary adenoma), neurosurgical procedures, and neurotoxic drugs; sensory olfactory loss can occur after viral infections and can be familial

TABLE 10-3: The Cranial Nerves—cont'd

Number of Nerve	Function	Tests to Evaluate	Interpretation of Findings and Disorders Affecting Function
II—Optic	Vision	• Examine the fundi with an ophthalmoscope, noting optic nerve color, disc margins, presence of hemorrhage or exudates • Check visual acuity by using eye chart or asking patient to read newsprint • Check visual fields by confrontation (see Chapter 2) • Check pupillary reaction to light	• Amaurosis fugax or transient painless loss of vision in one eye indicates retinal ischemia, which is most commonly caused by ipsilateral internal carotid artery stenosis
III—Oculomotor	Motor nerve to five extrinsic eye muscles • Medial rectus: abduction • Superior rectus: elevation and internal rotation • Inferior rectus: depression and external rotation • Inferior oblique: elevation and external rotation • Levator palpebrae	• For a detailed description of the evaluation of the extraocular movement, see Chapter 2 • Briefly, in evaluating cranial nerves III, IV, and VI, one checks the pupillary response to light and accommodation and notes whether the pupils are equal in size—check also for ptosis (drooping of the eyelid) and importantly, assess the range of movement of both eyes (see Chapter 2) • Check for involuntary jerking of the eyes (nystagmus) while examining lateral gaze and note whether or not it is sustained • Check pupillary response to accommodation	• Unilateral third nerve palsy should raise the questions of (1) subarachnoid bleed resulting from an aneurysm; (2) diabetes mellitus (pupil is spared); (3) atherosclerosis • Horner's syndrome is characterized by miosis, ptosis, and anhydrosis or impaired sweating over the face; the abrupt development of Horner's syndrome should raise the question of bronchogenic carcinoma with involvement of the superior cervical ganglion
IV—Trochlear	• Superior oblique eye muscle; depression and external rotation	• See above and Chapter 2	
V—Trigeminal	• Sensory root —Ophthalmic branch to cornea, conjunctiva, nasal cavity and sinuses, skin, forehead, eyebrows, nose —Maxillary branch to nose, lower eyelid, upper lip —Mandibular branch to lower face, lower lip, anterior two-thirds of the tongue, gums, teeth • Motor root innervates face and jaw muscles and masseters (mastication)	• Check corneal reflex by having patient look upward and touch cornea at the limbus with a wisp of cotton; normally, involuntary blinking occurs • With the eyes closed, test sensation over the face with a wisp of cotton • Check motor root by having patient clench his teeth while palpating masseter and temperal muscles bilaterally • Check the jaw jerk, which tests both the sensory and motor components	• Loss of corneal reflex with/without impaired sensation over upper face is seen with cerebellopontine angle tumors • Irritative lesions of sensory root may cause tic douloreux • Trismus or spasm of muscles of mastication should raise the question of tetanus or adverse reaction to phenothiazines • Unilateral masseter weakness or deviation of mandible to weak side may be seen with unilateral paralysis after a CVA

Continued.

TABLE 10-3: The Cranial Nerves—cont'd

Number of Nerve	Function	Tests to Evaluate	Interpretation of Findings and Disorders Affecting Function
VI—Abducens	• Lateral rectus eye muscle: abduction of the eye	• See above and Chapter 2	• Isolated sixth nerve palsy is frequently caused by diabetes mellitus, neoplasm, atherosclerosis or increased ICP
VII—Facial	• Sensory fibers to anterior two-thirds of tongue (taste), ear canal, and postauricular urea • Motor fibers to muscles of face	• Taste not routinely tested, but if indicated, add sugar, salt, and vinegar to extended tongue; assess with mouth rinsed between tests • Test motor functions by noting how patient: —Smiles and blinks naturally —Elevates eyebrows and wrinkles forehead —Forcibly closes eyelids against resistance —Shows his teeth —Puffs cheeks out —Whistles • Check nasolabial folds	• The tests listed permit differentiation between a peripheral facial palsy (lower motor neuron lesion) and a central facial palsy (upper motor neuron lesion). In general, in upper motor neuron lesions (for example following a CVA), the forehead muscle and upper eyelid are spared, whereas the lower face is affected. This is caused by bilateral innervation of forehead muscles from the cerebral cortex. By contrast, in a peripheral facial palsy caused by involvement of the seventh cranial nerve or its nucleus, all the muscles of one side of face are affected. The most common isolated seventh nerve palsy, cause unknown, is Bell's palsy.
VIII—Acoustic	• Cochlear portion subserves auditory function or hearing	• Obvious defects in hearing may be detected by responses to a ticking watch, rubbing of the thumb and index finger together next to the patient's ear, a tuning fork, or the whispered voice	• Impaired hearing can result from lesions in the external auditory canal, middle ear, inner ear, or central auditory pathways. Always check for obstruction of the external canal by cerumen. Perforated tympanic membrane, fixation of ossicles as in otosclerosis, damage to the organ of Corti by intense noise, ototoxic drugs, and neoplasms all can result in hearing loss.
	• Vestibular portion subserves spatial orientation, balance of equilibrium, and posture	• See Chapter 2 for a detailed analysis of the tests of labyrinthine function	• Vertigo can result from lesions of the vestibular, visual, or somatosensory system, vestibular dysfunction being the most common. Such labyrinthine dysfunction can be caused by infarction, trauma, ischemia, or toxins and may be recurrent

TABLE 10-3: The Cranial Nerves—cont'd

Number of Nerve	Function	Tests to Evaluate	Interpretation of Findings and Disorders Affecting Function
VIII—Acoustic—cont'd		• Weber's test—place vibrating tuning fork over vertex of skull and assess whether it is heard equally in both ears	• If a disease affects the auditory apparatus, the tuning fork will be heard best in the nonaffected ear. If the ear canal is obstructed, the tuning fork will appear louder on the affected side.
		• Rinne test—place vibrating tuning fork near auditory canal (air conduction) and then over mastoid process (bone conduction) and assess response	• Air-conducted (AC) sound is better appreciated then bone-conducted (BC) sound. A reversal whereby BC is greater than AC implies organ damage rather than nerve impairment.
IX—Glossopharyngeal	• Sensory —Sensation in posterior one third tongue and oropharynx, soft palate, vocal cords, and epiglottis —Taste in posterior one third of tongue • Motor: innervates the stylopharyngeus muscle	• This is tested with the vagus nerve as detailed below	• See below under vagus • Glossopharyngeal neuralgia resembles trigeminal neuralgia and is characterized by recurrent paroxysms of intense pain in the throat, often triggered by swallowing
X—Vagus	• Carries sensory and motor fibers to the muscles of the palate and oropharynx • Gives rise to the superior and inferior laryngeal nerve	• Have patient open mouth and say "aah," which normally causes contraction of the soft palate and *elevation* of the uvula in the midline • Touch the back of the tongue with a tongue blade to check the gag reflex.	• Movement of the uvula towards one side (i.e., the strong side) can be seen after CVAs. The voice is often hoarse and nasal in quality. Pharyngeal branches of the vagus may be involved in diphtheria. The recurrent laryngeal nerve can be damaged by intrathoracic lesions (aortic aneurysm, bronchogenic carcinoma) or as a result of thyroid surgery.
XI—Spinal accessory	• Innervates sternocleidomastoid and trapezius muscles	• Have patient lift shoulders or turn chin to either side against pressure of examiner's hand	• Can be abnormal with disorders such as polymyositis
XII—Hypoglossal	• Innervates the tongue	• Have patient open mouth and extend tongue and note any deviation from the midline	• Tongue may deviate to the affected side in a patient with hemiparesis caused by a CVA. Fasiculations of the tongue indicate a lower motor neuron lesion involving the hypoglossal nerve

Components of the Mental Status Examination

- State of consciousness
- Orientation
- Ability to cooperate
- Mood appropriateness
- Thought processes (content, stream, coherence and relevance of thought)
- Memory for recent and remote events
- Ability to handle concepts and proverbs
- Practical skills (reading, counting, writing)
- Speech problems and recognition of aphasia

Classification of Coma and Differential Diagnosis

I. Diseases that cause no focal or lateralizing neurologic signs or alteration of the cellular content of the CSF; usually brainstem functions and CT are normal
   A. Intoxications: alcohol, barbiturates, opiates
   B. Metabolic disturbances: anoxia, diabetic acidosis, uremia, hepatic coma, hypercapnia, hypernatremia, myxedema coma
   C. Severe systemic infections: pneumonia, typhoid fever, malaria, septicemia, Waterhouse-Friderichsen syndrome
   D. Circulatory collapse from any cause, and cardiac decompensation in the aged
   E. Epilepsy: postictal states
   F. Hypertensive encephalopathy and eclampsia
   G. Hyperthermia or hypothermia
   H. Concussion

II. Diseases that cause meningeal irritation with blood or an excess of white cells in the CSF, usually without focal or lateralizing cerebral or brainstem signs; the CT scan may be normal or abnormal
   A. Subarachnoid hemorrhage from ruptured aneurysm, AV malformation, occasionally trauma
   B. Acute bacterial meningitis
   C. Some forms of viral encephalitis

III. Diseases that cause focal brainstem or lateralizing cerebral signs, with or without changes in the CSF; CT scan is usually abnormal
   A. Brain hemorrhage
   B. Cerebral infarction caused by thrombosis or embolism
   C. Brain abscess, subdural empyema
   D. Epidural and subdural hemorrhage and brain contusion
   E. Brain tumor
   F. Miscellaneous—thrombophlebitis, some forms of viral encephalitis, focal embolic encephalomalacia caused by bacterial endocarditis, acute hemorrhagic leukoencephalitis, disseminated (postinfectious) encephalomyelitis

Modified from Adams R, Victor M: *Principles of neurology,* ed 3, New York, 1985, McGraw-Hill, p 267.

The Mental Status Examination

In the course of the routine physical examination, you will have had an opportunity to observe the patient's state of consciousness, orientation, ability to cooperate in the examination summary, and language ability. However, more formal testing of mental status is an integral part of the neurologic examination. Key elements in the mental status examination are listed in the top box opposite.

STATE OF CONSCIOUSNESS

You can readily ascertain whether a patient is alert, obtunded, or unconscious. For a detailed discussion of unconsciousness, see the section on the approach to the comatose patient (see bottom box opposite and Table 10-4).

ORIENTATION

The patient should be able to state correctly the date, place, and time as well as his own name.

ABILITY TO COOPERATE

You should have noted whether the patient is able to respond to questions and respond to requests in an appropriate manner. Failure to cooperate should raise several questions, including the state of consciousness, intrinsic CNS disease with a receptive aphasia (see below), underlying psychiatric problems, or whether you are dealing with an antagonistic and/or uncooperative patient.

TABLE 10-4: Glasgow Coma Scale to Assess the Level of Coma

Response	Points
Verbal responses	
• Oriented	5
• Confused	4
• Inappropriate words	3
• Incomprehensible	2
• None	1
Eye Opening	
• Spontaneously	4
• In response to speech	3
• In response to pain	2
• None	1
Motor Responses	
• Obeys commands	6
• Localizes pain	5
• Withdrawn	4
• Abnormal flexion	3
• Abnormal extension	2
• None	1

From Teasdale G, Jennette B: Assessment of coma and impaired consciousness: a practical scale, *Lancet* 2:81-84, 1974.

MOOD

Note the appropriateness of the patient's mood (i.e., whether he is anxious, angry, euphoric, or worried and especially if symptoms and signs suggestive of depression are present). For a more detailed discussion of depression and its recognition, see Chapter 11.

THOUGHT PROCESSES

Note the patient's thought processes, in particular the content and stream of thought, and whether it is coherent and relevant. The relating of information and reiteration of symptoms as well as any ideas and concepts should be understandable. Note whether he exhibits flight of ideas or discontinuous and inappropriate expression, and whether the patient has had any delusions or hallucinations. The presence of delusions or hallucinations may indicate a serious disturbance in thought processes, as may occur in schizophrenia, alcohol withdrawal syndromes, and toxic deliriums. For further details, see Chapter 11.

MEMORY FOR RECENT AND REMOTE EVENTS

The patient should be able to recall his past medical history in reasonable detail. The examiner can also check remote memory by asking questions about presidents and important world events. Short-term memory and the ability to retain new information can be tested by having the patient remember a set of digits, several objects, names of three or more people, or a simple sentence. The Babcock sentence is frequently used: "One thing a nation must have to be rich and great is a large secure supply of wood." A short memory span, arbitrarily defined as the inability to remember the type of information described above after a few minutes, should raise the question of intrinsic CNS disease as exemplified by the dementias. For further details on dementia, see Chapter 11.

ABILITY TO HANDLE CONCEPTS AND PROVERBS

Ask the patient to interpret some well-known proverbs such as the following:

- "Don't cross your bridges until you come to them."
- "A rolling stone gathers no moss."
- "People who live in glass houses should not throw stones."

Patients may be unable to interpret such proverbs or they may give very concrete answers. Their response may indicate either a dull normal patient, an uncooperative patient, organic CNS disease, or psychosis.

PRACTICAL SKILLS

Ask the patient to do any or all of the following:

- Read from a newspaper
- Write his name
- Spell some common five-letter words
- Do serial math by subtracting 7 from 100, then from the sum, and so on
- Delete all examples of the capital letter *A* from one or two paragraphs of newsprint

The above tests may be abnormal in patients with subtle disorders such as subclinical hepatic encephalopathy, Wernicke-Korsakoff syndrome, early Alzheimer's disease, and dementia caused by multiple small cerebral infarcts.

SPEECH PROBLEMS AND RECOGNITION OF APHASIA

In the course of the routine examination as well as neurologic assessment, you should have noted the rhythm of speech, ability to enunciate, the appropriate use of words, and any abnormal speech. *Dysarthria* (difficulty in articulating words) occurs with impaired movement of the palate, tongue, or lips, most frequently as a consequence of CNS lesions. Difficulty in speaking can result from impaired function of the vocal cords or larynx *(dysphonia);* with laryngitis, dysphonia is painful.

Aphasia (the inability to either produce or understand the spoken and/or written word) can be either receptive or expressive. A receptive aphasia is usually recognized by the patient's inability to understand questions or instructions and respond appropriately. Thus a patient may be unable to identify objects such as coins, paper clips, notebooks, a pen, a newspaper, or eyeglasses when asked to do so after they are placed in front of him. The patient can also be asked to write his own name or some simple phrases. An expressive aphasia often results in a broken or halting speech pattern. This can be elicited by asking the patient to read aloud from a newspaper.

Recognition of Some Common Neurologic Problems

Identifying a constellation of clinical findings that may well point to a specific diagnosis is often useful. The accompanying box lists some common neurologic problems and the key findings in the neurologic examination that support the diagnosis (Figs. 10-27 to 10-30).

Recognition of Some Common Neurologic Problems

Middle Cerebral Thrombosis/Embolism (see Figs. 10-27 and 10-28)

- Contralateral hemiparesis, arm > leg
- Contralateral pyramidal tract signs
- Spasticity
- Hyperactive DTRs
- Positive Babinski's/Chaddock's signs
- Contralateral hypalgesia and hypesthesia
- Contralateral loss of abdominal reflexes
- Aphasia if dominant hemisphere involved
- Contralateral central facial weakness (CN VII)

Common Carotid or Internal Carotid Artery High-Grade Stenosis

- Clinical picture varies depending on thrombosis propagation, embolic events, and markedly decreased flow; may be asymptomatic
- Transient monocular blindness (amaurosis fugax)
- Dimness of vision with exercise
- Headache
- Bruit present over carotid artery and/or over the eye
- Decreased or absent carotid pulsation

Continued.

Recognition of Some Common Neurologic Problems—cont'd

Transient Ischemic Attacks (TIAs) from Vertebral-Basilar Artery Insufficiency

- Dizziness
- Vertigo
- Diplopia
- Dysarthria
- Dysphagia
- Numbness of ipsilateral face and contralateral limbs

Signs of Cerebellar Dysfunction (i.e., Alcoholic Cerebellar Degeneration of Multiple Sclerosis)

- Dysnergia
- Dysmetria
- Dysdiadochokinesia
- Ataxia
- Intention tremor
- Scanning and slurring of speech

Signs of Lower Motor Neuron Lesions as Exemplified by

Poliomyelitis	and	*Guillain-Barré syndrome*
Areflexia		Areflexia
Motor paralysis		Motor paralysis
Hypotonia		Hypotonia
Sensation intact		Mild sensory disturbance
		↑ CSF protein without pleocytosis

Multiple Sclerosis (Prototype Demyelinating Disease)

- Optic neuritis (partial or total loss of vision with eye pain)
- Neurologic dysfunction disseminated in time and space*
  Brainstem—diplopia, intranuclear ophthalmoplegia, tic doloureux, Bell's palsy
- Cerebellar—nystagmus, ataxia, intention tremor, gait disturbances
- Spinal cord—weakness, spasticity, hyperreflexia clonus, (+) Babinski's sign, bladder dysfunction, incontinence, paraparesis

Parkinson's Disease

- Stooped posture
- Stiffness and slowness of movement
- Fixed, immobile facial expression
- Rhythmic tremor of limbs (especially pill-rolling tremor of fingers)
- Festinating gait (quick, shuffling steps at an accelerated pace)
- Cogwheel rigidity of arms
- Dementia insidiously progressive
- Dysarthria
- Excessive salivation

Peripheral Neuropathy (see box on pg. 389)

- Paresthesia (tingling, prickling, burning sensation)
- Hypesthesia
- Dysesthesia
- Hypalgesia

*Symptoms reflecting disease in different parts of the nervous system occurring at different times.

Recognition of Some Common Neurologic Problems—cont'd
Peripheral Neuropathy—cont'd
- Motor weakness in extremities
- Loss of deep tendon reflexes
- Unsteadiness of gait

Common causes of predominantly sensory neuropathy
- Diabetes
- Alcoholism
- Heavy metal exposure (arsenic)
- Hypothyroidism

Common causes of predominantly motor neuropathy
- Lead poisoning
- Guillain-Barré syndrome
- Acute intermittent porphyria
- Hypoglycemia (insulinoma)

Neuropathy with mixed sensory and motor features
- Carcinoma, lymphoma (paraneoplastic syndrome)
- Anemia
- Chronic liver disease
- Multiple myeloma
- Macroglobulinemia, cryoglobulinemia |

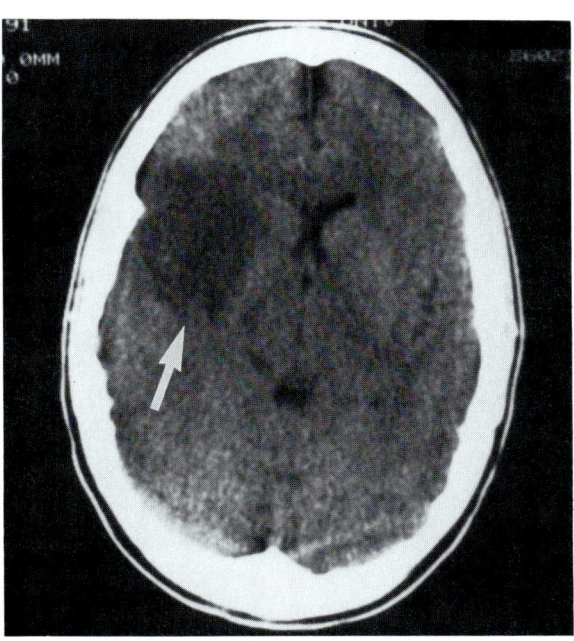

Fig. 10-27 CT scan of head shows a lesion caused by a right middle cerebral artery thrombosis.

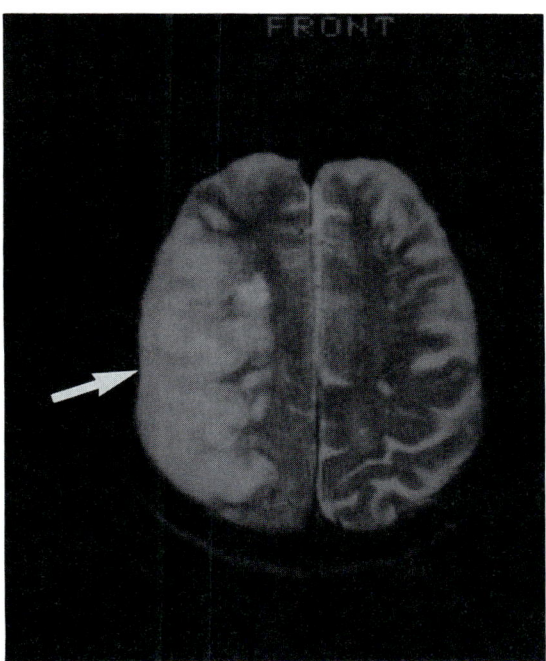

Fig. 10-28 MRI scan of head shows a large right hemisphere lesion caused by middle cerebral artery thrombosis.

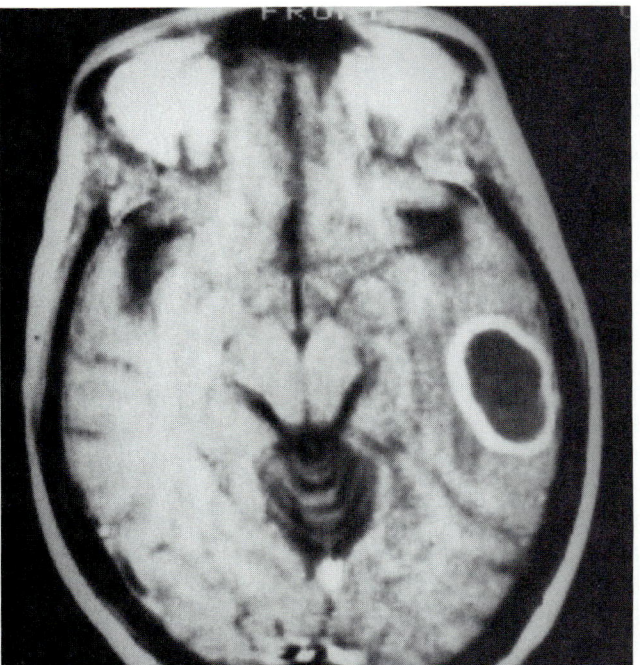

Fig. 10-29 MRI scan of head shows a mass lesion (tuberculoma) that enhances with contrast.

Fig. 10-30 MRI scan of head showing a large mass lesion (i.e., a tumor subsequently proven to be a meningioma).

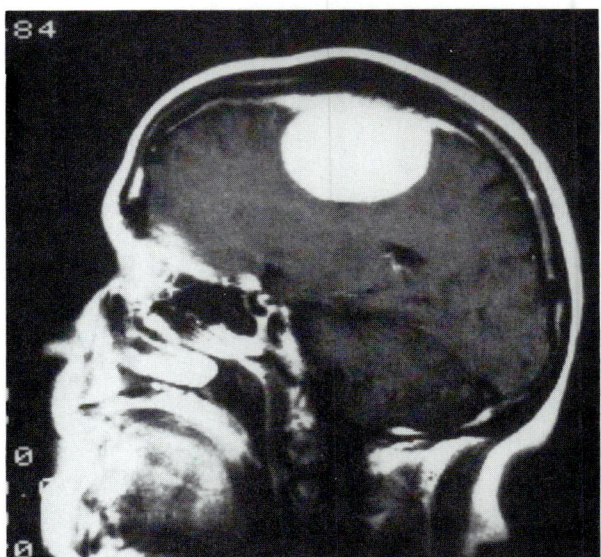

Approach to the Comatose Patient

Coma can be defined as pathologic loss of consciousness. The examination of the comatose patient requires a well-organized approach because a history cannot be elicited and the patient is obviously not in a position to cooperate in the physical examination. The examiner must have a workable classification of coma so that the findings on physical examination and basic investigations either point directly to the correct diagnosis or to further tests or procedures to establish the diagnosis. The bottom box on pg. 414 provides a classification of coma and a means of formulating the differential diagnosis. Table 10-4 provides information on the Glasgow Coma Scale, which is used to assess the level of coma.

1. Be sure to interview relatives as well as individuals who may have brought the patient to the hospital.
2. Check vital signs for evidence of hypertension, hypotension, hyperthermia, hypothermia, tachyarrhythmia, bradyarrythmia, tachypnea, and bradypnea. Each of these may be diagnostically important.
3. Because drug overdose is a very common cause of coma, review the patient's medication history or access to the medication of others. In addition, send blood and urine samples for a drug screen.
4. Because metabolic disturbances often cause coma, promptly send blood samples for testing to exclude most of the metabolic disorders listed in the bottom box on pg. 414.
5. Recall that many comatose patients have been given an intravenous injection of 50% glucose and naloxone by rescue squads before arrival at an emergency room to try and reverse coma resulting from hypoglycemia or overdosage of narcotics.
6. Based on the routine physical examination, exclude hypertensive encephalopathy (blood pressure determinations and funduscopic examination), COPD, tachyarrhythmia and bradyarrythmia (cardiac examination and ECG), and frank uremia. Carefully check the neck for signs of meningeal irritation.
7. A useful grading system for staging coma is the Glasgow Coma Scale (see Table 10-4). Using this scale along with an assessment of brainstem function provides important prognostic information. Assess the level of consciousness by noting verbal responses, eye opening, and motor responses. Assess brainstem function by noting eye movements at rest and after stimulation, pupillary responses, corneal reflexes, and oculocephalic and oculovestibular responses. The presence of doll's eye movements (which do not occur in alert persons) and eye movements in response to instillation of cold and/or warm water in one or both eyes indicate preservation of brainstem function. Conversely, absence of oculocephalic and oculovestibular responses indicates a brainstem abnormality.
8. Although motor and sensory function cannot be fully evaluated in a comatose patient, examinations of the cranial nerves, normal and abnormal reflexes, and other signs (e.g., Babinski's sign) often suffice to indicate whether localizing or lateralizing signs are present.

On completion of the neurologic examination, the examiner should be able to recognize which of three patterns is present.

- No *focal* or *lateralizing neurologic signs* are present.
- Evidence of *meningeal irritation* either does or does not exist.
- *Focal brainstem* or *lateralizing signs* are present.

The above breakdown will point the way for additional studies. In clinical practice, however, unless the cause of coma is quickly identified and reversed, the vast majority of patients undergo a CT scan of the head. A CT scan also frequently precedes the performance of a lumbar puncture.

Approach to the Patient with Delirium and Acute Confusional States

The box on pg. 422 provides a classification of delirium and acute confusional states. As with the comatose patient, you must have a usable classification and adopt a carefully organized approach to patients with delirium and confusional states.

Classification of Delirium and Acute Confusional States

I. Delirium
   A. In a medical or surgical illness (no focal or lateralizing neurologic sign; CSF usually clear)
      1. Typhoid fever
      2. Pneumonia
      3. Septicemia, particularly erysipelas and other streptococcal infections
      4. Rheumatic fever
      5. Thyrotoxicosis and ACTH intoxication (rare)
      6. Postoperative and postconcussive states
   B. In neurologic disease that causes focal or lateralizing signs or changes in the CSF
      1. Vascular, neoplastic, or other diseases, particularly those involving the temporal and parietal lobes and upper part of the brainstem
      2. Cerebral contusion and laceration (traumatic delirium)
      3. Acute purulent and tuberculous meningitis
      4. Subarachnoid hemorrhage
      5. Encephalitis resulting from viral causes (e.g., herpes simplex, infectious mononucleosis) and from unknown causes
   C. The abstinence states, exogenous intoxications, and postconvulsive states; signs of other medical, surgical, and neurologic illnesses absent or coincidental
      1. Withdrawal of alcohol (delirium tremens), barbiturates, and nonbarbiturate sedative drugs following chronic intoxication
      2. Drug intoxications: drugs such as scopolamine, atropine, amphetamine
      3. Postconvulsive delirium
II. Acute confusional states associated with psychomotor underactivity
   A. Associated with a medical or surgical disease (no focal or lateralizing neurologic signs; CSF clear)
      1. Metabolic disorders: hepatic stupor, uremia, hypoxia, hypercapnea, hypoglycemia, porphyria
      2. Infective fevers, especially typhoid
      3. Congestive heart failure
      4. Postoperative, posttraumatic, and puerperal psychoses
   B. Associated with drug intoxication (no focal or lateralizing signs; CSF clear): drugs such as opiates, barbiturates and other sedatives, trihexyphenidyl
   C. Associated with diseases of the nervous system (with focal or lateralizing neurologic signs and/or CSF changes)
      1. Cerebral vascular disease, tumor, abscess
      2. Subdural hematoma
      3. Meningitis
      4. Encephalitis
III. Beclouded dementia (i.e., senile or other brain disease in combination with infective fevers, drug reactions, heart failure, or other medical or surgical diseases)

Modified from Adams R, Victor M: *Principles of neurology*, ed 3, New York, 1985, McGraw-Hill, p 309.

Approach to the Patient with a Peripheral Neuropathy

The major symptoms and signs that should raise the question of a peripheral neuropathy include weakness, numbness, paresthesias, and pain, which can affect all extremities, as well as the trunk, or just one extremity. The last is termed *mononeuritis multiplex*. A detailed examination of motor and sensory function is indicated in patients with the above complaints. Physical findings often observed include weakness, hypalgesia, hypesthesia, and decreased deep tendon reflexes. As noted above, these effects can be localized or generalized. The box on pg. 389 lists the disorders that should be considered in the differential diagnosis of a peripheral neuropathy. Not infrequently, a peripheral neuropathy is the harbinger of a systemic disorder. In addition, in many cases, the cause of peripheral neuropathy remains unidentified.

Approach to the Patient with Signs of Meningeal Irritation

Signs of meningeal irritation must be checked in any patient complaining of headache or visual disturbances and/or found to be obtunded, semicomatose, or comatose. First, check for nuchal rigidity by passively flexing the neck and noting whether movement is limited by involuntary spasm or is painful. Alternatively, ask the patient to touch his chin to the chest; inability to do so also suggests meningeal irritation. *Kernig's sign* is checked by passively flexing the hip to a 90-degree angle and the knee to a 90-degree angle and then extending the knee. With a positive test, the extension of the leg on the flexed hip elicits resistance to further extension and pain in the hamstrings. *Brudzinski's sign* is elicited by passively flexing the neck while the patient is supine; a positive test involves flexion of the hips.

If any of the above signs of meningeal irritation are elicited, it is imperative to rule out meningitis or a subarachnoid hemorrhage by examination of CSF because prompt treatment is urgent. The box on pg. 424 lists the causes of meningitis. Other disorders that can cause meningeal irritation include posterior fossa tumors, meningeal carcinomatosis, CNS sarcoidosis, and intracranial mass lesions causing increased ICP.

Summary

A summary checklist for the neurologic examination is shown in the box on pg. 425.

Suggested readings

Adams RD, Victor M: *Principles of neurology*, ed 4, New York, 1989, McGraw-Hill. *A fine overall textbook of neurology.*

Brown MB, Hachinski VC: Acute confusional status, amnesia, and dementia. In Wilson JD, et al: *Harrison's principle of internal medicine*, ed 12, New York, 1991, McGraw-Hill 1991, pp 183-193. *A well-written brief treatise on an important set of problems.*

Charles BR, et al: Outcome in patients with asymptomatic neck bruits, New Engl J Med 315:860, 1986. *A key article on the natural history of neck bruits and their correlation with cerebrovascular disease and subsequent morbid events.*

Martin NB: Headache. In Wilson JD, et al: *Harrison's principles of internal medicine*, ed 12, New York, 1991, McGraw-Hill, pp 108-115. *A useful chapter on a very important symptom that is often indicative of a serious underlying disorder.*

Differential Diagnosis of Meningitis

Bacterial Meningitis

- *Neisseria meningitidis*
- Hemophilus influenzae
- Streptococcus pneumoniae
- Staphylococcus aureus and *S. epidermidis*
- Gram-negative bacteria
  Escherichia coli
  Klebsiella species
  Proteus species
  Pseudomonas species
- Mycobacterium species
- Leptospira species
- Rare
  Listeria monocytogenes
  Acinetobacter calcoaceticus

Viral (Aseptic) Meningitis

- Enteroviruses
  Coxsackieviruses
  Echoviruses
- Herpes simplex
  Meningitis or meningoencephalitis
- Cytomegalovirus
- Epstein-Barr virus
- Measles
- Mumps
- Influenza
- Varicella zoster
- Rubella
- Adenovirus

Nonviral Agents that may cause Encephalitis/Aseptic Meningitis Syndromes

- *Rickettsia species*
  Rocky Mountain spotted fever
  Q fever
- Psittacosis
- *Mycoplasma pneumoniae*

From Greenberger NJ, et al: *The medical book of lists: a primer of differential diagnosis in internal medicine,* ed 3, Chicago, 1990, Mosby–Year Book, p 265.

Summary Checklist for the Neurologic Examination

Examination of the Motor System

- Assessment of muscle strength (deltoids, biceps, triceps, wrist flexion and extension, fingers, hip flexion, extension, deduction, adduction, leg flexion and extension, ankle flexion and extension)
- Assessment of muscle time (spasticity, rigidity, flaccidity, atrophy)
- Abnormal motor functions (fasciculations, tics, tetany, tremors)

Examination of the Sensory System

- Pain (pin prick)
- Light touch (cotton)
- Position sense
- Vibration sense
- Stereognosis
- Two-point discrimination
- Sensory extinction
- Temperature

Cerebellar Function

- Dysergia, dysmetria, intention tremor
- Dysdiadochokinesia
- Gait and station
- Speech

Reflexes

- Normal reflexes, DTRs, superficial reflexes, brainstem reflexes
- Abnormal reflexes (pyramidal tract signs; i.e., hyperactive DTRs)
- Primitive reflexes (snout, grasp, palmomental)

Cranial Nerves

- I to XII

Mental Status Examination

- State of consciousness
- Orientation
- Mood
- Thought processes
- Memory for recent and remote events
- Judgement and practical skills
- Speech

Recognition of Some Common Neurologic Problems

- Thrombosis, embolism affecting the middle cerebral artery
- Transient ischemic attacks affecting the carotid or vertebral basilar arteries
- Cerebellar dysfunction
- Multiple sclerosis (prototype demyelinating disease)
- Parkinson's disease
- Alzheimer's disease
- Peripheral neuropathy
- Lower motor neuron disorders (Guillain-Barré syndrome)

CHAPTER ELEVEN

The Psychiatric Examination

CHAPTER OUTLINE

Psychiatric Interview

Recognition of Common Psychiatric Disorders
Major depression
Manic and hypomanic episodes
Generalized anxiety disorders
Panic disorders
Agoraphobia
Obsessive/compulsive disorder
Somatization disorder
Schizophrenic disorders
Delusional disorders
Dementia

Summary

Several studies have indicated that significant psychiatric problems are more common than is generally appreciated and that such problems are often not diagnosed promptly. In this connection, it has been estimated that approximately 5% of U.S. women and 3% of U.S. men have a major depressive episode sometime during their adult life. Further, it has been estimated that about 1% of the U.S. population, or approximately 2 million individuals, are schizophrenic. A major reason for the underdiagnosis of psychiatric disorders is the tendency for physicians to think more often in terms of organic cause of symptoms and thus to diagnose psychiatric problems, often erroneously termed "nonorganic," by exclusion. Accordingly, the examiner should be alert to both verbal and nonverbal clues suggesting a psychiatric problem and should be able to recognize common psychiatric disorders.

In this chapter we discuss the interview process, the psychiatric history, and major categories of psychiatric disorders. Special emphasis is placed on neuroses such as anxiety states, somatization disorder, depression and manic-depressive disease, and psychotic disorders such as schizophrenia. To reiterate, a detailed mental status examination should be carried out in all patients in whom a psychiatric disorder is suspected.

Psychiatric Interview

The basic patient interview has been presented in Chapter 1, and the fundamentals of the neurologic examination and the mental status examination have been discussed in Chapter 10 and is not reiterated in detail here. The reader should review the information that is essential for the discussion that follows. Ideally, the psychiatric interview should occur in a quiet, private, and comfortable setting. Introduce yourself and explain the reason or purpose for the interview. Initially, let the patient relate his story without frequent interruptions. Importantly, avoid asking too many questions that fit your preconceived notion of the problem; such questioning may well inhibit the patient from providing pertinent information. Questions are more likely to be answered freely if the examiner proceeds from the general to the particular and from emotionally neutral to more sensitive questions. Open-ended questions are often more helpful than direct questions. To illustrate, instead of asking directly, *Are you a chronic alcoholic?* you might get a more meaningful answer if you said *Tell me about your use of alcoholic beverages.* The latter query has a more permissive tone and may well evoke a different reply.

The psychiatric history should include much if not all of the following information and should be elicited by asking open-ended questions:

- Childhood illnesses and general health
- Adolescence (stresses, problems)
- Education
- Adult illnesses and general health
- Family history of mental illness
- Sexual history and practices
- Marital history
- Occupational history
- Previous mental health
- Medication use; drug abuse
- Antisocial behavior
- Current life situation (e.g., home, spouse, job)
- Time course of current complaints or problems and whether they are recurrent or cyclical
- Triggering or precipitating event
- Patient's interpretation of symptoms (insight)

To illustrate the applicability of the above information, recurrent problems are especially common with depressive disorders. A patient prone to recurrent neurotic problems frequently can relate their onset in adolescence or young adulthood.

Assess all of the following areas:

- Appearance and general behavior—note the patient's dress, hygiene, facial expressions, alertness, spontaneous speech and motor activity, eye contact, gestures, posture, tics.
- Mood—note appropriateness of mood and affect, attitudes, and especially if the patient is in a state such as somber, euphoric, or flat.
- Speech and answers to questions—note whether speech is coherent and relevant, spontaneous, and fast or slow.

- Content of thought — note whether the patient reports hypochondriacal or trivial complaints, depressed or suicidal thoughts, delusions, hallucinations, phobias, or undue fears.
- Cognitive function — note memory for recent and remote events, language skills, conceptual skills, computational and practical skills, attentiveness, and concentration.

Recognition of Common Psychiatric Disorders

Major Depression

The diagnostic criteria for a major depressive episode are detailed in the accompanying box. In addition to direct observation and interview with the patient, interviewing the patient's family and/or close friends is often useful. For example, ask them whether the patient has exhibited increasing despondency, lability of mood, irritability, indecisiveness, avoidance of social contact, and inappropriate anger and resentment. In observing the patient, also check for the following: (1) avoidance of eye contact; (2) slowness in responding to questions and instructions (psychomotor retardation); and (3) dress and personal hygiene, which may reflect regressive behavior.

Two important caveats must be emphasized. First, in any depressed patient, asking about suicidal ideas and intentions is crucial. Second, because psychiatric and organic disease may coexist, an organic disease (e.g., carcinoma of the pancreas) may trigger or be associated with a frank depression. Further, symptoms such as abdominal pain, anorexia, weight loss, and lability of mood are characteristic of both disorders.

Episodes of depression can occur independent of or related to manic disorders. The former is termed a *unipolar depression* and the latter is *bipolar depression*. (See box opposite and box on pg. 430.)

CASE 11-1 Depression

A 75-year-old woman was referred for evaluation of a 25-pound weight loss occurring over an 8-month period. She also complained of vague abdominal pain without symptoms such as nausea, vomiting, diarrhea, or hematochezia. She had undergone a detailed evaluation that included complete blood count, serum chemistries, upper GI endoscopy, colonoscopy, upper GI x-ray studies with small bowel follow-through, and a barium enema. Further, a CT scan of the abdomen had been done and all the above tests were either normal or unremarkable.

On observing the patient, a second examiner noted that she appeared somewhat withdrawn, spoke slowly, appeared tearful, and seemed fixated on her abdominal complaints. Further questioning revealed that she had early morning insomnia, significant anorexia, and she expressed feelings of "hopelessness." This constellation of features permitted the second examiner to arrive at a diagnosis of depression. The GI symptoms were somatic equivalents of the patient's underlying depressive disorder.

Institution of treatment with antidepressant medication resulted in amelioration of all the above symptoms and a weight gain of 15 pounds.

Diagnostic Criteria for a Major Depressive Disorder

I. At least five of the following symptoms have been present during the same 2-week period and represent a change from previous functioning; at least one of the symptoms is either (A) depressed mood, or (B) loss of interest or pleasure. (Do not include symptoms that are clearly caused by a physical condition, mood-incongruent delusions or hallucinations, incoherence, or marked loosening of associations.)
   A. Depressed mood (or can be irritable mood in children and adolescents) most of the day, nearly every day, as indicated either by subjective account or observation by others.
   B. Markedly diminished interest or pleasure in all, or almost all, activities most of the day, nearly every day (as indicated by either subjective account or observation by others of apathy most of the time).
   C. Significant weight loss or weight gain when not dieting (e.g., more than 5% of body weight in a month), or decrease or increase in appetite nearly every day (in children, consider failure to make expected weight gains).
   D. Insomnia or hypersomnia nearly every day.
   E. Psychomotor agitation or retardation nearly every day (observable by others, not merely subjective feelings of restlessness or being slowed down).
   F. Fatigue or loss of energy nearly every day.
   G. Feelings of worthlessness or excessive or inappropriate guilt (which may be delusional) nearly every day (not merely self-reproach or guilt about being sick).
   H. Diminished ability to think or concentrate, or indecisiveness, nearly every day (either by subjective account or as observed by others).
   I. Recurrent thoughts of death (not just fear of dying), recurrent suicidal ideation without a specific plan, or a suicide attempt or a specific plan for committing suicide.
II. A. It cannot be established that an organic factor initiated and maintained the disturbance.
    B. The disturbance is not a normal reaction to the death of a loved one (uncomplicated bereavement).

NOTE: Morbid preoccupation with worthlessness, suicidal ideation, marked functional impairment or psychomotor retardation, or prolonged duration suggest bereavement complicated by major depression.

III. At no time during the disturbance have there been delusions or hallucinations for as long as 2 weeks in the absence of prominent mood symptoms (i.e., before the mood symptoms developed or after they have remitted).
IV. Not superimposed on schizophrenia, schizophreniform disorder, delusional disorder, or psychotic disorder.

NOTE: A *major depressive syndrome* is defined as criterion I above.

Modified from *Diagnostic and statistical manual for mental disorders*, ed 3, revised, Washington, DC, 1987, American Psychiatric Association.

Manic and Hypomanic Episodes

Manic disorders are characterized by one or more distinct periods with a predominantly elevated, expansive, or unstable mood. The diagnostic criteria for a manic episode are detailed in the box below. The key abnormalities are obvious alterations in mood, speech, and behavior. The mood is elevated, euphoric, expansive, or irritable, as noted above. The mood can alternate or intermingle with a depressive mood.

The term *hypomanic* refers to a disturbance that is similar to but not as severe as a full-blown manic episode. Such behavior is also likely to be more transient.

Generalized Anxiety Disorders

The diagnostic criteria for generalized anxiety disorders are detailed in the box opposite. Interestingly, the recent characterization of a benzodiazepine-receptor complex supports the concept that the antianxiety actions of the benzodiazepines are mediated through this receptor. Note also that symptoms indicative of

---

Diagnostic Criteria for a Manic Episode

I. A distinct period of abnormally and persistently elevated, expansive, or irritable mood.

II. During the period of mood disturbance, at least three of the following symptoms have persisted (four if the mood is only irritable) and have been present to a significant degree
   A. Inflated self-esteem or grandiosity.
   B. Decreased need for sleep (e.g., feels rested after only 3 hours of sleep).
   C. More talkative than usual or pressure to keep talking.
   D. Flight of ideas or subjective experience that thoughts are racing.
   E. Distractibility (i.e., attention too easily drawn to unimportant or irrelevant external stimuli).
   F. Increase in goal-directed activity (either socially, at work or school, or sexually) or psychomotor agitation.
   G. Excessive involvement in pleasurable activities that have a high potential for painful consequences (e.g., the person engages in unrestrained buying sprees, sexual indiscretions, or foolish business investments).

III. Mood disturbance sufficiently severe to cause or necessitate the following.
   A. Marked impairment in occupational functioning or in usual social activities or relationships with others.
   B. Hospitalization to prevent harm to self or others.

IV. At no time during the disturbance have there been delusions or hallucinations for as long as 2 weeks in the absence of prominent mood symptoms (i.e., before the mood symptoms developed or after they have remitted).

V. Not superimposed on schizophrenic, schizophreniform disorder, delusional disorder, or psychotic disorder.

VI. It cannot be established that an organic factor initiated and maintained the disturbance. NOTE: Somatic antidepressant treatment (e.g., drugs, electroconvulsive therapy [ECT]) that apparently precipitates a mood disturbance should not be considered an etiologic organic factor.

NOTE: A *manic syndrome* is defined as including criteria I, II, and III above. A *hypomanic syndrome* is defined as including criteria I and II but not III (i.e., no marked impairment).

Modified from *Diagnostic and statistical manual for mental disorders*, ed 3, revised, Washington, DC, 1987, American Psychiatric Association.

autonomic hyperactivity (especially adrenergic-mediated activity) are quite common. This explains, at least in part, why such patients often respond to treatment with beta-adrenergic blockers.

Diagnostic Criteria for a Generalized Anxiety Disorder

I. Unrealistic or excessive anxiety and worry (apprehensive expectation) about two or more life circumstances—for example, worry about possible misfortune to one's child (who is in no danger) and worry about finances (for no good reason)—for a period of 6 months or longer, during which the person has been bothered more days than not by these concerns. In children and adolescents, this may take the form of anxiety and worry about academic and social performance.

II. If another axis I disorder is present, the focus of the anxiety and worry in I is unrelated to it (e.g., the anxiety or worry is not about having a panic attack [as in panic disorder], being embarrassed in public [as in social phobia], being contaminated [as in obsessive compulsive disorder], or gaining weight [as in anorexia nervosa]).

III. The disturbance does not occur only during the course of a mood disorder or a psychotic disorder.

IV. At least 6 of the following 18 symptoms are often present when anxious (do not include symptoms present only during panic attacks).

Motor Tension
1. Trembling, twitching, or feeling shaky
2. Muscle tension, aches, or soreness
3. Restlessness
4. Easy fatigability

Autonomic Hyperactivity
5. Shortness of breath or smothering sensations
6. Palpitations or accelerated heart rate (tachycardia)
7. Sweating or cold clammy hands
8. Dry mouth
9. Dizziness or lightheadedness
10. Nausea, diarrhea, or other abdominal distress
11. Flushes (hot flashes) or chills
12. Frequent urination
13. Trouble swallowing or having sensation of lump in throat

Vigilance and Scanning
14. Feeling keyed up or on edge
15. Exaggerated startle response
16. Difficulty concentrating or "mind going blank" because of anxiety
17. Trouble falling or staying asleep
18. Irritability

V. It cannot be established that an organic factor initiated and maintained the disturbance (e.g., hyperthyroidism, caffeine intoxication).

Modified from *Diagnostic and statistical manual for mental disorders*, ed 3, revised, Washington, DC, 1987, American Psychiatric Association.

Panic Disorders

The diagnostic criteria for panic disorder are listed in the box below. Again note that many of the symptoms appear to be mediated by autonomic nervous system hyperactivity.

Agoraphobia

Agoraphobia is a marked fear of being alone or being in public places from which escape might be difficult or where help would not be available in case of sudden incapacitation. The diagnostic criteria for agoraphobia are detailed in the top box opposite.

Obsessive/Compulsive Disorder

Although obsessive-compulsive behavior is common, such behavior generally does not cause significant distress to the individual or interfere with social or role functioning. A frank obsessive-compulsive disorder, however, does cause significant distress; the diagnostic criteria for this disorder are listed in the bottom box opposite.

Diagnostic Criteria for Panic Disorder

I. At some time during the disturbance, one or more panic attacks (discrete periods of intense fear or discomfort) have occurred that were (1) unexpected (i.e., did not occur immediately before or on exposure to a situation that almost always caused anxiety), and (2) not triggered by situations in which the person was the focus of others' attention.

II. Either four attacks, as defined in criterion I, have occurred within a 4-week period, or 1 or more attacks have been followed by a period of at least a month of persistent fear of having another attack.

III. At least four of the following symptoms developed during at least one of the attacks.
  A. Shortness of breath (dyspnea) or smothering sensations
  B. Dizziness, unsteady feelings, or faintness
  C. Palpitations or accelerated heart rate (tachycardia)
  D. Trembling or shaking
  E. Sweating
  F. Choking
  G. Nausea or abdominal distress
  H. Depersonalization or derealization
  I. Numbness or tingling sensations (paresthesias)
  J. Flushes (hot flashes) or chills
  K. Chest pain or discomfort
  L. Fear of dying
  M. Fear of going crazy or of doing something uncontrolled

NOTE: Attacks involving four or more symptoms are panic attacks; attacks involving fewer than four symptoms are limited symptom attacks (see section on agoraphobia, above).

IV. During at least some of the attacks, at least four of the symptoms listed above developed suddenly and increased in intensity within 10 minutes of the beginning of the first symptom noticed in the attack.

V. It cannot be established that an organic factor initiated and maintained the disturbance (e.g., amphetamine or caffeine intoxication, hyperthyroidism).

NOTE: MVP may be an associated condition but does not preclude a diagnosis of panic disorder.

Modified from *Diagnostic and statistical manual for mental disorders,* ed 3, revised, Washington, DC, 1987, American Psychiatric Association.

Diagnostic Criteria for Agoraphobia

I. Agoraphobia is the fear of being in places or situations from which escape might be difficult (or embarrassing) or in which help might not be available in the event of suddenly developing a symptom(s) than could be incapacitating or extremely embarrassing. Examples include: dizziness or falling, depersonalization or derealization, loss of bladder or bowel control, vomiting, or cardiac distress. As a result of this fear, the person either restricts travel or needs a companion when away from home, or else endures agoraphobic situations despite intense anxiety. Common agoraphobic situations include being outside the home alone, being in a crowd or standing in a line, being on a bridge, and traveling in a bus, train, or car.

II. Has never met the criteria for panic disorder.

Modified from *Diagnostic and statistical manual for mental disorders,* ed 3, revised, Washington, DC, 1987, American Psychiatric Association.

Diagnostic Criteria for Obsessive/Compulsive Disorder

I. Either obsessions or compulsions:
   A. Obsessions
      1. Recurrent and persistent ideas, thoughts, impulses, or images that are experienced, at least initially, as intrusive and senseless (e.g., a parent's having repeated impulses to kill a loved child, a religious person's having recurrent blasphemous thoughts).
      2. The person attempts to ignore or suppress such thoughts or impulses or to neutralize them with some other thought or action.
      3. The person recognizes that the obsessions are the product of his own mind, not imposed from without (as in thought insertion).
      4. If another axis I disorder is present, the content of the obsession is unrelated to it (e.g., the ideas, thoughts, impulses, or images are not about food in the presence of an eating disorder, about drugs in the presence of a psychoactive substance use disorder, or guilty thoughts in the presence of a major depression).
   B. Compulsions
      1. Repetitive, purposeful, and intentional behaviors that are performed in response to an obsession, according to certain rules, or in a stereotyped fashion.
      2. The behavior is designed to neutralize or to prevent discomfort of some dreaded event or situation; however, either the activity is not connected in a realistic way with what it is designed to neutralize or prevent, or it is clearly excessive.
      3. The person recognizes that his behavior is excessive or unreasonable (this may not be true for young children; it may no longer be true for people whose obsessions have evolved into overvalued ideas).

II. The obsessions or compulsions cause marked distress, are time-consuming (take more than an hour a day), or significantly interfere with the person's normal routine, occupational functioning, or usual social activities or relationships with others.

Modified from *Diagnostic and statistical manual for mental disorders,* ed 3, revised, Washington, DC, 1987, American Psychiatric Association.

Somatization Disorder

The essential features of a somatization disorder are recurrent and multiple somatic complaints of several years' duration that apparently are not caused by any physical disorders. The disorder begins before the age of 30 and has a chronic but fluctuating course. This disorder was previously referred to as either hysteria or Briquet's syndrome. The diagnostic criteria are detailed in the accompanying box. A floridly positive review of systems with numerous symptoms should raise the question of somatization disorder.

Diagnostic Criteria for Somatization Disorder

I. A history of many physical complaints or a belief that one is sickly, beginning before the age of 30 and persisting for several years.

II. At least 13 symptoms from the list below are present. To count a symptom as significant, the following criteria must be met.
 A. No organic pathology or pathophysiologic mechanism (e.g., a physical disorder or the effects of injury, medication, drugs, or alcohol) to account for the symptom or, when there is a related organic pathologic condition, the complaint or resulting social or occupational impairment is grossly in excess of what would be expected from the physical findings.
 B. Has not occurred only during a panic attack.
 C. Has caused the person to take medicine (other than over-the-counter pain medication), see a doctor, or alter life-style.

SYMPTOM LIST

GI symptoms

1. **Vomiting (other than during pregnancy)**
2. Abdominal pain (other than when menstruating)
3. Nausea (other than motion sickness)
4. Bloating (gassy)
5. Diarrhea
6. Intolerance of (gets sick from) several different foods

Pain Symptoms

7. **Pain in extremities**
8. Back pain
9. Joint pain
10. Pain during urination
11. Other pain (excluding headaches)

Cardiopulmonary Symptoms

12. **Shortness of breath when not exerting oneself**
13. Palpitations
14. Chest pain
15. Dizziness

> **Diagnostic Criteria for Somatization Disorder—cont'd**
>
> Conversion of Pseudoneurologic Symptoms
>
> 16. **Amnesia**
> 17. **Difficulty swallowing**
> 18. Loss of voice
> 19. Deafness
> 20. Double vision
> 21. Blurred vision
> 22. Blindness
> 23. Fainting or loss of consciousness
> 24. Seizure or convulsion
> 25. Trouble walking
> 26. Paralysis or muscle weakness
> 27. Urinary retention or difficulty urinating
>
> Sexual Symptoms for the Major Part of the Person's Life After Opportunities for Sexual Activity
>
> 28. **Burning sensation in sexual organs or rectum (other than during intercourse)**
> 29. Sexual indifference
> 30. Pain during intercourse
> 31. Impotence
>
> Female Reproductive System Symptoms Judged by the Person to Occur More Frequently or Severely than in Most Women
>
> 32. **Painful menstruation**
> 33. Irregular menstrual periods
> 34. Excessive menstrual bleeding
> 35. Vomiting throughout pregnancy
>
> NOTE: The seven items in boldface may be used to screen for the disorder. The presence of two or more of these items suggest a high likelihood of the disorder.

Modified from *Diagnostic and statistical manual for mental disorders,* ed 3, revised, Washington, DC, 1987, American Psychiatric Association.

Schizophrenic Disorders

Schizophrenic disorders are serious mental illnesses that are difficult to define, identify, and treat. The diagnostic criteria for schizophrenic disorders are detailed in the box on pp. 436-437. The term *schizophreniform disorder* refers to an illness in which the essential features are identical to those of schizophrenia except that the duration is less than 6 months but more than 2 weeks.

The first clue to a schizophrenic disorder may be the patient's inability to answer questions and speak appropriately. A second clue may be the bizarre nature of the patient's complaints. A mnemonic for conceptualizing schizophrenia consists of the five *A*'s:

- *Affect* — inappropriate and often flat
- *Autism* — thinking is self-centered and often meaningful only to the patient
- *Antisocial behavior*
- *Ambivalence*
- *Associations* — often loose and disjointed

Diagnostic Criteria for a Schizophrenic Disorder

I. Presence of characteristic psychotic symptoms in the active phase: either A, B, or C for at least 1 week (unless the symptoms are successfully treated).
   A. Two of the following.
      1. Delusions
      2. Prominent hallucinations (throughout the day for several days or several times a week for several weeks, each hallucinatory experience not being limited to a few brief moments)
      3. Incoherence or marked loosening of associations
      4. Catatonic behavior
      5. Flat or grossly inappropriate affect
   B. Bizarre delusions (i.e., involving a phenomenon that the person's culture would regard as totally implausible; e.g., thought broadcasting, being controlled by a dead person).
   C. Prominent hallucinations (as defined above) of a voice with content having no apparent relation to depression or elation, or a voice keeping up a running commentary on the person's behavior or thoughts, or two or more voices conversing with each other.
II. During the course of the disturbance, functioning in such areas as work, social relations, and self-care is markedly below the highest level achieved before onset of the disturbance (or, when the onset is in childhood or adolescence, failure to achieve expected level of social development).
III. Schizoaffective disorder and mood disorder with psychotic features have been ruled out (i.e., if a major depressive or manic syndrome has ever been present during an active phase of the disturbance, the total duration of all episodes of a mood syndrome has been brief relative to the total duration of the active and residual phases of the disturbance).
IV. Continuous signs of the disturbance for at least 6 months. The 6-month period must include an active phase (of at least 1 week, or less if symptoms have been successfully treated) during which there were psychotic symptoms characteristic of schizophrenia (symptoms in I), with or without a prodromal or residual phase, as defined below.
   A. *Prodromal phase* — a clear deterioration in functioning before the active phase of the disturbance that is not caused by a disturbance in mood or by a psychoactive substance use disorder and that involves at least two of the symptoms listed below.
   B. *Residual phase* — following the active phase of the disturbance, persistence of at least two of the symptoms noted below, these not being caused by a disturbance in mood or by a psychoactive substance use disorder.
   C. Prodromal or residual symptoms.
      1. Marked social isolation or withdrawal
      2. Marked impairment in role functioning as wage-earner, student, or homemaker

> **Diagnostic Criteria for Schizophrenic Disorder — cont'd**
>
> 3. Markedly peculiar behavior (e.g., collecting garbage, talking to self in public, hoarding food)
> 4. Marked impairment in personal hygiene and grooming
> 5. Blunted or inappropriate affect
> 6. Digressive, vague, overelaborate, or circumstantial speech; poverty of speech; or poverty of content of speech
> 7. Odd beliefs or magical thinking influencing behavior and inconsistent with cultural norms (e.g., superstitiousness, belief in clairvoyance, telepathy, "sixth sense," "others can feel my feelings," overvalued ideas, ideas of reference)
> 8. Unusual perceptual experiences (e.g., recurrent illusions, sensing the presence of a force or person not actually present)
> 9. Marked lack of initiative, interests, or energy
>
> EXAMPLES: Six months of prodromal symptoms with 1 week of symptoms from I; no prodromal symptoms with 6 months of symptoms from I; no prodromal symptoms with 1 week of symptoms from I and 6 months of residual symptoms.
>
> V. It cannot be established that an organic factor initiated and maintained the disturbance.
> VI. If there is a history of autistic disorder, the additional diagnosis of schizophrenia is made only if prominent delusions or hallucinations are also present.

Modified from *Diagnostic and statistical manual for mental disorders,* ed 3, revised, Washington, DC, 1987, American Psychiatric Association.

Delusional Disorders

The paranoid disorders include paranoia, paranoid disorder, and paranoid personality disorder. The boundaries of this group of disorders and their differentiation from schizophrenia of the paranoid type are still incompletely understood. The diagnostic criteria for frank paranoid disorder are listed in the box on pg. 438. The term *paranoid personality disorder* refers to a disorder in which the patient has paranoid ideation or pathologic jealousy but not delusions.

Dementia

The term *dementia* refers to a clinical state characterized by a progressive loss of intellectual capacities and a decline from previously attained intellectual levels. In almost all cases, intellectual functions deteriorate, including memory for recent and remote events, judgment, thinking, speech, abstract thought, spatial or temporal orientation, and responsiveness. The history is the most important part of the initial evaluation and should be obtained from both the patient and the family. In addition to a detailed chronologic account of the patient's current illness, ask specifically about any previous psychiatric problems, alcohol and substance use and abuse, medications, exposure to environmental toxins, trauma, surgery, and systemic diseases. Inquire about any changes in the patient's

Diagnostic Criteria for Delusional Disorder

1. Nonbizarre delusion(s) (i.e., involving situations that occur in real life, such as being followed, poisoned, infected, loved at a distance, having a disease, being deceived by one's spouse or lover) of at least 1 months' duration.
2. Auditory or visual hallucinations, if present, are not prominent (as defined in the box on pp. 436-437).
3. Apart from the delusion(s) or its ramifications, behavior is not obviously odd or bizarre.
4. If a major depressive or manic syndrome has been present during the delusional disturbance, the total duration of all episodes of the mood syndrome has been brief relative to the total duration of the delusional disturbance.
5. Has never met criterion I for schizophrenia (see box on page pp. 436-437), and it cannot be established that an organic factor initiated and maintained the disturbance.

Specify type: The following types are based on the predominant delusional theme. If no single delusional theme predominates, specify as **Unspecified Type.**

Erotomanic Type

Delusional disorder in which the predominant theme of the delusion(s) is that a person, usually of higher status, is in love with the subject.

Grandiose Type

Delusional disorder in which the predominant theme of the delusion(s) is one of inflated worth, power, knowledge, identity, or special relationship to a deity or famous person.

Jealous Type

Delusional disorder in which the predominant theme of the delusion(s) is that one's sexual partner is unfaithful.

Persecutory Type

Delusional disorder in which the predominant theme of the delusion(s) is that one (or someone to whom one is close) is being malevolently treated in some way. People with this type of delusional disorder may repeatedly take their complaints of being mistreated to legal authorities.

Somatic Type

Delusional disorder in which the predominant theme of the delusion(s) is that the person has some physical defect, disorder, or disease.

Unspecified Type

Delusional disorder that does not fit any of the previous categories (e.g., persecutory and grandiose themes without a predominance of either; delusions of reference without malevolent content).

From *Diagnostic and statistical manual for mental disorders,* ed 3, revised, Washington, DC, 1987, American Psychiatric Association.

functional abilities, such as eating, dressing, grooming, toileting, housekeeping, shopping, and managing finances.

The neurologic examination should be geared to detect focal lesions and signs of any brain dysfunction. Obviously it must include a detailed mental status examination. The patient often appears apathetic and disinterested, so superficially the patient appears depressed. However, closer evaluation usually reveals the loss of basic intellectual functions.

Several disorders associated with dementia can be treated effectively, with subsequent stabilization of, improvement in, or amelioration of dementia. Such treatable causes of dementia include:

- Myxedema
- Cushing's syndrome
- Chronic CNS infection
- Intoxications
- Wilson's disease
- CNS mass lesions (tumor, abscess)
- Subdural hematoma
- Communicating (normal-pressure) hydrocephalus

The last diagnosis should always be considered if a triad of findings (dementia, ataxia, and urinary incontinence) is present. Dementia resulting from other disorders, such as Wernicke-Korsakoff syndrome (caused by thiamine deficiency), can stabilize and even improve if the disorder is recognized and treated appropriately. A classification of disorders causing dementia is detailed in the box below. Three broad categories are emphasized:

Classification of Dementia

I. Diseases in which dementia is associated with clinical and laboratory signs of other medical disease.
   A. Hypothyroidism
   B. Cushing's syndrome
   C. Nutritional deficiency states such as pellagra, Wernicke-Korsakoff syndrome, and subacute combined degeneration of spinal cord and brain (vitamin B_{12} deficiency)
   D. Chronic meningoencephalitis: general paresis, meningovascular syphilis, and cryptococcosis
   E. Hepatolenticular degeneration, familiar and acquired
   F. Chronic barbiturate intoxication; bromidism
II. Diseases in which dementia is associated with other neurologic signs but not with other obvious disease
   A. Invariably associated with other neurologic signs
      1. Huntington's chorea (choreoathetosis)
      2. Schilder's disease and related demyelinative diseases (spastic weakness, pseudobulbar palsy, blindness, deafness)
      3. Amaurotic familial idiocy and other lipid-storage diseases (myoclonic seizures, blindness, spasticity, cerebellar ataxia)

Continued.

> ### Classification of Dementia—cont'd
>
>   4. Myoclonic epilepsy (diffuse myoclonus, generalized seizures, cerebellar ataxia)
>   5. Subacute spongiform encephalopathy or one type of Creutzfeldt-Jakob disease (myoclonic dementia)
>   6. Cerebrocerebellar degeneration (cerebellar ataxia)
>   7. Cerebrobasal ganglionic degenerations (apraxia-rigidity)
>   8. Dementia with spastic paraplegia (spastic legs)
>   9. Progressive supranuclear palsy
>   10. Certain hereditary metabolic diseases
>   B. Often associated with other neurologic signs
>   1. Thrombotic or embolic cerebral infarction
>   2. Brain tumor (primary or metastatic) or abscess
>   3. Brain trauma such as cerebral contusion, midbrain hemorrhage, or chronic subdural hematoma
>   4. Marchiafava-Bignami disease (often with apraxia and other frontal lobe signs)
>   5. Communicating (normal-pressure) or obstructive hydrocephalus (usually with ataxia of gait)
> III. Diseases in which dementia is usually the only evidence of neurologic or medical disease
>   A. Alzheimer's disease
>   B. Pick's disease
>   C. Degenerative disease of unspecified type

Modified from Adams R, Victor M: *Principles of neurology,* ed 3, New York, 1985, McGraw-Hill.

1. Diseases in which dementia is associated with clinical and laboratory signs of other medical disease
2. Diseases in which dementia is associated with other neurologic signs but not with other obvious medical diseases
3. Diseases in which dementia is usually the only evidence of neurologic or medical disease

Summary

A summary checklist for the psychiatric examination is shown in the box opposite.

Suggested readings

American Psychiatric Association: *Diagnostic and statistical manual for mental disorders,* edition 3, revised, Washington, DC, 1987, American Psychiatric Association. *The standard reference manual for psychiatric disorders.*

Brown MM, Hachenski VL: Acute confusional states, amnesia, and dementia. In Wilson JE, et al, editors: *Harrison's principles of internal medicine,* edition 12, New York, 1991, McGraw-Hill, pp 183-193. *A brief but informative chapter, very readable, dealing with an important topic.*

Judd LL, Broff DL, Bretton KT: Psychiatric disorders. In Wilson JE, et al, editors: *Harrison's principles of internal medicine,* edition 12, New York, 1991, McGraw-Hill, pp 2123-2146. *A useful, concise treatise of major psychiatric disorders and the therapeutic use of psychotropic medications.*

Summary Checklist for the Psychiatric Examination

General Information
- Adolescence (stresses, problems)
- Education
- Adult illnesses and general health
- Family history of mental illness
- Sexual history, marital history, occupational history
- Medication use, drug and alcohol use and abuse
- Current life situations (e.g., home, spouse, job)

Appearance and General Behavior
- Dress, hygiene
- Alertness, spontaneity of speech, motor activity
- Eye contact, gestures, postures, tics
- Oriented to time, place, person, situation

Mood
- Appropriateness of mood and affect

Speech and Answers to Questions
- Coherent, relevant, spontaneous

Content of Thought
- Depressed or suicidal thoughts
- Delusions, hallucinations, phobias, undue fears
- Hypochondriacal or trivial complaints

Cognitive Function
- Memory for recent and remote events
- Language skills
- Computational and practical skills
- Judgements
- Attentiveness and concentration

CHAPTER TWELVE

The Skin

CHAPTER OUTLINE

History Taking
Cardinal symptoms of skin diseases

Physical Examination of the Skin
Skin lesions characteristically involving specific areas
Pustular diseases
Miliaria
Eczematous diseases
Connective tissue diseases
Fungal infections
Purpura and petechiae
Macules, papules, and maculopapular diseases
Papulosquamous diseases
Tumors
Ichthyosis
Urticaria
Bullous and vesicular diseases
Viral infections of the skin
Bacterial infections of the skin
Dermal manifestations of systemic bacterial infections
Skin abnormalities in AIDS

Summary

Studies on the prevalence of skin disease in the community show that 25% of the population has a worrisome skin disorder. Most people will not seek medical attention. Many will self-medicate or try to ignore the condition. Nevertheless, skin complaints constitute about 10% of chief complaints to personal physicians.

The dermatologic evaluation requires a skillful history and an exacting examination of minute details. Skin lesions may affect the skin alone, or they may be a manifestation of a systemic illness. Difficulties encountered in diagnosis result from (1) the large number of diseases affecting the skin, (2) the fact that different etiologic causes can cause similar skin lesions, and (3) the fact that a single disease may result in various skin manifestations. Furthermore, individual lesions often change appearance with time.

Although we begin by describing the history-taking procedure for skin diseases and proceed to description and diagnosis of skin lesions, the examination is important in identifying most skin lesions.

History Taking

History usually provides clues to the diagnosis of skin lesions. The mode of onset, the ambient temperature and season, and the duration may be clues. The rapidity of onset of individual lesions, the expansion of individual lesions, the time required to develop new lesions, and initial distribution may provide important information.

In usual practice, we take the history and then perform the examination. In evaluating skin lesions, we begin by taking part of the history, then we examine the lesions, and finally we proceed to the rest of the history. In this way, historical questions may be guided by the probable differential diagnosis of the type of skin lesions.

Initial questions often include ones similar to the following:

- *Tell me about your skin condition.* An open-ended question so patient can express his own history and concerns.
- *When and where did this begin?* Establish onset to determine factors such as whether condition is acute or chronic, if relapse has occurred, etc. The site of the initial lesion may be helpful.
- *How has it changed?* The distribution and development of individual lesions is often characteristic. Whether they come and go is a good clue. *Has the condition involved any other sites?* Patients may fail to mention how it has spread unless prompted.
- *Have you had any other symptoms with it?* This helps to distinguish systemic and localized conditions (see accompanying box).
- *What have you done to treat it?* Many types of lesions are altered by therapies, some better, some worse. Others are just different.
- *Does sunlight have any effect?* Several disorders may result from photosensitivity.

Symptoms of Skin Lesions

Local Symptoms
- Swelling
- Pain
- Ulceration
- Draining
- Scaling
- Itching

Constitutional Symptoms (Systemic Illness)
- Chills
- Headache
- Nausea or vomiting

Chronic Illness
- Weight loss
- Night sweats
- Anorexia
- Malaise
- Fatigue
- Weakness

- *Do you know anyone with a similar rash?* This helps elicit information on contagious illness.
- *Do you have any idea what may be causing this?* Patients may have some insight into possible causes. Often, however, they also guess incorrectly.

The past medical history may be useful, and questions to ask should include the following:

- *Have you had anything similar before?* This question may reveal a recurrent condition.
- *Any other types of skin lesions or rashes?*
- *What about other illnesses you now have or have had?*
- *Are you allergic to anything?*
- *Do you use any medicine or any products from health food stores?* Patients may not think of nonprescription products as medicine.

The family history of eczema, asthma, hay fever, or allergies may be important in atopic dermatitis. Café-au-lait spots are findings typical in families with von Recklinghausen's disease (neurofibromatosis).

The social history of exposure to chemicals at work or at home and exposure to animals or plants may give a diagnostic tip. Ask about hobbies, travel (where and what was done), and other activities undertaken shortly before onset of the skin condition.

The review of systems may suggest a viral rash, hepatitis, SLE, rheumatoid disease, STDs, and other causes.

Before considering examination of the skin, it is important to understand terms. Tables 12-1 to 12-3 show some common terms that will enable you to communicate regarding skin lesions. Skin lesions may be described as *primary lesions* (Table 12-1), which are those present near the onset of illness.

TABLE 12-1: Descriptive Terms for Primary Skin Lesions

Terms Used to Describe Lesion	Definition	Examples
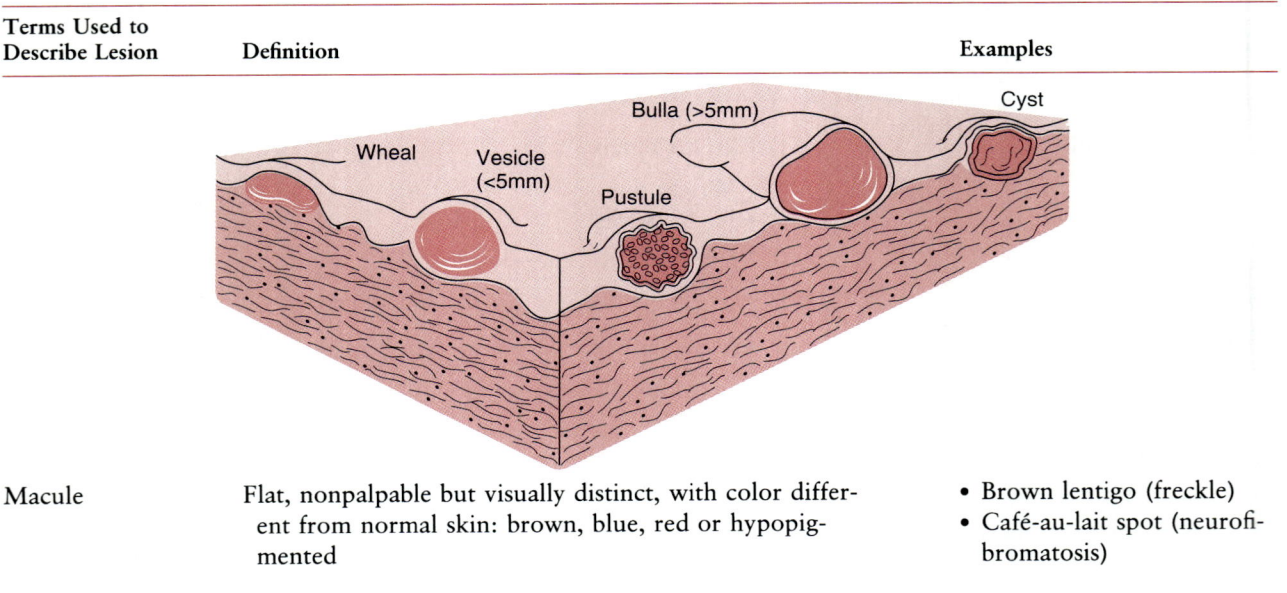		
Macule	Flat, nonpalpable but visually distinct, with color different from normal skin: brown, blue, red or hypopigmented	• Brown lentigo (freckle) • Café-au-lait spot (neurofibromatosis)

TABLE 12-1: Descriptive Terms for Primary Skin Lesions—cont'd

Terms Used to Describe Lesion	Definition	Examples
Macule—cont'd		• Viral exanthem (blanches) • Drug rash (red, may be papular) • Secondary syphilis • Hypopigmented (vitiligo) • Purpura (does not blanch)
Papule	Raised, solid lesion no larger than 5 mm in diameter	• Usual skin color or slightly yellow, white, pink: warts, skin tags • Brown color: melanoma, nevi, warts • Red: acne, eczema, insect bites, psoriasis • Blue: angiokeratoma
Plaque	Raised, solid lesion greater than 5 mm in diameter, may be formed by confluence of papules	• Seborrheic keratosis • Tinea versicolor • Pityriasis rosea • Psoriasis
Nodule	Raised, solid lesion more than 5 mm in diameter with edges well demarcated; a nodule is differentiated from a plaque in that the plaque tends to be superficial, whereas the nodule may involve deeper tissues	• Erythema nodosum • Rheumatoid nodules • Kaposi's sarcoma • Lipoma • Carcinoma
Wheal	A transient plaque caused by fluid transudation into the dermis, usually with erythema; central pallor may be present	• Hives • Dermographism • Urticaria pigmentosa (mastocytosis)
Vesicle	A well-demarcated collection of free fluid (blisterlike) between layers of skin up to 5 mm in diameter	• Small burn • Herpes simplex • Herpes zoster or varicella • Contact dermatitis • Dyshidrotic eczema
Pustule	A vesicle filled with purulent fluid (fluid with leukocytes), usually resulting from bacterial causes but not always	• Acne • Folliculitis • Candidiasis • Pustular psoriasis
Bulla	A well-demarcated collection of free fluid (blisterlike) in the skin larger than 5 mm in diameter	• Herpes zoster • Pemphigoid • Pemphigus • Bullous impetigo
Cyst	A nodule that contains fluid, either liquid or semisolid; usually has a defined lining	• Acne • Epidermal inclusion cyst

Dermatologic diagnoses rely heavily on these primary lesions. *Secondary lesions* (Table 12-2) occur when primary lesions have been altered, perhaps by scratching, treatment, or secondary infection, or when newer lesions have appeared. Certain special lesions have important diagnostic impact equivalent to that of primary lesions (Table 12-3).

TABLE 12-2: Descriptive Terms for Secondary Skin Lesions

Terms Used to Describe Lesions	Definition	Examples
Scales	Shedding, dead epidermal cells that have a whitish color and are dry	Fine scales • Pityriasis rosea • Psoriasis • Scarlet fever • Tinea Sheets of scales • Scarlet fever • Toxic shock syndrome • Scalded skin syndrome
Crusts—also called scabs	Superficial loss of epidermis with fluid that has dried on the surface; the dermal-epidermal junction is intact so no scar occurs with healing	Impetigo
Ulcers	Loss of epidermis and dermis below dermal-epidermal junction; these heal with scars	• Decubitus ulcers • Severe varicella • Diabetic ulcers • Pyoderma gangrenosum
Fissure	A line-shaped break in the epidermis with vertical walls through the dermal-epidermal junction.	• Chapped hands or lips • Split lip
Atrophy	Depressed area of skin resulting from thinning of skin layer because of loss of tissue; normal skin markings are lost giving increased transparency	• Striae • Aging • Following prolonged topical use of potent steroids
Scar	Formation of connective tissue that indicates the dermal-epidermal junction has been disrupted; initially pink, later white; scars may be depressed (atrophic) or heaped-up (hypertrophic)	• After acne (atrophic scar) • Hypertrophic scar (keloid)
Keloid	Overproduction of connective tissue in a scar, especially in black-pigmented races	May follow surgical procedures, cuts, or burns
Excoriation	A linear erosion or ulcer caused by scratching	• Urticaria • Neurodermatitis

TABLE 12-3: Descriptive Terms for Special Skin Lesions

Term Used to Describe Lesion	Definition	Examples
Petechia	Well-demarcated deposit of blood smaller than 5 mm in diameter caused by bleeding into the dermis; in contrast to macule, does not blanch when pressure is applied	• Thrombocytopenia • Meningococcemia • Rocky Mountain spotted fever
Purpura	A demarcated deposit of blood in the skin greater than 5 mm in diameter; well-defined edges as opposed to bruises, which blend with normal tissues at the margins	• Idiopathic thrombocytopenic purpura • Meningococcemia • Pneumococcemia • Rocky Mountain spotted fever
Comedo (plural comedomes)	A plug of sebum and keratin in the opening of a hair follicle; the opening to the follicle may be dilated, forming a blackhead; the opening of the hair follicle that remains closed is called a whitehead or closed comedone	• Open comedo (blackhead) • Closed comedo (whitehead)
Milia	A very small subepidermal cyst with no visible opening; usually multiple	Milia seen in babies
Burrow	A channel under the skin produced by a parasite	• Scabies • Creeping eruption (animal hookworm larvae)
Lichenification	Thickened, roughened skin produced by scratching	• Neurodermatitis • Atopic dermatitis
Telangiectases	Superficial enlarged visible blood vessels	• At proximal nail fold (lupus) • Cirrhosis
Target lesions	Usually on the palms, have three zones of color change when compared with normal color.	Erythema multiforme

Cardinal Symptoms of Skin Diseases

Key symptoms of skin conditions that patients bring to medical attention are discussed in the boxes on pp. 443 and 448.

RASH OR SKIN LESION

Because examination of a skin lesion can greatly reduce the number of words needed in description, examination accompanies history taking. Patients are

Key Symptoms in the Examination of the Skin	
• Skin rash	• Changes in color
• Acne	• Itching
• Nodule	• Hives
• Eczema	• Changes in hair
• Nonhealing ulcers	• Changes in nails

usually at a loss to make the subtle points that differentiate primary, secondary, and special skin lesions until answering perceptive questions of the examiner.

SKIN ULCERS

Ulceration may be caused by the original skin problem, be a complication of trauma or rescratching or picking at the skin, or be caused by therapy the patient has used.

Leg ulcers and foot ulcers are two common problems that may be related to arterial or venous compromise in the legs. Patients with diabetes mellitus and peripheral neuropathy may sustain trauma or injury to the feet (e.g., poorly fitting shoes) that may result in ulcers that become secondarily infected and heal poorly.

CHANGES IN COLOR

More frequently a complaint about a change in skin color regards a specific lesion. A "mole" has become darker than usual. The patient's concern is, "Could this be cancer?"

Other patients seek treatment for newly recognized spots of hyperpigmentation, sometimes caused by sunlight exposure or related to aging. Hypopigmented areas may be vitiligo.

Telangiectasia refers to permanently dilated tiny venules. These vessels blanch when firm pressure is exerted directly over them. When examined closely, individual vessels are apparent.

Periungual telangiectasia (usually along the proximal nailfold) may be found in collagen diseases such as lupus, scleroderma, or dermatomyositis. Telangiectasias ordinarily do not involve the palms or soles.

Spider angiomas, or arterial spiders, consist of a central artery feeding small dilated vessels. Pressure on the central arteriole produces blanching. Spider angiomas are characteristic of chronic liver disease, pregnancy, and the use of estrogens.

ITCHING OR HIVES

Itching *(pruritus)* may be present either because of a skin disorder or a systemic abnormality. Urticaria *(hives)* are itchy wheals that are occasionally associated with more diffuse swelling.

More specific questions to ask patients about pruritus or urticaria are the following:

When do you itch? Do you ever see hives with the itch? Separate localized from systemic problems. Establish whether this may be urticaria.

Do you itch in the same place each time? Patients who itch in the same place, scratching repeatedly, develop thickened skin and are prone to develop neurodermatitis.

Do you have itching around the anus? Around the vulva? Pruritus ani and pruritus vulvae are rather common and have many etiologic causes. *Any rash behind the knees, neck, or antecubital fossa?* Patients with atopy typically develop generalized itching in several places.

Do you have any other illnesses? Patients with cirrhosis (bile-salt induced) or lymphomas are at risk for generalized itching.

Any exposure to someone with itching? This question seeks communicable causes of itching such as scabies.

What about recent travel? Parasitic causes include swimmer's itch caused by schistosomiasis.

Is your skin dry? Patients with chronically dry skin may feel pruritic.

CHANGES IN HAIR OR NAILS

Patients complain of increased hair growth *(hirsutism)* in abnormal places, lack of hair caused by falling out *(alopecia)*, changes in texture of the hair (coarser than usual), thinning of the hair, hair breaking off, and premature graying.

Androgenic steroids may cause hirsutism in women. Other causes include (1) use of oral contraceptives or corticosteroids and (2) adrenal or ovarian abnormalities. Patchy alopecia may be caused by syphilis or fungal infection, or it may be idiopathic.

Nail changes include splitting, ridging, discoloration, pitting, separation from the nailbed, splinter hemorrhage, and abnormal transverse lines. These are described in the section on physical examination.

Physical Examination of the Skin

Begin the examination by examining the affected area. Proceed to examine the entire skin and mucous membrane surface (see box on pg. 450). This requires good lighting, a patient clothed only in an examining gown, and a draw sheet to cover sections for modesty. Patients occasionally object, wanting examination of only the affected area. However, several discoveries may result from a complete examination (Table 12-4):

- Other related skin lesions may be present that will help in diagnosis
- Abnormalities besides skin lesions may be present and guide diagnosis
- Unanticipated skin lesions may be found

The light sources most useful include natural sunlight (usually not available), overhead fluorescent lights (better than gooseneck incandescent), a pen flashlight (good for side lighting to show raised lesions), and the Wood's light (for some fungal infections or erythrasma).

Color of skin lesions may be the same as the patient's normal skin or may be red, erythematous, pink, violaceous, brown, black, blue, gray, or depigmented. Use direct pressure over a lesion to produce blanching, placing a glass microscopic slide over the lesion and exerting gentle pressure. Don't press too hard or cut the skin with the sharp edges of the slide.

Biology of the Skin

The skin consists of three layers: epidermis, dermis, and *hypodermis,* the subcutaneous fatty layer.

The *epidermis* is generated in the basal cell layer, moves up into the prickle cell layer, followed by the granular cell layer, to finally become the horny, or keratin, layer. Cells are scaled off as squames. The horny layer is protective and, if it is defective because of water content (caused by chapped skin), not produced well (psoriasis), or damaged (burns), the protection is defective.

Certain cells in the epidermis are important. The Langerhans cells function as antigen-presenting cells and can migrate to lymph nodes. They are important in allergic reactions. Melanocytes are found mainly in the basal layer. They function to produce melanin and transfer it to keratinocytes, which deposit it over the surface of the nucleus on the side facing the sun.

The *dermis* is a rich network of collagen, blood vessels, neural elements, hair follicles and sebaceous glands, and sweat glands.

Hair follicles (pilosebaceous glands) have sebaceous glands opening into them. Eccrine sweat glands occur over much of the body and produce the bulk of the fluid loss daily. Apocrine sweat glands open into hair follicles in certain body sites. Bacteria grow on their secretions and yield characteristic odors.

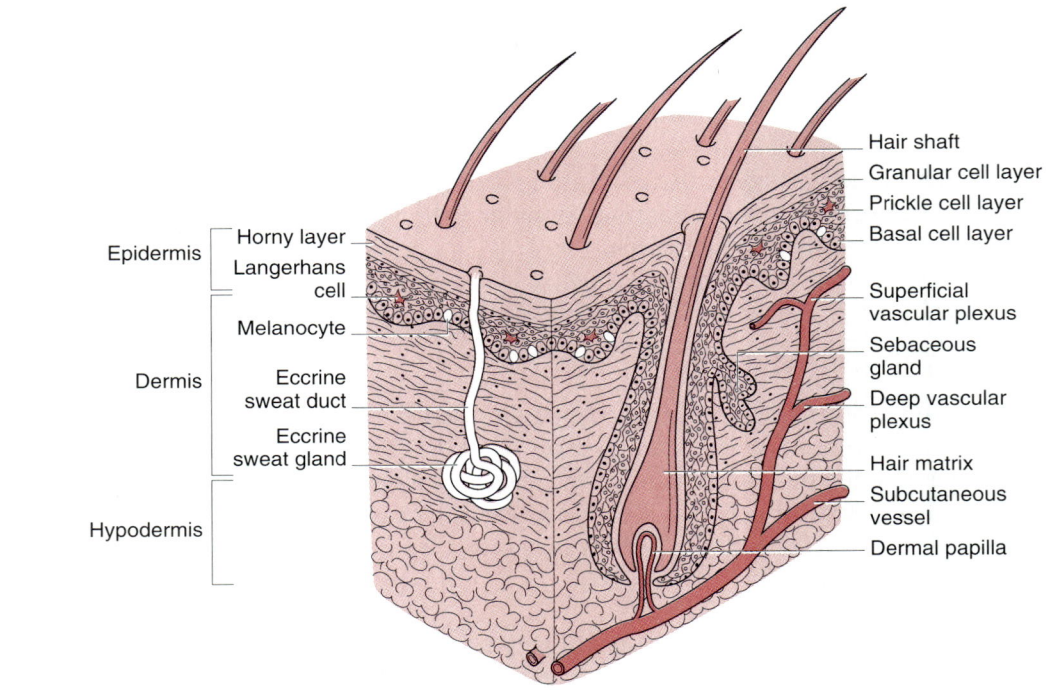

In evaluating each skin lesion, observe the following approach:

- Begin history with questions above
- Inspect the skin lesion(s) and note the following:
    1. Type of individual lesion (e.g., macule, papule, vesicle, petechia)
    2. Shape and margin of individual lesions
    3. Anatomic distribution of lesions
    4. Arrangement of lesions with respect to one another
- Evaluate primary lesions, secondary changes, special lesions, and associated findings

TABLE 12-4: Examining Forgotten Sites of Integument for Completeness

Site	Reason/Clues
Head and neck	
• Hair	• Individual hairs for color, texture, breaking
	• Distribution—loss (balding, alopecia) or excessive growth (hirsutism)
• Eyebrows	• Lateral thinning in hypothyroidism
• Eyelids and oral membranes	• Edema, ulcers, thrush
Hands	
• Palms	• Many lesions here can easily be missed (see Table 12-5)
• Nail and proximal nail folds	• Nail disorders
	• Telangiectasis of folds (collagen diseases)
Arms, chest, back, abdomen, legs	• Usually routinely examined
Feet	
• Soles	• Similar lesions to palms, but may not be on both soles and palms
• Nails	• Similar to finger nails but more fungal problems
Genitalia and perianal areas	• Sexually transmitted diseases and other special problems

After inspection, palpate the lesion for *induration* (firmness), *fluctuance* (firmness with soft top about ready to break open), depth, texture, and consistency. Is surgical drainage of purulence needed? Use the back of the fingers to palpate for temperature. Estimate the depth of a lesion to help differentiate between a plaque or a tumor. Gloves are not needed unless an ulcer, bleeding, drainage, or infection is suspected.

The shape and configuration of the individual lesion may provide a clue to the cause (Table 12-5). An oval shape is characteristic of the herald patch of pityriasis rosea, a ring *(annular)* shape of tinea corpus, and a *serpiginous* (snakelike) shape of visceral larval migrans. Likewise, the contour of lesions may be significant. Individual vesicles of chickenpox initially have smooth margins. Later, the margins become serrated. The margins of the lesions of smallpox remain smooth. Central clearing of some lesions (blastomycosis) may yield relatively normal-colored skin. Concentric erythema in the configuration of a bull's eye or target is characteristic of erythema multiforme.

Arrangement of lesions may be in groups, as are herpes simplex virus vesicles on the lips or genitalia (Plate 7). Vesicles, crusts, and later depigmented scars of herpes zoster follow a single dermatome distribution, usually on one side of the body. Vesicles of poison ivy may follow a linear distribution, usually not dermatomal. Either livedo reticularis or erythema infectiosum (fifth disease) may produce a *reticulated* (netlike) pattern on the skin.

Furthermore, the anatomic distribution may be characteristic (Table 12-6). Certain lesions may be found over extensor surfaces (e.g., psoriasis). Others are limited to hairy areas (e.g., folliculitis). The intertriginous areas with skin to skin contact (e.g., under large pendulous breasts) may be erythematous and pruritic

TABLE 12-5: Configuration of Dermatologic Lesions

Name	Configuration	Example
Annular	Ring shaped	Tinea (ringworm)
Circinate	Circular	Circinate balanitis (Reiter's syndrome)
Confluent	Lesions fusing together	Childhood exanthems
Discoid	Disc-shaped without central clearing	Discoid lupus
Discrete	Lesions separate	
Eczematoid	A tendency to erosion and crusting	Eczema
Generalized	Widespread, much of body	
Grouped	Lesions clustered together	Herpes simplex
Iris	A target, a bull's-eye lesion	Erythema multiforme
Keratotic	Thickened like a horn	Psoriasis
Linear	Line shaped	Poison ivy
Multiforme	More than one type of shape or form	Erythema multiforme
Papulosquamous	Papules and scaling plaques	Psoriasis
Reticulated	Lacelike	Erythema infectiosum
Serpiginous	Snakelike form	Cutaneous larva migrans
Telangiectatic	Dilated superficial blood vessels	Osler-Weber-Rendu disease
Totalis	Total body involved	Collagen disorders Alopecia totalis
Zosteriform	Dermatome distribution	Herpes zoster

(e.g., candidiasis). Sites of pressure over prominent bones of the back may contribute to skin necrosis (e.g., decubitus ulcers).

Skin Lesions Characteristically Involving Specific Areas

THE NAILS

Examination of fingernails or toenails often gives clues to skin lesions (Table 12-7). *Beau's lines* are transverse grooves across the nail caused by decreased growth during a severe illness. Tiny *pits* in the nails are characteristic of psoriasis.

Discoloration of the nails includes normal, dark brownish longitudinal lines in nails of black persons, and even darker color distributed diffusely in nails of persons taking azidothymidine (AZT). Yellow-nail syndrome includes nail changes along with pulmonary bronchiectasis, or pleural effusion. Sometimes fungal infections may produce slightly yellowish nails.

Nails may separate from the nailbed *(onycholysis)*. The most common reason is trauma to long nails, but psoriasis also produces this condition. *Terry's nails,* found in cirrhosis, show a ground-glass, whitish appearance on the proximal portion of the nails, with only the distal 1 to 2 mm being normal in color.

Mees' lines are horizontal white bands frequently present in chronic arsenic poisoning.

TABLE 12-6: Distribution of Skin Lesions as Clue to Disease

Disease	Appearance of Lesion	Characteristic Distribution	Other Clues
Atopic dermatitis	• Scratch marks • Red • Lichenification	Popliteal and antecubital fossas on face, neck, and upper chest	• Skin itches, chronic scratching, eczema, and lichenification • May have hay fever, asthma, urticaria
Contact dermatitis	• Swelling or redness of site • Edema of eyelids	Rash at site of contact; e.g., elastic—waist band; rubber—shoes; nickel—jewelry (fingers, neck); photoallergens—cheeks; perfumes—neck; nail polish—upper eyelids; detergent—hands	Find and remove offending agent to resolve skin lesions
Dermatitis herpetiformis	• Itchy red papules	Mostly on backside: arms and elbows, scapular areas, over sacrum, buttocks, and anteriorly below knees; usually spares mucous membranes	HLA-B8, gluten sensitivity
Erythema multiforme	• Target lesions • Central vesicles	Distal involvement: elbows, knees, and below to hands and feet; mucous membrane involvement with bulla in Stevens-Johnson syndrome	• Look for offending drug (e.g., sulfa). • Culture for mycoplasma, herpes
Pityriasis rosea	• Red, scaly herald patch about 10 days before later lesions, oval patches, pink	First lesion usually an oval-shaped "herald" patch; later, small scaling patches appear over trunk, front and back, and upper arms and upper legs; both the head and most of the arms and legs are spared.	• No lesions on palms or soles • Presumed viral etiology
Psoriasis	• Red scaly lesions	• Typically scalp and extensor surfaces of elbows and knees involved • Any part of body may be involved; fingernails develop tiny pits, and debris may be present under ends of nails	Chronic with exacerbations and remissions; arthritis may accompany, especially of DIP joints
Seborrhea	• Oily scales look like dandruff	Scalp, eyebrows, eyelids, nasolabial folds, and presternal areas are typically involved	
Secondary syphilis	• Many forms • Especially nummular, copper colored, about 10 mm; may be scaly like tinea	Eruption on face, trunk, palms, and soles Lesions of trunk may resemble pityriasis rosea; when face, palms, and soles are involved, syphilis is more likely	VDRL and FTA-ABS confirm unless in AIDS Benzathine penicillin is drug of choice

TABLE 12-7: Abnormalities of Fingernails

Name	Descriptions	Examples of Disease
Beau's lines	Transverse grooves	Severe illness
Pits in nails	Tiny pits	Psoriasis
Terry's nails	Proximal white ground glass appearance; distal 1 to 2 mm is pink	Cirrhosis
Mees' lines	Horizontal white bands	Arsenic poisoning
Splinter hemorrhages	Looks like splinter longitudinally under distal end of nail	Endocarditis (or nail trauma)
Yellow nail syndrome	Yellow color	Lung disease as pleural effusion
Koilonychia	Spoon-shaped depression in nails	Iron deficiency
Periungual telangiectasis	Telangiectasis of proximal nailfold	LE, dermatomyositis
Fungal infection	Distal portion of nail thickened or eroded	Fungal involvement—candida, tinea unguium

Splinter hemorrhages look somewhat like splinters under the nailbed. These may be caused by trauma or found in endocarditis.

THE MUCOUS MEMBRANES

Mucous membrane lesions of the mouth may give clues to an otherwise obscure diagnosis. Such lesions would include Koplik spots in measles (rubeola), thrush in AIDS, vesicles on the palate in hand-foot-and-mouth disease (coxsackievirus A-16), and ulcers in the mouth in lupus or in the vagina in Behçet's syndrome.

THE PALMS AND SOLES

Examination of palms and soles occasionally yields valuable clues. Many skin disorders have the potential to involve the palms or soles, but only a few do so regularly. Certain systemic diseases exhibit lesions on the palms and soles (Table 12-8). A few skin disorders localize to palms and soles. Thus examination of palms and soles is integral.

TABLE 12-8: Systemic and Some Local Diseases Manifested by Lesions found on Palms and Soles

Disease	Clinical Clues	Diagnostic Tests
Petechiae		
Rocky Mountain spotted fever (RMSF) (Plate 8)	• May have tick exposure • Fever, headache, delirium • Rapid progression usual	• Immediate: fluorescent antibody-staining skin biopsy for RMSF • Proteus OX-2, OX-19 titer • RMSF complement fixation titer
Meningococcemia (Plate 9)	• Sepsis or meningitis • Can cause death in hours • Patient appears septicemic	• Blood and CSF cultures for *Neisseria meningitidis* • Posterior nasopharyngeal cultures
Bacterial endocarditis (or sepsis) (Plate 10)	• Heart murmur, fever, and other signs of sepsis	• Blood cultures • Echocardiogram of cardiac valves for vegetations
Hemorrhagic varicella (Plate 11)	• Patient has exposure to chickenpox and exhibits vesicles of chickenpox	• Culture of lesions and throat
Hemorrhagic measles (Plate 12)	• Exposure to measles (rubeola) • Other manifestations of measles (cough, coryza, conjunctivitis, and Koplick spots)	• Culture of throat • Measles antibody titers, acute and convalescent
Macules		
RMSF (see Plate 8)	• Macules rather than petechiae in more slowly progressive disease	• As above
Meningococcemia (see Plate 9)	• Usually transient and early in course of illness, if at all	• As above
Secondary syphilis (Plate 13)	• Larger coin-shaped (nummular) lesions several mm in diameter	• VDRL, FTA-ABS
Measles (see Plate 12)	• Typical measles (rubeola) rash is morbilliform	• As above
Vesicles		
Varicella or zoster (Plate 14)	• Chickenpox (varicella) childhood illness; vesicles are widespread and appear in crops and are in different stages of development • Herpes zoster (shingles) virus, a dermatomal or disseminated reactivation of same virus	• As above
Hand-foot-and-mouth disease	• Coxsackievirus such as A-16 or other strain causes disease • Usually confined to hands, feet, and mouth	• Virus culture of throat, lesions, stool
Smallpox (no cases have occurred worldwide for several years)	• All vesicles appear in one crop and are at same stage • Widely spread over body	• Virus culture

Continued.

TABLE 12-8: Systemic and Some Local Diseases Manifested by Lesions found on Palms and Soles—cont'd

Disease	Clinical Clues	Diagnostic Tests
Papules		
Drug reactions (Plate 15)	• Rashes generalized, with palm and sole lesions, too; usually itchy	• Eosinophil count • Withdraw drug
Gonococcemia (Plate 16)	• Triad of migratory arthralgia, papules (or pustules), and tenosynovitis • May have urethral or vaginal discharge	• Culture of urethra, anus, and throat on Thayer-Martin media
Dishidrosis	• Pompholyx or dishidrotic eczema is confined to the palms and soles • Sweaty palms and severe itching are characteristic • Vesicles resolve to small dark brown spots, peeling	
Idiophytid reaction	• Allergic reaction to a fungal infection • Small, hard vesicles on the sides of fingers or the feet itch intensely	• Treat fungal infection and lesions disappear
Bacterial endocarditis (see Plate 10)	• Papules (pustules) of distal finger tufts (Osler's nodes) or of palms (Janeway lesions)	• Culture of blood • Echocardiogram of cardiac valves for vegetations
Scales and exfoliation		
Toxic shock syndrome (Plate 17)	• *Staphylococcus aureus* toxin causes systemic illness, diarrhea, delerium, sunburnlike rash that later peels off fingertips • Often associated with use of tampons	• Culture of urine, vagina for *S. aureus* • May have abnormal liver and kidney function studies
Scarlet fever	• Group A streptococcal infection may be severe and cause systemic dysfunction • Later peels	• Culture throat for streptococcus • ASO titer, streptozyme titer
Reiter's syndrome	• Characteristic rash on palms and soles is called keratoderma blenorrhagicum	• HLA B27
Dyshidrosis	• Pompholyx • Dishidiotic eczema • See above	• As above
Tinea (Plate B)	• Tinea pedis (athlete's foot), tinea corporis, or tinea capitis (ringworm of body or head), characteristically scales	• Culture
Erythema multiforme (Plate 19)	• Inflammation of skin and mucous membranes with iris or target lesions • Concentric rings • Inner ring may form bullous lesions • If exfoliation occurs, especially in mouth, called Stevens-Johnson syndrome	• Mycoplasma complement fixation titer • Herpes simplex titer • Withdraw offending medicines

TABLE 12-9: Pustular Diseases

	Age Range	Anatomic Defect	Microbes	Appearance	Healing	Therapy
Acne vulgaris	16 to 24 years	Blocked pilosebaceous follicle	*Propionibacterium acnes*	Comedones, pustules	Pitted scars	Tetracycline
Rosacea	35 to 60 years	Not known	None	Pustules, telangiectasia	Rhinophyma	Tetracycline
Hidradenitis suppurativa	After puberty	Blocked apocrine glands	Gram-negative bacilli	Pustules, tracts tunneling under skin	Depressed scars	Specific antibiotics

Pustular Diseases (Table 12-9)

ACNE VULGARIS

Acne vulgaris is a common skin disease. It begins after puberty and subsides after a few years, only to recur in later adult years in some people.

Acne begins in the pilosebaceous glands. Keratin plugs the ducts (comedomes) of the sebaceous gland—the hair follicle. Both open comedomes (blackheads) and closed comedomes (whiteheads) begin with the keratin plug in the sebaceous follicle. Lipases from *Propionibacterium acnes,* which colonize the follicles, break down sebum and form keratin plugs. Papules, pustules, nodules, and pus-filled cysts result progressively. Healing of deeper lesions leave scars, especially if crude attempts to squeeze or drain lesions have been used.

The history may show that summertime exposure to sunlight has beneficial effects. Diet choices, chocolate, soft drinks, or greasy foods apparently make acne worse in some persons. Exacerbations may cycle with menses, and acne may become worse or better with pregnancy or contraceptives. Greasy cosmetics also exacerbate acne in some people.

ROSACEA

Rosacea is a chronic inflammatory disorder localized to the face and nose, especially in people between ages 30 and 50 years. Papules, pustules, erythema, and telangiectasia are common, especially on the nose and the middle third of the face. In rosacea, papules are not caused by keratin in follicles. Untreated rosacea may lead to granuloma formation or cutaneous hyperplasia. *Rhinophyma,* an enlarged, red, nodular nose, sometimes with thickened adjacent face, may result.

HIDRADENITIS SUPPURATIVA

Hidradenitis suppurativa is a chronic inflammatory pustular disorder caused by blocked apocrine glands (Plate 20). Chronic purulent papules, pustules, and sinus tracks result in scarring of axillae, breasts, and the pubic and perineal areas. The disease may be found in males but more commonly occurs in obese females. A hallmark has been comedones with two openings. This allows the formation of epithelialized tunnels under the skin with abscesses and sinus tracts. A defect in polymorphonuclear leukocyte–killing activity resulting in reduced ability to kill infecting gram-negative bacilli (*Escherichia coli, Proteus* sp.) has been described in a small percentage of people with this disorder.

CASE 12-1 Hidradenitis Suppurativa

A 62-year-old retired engineer was seen for draining abscesses in both axillary areas, the pubic area, and the perineum. He had had these chronically for 4 years and wore a diaper inside of his underwear to catch the purulent, foul-smelling drainage.

He had no other complaints and was taking only antibiotics for the drainage. Antibiotics, however, were only transiently helpful.

On examination he was a pleasant, well-groomed man appearing older than his stated age. Vital signs were normal, and no adenopathy was present. The general examination was normal except for the skin. Both axillae had scars from old draining sites. Firm, red, raised tender nodules were present in close proximity to draining sinuses. Similar lesions were found in the pubic and peritoneal areas (see Plate 20).

A clinical diagnosis of hidradenitis suppurativa with abscesses, sinus tracts, and tunnels was made.

A needle aspirate and culture of one of the abscesses was taken. This grew *Proteus mirabilis*. He was treated with a new, investigational antibacterial agent and improved for a brief time.

Miliaria (Plate 21)

Miliaria crystallina is initially a condition where sweat is trapped in the epidermis layer. This causes a tiny, clear sweat retention vesicle under the skin surface. These 0.5 to 1.0 mm vesicles look like tiny drops of water on normal-appearing skin. These may cause irritation and may become infected. Miliaria occurs in older bedridden patients who are kept too warm. Miliaria crystallina does not have surrounding erythema, inflammation, or other symptoms.

Miliaria rubra, prickly heat rash in babies or adults in the tropics, consists of tiny red spots that have a tingling, prickling, itching sensation (Plate 21). The eccrine duct obstruction is deeper in miliaria rubra than in miliaria crystallina. If the patient continues to sweat and form miliaria, bacterial secondary infection may cause pustules.

Eczematous Diseases

Eczema is a common inflammatory skin disorder. Some lay people refer to many skin disorders as eczema. *Eczema* is characterized by superficial inflammation of the skin accompanied by itching, erythema, vesicles, edema, oozing, excoriation, crusting, and scaling. After chronic scratching, the tissues become thickened *(lichenification)*. Look carefully to identify features to assist in the differential diagnosis: (1) individual lesions—erythema, scales, or vesicles, and (2) distribution pattern of lesions.

ATOPIC DERMATITIS (PLATE 22)

The term *atopy* was coined to refer to the hereditary tendency to have hay fever, asthma, urticaria, and a distinct dermatitis. People with atopy tend to develop pruritus (itching) under stress. The earliest rash may be a red papule or a scratch. With scratching, erythema occurs, then weeping, scaling, and lichenification.

The typical distribution involves the face and extensor surfaces in infants and flexion creases in adults. Itching may be severe and involve the head, neck, and shoulders. Some patients have only hand eczema. The backs of the fingers near the webs may be affected, especially following exposure to irritants.

Age-Related Atopic Dermatitis

The infant commonly has eczema with erythematous patches, either dry or oozing, usually on the cheeks. Adolescents have atopic eczema on the back of the neck, at the flexor areas at elbows, knees, and wrists, on the eyelids, and behind the ears. The skin becomes dark red because of excoriations. Infection, lichenification, and hyperpigmentation occurs later. Still later, chronic inflammation may result in depigmentation. After age 30 years, chronic hand or foot eczema may begin and last for years.

Factors in the pruritus include rapid changes in atmospheric temperature or humidity. Hot baths may make itching worse. Fabrics such as wool or nylon may cause pruritus resulting from heightened tactile sensitivity.

Other characteristic examination findings may suggest atopic dermatitis. Frequent, intense pruritus of eyelids leads to rubbing and scratching. A double medial lower eyelid fold develops. Cataracts (opaque lens) occur in 5% to 10% of those affected. Broken hairs resulting from scratching and alopecia areata occur more frequently in atopic patients. Serum IgE may be increased.

CONTACT DERMATITIS

The term *contact dermatitis* is used for a rash resulting from contact between a substance and skin. It is used for allergic contact dermatitis and also for nonallergic mechanisms.

Irritant dermatitis occurs after a single contact with a strong irritant (e.g., some acids), or after repeated exposures to milder irritants (e.g., some detergents).

Allergic contact dermatitis requires first that the skin has been altered in its reactivity, usually by previous contact. Following that, skin contact with the substance or a closely related substance is required to produce reaction.

Contact urticaria refers to urticaria (hives) that occurs at a site distant from the contact between skin and the allergen (Plate 22). Both the amount of allergen and the patient's own reaction to it determine whether localized or generalized hives, asthma, or even anaphylaxis will result.

Common substances that produce contact dermatitis include plants (poison ivy), jewelry (containing nickel), adhesive tape, shoe leather, elastic, rubber, cosmetics, and perfumes.

On examination, the anatomic distribution of rash is likely to suggest a possible cause. The rash may take one of several forms: erythema, lichenification caused by scratching, patches of vesicles, or oozing superficial ulcers.

Connective Tissue Diseases

The name *connective tissue diseases* is used because the collagenous connective tissues distributed throughout the body may be affected. Skin abnormalities are prominent in these disorders: SLE, RA, scleroderma, and dermatomyositis. These are discussed in more detail in Chapter 9, musculoskeletal diseases.

SYSTEMIC LUPUS ERYTHEMATOSUS

Criteria for classifying SLE have been proposed for research purposes. Patients who manifest 4 criteria from a list of 11 and do not have other diagnoses as the

TABLE 12-10: Skin Lesions Found in SLE

Lesion	Frequency
Alopecia	50%
Telangiectasia	50%
Raynaud's phenomenon	15%
Mucous membrane lesions	10%
Pigment changes	10%
Sclerodactyly	10%
Urticaria	10%
Livedo reticularis	8%
Thrombophlebitis	7%
Chronic ulcers	5%
Rheumatoid nodules	5%
Bullous lesions	3%

cause are quite likely to have SLE (see pg. 344). There is no time restriction on the duration over which patients must be followed to see if they exhibit four of the criteria. These criteria are not an exhaustive listing of every possible finding in lupus, but they do show that SLE involves multiple systems. Skin lesions characteristic of, but not specific for, SLE are listed in Table 12-10.

Discoid lupus erythematosus (LE) skin lesions consist of erythematous or violaceous plaques with a scale that extends deep into skin follicles. They expand slowly at the margins. As these heal, the skin develops an atrophic scar, central depigmentation, and telangiectasia. Discoid LE lesions are usually on the head: forehead, cheeks, nose, or ears. The scalp may be involved in over 50% of patients. Progression of discoid LE to SLE is uncommon, but patients with SLE may have discoid lesions.

RHEUMATOID ARTHRITIS

RA is discussed in Chapter 9. Skin lesions include subcutaneous nodules, thin skin caused by steroid use, red eyes caused by dryness, and telangiectasias.

SCLERODERMA

Scleroderma (systemic sclerosis) is an uncommon disorder of fibrosis of connective tissue throughout the body. *Scleroderma* is the term applied to the tight thickening of the skin. Other manifestations include *Raynaud's phenomenon* (triphasic color change of the fingers or toes in response to cold exposure), telangiectasias, and involvement of the esophagus (dysphagia and dysmotility), heart (hypertension and conduction delays), lungs (interstitial fibrosis and pulmonary hypertension), and kidneys (renal failure). Such patients may have a progressive downhill course.

In the absence of visceral involvement, the patient may have the benign CREST syndrome (*c*alcinosis, *R*aynaud's phenomenon, *e*sophageal dysmotility, *s*clerodactyly, and *t*elangiectasias). Anticentromere antibodies are common in CREST but not scleroderma.

Skin involvement with scleroderma often passes through stages: edema, induration, and atrophy. In the beginning, the skin of the face and digits appears tense and exhibits nonpitting edema for weeks or months. Later the skin of the face and fingers becomes hard and is bound to underlying tissues. The fingers cannot be extended. Increased or decreased pigmentation may occur. Finally, the atrophic phase results in shiny skin. The fingertips are small and pointed. Ulcerations develop and may become infected. The face loses normal lines and wrinkles and looks more like a mask.

DERMATOMYOSITIS

Proximal muscle weakness *(polymyositis)* and chronic skin inflammation may occur alone, or, if together *(dermatomyositis)*, as an inflammatory disease of uncertain etiologic cause. This also is an uncommon disorder.

Criteria for diagnosis include weakness of the proximal muscles, increased concentration of creatine phosphokinase (CPK), EMG evidence, muscle biopsy showing myocyte necrosis with phagocytosis and regeneration, and skin changes.

Typical skin findings include heliotrope, periorbital violaceous skin, and edema of the eyelids. Gottron's papules are flat 2 to 10 mm violaceous papules over the dorsum of the interphalangeal joints, on the sides of the fingers, and on the hands, elbows, patellas, and medial malleoli. They are considered pathognomonic. Telangiectasias are common along the proximal nail fold.

Fungal Infections (Plate 23)

DERMATOPHYTOSIS

Superficial fungal infections of the skin, hair, or nails are referred to as *tinea*, followed by a word indicating the anatomic site involved. *Tinea pedis* refers to foot infection, *tinea cruris* to groin, *tinea corporis* to body, *tinea barbae* to beard, *tinea manus* to hand, *tinea capitis* to scalp, and *tinea unguium* to fingernails or toenails.

Three genera of fungi, *Microsporum*, *Trichophyton*, and *Epidermophyton*, are known as dermatophytes. Each has the ability to digest keratin. These become invasive only rarely, even in the presence of immunosuppression. The microbial species is determined by culturing scrapings from the scales.

Tinea pedis may be transmitted by shared bathing facilities. Fungal growth is enhanced by warm, moist feet (see Plate 18). Men are more commonly affected than are women or children. Tinea pedis usually begins in the web between the fourth and fifth toes. Later, other toes and the arch and sides of the foot may be affected. The skin between the toes becomes itchy, inflamed, and macerated. Warm weather encourages acute episodes of vesicles on the toes, instep, and sides of the foot. Sometimes bacterial suprainfection occurs. Chronic infection produces fine white scales. Fungal involvement of toenails may result in thickened, distorted nails that collect large amounts of debris underneath the distal margins. Itching may be intense, especially when shoes and socks are removed. When the foot is infected with *T. rubrum,* a "moccasin" distribution commonly involves the edge of the sole of the foot and the plantar surface.

An idiophytid (or "id") reaction is an allergic reaction, usually caused by tinea pedis. Small, hard vesicles 1 to 2 mm in diameter appear on the sides of the fingers or on the feet. These may itch intensely.

Tinea corporis, *ringworm* of the body, exhibits characteristic rounded pink macules with white scales and slightly raised borders. The lesions enlarge by expanding at the periphery while clearing in the center. Tinea corporis is often self-limited.

Tinea capitis, ringworm of the scalp, is predominantly found in prepubertal children and is usually caused by *T. tonsurans.* Highly contagious in this age group, it sometimes causes epidemics. A consistent sign is the broken-off "stub" hair. This gives patches of partial baldness. *M. canis* from puppies and kittens and *M. audouinii* from humans also cause broken-off hairs. Patchy baldness may be caused by broken-off hairs with some fungi and black dots with others.

Patchy alopecia (hair loss) may be caused by several agents: tinea capitis, secondary syphilis, or idiopathic bald patches *(alopecia areata).* The last does not exhibit broken hairs or black dots.

Onychomycosis (tinea unguium) often involves the toenails in people who have had longstanding tinea pedis (Plate 23). Affected nail(s) appear dull and thick, and the distal edge becomes separated from the nailbed *(onycholysis).*

Characteristic features help to differentiate other forms of nail involvement. Psoriasis of the nails produces tiny (1 mm) pits in the nails. *Candida albicans* infection of the nails commonly gives changes distally, whereas *Trichophyton* sp. may cause swelling of the nailplate attachment.

Tinea versicolor is caused by *Malassezia furfur (Pityrosporum orbiculare).* The macular lesions of tinea versicolor may be pale, pink, or brown in white persons or dark in black persons (Plate 24). The term *versicolor* (changes color) comes from the appearance of a change in color of lesions when the patient gets a suntan. Infected sites remain hypopigmented. Thus the name "versicolor" because lesions seem to change color. Actually, they remain unchanged when the surrounding skin darkens.

CANDIDIASIS

Candida albicans, a yeast, not a dermatophyte, normally inhabits the gut. Predisposition to candidal infections occurs in people treated with antibiotics, women taking oral contraceptives, those who have undergone corticosteroid therapy or cancer chemotherapy, and in people who have diabetes mellitus or AIDS. Intertriginous skin sites, the mouth, and the vagina are common sites for infection.

Under breasts and in the groin, perianal areas, or vulva, *C. albicans* forms elongated yeast cells that resemble hyphae. These penetrate between epithelial cells to form small papules. With candidal growth, the skin may be denuded, leaving a glistening raw base. Scattered away from the margins of the raw areas, red papules termed *satellites* are found. They are useful in distinguishing candidiasis from tinea.

Candidiasis has a predilection for warm, moist sites. Candida organisms may infect the fingernails in people who have moist hands or who work with their hands in water. *Candidal vulvovaginitis* may result in a cottage-cheese–like discharge. The vulva become red, swollen, and pruritic. The inner aspects of the thighs and the anus may be involved.

Candidal balanitis (inflammation of the glans penis and prepuce) may occur in the circumcised or uncircumcised male. Tender, red, pinpoint papules may appear in diabetic men or in men who have had intercourse with a female who has candidal vulvovaginitis.

Patients with AIDS frequently develop oral thrush as the CD-4 lymphocyte count decreases. White patchy or confluent exudates appear on the buccal mucosa, tongue, or throat. If candidal esophagitis accompanies thrush, dysphagia results. Although the appearance is characteristic, cultures are necessary for confirmation because viral esophagitis can result in similar lesions.

TABLE 12-11: Palpable and Nonpalpable Purpura

Condition	Palpable Purpura	Description	Etiology
Purpura simplex (Schamberg's disease)	No	Brick or rust-colored instead of usual purple	Capillaritis, idiopathic
Connective tissue atrophy	No	Steroid purpura	Use of steroids
		Senile purpura	Aging and solar damage
Systemic diseases	No	Thrombocytopenic purpura	Decreased platelets
	No	Fragile capillaries	Scurvy
	No	Thrombosis (may be ecchymotic instead of petechial)	Disseminated intravascular coagulation
Vasculitis	Yes	Vasculitis	Leukocytoclastic vasculitis
	Yes	Vasculitis or emboli	RMSF
			Meningococcemia

Purpura and Petechiae (Plate 25)

Purpura signifies bleeding into the dermis. Tiny (1 to 2 mm) purpura are termed *petechiae*. Large (>0.5 cm) purpuric macules are called *ecchymoses*. Purpura may occur spontaneously or be caused by trauma. Damaged blood vessel walls, decreased platelet counts, reduced vitamin K–dependent clotting factors, or hypofibrinogenemia may cause petechiae or purpura.

In addition to observing the distribution of purpura, rub the examining fingers over the petechiae looking for induration (firmness or elevation). Palpable purpura indicates vasculitis (Table 12-11). Nonpalpable purpura may be caused by thrombocytopenia or benign purpura of the legs of the elderly.

Petechiae or ecchymoses are common in systemic illnesses, including Rocky Mountain spotted fever (RSMF), meningococcemia, and other less common diseases. The first two commonly have generalized rash. When petechiae are found on the palms and soles of a very sick patient (Plate 25), especially if petechiae are palpable on skin elsewhere, either RMSF or meningococcemia should be suspected. Because these may be fulminant, rapid diagnosis and initiation of therapy may prevent death. RMSF, caused by *Rickettsia rickettsii*, is transmitted by tick bite. One-sixth of patients deny tick exposure. Patients appear with fever and headache and may be delirious. The patient with mild or early illness may exhibit macules that blanch with pressure instead of with petechiae (see Plate 8). Both macules and petechiae may appear together. Rapid progression in untreated disease may result in ecchymoses.

Neisseria meningitidis is carried in the posterior nasopharynx and is transmitted by person-to-person spread, typically among people who eat, drink, or sleep in proximity. In those with septicemia or meningitis, rash is generalized and on the palms and soles. Although meningococcemia causes macules and petechiae, palpable petechiae predominate.

Chickenpox and measles may both be hemorrhagic, with some lesions appearing petechial (see Plates 11 and 12). They are diagnosed not because of the petechial lesions but because of other manifestations.

Persons with septicemia of bacterial endocarditis may exhibit petechiae on palms, soles, conjunctivae, or elsewhere (see Plate 10). Rat-bite fever resulting

TABLE 12-12: Macular, Papular, and Maculopapular Rashes

Parameter	Rubeola (Measles)	Drug Rash	Rubella (3-day Measles)	RMSF	Neisseria gonorrheae	Syphilis
Age	• 1 to 20 years	• Any	• 1 to 20 years	• 10 to 55 years	• After puberty	• After puberty
Sites	• Total body	• Total body	• Total body	• P and S, generalized	• Few lesions anywhere	• P and S and body
Lesion and color	• 0.5 to 1.0 mm in diameter macules and maculopapules • Morbilliform	• Papules more common • Maculopapular	• Pink maculopapules	• Macules early or in mild disease • Petechiae later or in severe disease	• Macules may become pustules	• Nummular, copper colored, but may have other appearance
Pruritus	• No	• Yes	• No	• No	• No	• No
Associated findings	• Cough, coryza • Conjunctivitis • Koplik's spots	• May be drug fever or eosinophilia	• Adenopathy • Arthralgia in teenagers • Petechiae on soft palate	• Petechiae and purpura if severe	• Rash • Arthritis • Tenosynovitis	• Rash • Adenopathy • Flulike syndrome
Palms and soles	• Yes	• Yes	• No	• Yes	• Yes	• Yes
Diagnosis	• CF titer • Virus isolation	• Stop drug	• Rubella titer	• FA on skin biopsy • Complement fixation and titer	• Culture from anus, throat, blood, urethra	• VDRL and FTA-ABS

from *Streptobacillus moniliformis* may cause fever, generalized symptoms, and a macular or petechial rash on the body, palms, or soles.

Macules, Papules, and Maculopapular Diseases (Plate 26)

A *macule* denotes a flat spot. A *papule* is a small, circumscribed, solid elevation of the skin. The combination word *maculopapular* indicates a combination of macules and papules. Some of the lesions may have a papule in the center of the macule. In contrast, *papulosquamous* indicates papules and scales in the eruption. There is overlap, and some papulosquamous disorders may be classified as maculopapular.

In examining macules, press with the fingertip and quickly remove to be sure they blanch. An alternate technique is to apply pressure with a glass slide or test tube. Petechiae, in contrast to macules, do not blanch when pressure is applied because they are caused by extravasated blood.

Macular, papular, and maculopapular rash associations are listed in Table 12-12. These lesions may be found predominately on palms and soles, be scattered, or be generalized.

TABLE 12-13: Rashes that May Occur in Drug Eruptions

Name of Rash	Appearance	Examples of Causes
Acneiform	Looks like acne	Steroids, SSKI, lithium
Erythema multiforme	Targetlike lesions	Sulfonamides, barbiturates
Exfoliative dermatitis	Red skin, scaling	Isoniazid, gold therapy
Fixed drug eruptions	Round, red placques that develop at same site if drug is given again	Tetracyclines, quinine, sulfonamides
Photosensitivity	Rash in areas exposed to sunlight	Quinolines, tetracyclines, sulfonamides, psoralens
Purpura	Purpura or ecchymoses	Coumadin with aspirin
Toxic epidermal necrolysis	Rash resembles scalded skin	Barbiturates, phenytoin, penicillin
Toxic erythema	Measleslike rash (morbilliform)	Antibiotics such as penicillin, sulfonamides and thiazides
Urticaria	Hives	Antibiotics, salicylates
Vasculitis	Palpable purpura	Sulfonamides

RUBEOLA (MEASLES)

Measles, the old-fashioned, hard, 8-day measles, once an illness of childhood, has become delayed until the high school or college years because of partial immunization of the population. Associated findings as listed (along with a history of exposure 7 to 14 days before onset) help to make the diagnosis: cough, coryza, conjunctivitis, and, early in the course, *Koplik's spots.* These blue-white spots have a red base on the buccal mucous membrane opposite the premolars. These spots appear 1 to 2 days before the rash and last 2 to 4 days.

The measles rash (see Plate 12) is 0.1 to 1 cm maculopapules, dark red to purplish. They frequently become confluent and may be termed morbilliform, meaning distinctively like measles.

Early the rash blanches, later it does not. The rash turns brownish and has a fine scale as it fades.

DRUG RASH

Drug eruptions take many forms and are caused by a variety of mechanisms (Table 12-13). A rather common form is a fine, reddish papular rash over the trunk or any part of the body (see Plate 15).

RUBELLA (GERMAN MEASLES)

Rubella (the 3-day measles) has also been greatly reduced in incidence by widespread immunization. It typically occurred a little later in childhood than did rubeola, into the teen years. Children may be relatively asymptomatic other than having the rash. Adults may have arthralgia. If the patient is pregnant and has rubella during the first trimester, the fetus may develop a number of congenital abnormalities.

Onset occurs after 14 to 21 days of incubation. Rubella is associated with a pink oval maculopapule. The rash fades in 1 to 2 days, but fine desquamation may occur.

CASE 12-2 Meningococcemia

An 18-year-old male high school senior was brought to the emergency department with a rash and fever.

The patient had not felt well for a few days but had attended school and continued extracurricular activities. On the morning of admission he had asked his mother to take his temperature because he had a bad headache. She noted a spotty red rash on his face. After breakfast, the rash had progressed to cover the chest and abdomen.

On examination he appeared ill, asking for the lights to be turned low (photophobia). His temperature was 39° C, and pulse was 115 beats/min.

Generalized nonblanching, palpable petechiae were present over the face, trunk, and legs to the knees (see Plate 9). Petechiae were also on the palate, palms and soles, and conjunctiva.

His neck was stiff, and he had a positive Kernig's sign.

Because this occurred in January, meningococcemia and meningitis were felt to be more likely than Rocky Mountain spotted fever. An IV line was inserted, and 2 million units of aqueous penicillin G were administered at once.

The CSF analysis showed a WBC of 605; 98% were polymorphonuclear cells. The glucose was reduced to 18 mg/dl, and the protein increased to 175 mg/dl. *Neisseria meningitidis* grew from cultures of the posterior nasopharynx, blood, and CSF. After therapy for 10 days, the patient recovered uneventfully.

OTHER

RMSF is caused by *R. rickettsii* transmitted by a tick bite. Patients typically become ill very quickly, with rapid progression of the rash to a petechial or hemorrhagic condition. Patients also typically have fever and headache and become delirious.

N. gonorrheae and *N. meningitidis* may cause rashes that look similar. Usually the rash of disseminated gonococcal disease is pustular (see Plate 16). Rash from meningococcal disease may be pustular, petechial, or, less often, begin as macular.

Gonococcemia may be suspected from the triad of migratory arthralgia, papular or pustular skin lesions involving the body, palms, or soles, and tenosynovitis. Tenosynovitis is characterized by pain along a tendon sheath, made worse if the tendon is moved along its course. A history of sexual contact with someone who might harbor *N. gonorrheae* lends support to the diagnosis, as do appropriate cultures.

Syphilis has been termed the great mimicker because it has such a great variety of appearances. The rash of primary syphilis (the chancre) is a painless ulcer with a firm, indurated margin (Plate 26). The rash of secondary syphilis commonly occurs on the palms and soles as a coin-shaped (nummular) coppery brown color. It is usually accompanied by systemic myalgia, fever, and generalized lymphadenopathy.

Papulosquamous Diseases (Plates 27, 28, and 29)

Papulosquamous diseases are characterized by papules with scaling of squames. These diseases include seborrheic dermatitis, psoriasis, pityriasis rosea, and lichen planus (Table 12-14). The differential diagnoses of papulosquamous diseases should always include secondary syphilis.

CASE 12-3 Secondary Syphilis

A 22-year-old man sought medical care for a fever reaching 103° F and a rash.

He had been sick for 4 or 5 days with generalized myalgia, lethargy, and daily afternoon temperatures as high as 104° F. He had taken some of his girlfriend's tetracycline, which was left over from a previous infection. He denied having a headache or stiff neck, being exposed to animals or ticks, or using intravenous drugs.

On examination, the temperature was 102.5° F and heart rate was 110 and regular. There was generalized adenopathy. The chest was clear, and no murmurs were present. Neither the liver nor spleen was palpable.

The skin examination showed a rash measuring 7 by 9 mm on the palms and soles, predominantly, but also on the rest of the body (see Plate 26). The individual lesions were copper-colored, circular, nonpalpable, nontender, not pruritic, and not draining.

The laboratory studies showed the VDRL to be reactive at 64 dilutions and a positive test for FTA-ABS. The HIV antibody test was negative. He was treated with benzathine penicillin, 2.4 million units.

TABLE 12-14: Papulosquamous Diseases

Parameter	Seborrheic Dermatitis	Psoriasis	Pityriasis Rosea	Lichen Planus
Age	In babies (cradle cap) and children, but especially adults and old age	15 to 40 years	10 to 35 years	Usually 30 to 70 years
Sites	Scalp, eyebrows, eyelashes nasolabial folds, external ear canal, behind ears, presternal area	Elbows, knees, scalp, gluteal cleft and nails (extensor surface)	Thorax or proximal extremities	Flexor surfaces—wrists, forearms, legs above ankles, lumbar area
Color	Inflamed base	Red to dark red	• Salmon pink • Hyperpigmented in blacks	• At first pink, later purple • Persists for months; becomes dark red.
Type of scales	Greasy white or yellow	Silvery scales	Fine scale attached in a ring around inside of pink lesion (collarete)	
Mechanism	Yeastlike *Pityrosporum ovale* may help perpetuate	Transit time of keratinocytes	Unproven viral etiology	Inflammatory
Associated findings	• Exacerbations and remission • May be prominent in AIDS patients or in those with parkinsonism	• Exacerbations and remissions • Pitting of nails • DIP arthritis	Rash on back follows skin lines in a Christmas tree distribution	Five P's—planar (flat) polyangular, purple papules, pruritic
Pruritis	Some	Variable	Sometimes	Yes
Diagnostic aids	Scrapings negative, unlike tinea versicolor	Auspitz's sign (fine bleeding points if scales scratched off)	Herald patch is first lesion appearing 7 to 10 days before others, and is larger	Wickham's stria (netlike pattern of whitish lines across top)

SEBORRHEIC DERMATITIS

Seborrhea is a skin disorder of unknown etiologic cause that affects hairy areas. The skin becomes red, scaly, and greasy-looking and often itches (Plate 27). Untreated patients may excoriate the skin, allowing a secondary bacterial infection. Although *Pityrosporum orbiculare* has been suggested as an organism that may help to perpetuate seborrhea, scrapings do not show fungus, as does tinea versicolor.

In babies, scalp seborrhea is called *cradle cap*. The scalp appears symmetrically red, with greasy-appearing white scales. In the adult, mild seborrhea may appear to be dandruff. Seborrhea may affect eyebrows, forehead, eyelashes, the folds along the nose, and the presternal area in a symmetric distribution. Patients with AIDS or parkinsonism may develop especially prominent seborrhea.

PSORIASIS

Psoriasis is a chronic papulosquamous disease that involves increased cell division in the basilar epidermal layer. Keratinocyte transit time through the epidermis is accelerated as much as 10-fold, which does not allow time for individual cell maturation.

Psoriasis may begin in childhood, but more often starts after puberty. Symmetric patches appear on extensor surfaces, knees, elbows, buttocks, or on the scalp (Plate 28). Initial papules coalesce into red plaques. Both papules and plaques are covered with silvery scales. The hair is not involved, but fingernails may exhibit tiny (less than 1 mm) pits. Individual papules or plaques of psoriasis may be quite pruritic. Removal of scales frequently leaves fine bleeding points called Auspitz's sign.

Lesions of psoriasis may appear in areas of skin trauma previously uninvolved by psoriasis *(Koebner's phenomenon)*. Pustules are not common, but they may appear during acute episodes.

Severe psoriasis can result in generalized exfoliative erythroderma. Psoriatic arthritis may appear between ages 30 and 50 years. Joints typically involved include the distal interphalangeal joints (compare with Heberden's nodes) and the spine. The joints involved are usually asymmetric, but symmetric arthritis may occur.

PITYRIASIS ROSEA

Pityriasis rosea is another papulosquamous disease, of putative viral origin, which occurs predominantly in females aged 10 to 35 years. Seasonal onset is typical during fall and spring. Application of ultraviolet light or sunlight may hasten resolution.

The first lesion (herald patch) of pityriasis rosea is oval, salmon-colored, covered with scales, 2 to 10 centimeters across, and on the trunk or proximal part of the extremities (Plate 29). Often it goes unnoticed by the patient until the generalized eruption occurs 7 to 10 days later. The generalized eruption exhibits 1 to 2 mm papules and 3 to 6 mm oval plaques that are salmon pink. The long axes of the oval lesions are parallel to the skin lines, especially on the back, trunk, and legs. On the back, distribution of the lesions resemble drooping pine tree branches. Individual lesions have a crinkly scale of exfoliation that begins near the center of each lesion. An oval ring of scale called the *collarette scale* remains attached inside the margins of the salmon-colored plaque. Lesions of pityriasis in darkly pigmented people may be dark instead of pink, and postinflammatory hyperpigmentation is the rule after the illness resolves.

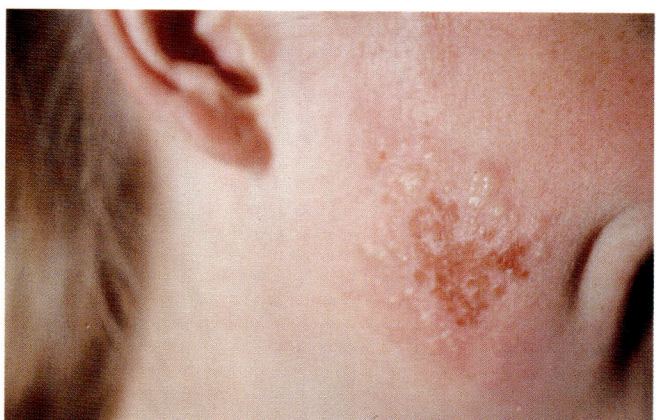

Plate 7 Herpes simplex virus arranged in groups.

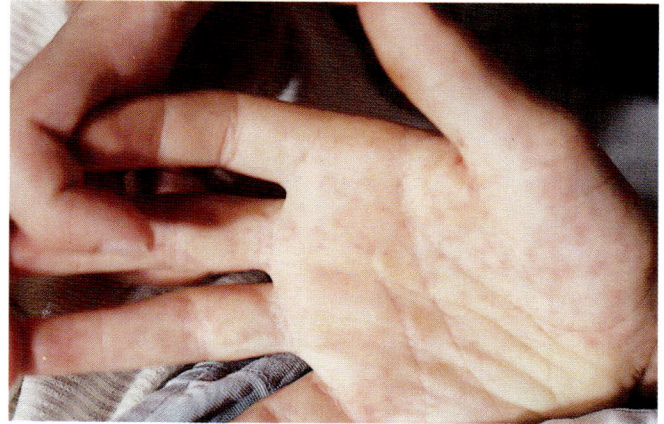

Plate 8 Rocky Mountain spotted fever.

Plate 9 Meningococcemia.

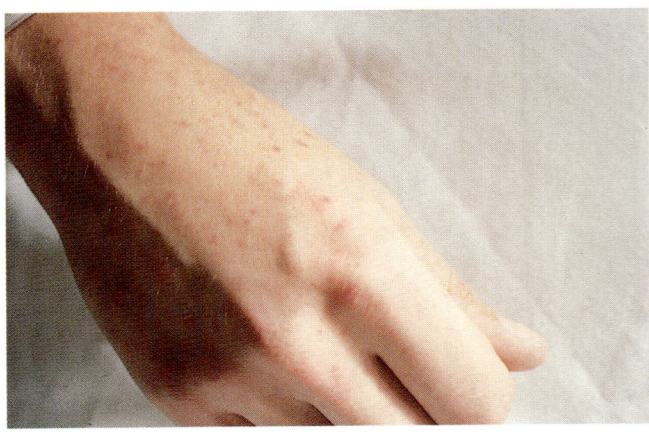

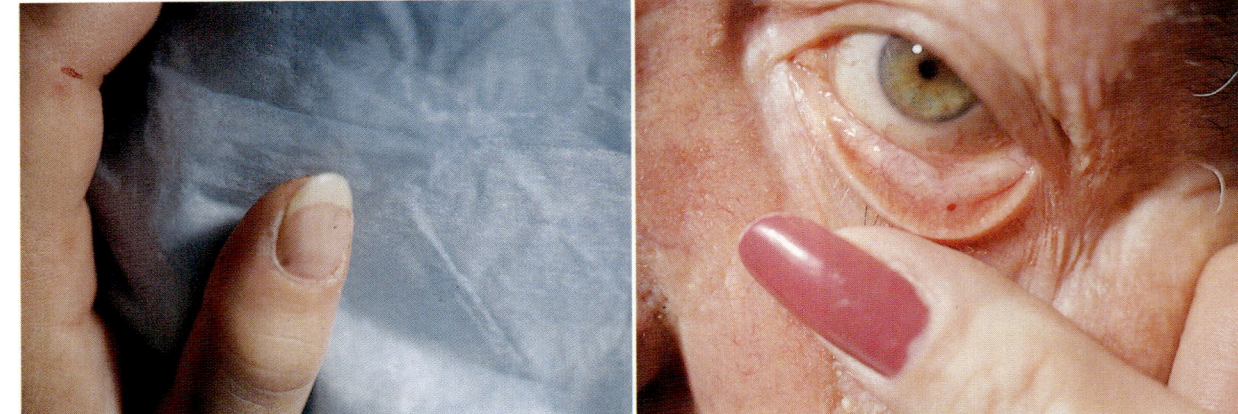

Plate 10 Bacterial endocarditis. **A,** Splinter hemorrhage under fingernail. **B,** Conjunctival petechiae.

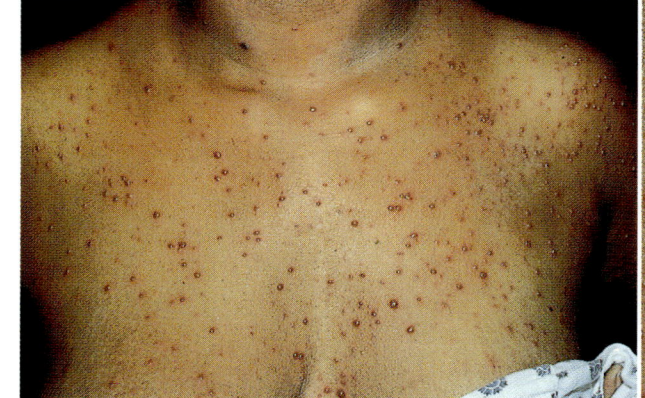
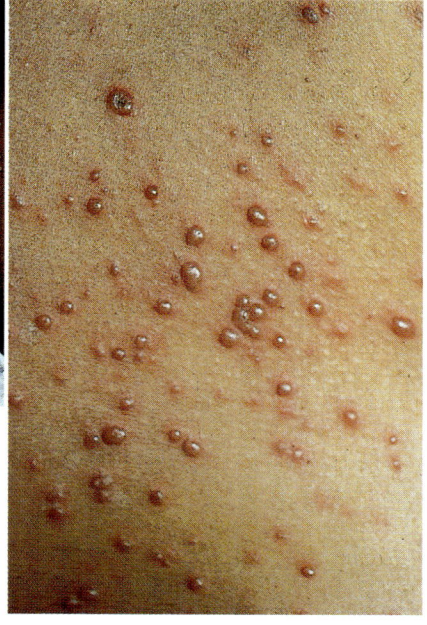

Plate 11 Chickenpox in an adult. **A,** View of the affected area. **B,** Close up of vesicles.

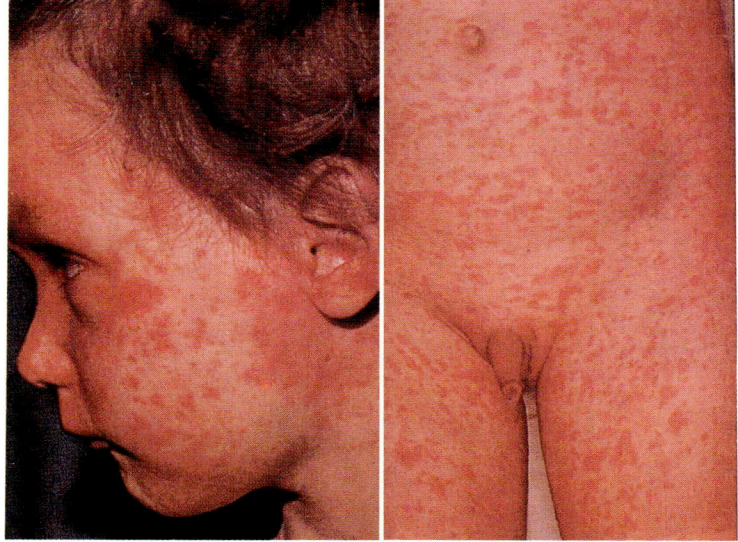

Plate 12 Measles. **A,** Rubella. **B,** Rubeolla. (Courtesy Dr. Loren H. Amundson, University of South Dakota, Sioux Falls.)

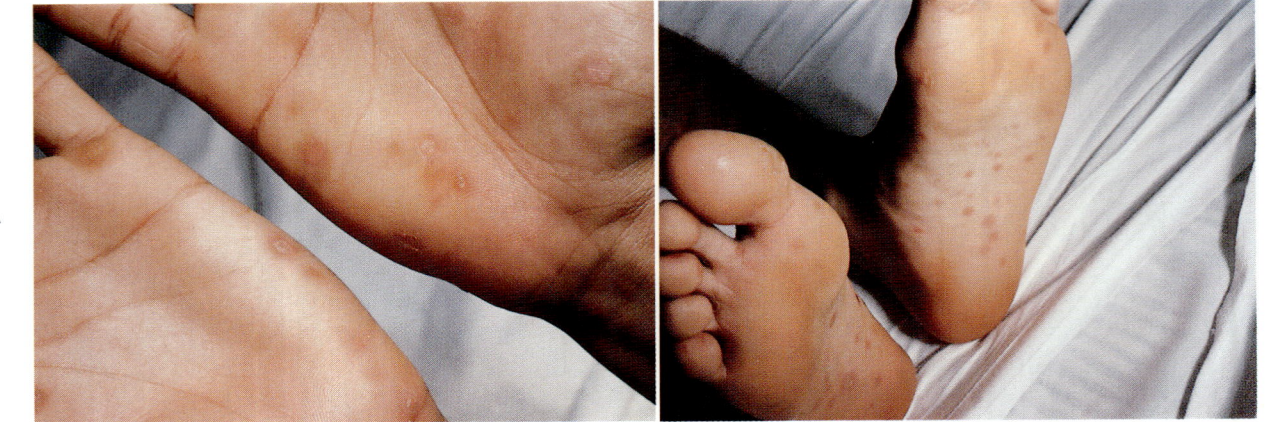

Plate 13 Secondary syphilis. **A,** On hands. **B,** On soles.

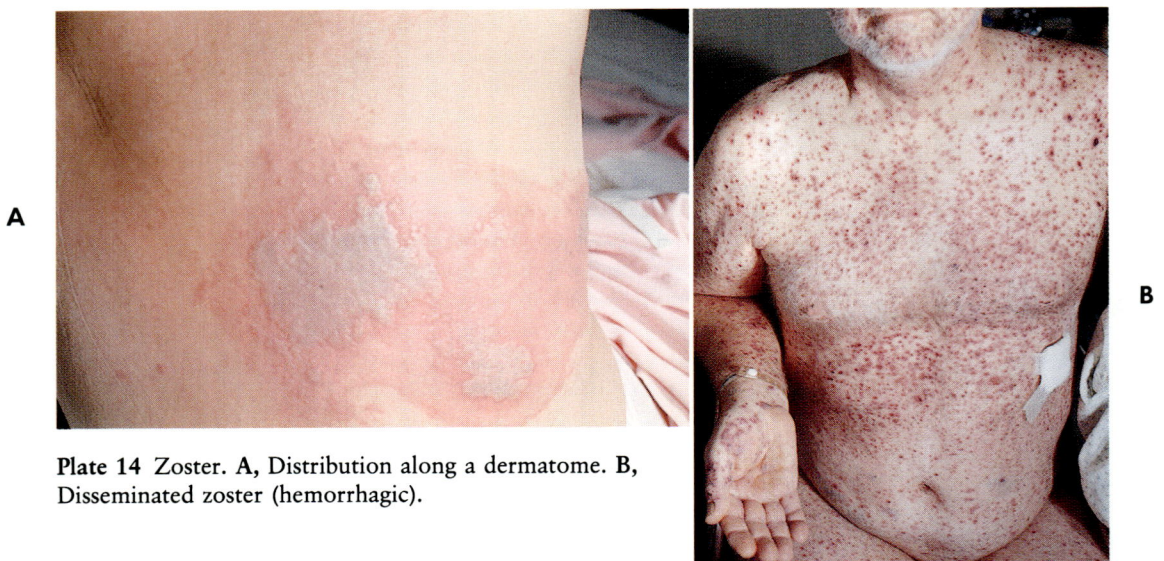

Plate 14 Zoster. **A,** Distribution along a dermatome. **B,** Disseminated zoster (hemorrhagic).

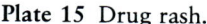

Plate 15 Drug rash.

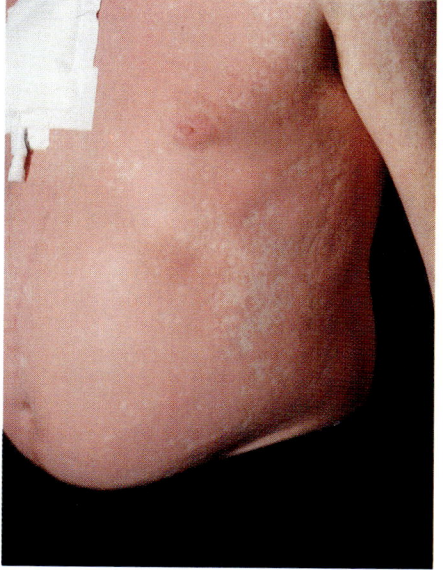

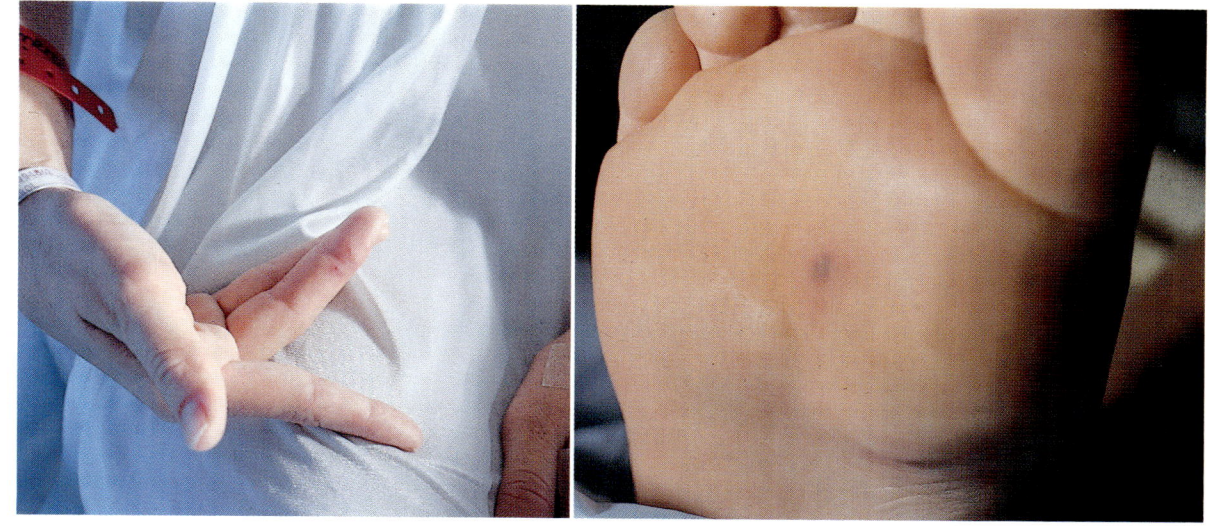

Plate 16 Disseminated gonococcemia. **A,** On hands. **B,** On soles.

Plate 17 Toxic shock syndrome: hand peeling.

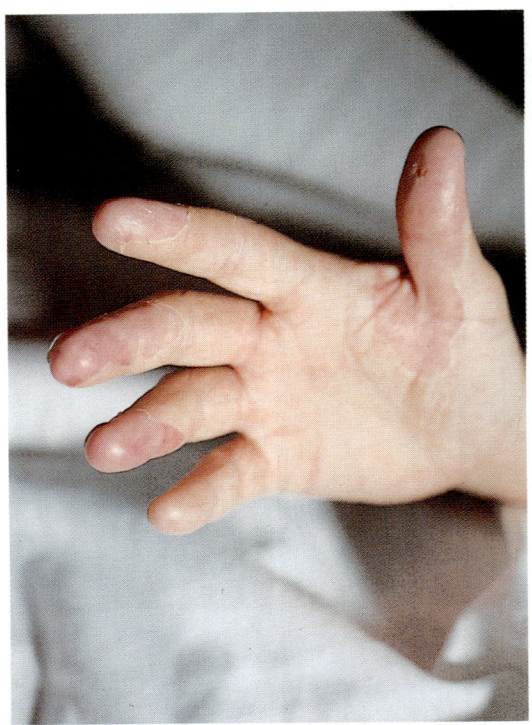

Plate 18 Tinea pedis. (Courtesy Dr. Loren H. Amundson, University of South Dakota, Sioux Falls.)

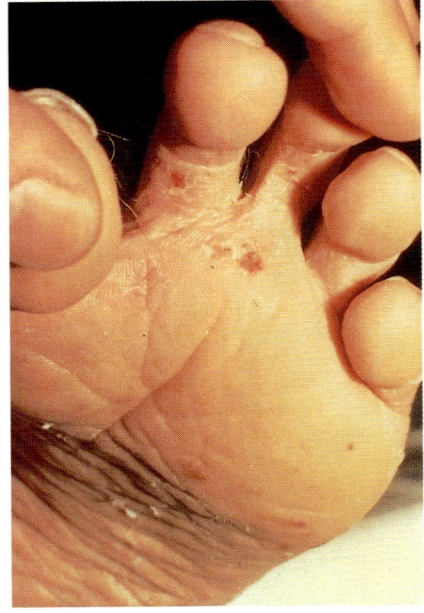

Plate 19 Erythema multiforme. **A,** On palm. **B,** In mouth (Stevens-Johnson syndrome). (Courtesy Dr. Loren H. Amundson, University of South Dakota, Sioux Falls.)

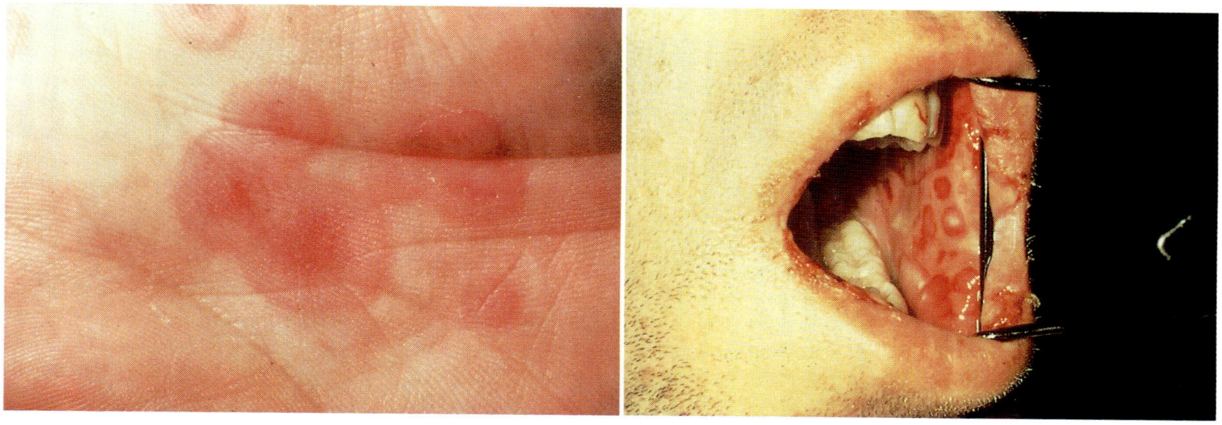

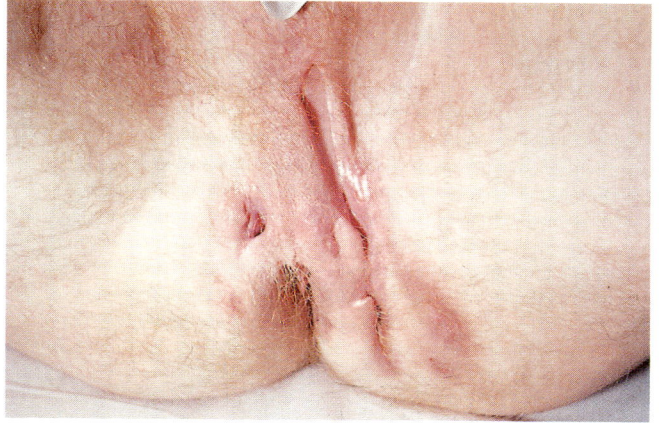

Plate 20 Hidradenitis suppurativa.

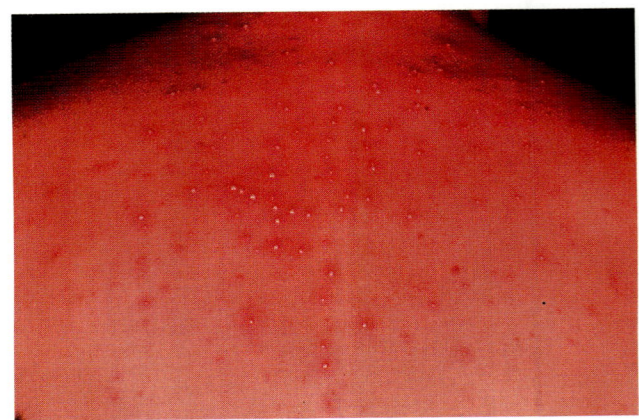

Plate 21 Miliaria. (Courtesy Dr. Loren H. Amundson, University of South Dakota, Sioux Falls.)

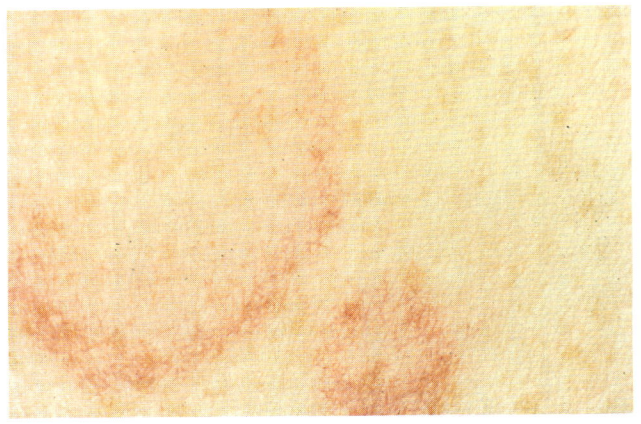

Plate 22 Urticaria (hives). (Courtesy Dr. Loren H. Amundson, University of South Dakota, Sioux Falls.)

Plate 23 Onchomycosis. **A,** On hands. **B,** On feet. (Courtesy Dr. Loren H. Amundson, University of South Dakota, Sioux Falls.)

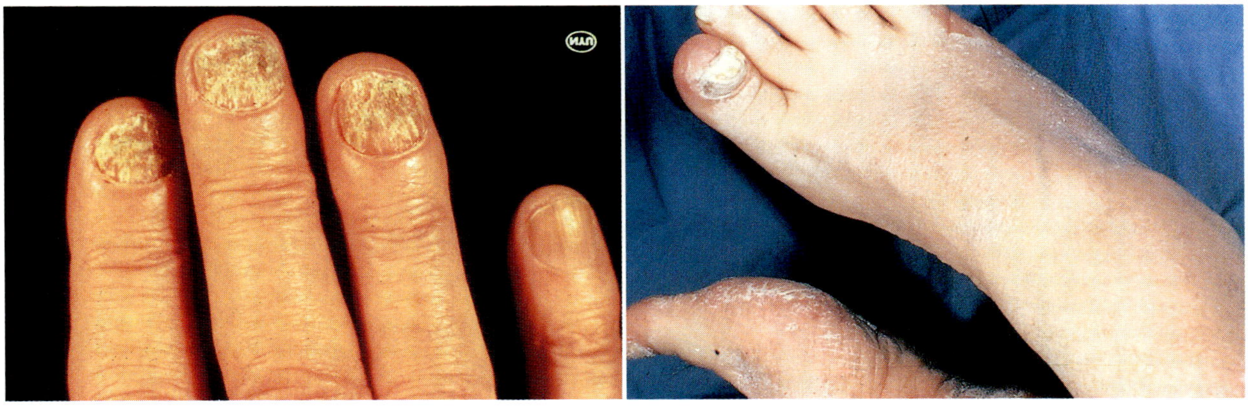

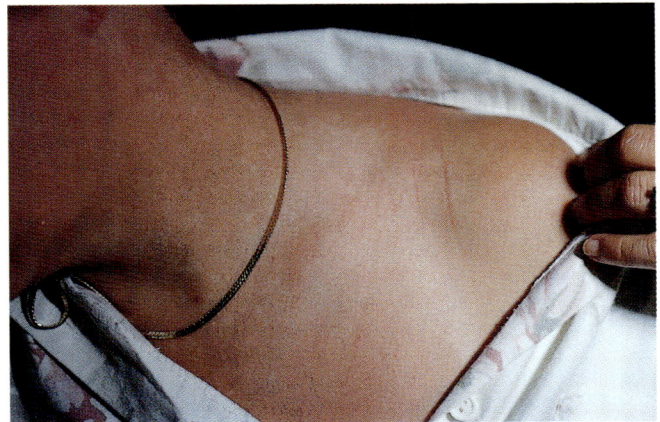

Plate 24 Tinea versicolor.

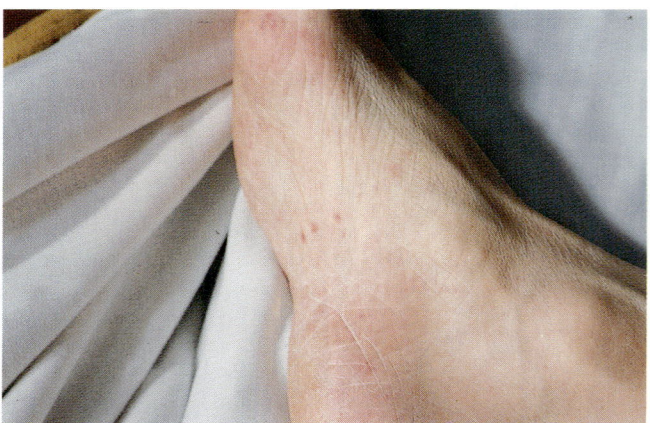

Plate 25 Petechiae of sepsis.

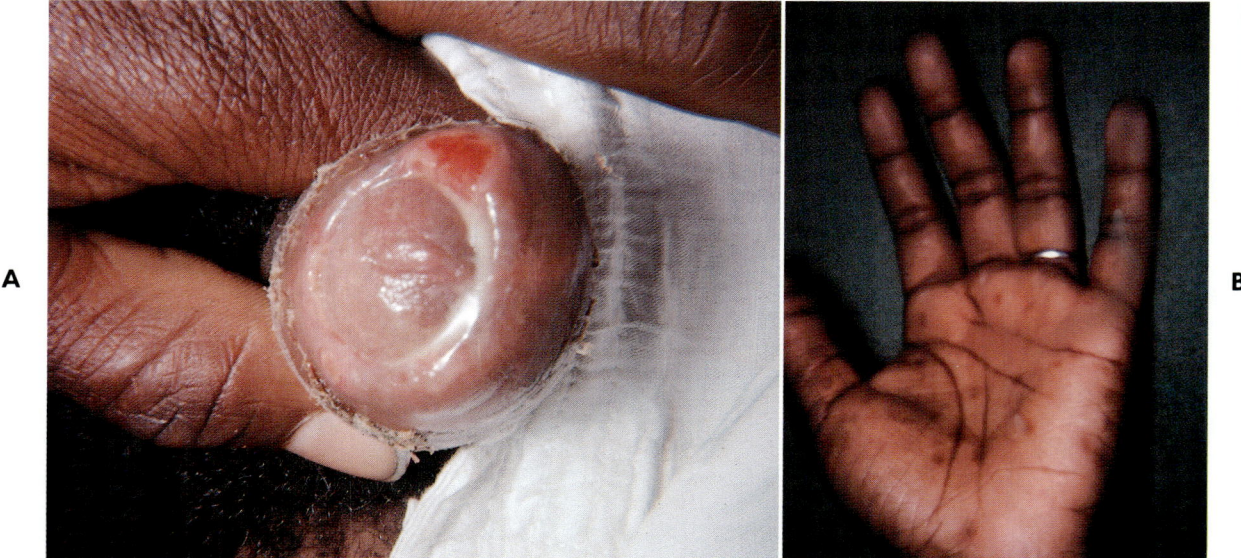

Plate 26 Syphilis. **A,** Primary chancre. **B,** Secondary lesion on palm of black patient. (Courtesy Dr. W.S. Royster, U.S. Public Health Service, Kansas City, Missouri.)

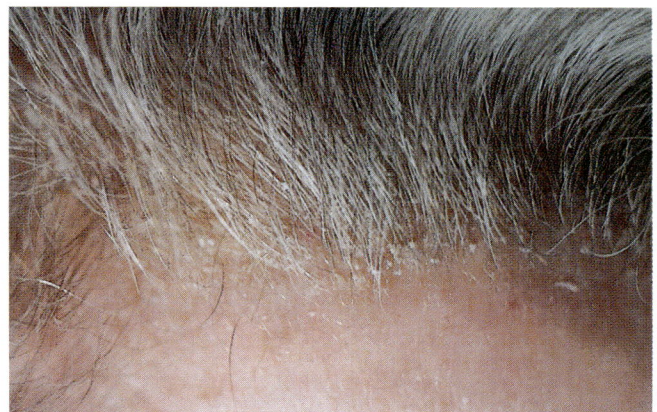

Plate 27 Seborrhea.

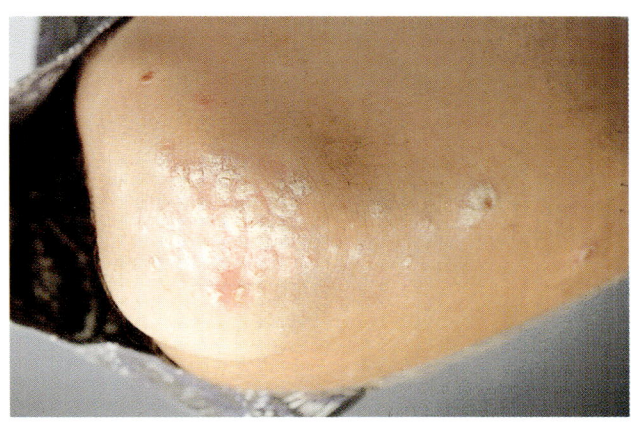

Plate 28 Psoriasis. (Courtesy Dr. James Kalivas, Division of Dermatology, University of Kansas.)

Plate 29 Herald patch of pityriasis rosea.

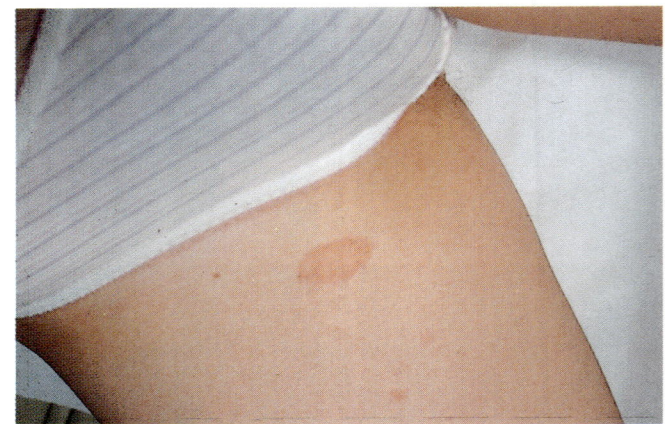

Plate 30 Benign nevus. (Courtesy Dr. Loren H. Amundson, University of South Dakota, Sioux Falls.)

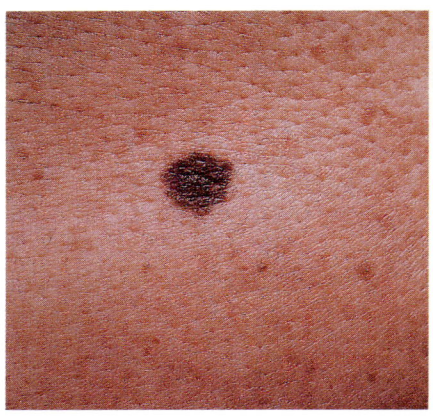

Plate 31 Superficial spreading melanoma. (Courtesy Dr. Loren H. Amundson, University of South Dakota, Sioux Falls.)

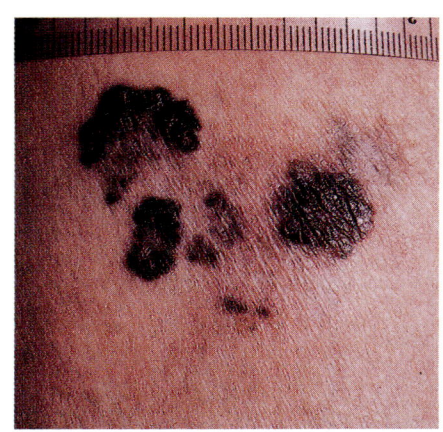

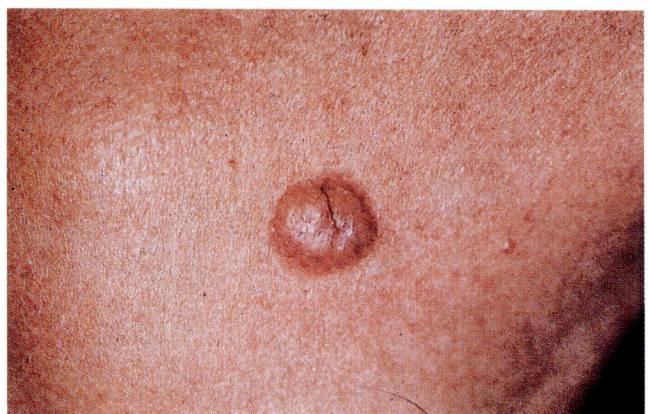

Plate 32 Basal cell carcinoma. (Courtesy Dr. Loren H. Amundson, University of South Dakota, Sioux Falls.)

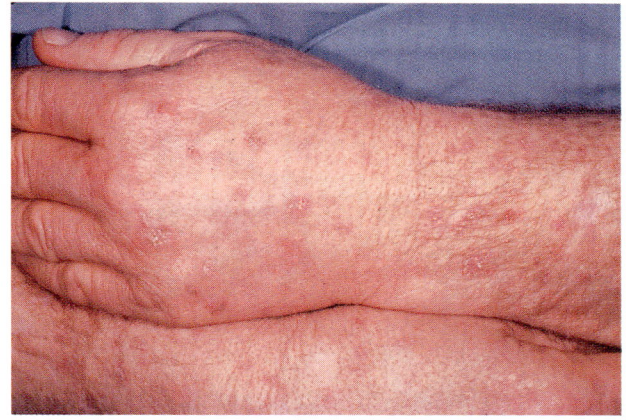

Plate 33 Actinic keratosis. (Courtesy Dr. Loren H. Amundson, University of South Dakota, Sioux Falls.)

Plate 34 Squamous cell carcinoma. (Courtesy Dr. Loren H. Amundson, University of South Dakota, Sioux Falls.)

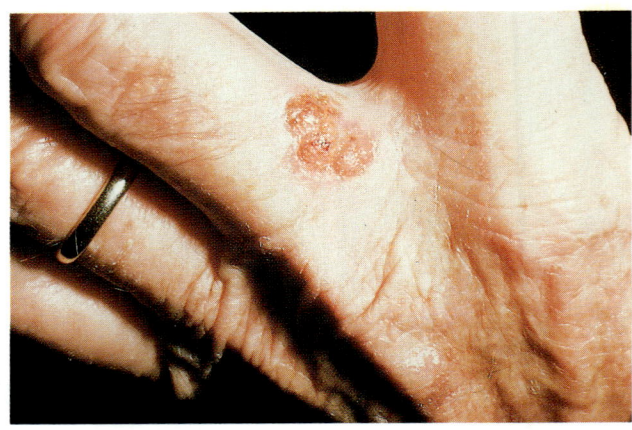

Plate 35 Cherry angioma. (Courtesy Dr. Loren H. Amundson, University of South Dakota, Sioux Falls.)

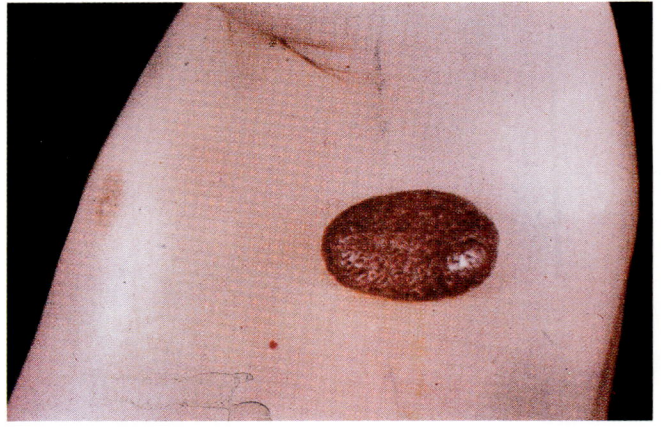

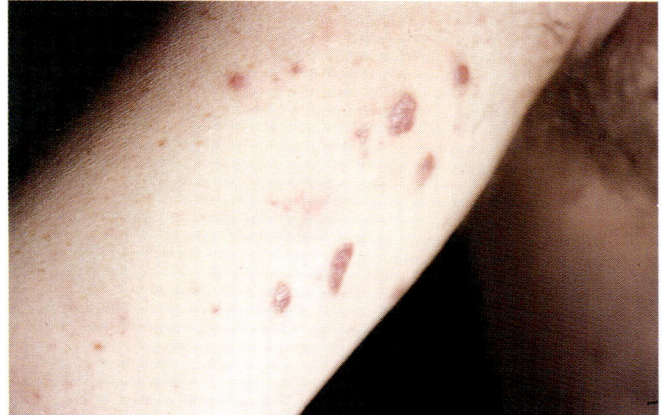

Plate 36 Kaposi's sarcoma of forearm.

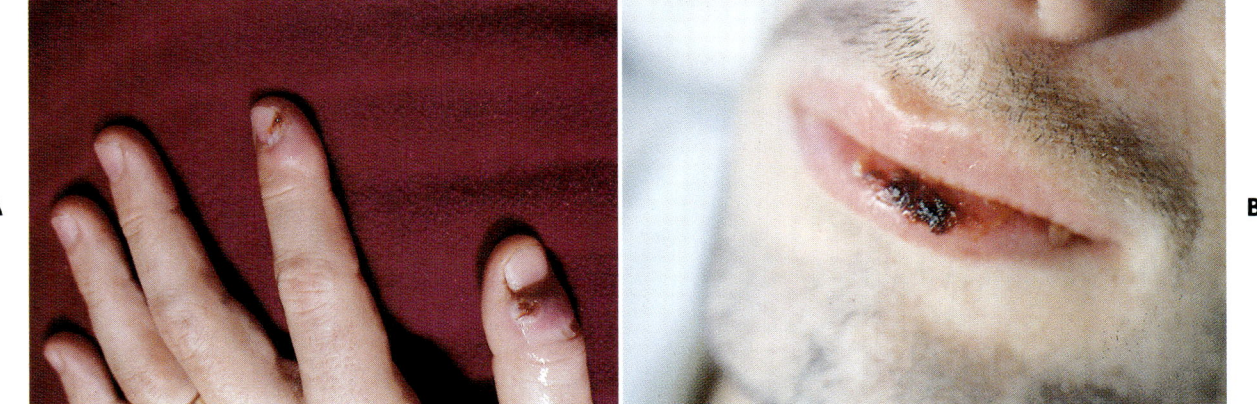

Plate 37 Herpetic whitlow. **A,** Of fingernail. **B,** Of mouth.

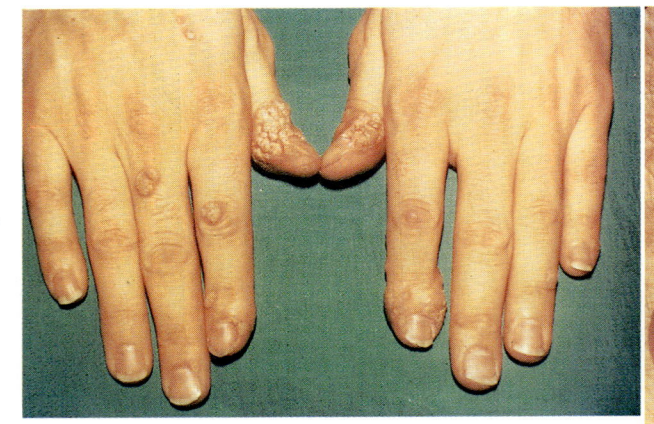
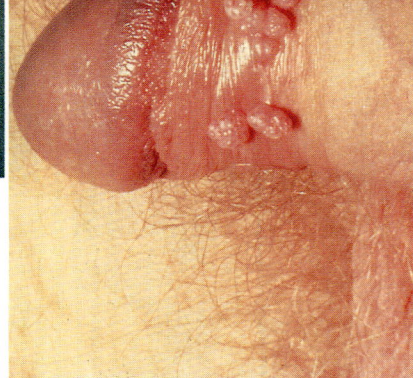

Plate 38 Warts. **A,** On hands. **B,** Condyloma acuminata of penis. (Courtesy Dr. Loren H. Amundson, University of South Dakota, Sioux Falls.)

Plate 39 Erysipelas of nose.

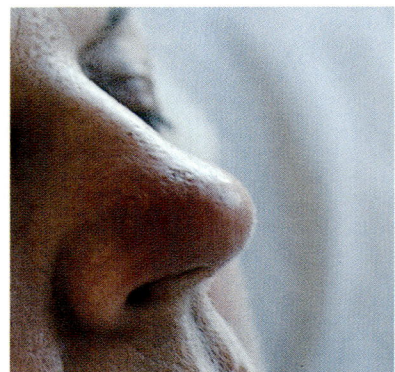

Pityriasis rosea may be asymptomatic or associated with transient itching. Pityriasis does not involve the palms or soles, as syphilis may. Care must be taken to exclude secondary syphilis by obtaining a screening test such as the VDRL or the RPR.

LICHEN PLANUS

Lichen planus is a papulosquamous skin disease, with onset between 30 and 70 years of age.

Lesions of lichen planus are flat, purple, 2 to 8 mm papules, the borders of which are not rounded but polygonal. The surface of such a lesion is criss-crossed with white or silver lines called *Wickham's striae*. These produce a lacy netlike appearance. Clinical aspects of lichen planus may be recalled by the rule of "5 P's"—*p*ruritic, *p*lanar (flat), *p*olyangular *p*urple *p*apules. The papules may be discrete, but they often aggregate.

Lesions of lichen planus usually first appear on the flexor surfaces of the wrists and forearm, but also on legs above the ankles, the sacral area, the penis, or on mucous membranes. Koebner's phenomenon may also occur in lichen planus with lesions appearing along scratch marks. Immunofluorescent staining of a skin biopsy may show nonspecific deposits of immunoglobulins and complement.

Tumors (Plates 30 to 36)

Because of the many types and varied appearances of skin tumors, the student of physical diagnosis will not be expected to learn to differentiate each of these. However, some of the more common or more important benign and malignant tumors do deserve attention, so the student can develop an approach to physical diagnosis that will entertain the possibility of a malignant lesion.

Selected for discussion here are the following:

- Benign nevi
- Malignant melanoma
- Basal cell carcinoma
- Actinic keratosis
- Squamous cell carcinoma
- Cherry angiomas
- Kaposi's sarcoma

NEVI

Nevi, commonly referred to as moles, exhibit a variety of colors, sizes, and shapes. They may be yellow, brown, black, or flesh-colored (Plate 30). Some are raised, others are pedunculated, warty, or hairy. Most appear during childhood, puberty, or pregnancy.

Nevi are benign tumors composed of cells derived from melanocytes. Nevi are so common that nearly everyone has one or more. The number tends to increase with sun exposure. Several pigmented spots merit description:

- *Freckles* are slightly pigmented spots, 1 to 3 mm in diameter, which increase in number and darken with sun exposure. The epidermis is microscopically normal but has increased melanin. Persons with light complexions develop these more often.
- The *lentigo (lentigines)* is darker and sparser than freckles. This brown macule is similar to a freckle, but with an irregular border. These do not increase in number with sun exposure but do appear with aging.

> **Suspicious Symptoms and Signs in a Nevus**
>
> **Symptoms**
> - Itching
> - Enlargement
> - Changes in pigmentation—either increased or decreased
> - Spread of pigmentation to adjacent skin
> - Inflammation
> - Bleeding
> - Ulceration
>
> **Signs (Use ABCDE Criteria)**
> - Asymmetric
> - Border is irregular
> - Color is mixed
> - Diameter measures more than 5 mm
> - Elevation is irregular

- *Junctional nevi* are smooth, flat or slightly elevated light brown to black moles, 1 to 6 mm in diameter. They are uniformly pigmented. Nevus cells are at the dermal-epidermal junction. Junctional nevi rarely become malignant.
- *Compound nevi* are usually slightly elevated, at times dome-shaped. The color may be flesh or brown. They become more elevated with age. Occasionally these have a white halo around the base.
- *Dermal nevi* are initially brown or black but become lighter or flesh-colored. These are dome-shaped or warty and are 4 to 10 mm in diameter. They resemble certain melanomas, but dermal nevi of long duration do not usually become malignant.
- *Dysplastic nevi* differ from common nevi or moles in the likelihood of becoming malignant (5% to 10%). These appear in sun-protected areas, the back, the legs, and the female breast. Individual lesions tend to be larger (greater than 5 mm as compared with under 6 mm for common moles), occasionally larger than 1 cm. Instead of being a uniform color, these have several colors in a single lesion such as, pink, brown, and black (see the accompanying box). Dysplastic nevi may be part of an autosomal dominant syndrome. If someone in the family has had melanoma, patients with dysplastic nevi should be examined carefully and followed closely for changes in moles. Dysplastic nevi also occur sporadically without a family pattern.

MALIGNANT MELANOMA

Melanomas cause more deaths than does any other skin cancer. Differentiating between the several types of melanoma is based on a combination of clinical and histopathologic criteria. The superficial spreading type is most common (Plate 31). Persons with light hair and fair skin that tans poorly, sunburns easily, and freckles have increased risk of developing melanoma. People who have had repeated sunburns or very severe sunburns are also at increased risk.

Distribution of superficial spreading melanoma is commonly on the back and chest of males and on the back or legs of females. The individual lesions have the characteristics listed in the box opposite.

The nodular melanoma is the type most often misdiagnosed. It occurs in the 40- to 60-year range, more often in males. It may be flesh-colored, brown, red-brown, or black, and it resembles a blood blister, hemangioma, or a polyp.

Acral-lentiginous melanomas tend to remain flat. This form occurs more in black and Oriental persons and is found on palms, soles, digits, and mucous membranes. These melanomas may produce the rapid appearance of a pigmented longitudinal band under a fingernail or toenail. They invade aggressively and metastasize early.

Depth of invasion of the melanoma is the most important single factor in patient outcome. Early excisional biopsy for suspicious lesions is indicated.

A classic history for the patient who has had relapse of melanoma is one who appears with a glass eye as a result of previous ocular surgery for melanoma and a large liver. Hepatic metastases can appear many years after resection of a primary melanoma of the eye.

BASAL CELL CARCINOMA

Basal cell carcinoma is the most common skin cancer among the white population. It usually occurs after age 40, typically on the face. Basal cell cancer is rare in black and Oriental persons. Risk factors include sun exposure and fair skin. The incidence at younger ages is increasing, probably because of sun exposure.

Basal cell carcinomas may take many clinical forms: nodular, pigmented, erosive, cystic, or sclerosing (Plate 32). Ulcerated basal cell carcinomas have been called rodent ulcers. Basal cell tumors characteristically enlarge slowly and rarely metastasize. Nonhealing ulcers should be evaluated as possibly being basal cell carcinoma.

ACTINIC KERATOSIS

These are discrete (1 cm or less) lesions with rough surfaces; they are especially found in sun exposed areas of skin. An adherent yellow crust or scale covers the lesion (Plate 33). Removing the crust may cause bleeding. An actinic keratosis may occur as a single papule or a plaque, or involve large patches of the face, forehead, or hands. Although transition to squamous cell carcinoma is uncommon, that should be considered for any area of actinic keratosis that enlarges, ulcerates, or bleeds.

SQUAMOUS CELL CARCINOMA

Squamous cell carcinomas are malignant tumors that invade locally and sometimes metastasize (Plate 34). They may arise from actinic keratosis or from other uncommon precursors, such as leukoplakia, coal tar exposure, ingestion of arsenic, along chronically draining sinus tracts, or in scars from thermal burns. The distribution of squamous cell carcinomas differs slightly from that of basal cell carcinomas. Squamous cell carcinomas are found on the scalp, the dorsum of the hands, the lower lip, and the ear. They are more commonly seen in middle-aged and elderly persons. Lesions may form plaques and nodules, and they may ulcerate or bleed. The tumors are usually firm but may be soft to palpation. Commonly the base is red and inflamed.

Some Causes of Pruritus	
Skin causes • Dry skin • Bites • Scabies Systemic illness • Uremia	• Biliary tract obstruction • Lymphoma • Polycythemia • Iron deficiency Pregnancy—during third trimester Drugs that cause allergic rash

CHERRY ANGIOMAS

Cherry angiomas are benign vascular malformations usually observed after age 30. The number increases with age. They are also called *senile hemangiomas*. These red papules are 0.5 to 3 mm in diameter and are usually located on the trunk (Plate 35). Some patients have as many as a hundred, others only a few. These are not malignant, though patients may ask.

KAPOSI'S SARCOMA

Before AIDS was prevalent, Kaposi's sarcoma was a rare vascular neoplasm found in elderly men of Italian, Greek, or Jewish ancestry. Now Kaposi's sarcoma is found most commonly in young persons infected with HIV. The incidence of Kaposi's sarcoma has been decreasing in those with AIDS for unknown reasons.

Kaposi's sarcomas begin as pink, red, or purple macules or papules (Plate 36). They progress to nodules and may become blue-black. Several lesions typically appear about the same time on the face, head, and neck and trunk. Oral and GI tract lesions are common.

Ichthyosis

Dry rectangular scales (fishlike) of the skin are responsible for the name "ichthyosis." Because of a disorder of shedding keratin, the horny layer produces scaly skin. Several varieties of ichthyosis have been described, but ichthyosis vulgaris is most common (1 in 100 people with ichthyosis). Ichthyosis vulgaris is commonly found in atopic patients. Dry scaling skin is prominent on the legs and arms, especially on the extensor surfaces. The antecubital and popliteal fossas are spared. The condition tends to worsen during winter months in northern climates.

Certain systemic illnesses may have acquired ichthyosis, including hypothyroidism, lymphoma, and AIDS.

Urticaria

Pruritus and urticaria are considered together because they are often associated. Pruritus (itching) is that sensation that we try to relieve by scratching, scraping, or rubbing. Urticaria (hives or wheals) may result from scratching or be caused by allergy without scratching. Wheals are a vascular reaction pattern, edema of the skin producing transient reddish or whitish skin swellings. Pruritus may be caused by dry skin and other causes (see the accompanying box).

Urticaria (hives) may be acute or chronic. The usual size of hives (wheals) is 2 to 4 mm, but some enlarge to several centimeters. A red or clear halo may surround the hive. Central clearing sometimes occurs. The distribution of hives over the body appears to be random.

Acute urticaria is defined as hives lasting shorter than 6 weeks; *chronic,* longer than 6 weeks. Most patients with chronic urticaria (80% or more) will not have a definite diagnosis found (idiopathic). Many possible diagnoses must be considered in evaluation.

Several characteristics of urticaria have been delineated. Immune-mediated urticaria is associated with atopy or allergies. These are IgE-mediated and may include exposure to mold, pollen, foods, additives, or drugs. Serum sickness with urticaria causes activation of immune complexes following injection of animal serum (e.g., for snakebite). Here urticaria is associated with fever, arthralgias, and lymphadenopathy. Infections, collagen diseases, and hereditary angioedema are other causes of urticaria. Urticaria may also be caused by mechanical means (e.g., pressure or vibration), heat or cold, or exposure to sun, or it may be idiopathic.

Bullous and Vesicular Diseases

Vesicles and bullae (sing. bulla) are superficial, clear, and fluid-filled. They are differentiated by size, with vesicles being less than, and bullae larger than, 5 mm.

VESICULAR DISEASES

Vesicles are the characteristic skin lesion on the body in varicella (chicken pox), varicella zoster (herpes zoster), and hand-foot-and-mouth disease (see Plates 11 and 14).

Chicken pox and zoster lesions have a similar appearance, both being caused by the same virus. Zoster is the relapse form of varicella, usually occurring in a dermatome distribution, after the virus has been sequestered in the dorsal root ganglia. The individual lesions have been described as a dew drop on a rose petal (clear vesicle with a red base).

Smallpox (variola) no longer exists because of the global eradication program of immunization. The lesions of smallpox differed from those of chickenpox. Each produced large vesicles over the entire body. Smallpox vesicles appeared in one crop. All vesicles, and later all crusts had the same age. Chickenpox vesicles appear in crops at different times. Vesicles and later crusts differ in stages of maturation. New vesicles appear in chickenpox up to 7 days into the illness, even after older lesions begin to crust. In smallpox, individual lesions remained round. In chickenpox, the edges of lesions become serrated. Lesions of smallpox began on the face and scalp and spread to the back, chest, and arms and legs, with more lesions on the arms and legs than on the trunk. In chickenpox, lesions spread peripherally, so that older lesions are on the trunk and more recently appearing lesions are on the extremities.

Hand-foot-and-mouth disease is characterized by a vesicular exanthem. The cause is usually a coxsackievirus, especially A-16. Small vesicles in the mouth may coalesce to form bullae. Vesicles on the palms and soles are surrounded by tender papules.

BULLOUS DISEASES

Blisters are bullae. Several disorders of sloughing of the skin or bullous diseases are considered below. Disorders of adherence of epidermis occur at various layers.

TABLE 12-15: Characteristics of Some Bullous Diseases

Parameter	Pemphigus Vulgaris	Bullous Pemphigoid	Dermatitis Herpetiformis
Age of patient	35 to 60 years	Over age 60	10 to 50 years
Initial lesion	Mouth or mucous membranes	Itchy plaque	Itchy papules or vesicles
Description	• Intraepidermal (bullae) • Flaccid blisters, easily ruptured	• Below basal cell layer • Tense blisters and hard to rupture	Basal cell layer
Distribution	Trunk, legs, sometimes face; occur in mouth	Abdomen, flexor surfaces, arms, and legs; palms and soles	Elbows, knees, neck, shoulders, buttocks; rare in mouth
Itching	No	Yes	Yes and burning
Duration	Chronic for years, lesions spread and heal slowly	Lasts years, does not spread, heals rapidly	Chronic for years
Special signs	Nikolsky's sign	Nikolsky's sign is negative	
Diagnostic tests	• Antibody titer • IgG-staining keratinocytes	• Basement membranes • IgG staining	Linear IgG

Staphylococcal Scalded Skin Syndrome

Staphylococcal scalded skin syndrome (SSSS) is not strictly a bullous disease but appears similar to these, may involve bullae, and is caused by sloughing of the superficial epidermis. The epidermal sloughing is caused by a split below the granular layer that is caused by a toxin of *Staphylococcus aureus*. Nikolsky's sign may be present (see pemphigus). The lesions are superficial enough to heal without scars.

Toxic Epidermal Necrolysis

Toxic epidermal necrolysis (TEN) appears similar to SSSS, but the epidermis is split at a deeper layer. Drug reactions, immunizations, or graft-versus-host disease cause TEN. Sheets of skin or mucous membranes separate from the body, leaving large, denuded, burnlike surfaces.

Pemphigus Vulgaris

Pemphigus (Table 12-15) is a rare bullous disease that was lethal before the advent of antibiotics and the use of corticosteroids. Flaccid bullae, or blisters, appear on the skin or mucous membranes and sometimes first in the mouth. Nikolsky's sign is present. The epidermis easily detaches from the skin. Demonstrate this by pressing and sliding the examining fingers over affected skin. This action separates the upper skin layers. In pemphigus, IgG antibodies are deposited in the intercellular substance of the skin and may be demonstrated by immunofluorescence. Pemphigus antibodies may be demonstrated in the serum.

Bullous Pemphigoid

Pemphigoid (see Table 12-15), occurring in the elderly, is a more benign disease than is pemphigus vulgaris. Pruritus often appears first, then tense bullae appear on the flexor surfaces, but seldom in the mouth. These may wax and wane for several years. Unlike pemphigus, pemphigoid does not denude large areas of skin. IgG antibodies are deposited in the skin, along with complement.

Erythema Multiforme

Erythema multiforme is an acute or chronic disorder of the skin and mucous membranes. Red or pink circular lesions have a target or bull's-eye appearance, caused by three colored rings and a pale center (see Plate 19). Central bullous formation may occur. Milder cases may exhibit macular, papular, or urticarial lesions without bullae. With bullous formation of erythema multiforme, massive amounts of skin may slough, and oral ulcerations develop (see Plate 19, *B*). *Stevens-Johnson syndrome* is the name applied to this condition. The etiologic causes of Stevens-Johnson syndrome include *Mycoplasma pneumoniae,* herpes simplex virus, sulfonamides, and penicillins, among others.

Dermatitis Herpetiformis

Dermatitis herpetiformis (see Table 12-15) is characterized by groups of vesicles located over the elbows, knees, shoulders, or sacrum that itch intensely. These lesions are about 3 to 6 mm in diameter and are located deep so that a firm nodule is apparent, rather than a bulla. Dermatitis herpetiformis may occur with small intestinal changes similar to adult celiac disease.

Viral Infections of the Skin (Plates 37 and 38)

Skin lesions are common in viral infections. They may be caused by replication of the virus in the skin, by immune responses of the host, or by both. Of the viral infections that may involve the skin, four are considered here: herpes zoster, herpes simplex, genital warts, and molluscum contagiosum.

HERPES ZOSTER

Herpes zoster, often called shingles, is caused by reactivation of the chickenpox virus, varicella, and was discussed under vesicles. After primary infection with varicella, the virus survives in a latent form in dorsal root ganglia. Certain stimuli allow the virus to traverse down the axon to the skin, where vesicles appear in a dermatome distribution. Pain, itching, or irritation precede the eruption by 48 to 72 hours. Onset begins with a red base, on which appears a small but enlarging clear vesicle (see Plate 14). Later it becomes white and then yellow before rupturing. Oozing fluid develops a crust that may require 7 to 10 days to heal. During zoster, patients may develop systemic symptoms. Pain in a dermatome distribution of the rash may be very severe, especially in older persons.

The pain may persist for weeks or months. It may be so severe as to prevent the patient from wearing any clothing that might touch the affected area. Pain may persist even after complete healing of the skin. Healed skin shows only mottled-appearing scars where the zoster lesions were located.

Disseminated zoster out of the primary dermatome occurs in some patients, particularly those who are immunosuppressed. The vesicles may resemble the rash of chickenpox.

Zoster vesicles seldom show a similarity to vesicles of poison ivy. A streak across the skin with poison ivy can cause vesicles in the line of the scratch. Poison ivy is more likely to itch and less likely to be painful than is zoster. Herpes simplex vesicles may at times resemble lesions of zoster or poison ivy.

HERPES SIMPLEX

Two herpes simplex viruses, referred to as HSV 1 and HSV 2, produce skin lesions that look similar. They usually cause different anatomic distributions of eruptions, but there are several characteristics common to both. After primary infection (gingivostomatitis for HSV 1 and genital herpes for HSV 2), each virus establishes latency in the dorsal root ganglia (as does varicella). Thus reactivation typically results in repeated episodes of herpes vesicles in the distribution of a particular neuron. HSV 1 may cause genital lesions if it is inoculated there. HSV 2 may cause oral, labial, or finger vesicles.

Primary herpetic gingivostomatitis usually occurs during childhood. The patient is systemically ill with fever, a sore mouth, a sore throat, and adenopathy (submental, anterocervical). Vesicles appear on the lips, tongue, palate, and pharynx, and the vesicles ulcerate. Healing is slow, often requiring as long as 2 weeks.

Reactivation of HSV 1 (cold sore or fever blister) occurs on the outer portion of the lips. Reactivation vesicles may be inside the mouth in patients who are immunosuppressed. Also, reinoculation of herpes virus inside the mouth can result in lesions there, even in patients who have a history of herpes vesicles.

Primary HSV 2 is characterized by herpetic vesicles on the penis, vulva, or vagina. In homosexuals, they may be in the perianal area or rectal mucosa. In either sex, vesicles in the urethra may make voiding painful or impossible. Other symptoms include headache, myalgia, fever, and inguinal lymphadenopathy. Parestheses may occur. HSV 2 may exhibit frequent relapses into vesicles over an extended time.

The typical time course of recurrent vesicles of HSV 1 or HSV 2 begins with local irritation, usually an itching. After about 1 day, a red base appears, and a clear, fluid-filled vesicle becomes apparent. This may remain intact for 2 or 3 days, during which the fluid becomes yellow and purulent looking (see Plate 7). Then the roof breaks, an ulcer forms, and a crust covers the sore, which often requires 5 to 7 days for healing. Typical total duration of lesions is 1 to 2 weeks.

Factors that promote the occurrence of herpes lesions include stress, sunburn, fever, menses, and trauma.

Special problems with herpes include locally invasive herpes in patients who have AIDS, herpes infection of the cornea, and herpes encephalitis or meningitis.

Herpetic whitlow (paronychia) is a purulent-looking infection near the fingernail (Plate 37). Health care workers typically acquire them by direct contact.

WARTS

Warts are rough-appearing skin elevations usually 2 to 5 mm in diameter (Plate 38). These are caused by papilloma viruses, which are also DNA viruses. The most common sites for warts are the hands, feet, face, around the knees, and perianal areas.

Warts, because of their presence, bring patients to medical attention. Except for plantar warts, most warts are painless. On examination, warts may exhibit a variety of sizes and shapes.

Warts are mildly contagious. Patients are advised to avoid scratching or shaving them to avoid autoinoculation to other parts of the body. Certain venereal warts have been associated with cervical cancer.

MOLLUSCUM CONTAGIOSUM

Molluscum contagiosum is caused by a DNA poxvirus. These contagious, shiny, dome-shaped skin lesions are flesh-colored, pink, or red. Palpation (use gloves) shows a firm margin. A central plug may be removed to leave an umbilicated central depression. Lesions may be single but are frequently multiple, especially in patients with AIDS.

Bacterial Infections of Skin (Plate 39)

Bacteria may cause skin lesions because of local invasion (impetigo) or as a result of an infection elsewhere (septicemia). Organisms may be inoculated below the superficial epidermis by trauma, even minor trauma, or by disturbances of normal anatomy (hair follicle, hangnail). Virulence of the organisms and host immune factors combine to determine whether infection will occur and the extent of infection.

IMPETIGO

Impetigo is a superficial skin infection, highly contagious, usually found in children. It is caused by *Streptococcus pyogenes* group A, *Staphylococcus aureus*, or both. Lesions typically involve exposed areas of skin, the face, scratching of insect bites, and trauma.

Early lesions of impetigo are often rapidly crusting clear vesicles; they are 2 or 3 mm to 2 cm in diameter. The honey-colored crusts (scabs) are moist and oozing. If the crusts are removed, the base is red and eroded. In contrast, *S. aureus* crusts are hard, dry, dark brown, and thin, especially at the margins. Patients who are infected with a nephritogenic strain of streptococcus may develop glomerulonephritis after impetigo.

ERYSIPELAS

Streptococcus pyogenes group A infection, which spreads superficially in the dermis with an advancing border—a line of demarcation between infected and uninfected skin—is characteristic of erysipelas. The affected skin is red, warm, tender, and slightly swollen (Plate 39). Adjacent skin not yet infected feels normal. Associated systemic symptoms include pain, malaise, chills, and fever. The portal of entry is often a minor fissure on the face or feet (e.g., tinea pedis).

Key to the diagnosis of erysipelas is the distinct line at the edge of infected skin. This infected margin progressively moves across uninfected skin, often quite rapidly. Show this by drawing a line along the margin of erythema. A few hours later the erythema extends beyond the original line. Only superficial skin layers are involved, as compared with deeper tissue involvement in cellulitis. Untreated, patients with erysipelas may develop streptococcal septicemia.

Dermal Manifestations of Systemic Bacterial Infections

Remote systemic bacterial infections may result in skin lesions caused by bacteremia itself, by toxins that have skin or mucous membrane effects, or by immune mechanisms (see the top box on pg. 478).

Skin Abnormalities in AIDS

Persons who have AIDS are particularly susceptible to a variety of dermatologic abnormalities. These are grouped by anatomic site in the bottom box on pg. 478.

Systemic Bacterial Infections with Dermal Manifestations

Bacterial endocarditis
  Osler nodes (finger tips)
  Janeway lesions (palms of hands)
  Roth's spots (fundus of eye)
  Splinter hemorrhages (nail beds)
  Conjunctival petechiae (conjunctiva)
  Palatal petechiae (palate)

Bacterial sepsis
  Staphylococcus aureus (petechiae)
  Pseudomonas aeruginosa (ecthyma gangrenosum [vasculitis])
  Meningococcus (petechiae on palms, soles, and elsewhere)
  Gonococcemia (pustules)

Toxin effects on skin from remote bacterial infection
  Toxic shock syndrome caused by *S. aureus* (sunburnlike rash with peeling of fingertips later)
  Scarlet fever caused by streptococcal infection (erythema, a "sandpaper rash"; also may peel later)
  Scalded skin syndrome caused by *S. aureus* (skin sloughs to look scalded)

Cutaneous Abnormalities In Persons with AIDS

Hair
  Premature graying
  Balding, thinning
  Alopecia areata
  Seborrhea

Face
  Premature aging
  Hypertrichosis of eyelashes
  Seborrhea of moustache
  Molluscum contagiosum
  Herpetic ulcers, erosive
  Kaposi's sarcoma

Mouth
  Cheilitis
  Herpes lesions
  Candidal infections
  Kaposi's sarcoma on palate, gingiva
  Hairy leukoplakia on sides of tongue
  Chronic severe gingivitis

Nails
  Pitting caused by psoriasis
  Dermatophyte damage
  Candidal damage
  Dark blue-brown discoloration caused by azidothymidine
  Yellow-colored nails

Palms and soles
  Lesions of secondary syphilis
  Kaposi's sarcoma
  Scabies on finger webs

Thorax
  Herpes zoster
  Tinea versicolor
  Psoriasis
  Papular eruptions caused by drugs (especially sulfonamides)
  Kaposi's sarcoma
  Telangiectasias, especially above clavicles
  Erythroderma caused by drugs

Genitalia
  Herpes simplex ulcers
  Molluscum contagiosum
  Venereal warts (condyloma acuminatum)
  Candidal vaginitis

Summary

A summary checklist for the evaluation of skin disorders is shown below.

Summary Checklist for Evaluation of Skin Disorders

Individual lesions
  Primary skin lesions
  Secondary skin lesions
  Special skin lesions
Configuration of individual lesions
Distribution of lesions
Special sites for examination of skin
  Hair
  Eyebrows
  Eyelids
  Nails and nailbeds
  Palms and soles
  Genitalia and perineum
  Mucous membranes
Types of skin lesions

Pustular lesions
Eczematous diseases
Atopic dermatitis
Connective tissue diseases
Microbial infections
  Fungi
  Bacteria
  Viruses
Macules, papules, and petechiae
Exanthems
Papulosquamous diseases
Tumors
Urticaria
Vesicles and bullae
Manifestations of AIDS

Suggested readings

Basset A, Liautaud B, Ndiaye B: *Dermatology of black skin,* translated from French by Andrew Pembroke. Oxford, England, 1986, Oxford University Press. *A pocket atlas that illustrates skin lesions in black patients. Differences from lesions in white patients may be significant.*

Ginder PA, et al: Hidradenitis suppurativa: evidence for a bactericidal defect correctable by cholinergic agonist in vitro and in vivo, *J Clin Immunol* 2:237, 1982. *An occasional patient with hidradenitis may have an identifiable cause besides the obvious bacteria.*

Habif TP: *Clinical dermatology: a color guide to diagnosis and therapy,* ed 2, St Louis, 1990, Mosby–Year Book. *A comprehensive guide to skin lesions. Loaded with excellent color photographs and accompanied by useful discussions.*

CHAPTER THIRTEEN

The Pediatric Patient

CHAPTER OUTLINE

History Taking
Physical Examination of the Pediatric Patient
Descriptive measurements
Observation
Head and neck
Chest
Abdomen
Genitalia
Musculoskeletal system
Neurologic examination

Summary

Pediatrics is the specialty of medicine dealing with patients ranging from the very low birth weight, preterm neonate to the young adult. The physical examination, therefore, needs to be adjusted for the age and size of the patient. Many of the variations noted during the physical examination can be explained by differences in the rate of growth of each organ system from birth to adulthood. These variations are noted in the discussion of each organ system.

Many pediatric patients are apprehensive because they do not feel well at the time of the examination. They are unfamiliar with the physical setting and with many of the instruments used during the examination. Spending some time talking and playing with the patient before initiating the examination will make it a more pleasant experience.

History Taking

By definition, the neonatal period lasts from birth to 28 days of age. The child is considered an infant until the age of 2 years and then enters the toddler stage until 6 years old. The adolescent period usually begins when the child becomes a teenager.

Before beginning the physical examination, record a careful, detailed history from the patient and/or other family members. For the pediatric patient being seen for the first time, ask about prenatal problems (e.g., maternal diabetes),

TABLE 13-1: Normal Ages for Attainment of Major Developmental Milestones

Age	Motor	Language	Adaptive Behavior
4 to 6 wks	Head lifted from prone position and turned from side to side	Cries	Smiles
4 mo	No head lag when pulled to sitting from supine position; tries to grasp large objects	Sounds of pleasure	Smiles, laughs aloud, and shows pleasure to familiar objects or persons
5 mo	Voluntary grasp with both hands; plays with toes	Primitive sounds ("ah, goo")	Smiles at self in mirror
6 mo	Grasps with one hand; rolls prone to supine; sits with support	Range of sounds greater	Expresses displeasure and food preferences
8 mo	Sits without support; transfers objects from hand to hand; rolls supine to prone	Combines syllables ("baba, dada, mama")	Responds to "no"
10 mo	Sits well; creeping; stands holding; finger-thumb apposition in picking up small objects		Waves "bye-bye," plays "patty-cake" and "peek-a-boo"
12 mo	Stands holding; walks with support	Says two or three words with meaning	Understands names of objects; shows interest in pictures
15 mo	Walks alone	Several intelligible words	Requests by pointing; imitates
18 mo	Walks up and down stairs holding; removes clothes	Many intelligible words	Carries out simple commands
2 yr	Walks up and down stairs by self; runs	Two- to three-word phrases	Organized play; points to some parts of body

From Rudolph AM, et al: *Rudolph's pediatrics*, ed 19, Norwalk, CT, 1991, Appleton & Lange.

history of family disorders (e.g., Marfan syndrome, neurosensory hearing loss), and problems previously identified during health care visits (e.g., delayed growth for age). The attainment of maturation milestones may be highly variable, depending on the specific milestones, but note especially the child who is always early or invariably late (Table 13-1). The present examination is important in determining the process occurring during the acute illness. A detailed record of the examination is also needed for comparison with past and subsequent visits. Because the pediatric patient will undergo continual, sometimes rapid, changes in physical characteristics such as height, weight, and organ size, noting the type and rate of change occurring over time is important.

Record the results of the physical examination in an orderly, logical fashion. Because many younger patients may not be able to cooperate with the examiner, you may need to perform first those components of the examination which require the infant to be quiet. For example, listen to the heart and lungs while the infant is resting quietly, often in a parent's lap. This should be followed by examination of the abdomen. Examination of the ears and oral cavity is best left for the end.

Physical Examination of the Pediatric Patient

Until the age of adolescence, it is not unusual for the parents to remain in the room during the physical examination. The adolescent patient will often prefer not to have the parent present, which may require the presence of a chaperone. The area to be examined must be fully exposed, but the modesty of the child of any age must be respected. If the room is cool, the patient may not be completely disrobed, but have each group of clothing removed and replaced in succession. If a potentially painful procedure is to be performed, discuss this with the patient and family members.

Descriptive Measurements

Before performing the physical examination, the measurements that are usually taken include height and weight, temperature, head circumference, respiratory rates, pulse, and blood pressure. Record height, weight, and head circumference on appropriate graphs to assess adequate and appropriate rates of growth (Figs. 13-1 to 13-12).

The infant is measured in the supine position, holding the end of the tape at the infant's foot and reading at the head to the nearest centimeter (Fig. 13-13). An alternative method is the use of a flat measuring board. The older child can be measured while standing on a scale.

For most children under 6 years of age, an axillary temperature reading is satisfactory. The axillary temperature is obtained by placing the thermometer in the axilla and putting the arm along the patient's body, holding it there for 3 minutes. These usually read 2° F lower than the rectal temperature and 1° F lower than the oral temperature. After the age of 6 years, an oral temperature can be taken.

Measure the head circumference for the infant less than 2 years old. Comparison with standard values (see Figs. 13-3 and 13-9) will reveal whether the growth is age-appropriate. The head is measured at its greatest circumference using a paper or steel tape.

As discussed further below, measure the pulse rate either by auscultation of the heart or by palpation of an arterial pulse. Obtain the respiratory rate by watching chest movement or by auscultating the chest.

Blood pressure should be measured while the child is calm, before the beginning of the examination. Allowing the child to pump the cuff will often relieve anxiety. The proper size cuff is between one-half to two-thirds the length of the upper arm, with similar sizes used in the leg. The cuff is inflated to higher than the suspected systolic pressure then released slowly, with the examiner listening for the first sound compatible with the systolic pressure. When the sounds disappear, the pressure recorded is compatible with the diastolic pressure. At birth, the systolic and diastolic pressures are 60 to 90 and 20 to 63 mm of mercury, respectively. These numbers will usually rise 2 to 3 mm per year of age until the adult levels are reached at approximately puberty. If the infant is crying or apprehensive, the pressures measured may be artificially elevated.

Observation

The impression obtained on initial observance of the child may contribute significantly to the ultimate diagnosis. Note whether the child appears ill, as well as the state of the sensorium. The normal child will usually offer some resistance

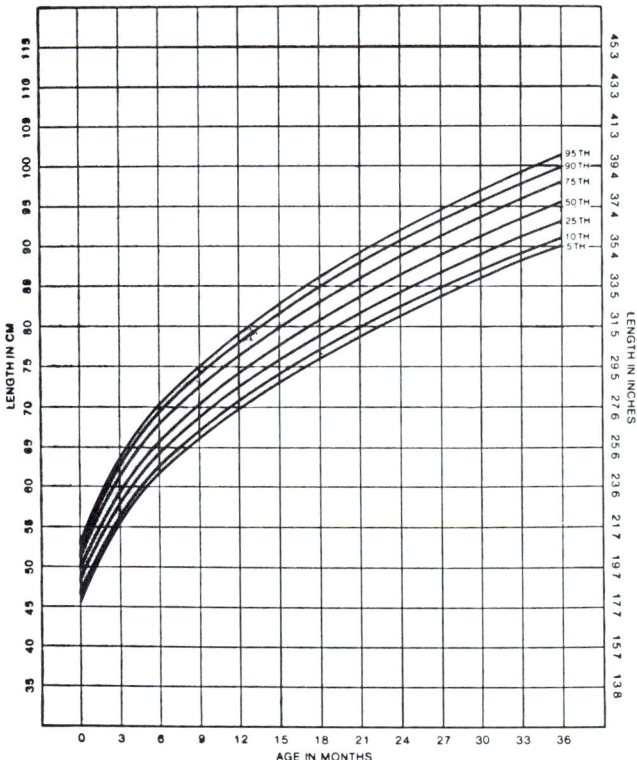

Fig. 13-1 Girls from birth to 36 months: length by age. From Hoeckelman RA, et al: *Primary pediatric care,* ed 2, St. Louis: 1992, Mosby–Year Book; modified from Hamill VV, et al: *Am J Clin Nutr* 32:607, 1979.

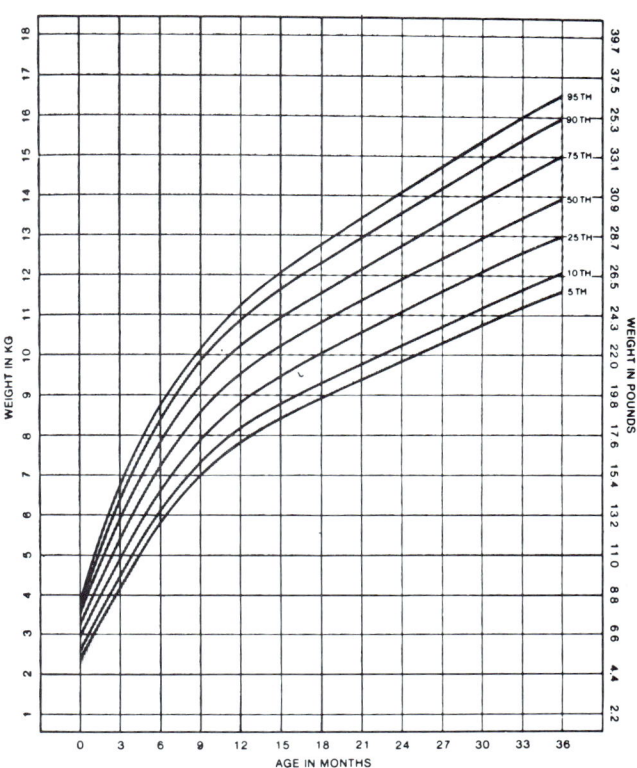

Fig. 13-2 Girls from birth to 36 months: weight by age. From Hoeckelman RA, et al: *Primary pediatric care,* ed 2, St. Louis: 1992, Mosby–Year Book; modified from Hamill VV, et al: *Am J Clin Nutr* 32:607, 1979.

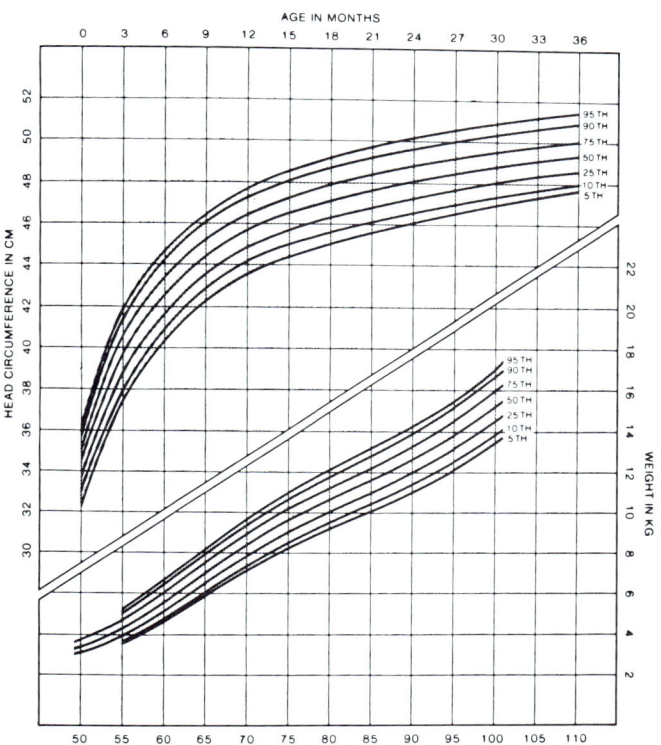

Fig. 13-3 Girls from birth to 36 months: head circumference by age and weight by length. From Hoeckelman RA, et al: *Primary pediatric care,* ed 2, St. Louis: 1992, Mosby–Year Book; modified from Hamill VV, et al: *Am J Clin Nutr* 32:607, 1979.

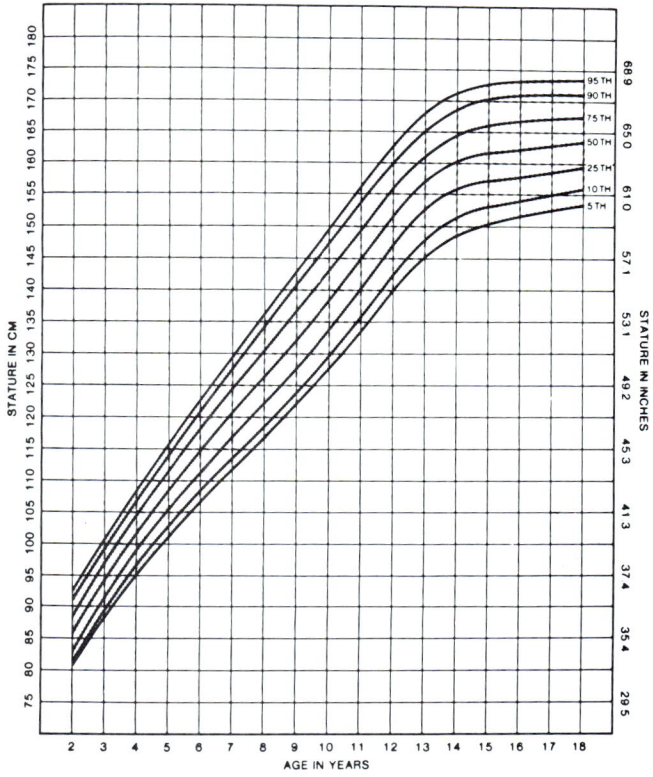

Fig. 13-4 Girls from 2 to 18 years: stature by age. From Hoeckelman RA, et al: *Primary pediatric care,* ed 2, St. Louis: 1992, Mosby–Year Book; modified from Hamill VV, et al: *Am J Clin Nutr* 32:607, 1979.

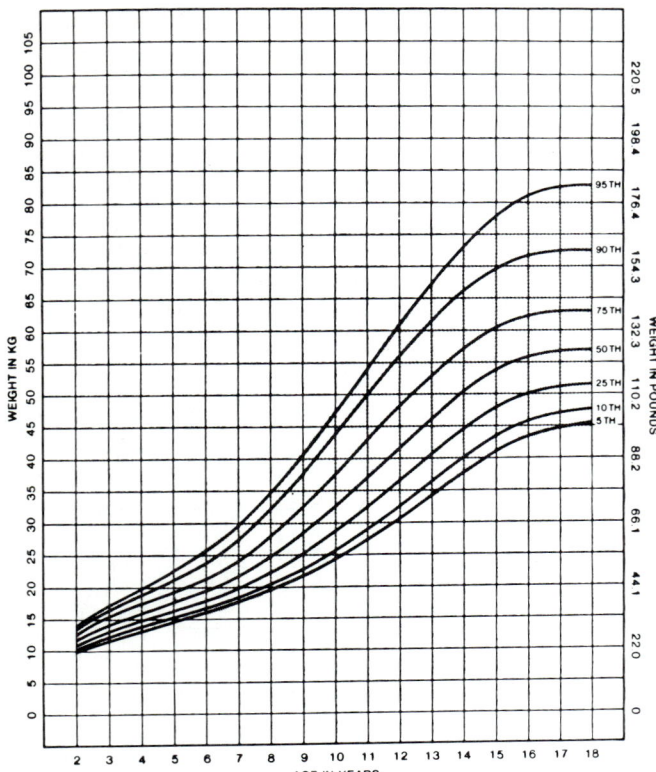

Fig. 13-5 Girls from 2 to 18 years: weight by age.
From Hoeckelman RA, et al: *Primary pediatric care,* ed 2, St. Louis: 1992, Mosby–Year Book; modified from Hamill VV, et al: *Am J Clin Nutr* 32:607, 1979.

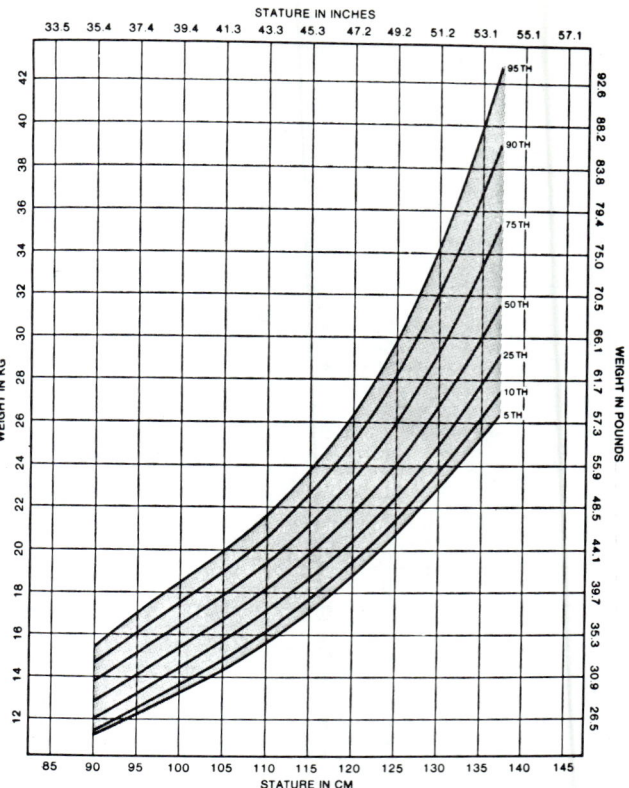

Fig. 13-6 Prepubertal girls: weight by stature.
From Hoeckelman RA, et al: *Primary pediatric care,* ed 2, St. Louis: 1992, Mosby–Year Book; modified from Hamill VV, et al: *Am J Clin Nutr* 32:607, 1979.

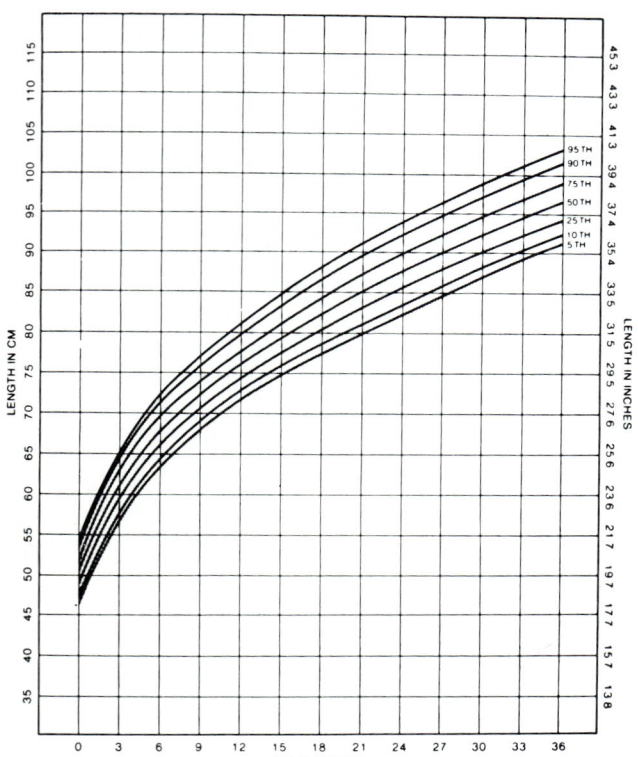

Fig. 13-7 Boys from birth to 36 months: length by age.
From Hoeckelman RA, et al: *Primary pediatric care,* ed 2, St. Louis: 1992, Mosby–Year Book; modified from Hamill VV, et al: *Am J Clin Nutr* 32:607, 1979.

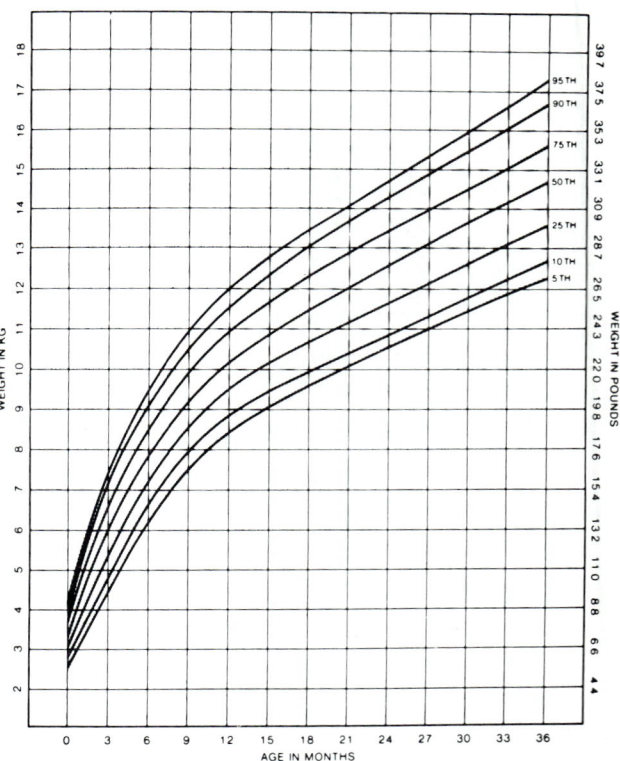

Fig. 13-8 Boys from birth to 36 months: weight by age.
From Hoeckelman RA, et al: *Primary pediatric care,* ed 2, St. Louis: 1992, Mosby–Year Book; modified from Hamill VV, et al: *Am J Clin Nutr* 32:607, 1979.

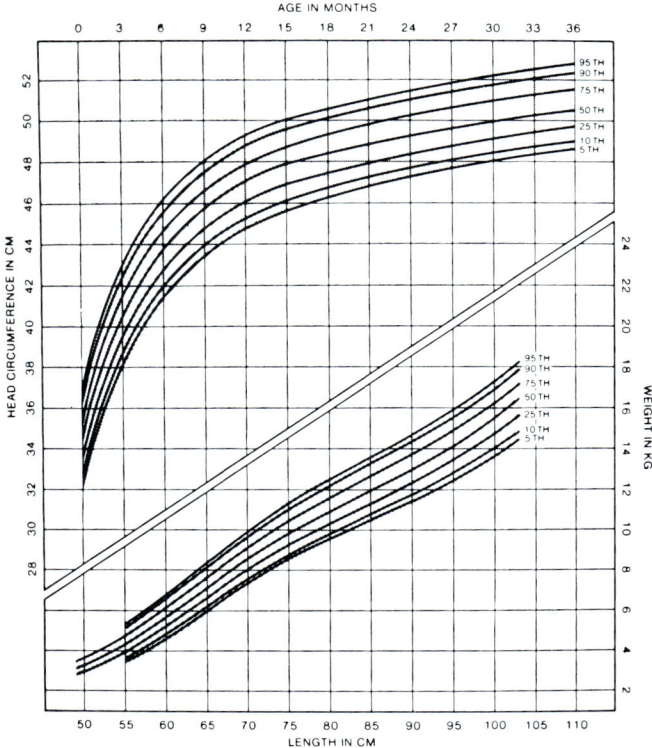

Fig. 13-9 Boys from birth to 36 months: head circumference by age and weight by length.
From Hoeckelman RA, et al: *Primary pediatric care,* ed 2, St. Louis: 1992, Mosby–Year Book; modified from Hamill VV, et al: *Am J Clin Nutr* 32:607, 1979.

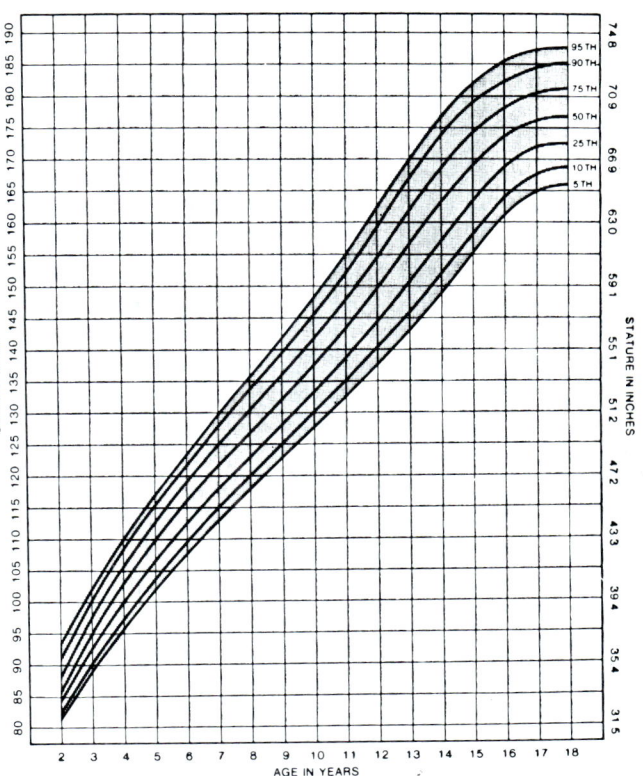

Fig. 13-10 Boys from 2 to 18 years: stature by age.
From Hoeckelman RA, et al: *Primary pediatric care,* ed 2, St. Louis: 1992, Mosby–Year Book; modified from Hamill VV, et al: *Am J Clin Nutr* 32:607, 1979.

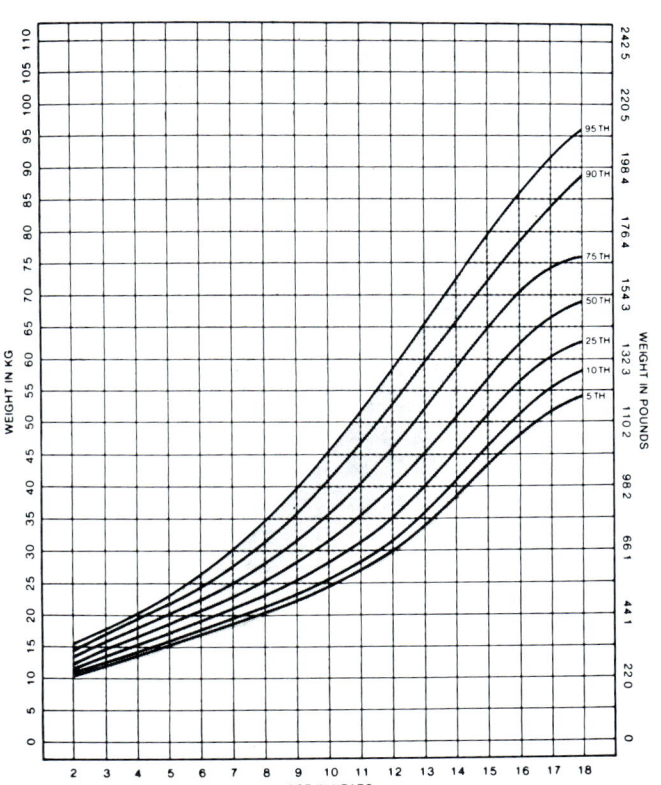

Fig. 13-11 Boys from 2 to 18 years: weight by age.
From Hoeckelman RA, et al: *Primary pediatric care,* ed 2, St. Louis: 1992, Mosby–Year Book; modified from Hamill VV, et al: *Am J Clin Nutr* 32:607, 1979.

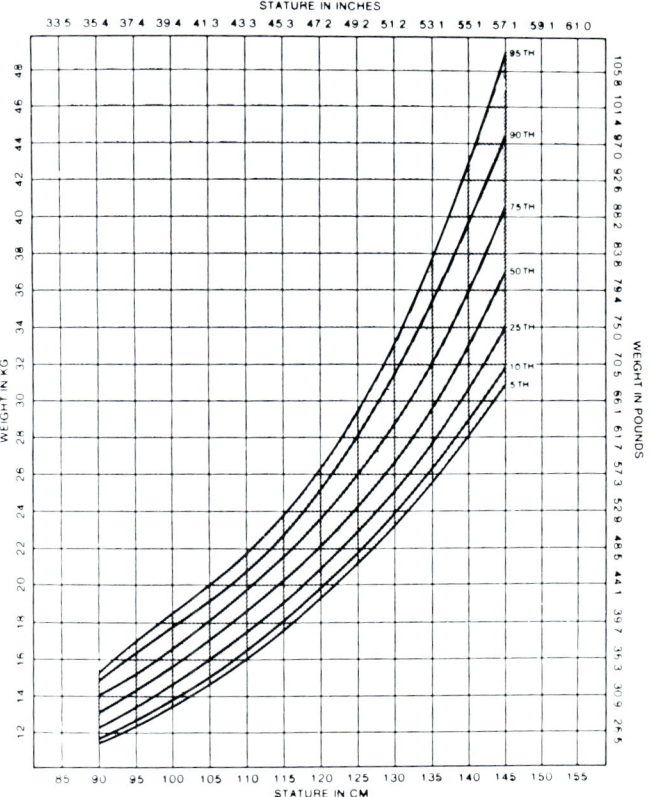

Fig. 13-12 Prepubertal boys: weight by stature.
From Hoeckelman RA, et al: *Primary pediatric care,* ed 2, St. Louis: 1992, Mosby–Year Book; modified from Hamill VV, et al: *Am J Clin Nutr* 32:607, 1979.

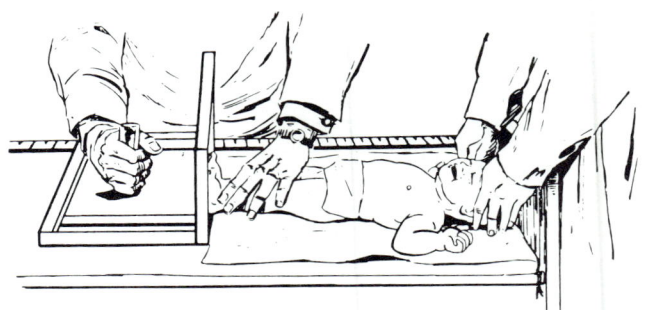

Fig. 13-13 Measurement of length in the infant. From *Evaluation of body size and physical growth in children,* The Maternal and Child Health Program, Rockville, MS, 1976, US Department of Health, Education, and Welfare.

to the examiner. The child who lies passively during the examination may be acutely ill. Observe the position of comfort as well as voluntary or involuntary movements. Certain diagnoses suggested by observation are listed in Table 13-2.

Estimate the patient's state of nutrition by observing skin turgor, bony prominences, and muscle wasting.

During the examination, observe the skin for abnormal pigmentation, nevi, and abnormal color such as cyanosis or jaundice. The color of the tongue will help differentiate peripheral from central cyanosis. With peripheral cyanosis, the tongue is pink, whereas with central cyanosis, the tongue is blue. Central cyanosis is usually associated with significant pulmonary or congenital heart disease. The presence of pallor is most easily determined by observing the nail beds, conjunctivae, or tongue.

The capillary refill time helps determine circulatory status. To determine the capillary refill time, pinch the abdominal skin. The color usually returns in less than 2 seconds. Skin turgor is helpful in determining the state of hydration. Edema can be determined by observing if impressions are left in the skin following finger pressure. Edema is first noted in the eyelids, followed by that seen in the dependent parts.

Rashes are common in children. The color, distribution, feeling to touch, elevation, and presence of fluid and/or pain are helpful in determining the etiologic cause of the rash. *Rashes* that are usually erythematous are common with viral diseases such as measles, rubella, and roseola. The erythematous eruption may also be caused by any type of irritation, such as diaper rash or exposure to wind and sun. *Macules* are discrete, nonraised lesions and are seen in children with a viral disease such as an echovirus or a coxsackievirus or with erythema

TABLE 13-2: Pediatric Diagnoses Suggested by Observing the Patient

Condition	Characteristics
Down syndrome	Prominent epicanthal folds, large tongue, high arched palate, simian crease
Prader-Willi syndrome	Obesity, hypotonia, mental retardation
Rickets	Growth retarded, legs bowed, costochondral junctions prominent
Turner's syndrome	Short stocky build, shieldlike chest, short webbed neck, low-set ears
Hypothyroidism	Delayed growth, short stature, large protruding tongue
Waardenburg's syndrome	White forelock, hearing loss, different colors of irises

infectiosum. The firm skin and subcutaneous elevations with discolorations following the macular stage of illness are called *papules*. Skin elevations containing fluid are vesicles commonly seen in chickenpox or herpes simplex. If the fluid is purulent, the elevations are called *pustules*, which are usually caused by bacterial infection or abscesses.

The patient with a chromosomal aberration may be identified by abnormal dermatoglyphics on the hands. *Dermatoglyphics* are ridges formed by the raised apertures of sweat glands. Examination of the nails for abnormal color, infection, hemorrhage, and shape is useful in determining the cause of disease. Note the hair distribution, density, and patterns.

While examining each portion of the body, observe the lymph nodes and palpate them for size, tenderness, and mobility. In the patient less than 12 years of age, cool to touch, movable, nontender nodes from 0.5 to 1 cm in diameter are not unusual. If enlarged nodes are identified, carefully examine the area drained by these nodes to determine the etiologic cause of the enlargement.

Head and Neck

Compared with that of the older child and adult, the head is a significant proportion of total body length during the first few years of life. After 3 months of age, the head is normally covered with smooth, fine hair. Symmetry of the head is caused by organized growth along the suture lines of the skull. An asymmetric head would indicate premature or irregular closure of the sutures (Fig. 13-14). Sutures are palpated as ridges until about 6 months of age.

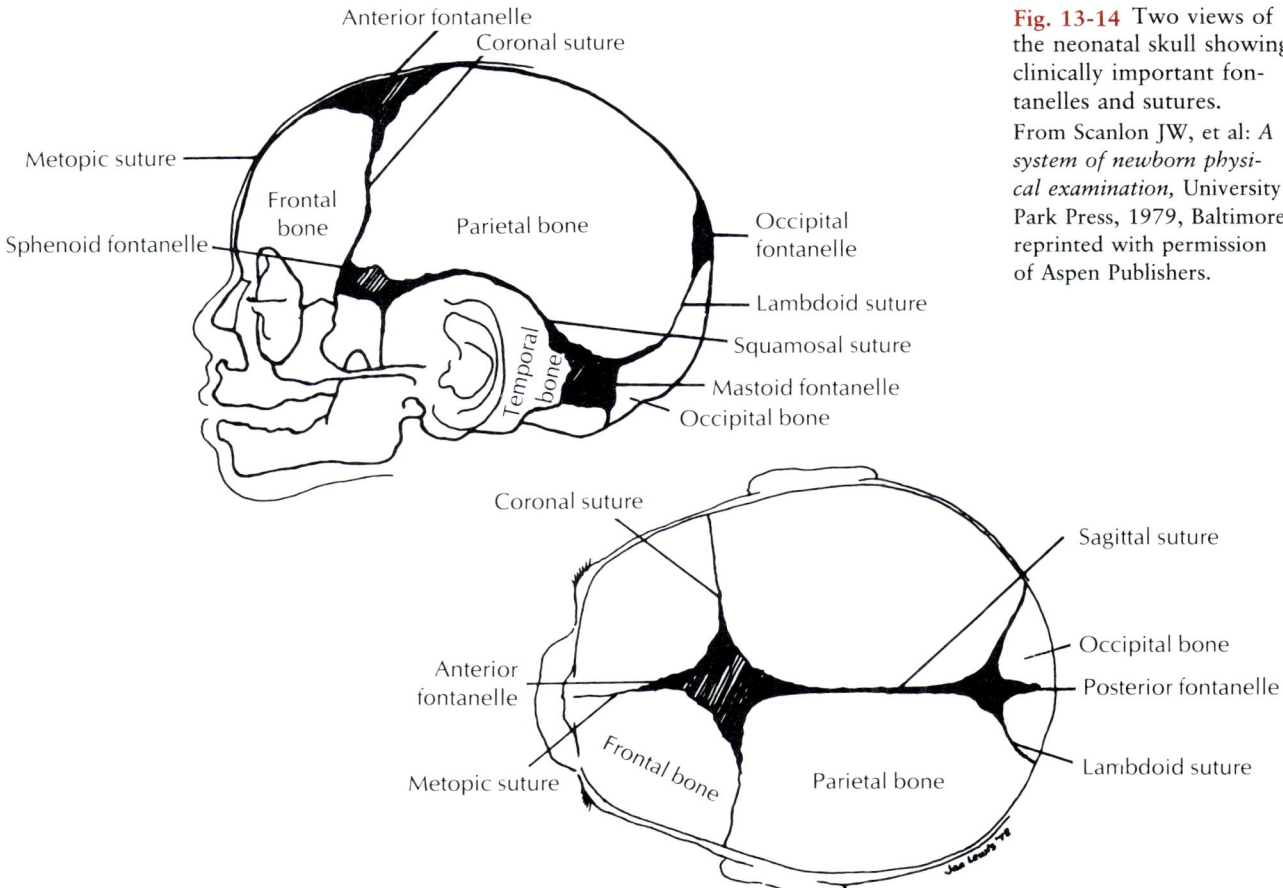

Fig. 13-14 Two views of the neonatal skull showing clinically important fontanelles and sutures. From Scanlon JW, et al: *A system of newborn physical examination,* University Park Press, 1979, Baltimore; reprinted with permission of Aspen Publishers.

The anterior fontanelle is a diamond-shaped area that is usually closed by 24 months of age (see Fig. 13-14). The posterior fontanelle is a triangular-shaped area that is usually closed by 2 months of age. Tenseness or bulging of the fontanelle is best evaluated with the infant in the sitting position. A bulging fontanelle may indicate increased ICP, whereas a depressed fontanelle may be associated with dehydration and malnutrition. Auscultate the fontanelle with the diaphragm of the stethoscope to determine if a bruit is present, as is found in the presence of an arteriovenous malformation.

Palpate the skull for bossing, craniotabes, and, in the older child, tenderness over the sinuses. *Bossing* is described as bulging of the frontal areas. *Craniotabes* is a snapping sensation elicited by pressing on the scalp just above and behind the ears. Observe the face to determine any area of weakness or paralysis, swelling caused by edema, or glandular enlargement. Palpate the angle of the jaw and submaxillary and submandibular areas to identify enlarged glands.

EYES

Vision in the infant less than 1 year old can be estimated by the patient's interest in a light or other bright object. Funduscopic examination may be difficult, especially in the infant or toddler less than 4 years of age. Observe the eyes for loss of upward gaze, nystagmus, or ptosis. Strabismus is usually not present after 6 months of age. Strabismus may be identified by alternately covering one of the patient's eyes and looking at the opposite eye for motion.

Note the color of the sclera. Observe the conjunctiva for evidence of conjunctivitis or hemorrhage. Sties must be differentiated from a chalazion, a nonpainful swelling of the lid edge caused by an inclusion cyst (see Chapter 2). Examine the cornea for ulcerations, discolorations, or haziness. Estimate the ocular interpupillary distance (OID) to identify the patient with hypotelorism or hypertelorism. *Hypotelorism* is a decreased OID, whereas *hypertelorism* is an increased OID. The pupils should be of equal size and shape and react appropriately to light. Test accommodation by having the patient look at an object at a distance and quickly bringing it toward the patient.

The iris develops its pigmented color within 6 months of age. Check the iris for *coloboma* (absence of part of the iris), *Brushfield's spots* (white spots in iris), and adhesions from the iris to the lens. Examine the lens with an ophthalmoscope for white or gray spots indicative of opacities such as cataracts. A red reflex indicates a normal vascularization of the retina. Attempt to identify the optic disc, which normally has a sharp border. The macula will appear cherry red in certain neurodegenerative disorders.

EARS

Anomalies of the ears are often associated with anomalies of other organ systems. For example, low-set ears are associated with renal anomalies. In these patients, the upper portion of the ear is located below the level of the eye. Evaluate the external ear canals for any discharge. To examine the eardrum, gently insert the otoscope into the ear canal (Fig. 13-15). By resting the hand that holds the otoscope on the infant's head, any motion made by the child will be accompanied by similar movement of the otoscope. The direction of the canal in infants is upwards, whereas in older children the canal goes downward and forward. Therefore, to view the drum, the auricle in the infant should be pulled downward, whereas in the older child it should be pulled upward and back.

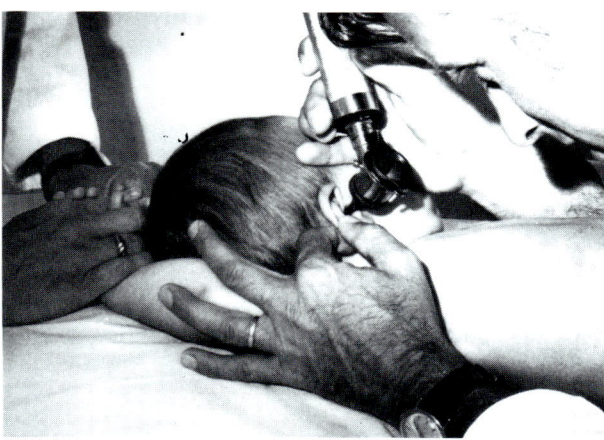

Fig. 13-15 Otoscopic examination of the child. From Hoeckelman RA, et al: *Primary pediatric care,* ed 2, St. Louis, 1992, Mosby–Year Book; photograph by P. Ruben.

The normal ear drum is gray-white and translucent with landmarks similar to those of adults. A slight redness may be caused by crying or manipulation. With acute otitis media, the drum usually bulges upward and becomes diffusely red and there is loss of the light reflex. With resolving otitis media or allergic conditions, an air fluid level with retraction of the drum may occur. Assess the mobility of the eardrum by insufflation of air through the otoscope.

Hearing should be routinely assessed in the older child. If hearing loss is suspected in a younger infant, refer the patient for appropriate testing.

NOSE

Note any unusual shape of the nose. Inspect the nasal mucosa with a light and note any type of secretion. A nasal speculum can be used in older patients at risk for nasal polyps, such as the child with allergies.

MOUTH

In the cooperative child, inspect the mouth and oral cavity for the presence of mucosal lesions and the number and status of teeth. Examine the gums for swelling and evidence of bleeding. Observe the tongue for tremors, unusual color, and texture. *Thrush* of the tongue is a coalescent white membrane that will not scrape off with a tongue blade.

Depression of the anterior half of the tongue with a depressor will allow inspection of the hard palate. If a cleft palate or defect in the palate is observed, it should be noted if the cleft involves the hard palate, the soft palate, uvula, or a combination. Advancing the tongue depressor causes the child to gag but allows a fleeting inspection of the tip of the epiglottis, uvulae, and posterior pharynx (Fig. 13-16). The tonsils are often larger during earlier childhood. Look for any exudates or membranes in the posterior pharynx.

It is important to listen to the infant's voice or cry for any hoarseness or stridor. The lesion causing inspiratory stridor is usually outside of the thorax, whereas the lesion causing expiratory stridor is usually within the thoracic cage. With inflammation in the supraglottic area, the patient's voice may be muffled, and he has difficulty swallowing. With glottis obstruction, a high-pitched crow is heard, and the voice is hoarse.

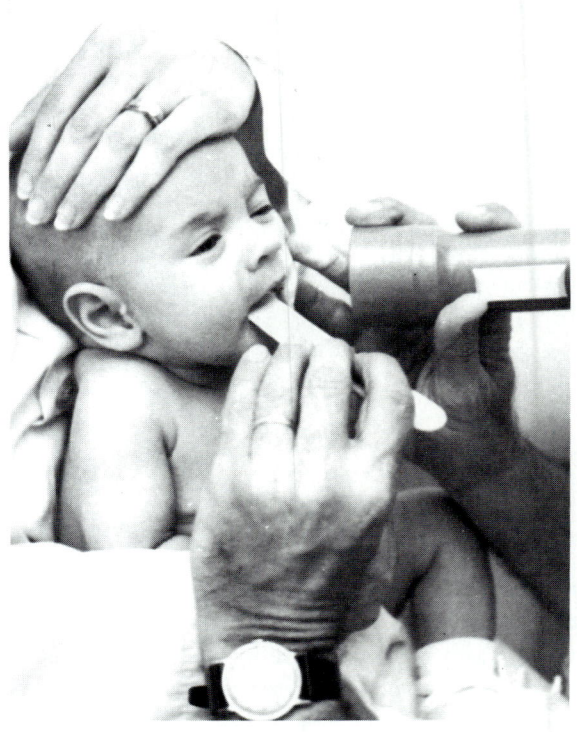

Fig. 13-16 Examination of the pharynx in the infant. From Hoeckelman RA, et al: *Primary pediatric care*, ed 2, St. Louis, 1992, Mosby–Year Book; photograph by P. Ruben.

NECK

During the first 4 years of life, the neck appears relatively short compared with the adult ratio. Examine the neck for webbing and edema. Webbing is associated with gonadal dysgenesis, whereas edema of the neck is associated with local infections, obstruction of the superior vena cava, and any of the causes of generalized edema. Within the neck, palpate the sternocleidomastoid muscles, trachea, and thyroid for any abnormalities. Check the vessels located in the neck for size or abnormal pulsations. The neck should be extended and flexed to identify resistance. *Torticollis,* or a shortening of a sternocleidomastoid muscle, causes the neck to be held at an angle and may or may not be associated with a muscle mass. Auscultation of the neck with the bell of the stethoscope will identify murmurs transmitted from the heart.

Chest

Observe the chest for symmetry and equal movements bilaterally. In children under 6 years of age, most respiratory activity is related to depression of the diaphragm and can be compromised by increased intraabdominal pressure. At a later age, air exchange is primarily caused by thoracic motion. A paradoxic motion of the chest and diaphragm will occur when the normal relationship between chest expansion and diaphragm movement is abnormal.

Palpate the chest wall on both sides and note the presence of axillary lymph nodes, areas of tenderness, and symmetry of movement. Percuss the chest wall, defining the heart and top of the liver (see Chapter 5).

In girls, breast development usually begins after the age of 8 to 10 years (see Chapter 8). Examine the breasts for any discharge, masses, or nodules. In the adolescent male, it is not unusual to have some breast development with a mass present immediately behind the areola.

LUNGS

The normal respiratory rate will vary from 30 to 40 breaths/min at birth, 20 to 30 breaths/min during infancy, and 15 to 25 breaths/min during childhood, dropping to 14 to 20 breaths/min during adolescence.

When auscultating the chest, listen with the patient both supine and sitting. Examine the entire chest, listening for equal breath sounds on both sides and abnormal extraneous sounds. Breath sounds may seem louder than in the adult; this is normal. Because of the small size of the chest in the very young infant, a chest x-ray film is often necessary to identify the area associated with abnormal physical findings.

HEART

In the newborn, the pulse rate is normally 120 to 160 beats/min, decreasing to 60 to 80 beats/min in the adolescent (see Table 4-6). The sleeping pulse rate is usually lower than the awake rate. Pathologic arrhythmias are unusual in childhood. Most children have sinus arrhythmia, and an occasional premature beat or extra systole is not unusual.

Palpate pulses in the neck, femoral area, and upper and lower extremities in all patients. The cardiac impulse may or may not be visible in the normal patient. In very young infants, palpating the point of maximal impulse may be difficult. In older children, it is usually located in the fifth intercostal space in the midclavicular line.

Examine the patient in both the supine and sitting position and note any thrills or rubs. In older infants and children, percussion is used to determine the size of the heart. Use both the bell and diaphragm of the stethoscope to listen to the heart sounds in the same areas as in the adult. At the more rapid heart rates of the younger infant, identifying the splitting of the second heart sound may not be possible. Describe any murmur that is identified in relationship to its intensity, location in relationship to the first and second heart sound, location of maximum intensity on the chest wall, and any changes in intensity that occur with a change in position (see Tables 4-2 and 4-5).

Abdomen

As stated previously, it is frequently necessary to examine the abdomen first while the child is quiet. Because of the normal lordotic stance of the child, the abdomen frequently appears to be protuberant. Because the abdomen is used for respiration in the younger child, the abdominal wall will move with respirations. It is normally flat when the child is in the lying position but may be depressed in the dehydrated infant.

Umbilical hernias are common in children under 2 years old and may be accentuated when the infant cries. Diastasis of the rectus muscles is usually a normal variant. The abdomen should be observed for visible peristalsis, which is always a sign of obstruction unless proven otherwise.

Auscultate the abdomen for peristaltic sounds, and percuss it for organ size and evidence of fluid. Palpate the abdomen gently and superficially. Identify any areas of tenderness, although these are often difficult to localize in the child. In the child who cannot respond to your questioning about abdominal tenderness, start your

Fig. 13-17 Standards for genitalia maturity ratings in boys.
From Tanner JM: *Growth at adolescence,* ed 2, Oxford, 1962, Blackwell Scientific Publications.

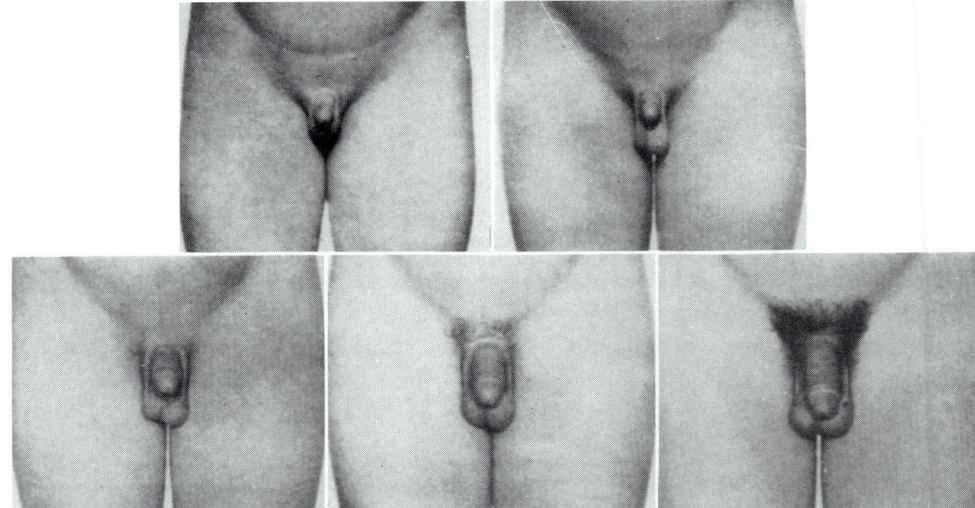

palpation in an area that you know is nontender. Gradually approach the suspected tender area and watch the child's face for evidence of grimacing or change in crying. The spleen is normally palpable 1 to 2 cm below the left costal margin in young infants and children, and the liver is palpable 1 to 2 cm below the right costal margin. On deeper palpation, a significant portion of the right kidney may be palpated, as well as the tip of the left kidney. Palpate the inguinal and femoral areas for evidence of hernias, adenopathy, and femoral pulses.

Genitalia

The distribution of pubic hair, if present, should be described according to the Tanner stage (Fig. 13-17; see also Fig. 7-2). In the young female, the vaginal orifice is easiest examined with the child in the knee-chest position, which allows adequate visualization of the area. Palpation of the vagina is usually omitted until puberty. In the postpubertal female, a complete pelvic examination should be performed on a regular basis.

In the male, examine the penis for the position of the urethral orifice. Adhesions of the prepuce to the glands are not unusual in the child less than 4 years of age. Inspect the scrotum for evidence of a hernia or hydrocele. Palpate to ensure that both testes have descended from the abdomen. Torsion of the spermatic cord first appears as an acute swelling of the scrotum with discoloration; it is a surgical emergency.

When either a male or a female child appears with injuries to the genitalia, genital irritations, or genital discharges, consideration must be given to sexual abuse as a possible etiologic cause.

Inspect the anus and perform an examination in patients with lower GI symptoms or abdominal pain. An anal fissure (a cut or tear in the mucosa) is not unusual in the child under 2 years of age. Observe the coccygeal area for a pilonidal dimple with a possible sinus. Frequently there is an associated tuft of hair at the sinus' opening. Carefully palpate the area to see if the sinus is occluded, forming an enlarged cyst.

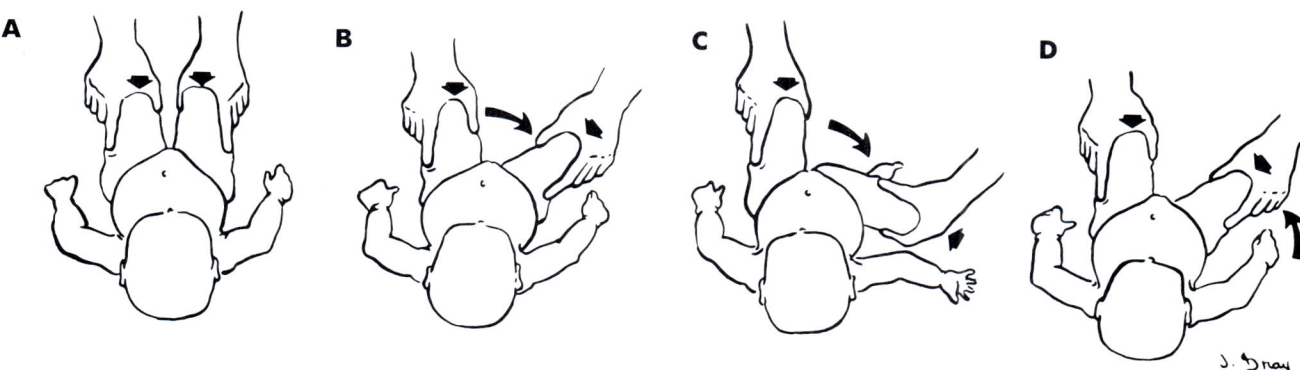

Fig. 13-18 Examination for congenital dislocation of the hip. **A,** Downward pressure of the hips to produce posterior dislocation. **B,** The hip to be examined is then abducted. **C** and **D,** Positive Ortolani's sign is elicited by feeling the head reenter the acetabulum with a click. Keep your finger on the baby's greater trochanter during all phases of the examination.
From Stanisavljevic S: *Diagnosis and treatment of congenital hip pathology in the newborn,* Baltimore, 1964, Williams & Wilkins.

Musculoskeletal System

Examine the extremities for shape, length, and presence of anomalies. Observe the fingers and toes for clubbing. Examine the extremities for evidence of pain or tenderness over a bone, muscle mass, or joint. If possible, the child should walk and run to help identify abnormalities in gait and coordination. Toe walking, which may be normal until 3 years of age, may be a sign of spasticity, muscular dystrophy, or muscle imbalance.

Passively examine all joints for adequacy of motion, effusions, erythema, tenderness, or heat. In the young infant, examine the hips for evidence of congenital dislocation or subluxation (Fig. 13-18).

At birth the feet are almost never straight but in a somewhat either varus or valgus attitude. If this was caused by in utero positioning, the foot will straighten to the midline with a minimal effort. More severe anomalies such as club feet or metatarsus varus require forceful manual stretching or may not be straightened at all by hand.

It is important to examine the spine on every routine examination. Check the midline for any dimpling with an overlying tuft of hair, masses, or discolorations. Examine motion of the spine with the patient in both the prone and supine positions. Abnormalities in posture such as lordosis, kyphosis, and scoliosis need to be identified early in childhood (see Chapter 9).

Examine all muscle groups for development, increased tone as evidenced by spasm, or decreased tone as evidenced by flaccidity. Identify any contraction with or without muscle atrophy by muscle groups.

Neurologic Examination

Much of the neurologic examination can be performed when examining other portion of the body. Reflex responses change with maturation between birth and 3 to 6 months of age (Table 13-3). Note the state of consciousness, position of the patient, and spontaneous movements. In the older child, coordination can be tested by playing with the patient. Tremors must be distinguished from choreiform movements and athetosis. Superficial and deep tendon reflexes should be equal in intensity bilaterally.

Evaluate the developmental motor activity according to age. In the child more than 6 years of age, an accurate sensory examination can be performed (see Chapter 10).

TABLE 13-3: Strength of Eight Reflexes for Infants Between 28 and 40 Weeks' Gestation

	28	30	32	34	36	38	40
Sucking*	Weak, not really synchronized with swallowing		Stronger and better synchronized with swallowing		Perfect		
Palmar grasp†	Present but weak			Stronger		Excellent	
Response to traction†	Absent		Begins to appear	Strong enough to lift part of body weight		Strong enough to lift all of body weight	
Moro reflex‡	Weak, obtained just once, incomplete		Complete reflex				
Crossed extension§	Flexion and extension in random pattern, purposeless reaction		Good extension but no tendency to adduction		Tendency to adduction but imperfect	Complete response with extension, adduction, fanning of toes	
Automatic walking‖	—	—	Begins tiptoeing with good support on sole and righting reaction of legs for a few seconds	Pretty good; very fast tiptoeing		A premature who reaches 40 weeks walks in toe-heel progression or on tiptoes A full-term newborn of 40 weeks walks in heel-toe progression on whole sole of foot	
Root¶	Good with reinforcement		Good (no reinforcement)	Good		Good	Good
Pupillary response			Present	Present		Present	Present

Modified from Rudolph AM, et al: *Rudolph's pediatrics*, ed 19, Norwalk, CT, 1991, Appleton & Lange.
*The examiner evaluates the sucking reflex by introducing a finger into the infant's mouth to observe the strength and rhythm of sucking. The synchrony of sucking and swallowing is observed during feeding.
†The examiner inserts the index fingers into the infant's hands from the ulnar side and gently presses against the palmar surface. The infant's fingers flex around the finger. When the index fingers are drawn upward, the palmar grasp spreads to the flexor muscles of the arm. The term infant can support his entire weight by this traction response.
‡The examiner grasps the infant's hands and lifts the shoulders a few cm while keeping the back of the head on the bed, then suddenly releases the hands. The normal reflex is a brisk abduction of the arms at the shoulder and extension of the forearms at the elbow, followed by adduction of the arms and flexion of the forearms. Complete opening of the hands occurs in the first phase.
§The examiner holds one of the infant's legs in extension and rubs the sole of the foot. The complete response has three components: (1) the opposite leg rapidly flexes or "retreats" followed by extension; then (2) the opposite leg adducts; and (3) the toes fan.
‖The examiner holds the infant by the trunk and lifts him slightly forward. The infant steps forward as each foot contacts the surface.
¶Stroking the cheek near the mouth causes the infant to turn the face to that side, open the mouth, and attempt to suck.

Summary

A summary checklist for the evaluation of the pediatric patient is shown on the opposite page.

Summary Checklist for Examination of the Pediatric Patient

Measurement
  Weight
  Height
  Temperature
  Heart rate
  Pulse rate
  Blood pressure
  Head circumference
    (less than 2 years old)
Observation
  Activity level
  Nutritional state
  Skin
    Pigmentation
    Color
    Rashes
  Nails
  Hair distribution
  Lymph nodes
Head and neck
  General
    Fontanelles, open or closed
    Sutures
    Symmetry
  Eyes
    Visual acuity
    Strabismus
    Scleral color
    Cornea
    Interpupillary distance
    Iris
    Funduscopic examination
  Ears
    Location
    Discharge
    Tympanic membrane
      (color and mobility)
  Nose
    Shape
    Mucosa
  Mouth
    Teeth
    Mucous membranes
    Cleft palate
    Voice
  Neck
    Webbing
    Edema
    Torticollis
Chest
  General
    Movement
    Symmetry
    Breast development
  Lungs
    Breath sounds
  Heart
    Rhythm
    Point of maximal impulse
    Heart sounds
Abdomen
  Organ size
  Tenderness
  Umibilical hernia
  Bowel sounds
Genitalia
  Pubic hair
  Testes
  Urethral orifice location
  Vagina
  Irritation
  Discharge
  Anal fissure
Musculoskeletal
  Symmetry
  Gait
  Joints
  Muscle strength
Neurologic
  Reflexes
  Coordination

Suggested readings

Behrman RE, et al: *Nelson Textbook of Pediatrics*, ed 14, Philadelphia, 1992, WB Saunders.

Hoekelman RA, et al: *Primary Pediatric Care*, ed 2, St Louis, 1992, Mosby–Year Book.

Rudolph AM, et al: *Rudolph's Pediatrics*, ed 19, East Norwalk, CT, 1991, Appleton & Lange.

APPENDIX A

Latin and Greek Roots

Word Roots	Root Meaning	Example
a	lack, without	a-pnea (lack of breathing)
ab	off, from, away from	ab-ductors (to lead away from)
acet	vinegar	acet-ic acid (constituent of vinegar)
ad	to, toward	ad-ductors (to lead or draw towards)
agog	lead away	secret-agogue (to cause secretions to flow)
album	the white of an egg	album-in (the white of an egg)
alis	pertaining to	intestin-alis (pertaining to the intestine)
alve	a cavity	bi-valve (two cavities)
amaur	dark, obscure	amaur-osis (blindness)
andr	a man	andro-gen (producing man)
anser	a goose	pes anserina (foot of a goose)
anti	against or opposite	anti-toxins (against a toxin or poison)
aphrodit	goddess of love and beauty	aphrodisiac (enhancing love)
aphtha	an ulcer	aphthous stomatitis (ulcer of the mouth)
aqua	water	aqua-tic (pertaining to water)
arachn	spider	arachno-dactyly (spider fingers)
areol	a little open space	areol-a (nipple)
asthen	weak	my-asthenia (muscle weakness)
astr	a star	astro-cyte (star cell)
ather	the silk of an ear of corn	ather-oma (corn silk–shaped tumor)
audi	hear	audi-tory nerve (hearing nerve)
azyg	unpaired	azygous vein (unpaired vein in chest)
bacill	a little stick	bacill-ary (a rod- or stick-shaped bacteria)
bact	a rod	bact-erium (a rod-shaped microbe)
balan	an acorn	balan-itis (inflammation of the glans penis)

Word Roots	Root Meaning	Example
bi	two or double	bi-ped (two feet)
bin	two	bin-ocular (using two eyes)
bili	bile, anger	bili-rubin (bile pigment)
blephar	eyelash, eyelid	blephar-ospasm (spasm of the eyelids)
bronch	windpipe	bronch-itis (inflammation of the windpipes)
bulim	hunger	bulim-ia (forced vomiting)
cac	bad	cac-ophony (bad sound)
calc	the heel, limestone	calci-tonin (helps deposits calcium salts)
calor	heat	calor-ic (dealing with heat or energy)
capr	a goat	capri-corn (goat horn)
card	the heart	cardio-pulmonary (heart and lungs)
carn	flesh	carn-ivorous (flesh or meat eating)
celib	unmarried	celib-acy (without sexual intercourse)
cent	a hundred	cent-imeter (measure into one hundred parts)
ceri	wax	cer-umen (ear wax)
chol	bile, anger	chole-stasis (bile standstill)
chondr	cartilage	costo-chondritis (rib/cartilage inflammation)
cide	kill	fratri-cide (to kill sibling)
cili	eyelash or small hair	cili-a (small hairlike projections)
cine	move or motion	cine-mascope (to look at motion pictures)
circ	ring	circ-cumsize (to cut around a ring)
cleid	key or clavicle	sterno-cleid-omastoid (muscle that goes from sternum and clavicle to mastoid)
coarct	pressed together	coarct-ation (condition of aorta and pulmonary artery being joined together with a patent tube)
coit	coming together	coit-us (the act of coming together in sexual intercourse)
conus	cone	conus medullaris (the end cone-shaped segment of the spinal cord)
cord	heart	ac-cord (to the heart)
corn	horn	corn-ified (made into horny tissue)
cruci	a cross	cruci-ate (cross-shaped ligaments in the knee)
crur	the leg	crur-is (leg between knee and ankle)
crypt	hidden	crypt-ogenic (a hidden beginning)

Word Roots	Root Meaning	Example
cune	a wedge	cune-iform (wedge form or shape)
cunn	the vulva	cunn-ilingus (pertaining to tongue and vulva)
dacry	tears	dacry-ocystitis (inflammation of the tear glands)
dactyl	finger or toe	dactyl-itis (inflammation of the finger or toe)
dehisc	split	dehisc-ence (splitting apart of the surgical incision)
dei	god	dei-ty (pertaining to a god)
demono	evil spirit	demon-iac (having to do with evil spirits)
deo	god	in excelsus deo (in highest, God)
dicrot	double-oared	dicrot-ic (double beating)
dipther	membrane	dipther-ia (disease with a membrane)
dolor	sorrow	dolor (used as a cardinal sign of inflammation meaning discomfort)
dulc	sweet	dulc-ify (to make sweet)
duo	two	duo-denum (the first division of small intestine)
dur	hard	dur-ess (enduring hardness)
dyn	power	a-dyn-amic ileus (lack of power resulting in lack of intestine motility)
dys	bad	dys-menorrhea (bad menses)
ebri	drunk	in-ebri-ated (referring to drunken state)
ec	out of	ec-toderm (referring to outer layer of skin)
ect	outside	ect-oderm (the outside skin)
ectomy	cut out	cyst-ectomy (cut out the bladder)
ectopy	displacement	ecto-pic (outside of, ectopic pregnancy)
edema	a swelling	pedal edema (a fluid swelling in the legs)
efferen	carrying away	efferent arteriole (arteriole carrying blood away from a structure)
ell	small	organ-elle (small organ)
emet	vomit	hemat-emet-esis (the condition of vomiting blood)
emphys	inflate	emphys-ema (air inflating the tissues)
en	in or into	en-anthem (blossoming or eruption in the mouth)

Word Roots	Root Meaning	Example
encephal	brain	encephal-itis (inflammation of the brain)
entero	intestine	entero-pathagon (a microbe of the intestines)
epi	upon, over	epi-scler-itis (upon sclera—inflammation of)
eros	love	ero-tism (sexual desire)
erythr	red	erythr-ocyte (red cell)
escha	scab	escha-r (a slough or scab)
etho	custom or habit	etho-logy (study of habits)
etiol	cause	etiol-ogy (study of causes)
eu	good	eu-capnia (good smoke, or normal carbon dioxide tension)
evolut	unrolling	evolut-ion (to roll out from)
ex	out, off, or from	ex-enteration (surgical removal of the bowel from the body cavity)
exi	go out	exi-tus (going out, death)
exo	outside	exo-cytosis (discharge from a cell to the outside)
falx	a sickle	falx cerebri (sickle-shape fold of dura separating the two cerebral hemispheres)
febr	fever	febr-ile (characterized by fever)
fecul	foul	fecul-ent (foul-smelling sediment)
feli	cat	feli-ne (catlike)
fem	thigh	fem-ur (thigh bone)
femin	female	femin-inity (qualities of a woman)
fenestr	window	fenestr-a (a windowlike opening)
ferous	carrying	semini-ferous (seed carrying)
feti	putrid smelling	feti-d (disagreeable smell)
fil	thread	fil-aria (threadlike parasites)
flagell	whip	flagell-iform (whip shaped)
fleur	flower	fleur-de-lis (flower of love)
flux	flowing	bloody flux (bloody diarrhea)
follicul	little bag	follicul-itis (inflammation of a follicle)
fract	to break	march fract-ure (broken bone caused by walking)
furfur	bran or dandruff	malassezia furfur (fungus producing scales resembling bran)
gam	marriage	gam-etocyte (a cell at the sexual stage especially used of malaria)
gangli	knot on a string	gangli-on (a knotlike mass)

Word Roots	Root Meaning	Example
gast	stomach	epi-gast-ric (over the stomach)
gemin	twin, double	bi-geminy (occurring in twos, or pairs)
gen	bear, produce	gene (the unit of heredity)
geni	chin or jaw	geni-ohyoid (chin and hyoid bone)
genicul	elbow or knee joint	genicul-ate (bent like a knee)
genit	beget	pro-genit-or (ancestor)
genu	knee	genu valgum (knock kneed)
geny	production	pro-geny (offspring)
geo	earth	geo-phagia (to eat earth)
gravid	pregnant	gravid-a (number of pregnancies)
guan	dung	guan-o (bird dung)
gymn	naked	gymn-astics (athletics)
gyr	turning a circle	gyr-ectomy (excision of gyrus of brain)
haem, hem	blood	haem-atidrosis (sweating blood)
halit	breathing	halit-osis (breathing out bad breath)
hemi	one-half	hemi-anopia (one half lack of vision)
hepa	liver	hepa-titis (inflammation of the liver)
hept	seven	hept-ose (a sugar containing seven carbons)
herpes	creeping	herpes simplex (herpes virus infection)
heter	other or different	heter-osexual (pertaining to the other or opposite sex)
hex	six	hex-ose (monosaccharide with six carbons)
hidro	sweat	an-hidrotic (lack of sweating)
humer	the shoulder	humer-us (the bone extending from shoulder to elbow)
hydat	water	hydat-id cyst (a cystlike water collection)
hydr	water	hydr-ocephalus (accumulation of water on the head)
hyp	under	hyp-oactive (under activity)
hyper	above	hyper-active (over activity)
hypo	beneath	hypo-thyroidism (condition of deficiency of thyroid activity)
iasis	condition of	trypanosom-iasis (condition of being infected by trypanosomes)
iatr	physician	iatr-ogenic (caused by physicians)
icter	jaundice	icter-us (jaundiced)

Word Roots	Root Meaning	Example
infer, infra	underneath, below	infra-clavicular (beneath a clavicle)
insect	insect	insect-icide (kill insect)
iso	equal	iso-coria (equal-sized pupils)
itis	inflammation	ir-itis (inflammation of iris)
juxta	near	juxta-position (placed near to)
labi	a lip	naso-labi-al groove (groove near nose and lip)
lano, leni	wool	lano-lin (wool oil)
leo	lion	leo-nine facies (lionlike facies of leprosy)
leuc, leuk	white	leuk-ocyte (white cell)
levo	left-hand	levo-rotatory (to turn to the left)
lith	stone	nephro-lith-iasis (kidney stone, condition of)
luc, lux	light	trans-luc-ent (light moves across)
lup	wolf	lup-us (wolf)
manu	hand	manu-al (pertaining to the hand)
mar	the sea	mar-ine (related to the sea)
marant	wither	marant-ic (wasting away)
marasm	waste	marasm-us (dying away, protein calorie malnutrition)
mene	month	men-arche (beginning month of menses)
meso	middle	meso-nephron (middle kidney)
meta	after, beyond	meta-chromatic (beyond the color, stains different with same dye)
metab	change	metab-olism (to turn about or change)
meter, metr	measure	centi-meter (one hundredth of a meter)
mictur	urinate	mictur-ition (urinate)
mid	middle	mid-foot (middle part of foot)
mon	one	mon-ochromatic (having only one color)
mort	death	mort-isemblant (apparently dead)
morul	a little mulberry	morul-atin (forming the morula)
muta	change	muta-tion (change in form or quality)
muti	cut off	muti-lation (to cut off an important part)
myo	a muscle	myo-cardial (heart muscle)
myco	a fungus	myco-logy (study of fungi)

Word Roots	Root Meaning	Example
myxo	mucus	myxo-virus (group of viruses, literally mucus virus)
necr, necros	dead	necro-lysis (dead and dissolution)
neo, novi	new	neo-logism (a new word)
neph	kidney	neph-rectomy (to cut out a kidney)
omni	all	omni-vorous (to eat all, both plants and animals)
ortho	straight	ortho-dontics (straight teeth)
ophthalm	the eye	ophthalm-ology (study of the eye)
os, ora	mouth	os cervix (opening of mouth of the cervix)
os	bone	os pubis (pubic bone)
osti	small opening	col-ostomy (small opening from colon to skin surface)
oto	ear	otitis (inflammation of the ear)
ove	egg	ovi-duct (to carry eggs)
paed	a child	ortho-pedics (straight child—skeletal)
parthen	a virgin	parthen-ogenesis (virgin birth)
patho	disease	patho-genic (disease producing)
pauc	few	pauc-ibacillary (a few bacteria)
ped	child	ped-erast (lover of a boy—sexually)
pedi, pedo	child	pedi-atrician (child's doctor)
pedi	foot	pedi-cure (foot care)
peri	around	peri-aortitis (inflammation around aorta)
pes	foot	pes anserinus (goose's foot)
phaco	lens or lentil shaped	a-phakia (no lens)
phago	to eat	phago-cyte (cell that ingests or eats)
phon	sound	phon-ocardiogram (writing sounds of heart)
phor	carry	phos-phorus (to carry light)
phos	light	phos-phorus (to carry light)
phren	a diaphragm	phren-ospasm (spasm of diaphragm)
pilus	hair	pili-form (hair-shaped)
pisc	fish	pisc-icide (fish killing or poison for fish)
pityr	bran	pityr-iasis (branlike scales condition)
plumb	lead	plumb-ism (lead poisoning)
pneuma	air	pneuma-turia (air in the urine)
poly	many, much	poly-microbial (many bacterial species)

Word Roots	Root Meaning	Example
pre, pro, pros	before	pre-morbid (before death)
proct	rectum	proct-itis (inflammation of rectum)
proto	first, original	proto-zoa (first animal)
pruri	itch	pruri-tis ani (perianal itching)
pseud	false	pseudo-cyst (false cyst)
psych	mind	psycho-analysis (analysis of mind)
puer	boy	puer-pera (child, to bear)
purg	cleanse	purg-ative (to cleanse bowels)
purpur	purple	purpur-a (petechial skin lesions)
pus	inflammation	pus-tular (pertaining to pustules)
pyo	pus	pyo-cyanin (blue pus)
pyro	fire	pyro-mania (fire madness)
raph	suture	raphe (a seam)
re	back again	re-action (to act again)
ren	a kidney	reno-cortical (cortex of kidney)
ret, reticul	a network	reticul-ar (resembling a net)
rheum	watery flow, flux	rheum-atogenic (to produce rheumatism)
rhino	nose	rhino-phyma (nose growth)
rhonch	snore	rhonch-us (rattling in throat or bronchial tubes)
ruct	belch	ruct-us hystericus (frequent noisy belching)
sacchar	sugar	poly-sacchar-ide (many sugars)
sacr	sacred	sacr-odynia (pain in the sacrum)
sali	salt	sali-ne (salty)
sapro	rotten	sapro-phyte (plant living on decaying vegetation)
sarc	flesh	sarc-omere (flesh part)
scler	hard	scler-oderma (hard skin)
scorbut	scurvy	scorbut-igenic (produces scurvy)
scot	darkness	scoto-chromogen (produce color in the dark)
scrot	a pouch	scrot-um (pouch containing testes)
selen	the moon	selen-oplegia (moon stroke)
semen	sperm	semen-uria (sperm in urine)
semi	half	semi-flexion (midway between flexion and extension)
sen	an old person	sen-escence (to grow old)

Word Roots	Root Meaning	Example
senil	of old people	senil-ity (physical and mental deterioration seen in old age)
sero	serum, whey	sero-negative (negative tests on the serum)
sinist	the left hand	sinist-rocular (left eye)
-sis, asis	condition of	mydri-asis (condition of dilated pupil)
sol, solar	sun	sol-unar (pertaining to sun and moon)
soma	body	soma-tic (pertaining to the body)
somn	sleep	somn-ambulation (sleep walking)
spect	look at	spectro-meter (method to measure light rays)
steth	chest	steth-oscope (used to examine chest)
sub	below	sub-acute (between acute and chronic)
succ	juice	succ-us entericus (intestinal juice)
sucr	sugar	sucr-osemia (sucrose in the blood)
sud	sweat	sud-amen (to sweat)
super	above—excess	super-acid (excessively acid)
supra	above—over	supra-infection (infection on top of another infection)
sys, syn	together	syn-chronous (together in time)
tachy	quickly	tachy-phagia (rapid eating)
tali	ankle	tali-pedic (ankle foot, club-footed)
tela	woven, web	tela-ngiectasia (woven vessel dilated)
tenesm	straining	tenesm-us (straining at stool)
thalass	sea	thalass-emia (sea blood, observed in people from around the Mediterranean)
theor	speculation	theor-em (principle determined by speculation)
therm	heat	therm-ometer (heat-measuring device)
tot	all	toti-potential (all power)
tox	poison	toxi-genic (poison producing)
trans	through	trans-fer (to carry through or across)
tri	three	tri-angle (three angles)
trichin	hair	trichi-asis (ingrowing eyelashes)
trivi	crossroads	tri-via (three roads, commonplace)
troch	wheel	troch-lea (wheel or pulley-shaped)

Word Roots	Root Meaning	Example
trop	turning	eso-trop-ia (inward-turning eye)
tuber	knob	tuber-ous sclerosis (condition having knobs, hard)
tumor	a swelling	tumori-genic (producing swellings)
tunic	a covering	tunica albuginea (dense white coat)
turb	tumult	turb-idity (disturbance causing cloudiness)
tuss	cough	per-tussis (intensive cough)
tympan	drum	tympanitic (drumlike sound)
uni	one	unisexual (one sex)
ule	little	pust-ule (little pus)
ultr	beyond	ultra-sound (beyond sound)
umbo	projecting knob	umbo-nate (knoblike)
un	not	un-fulfilled (not fulfilled)
uvea	iris, ciliary body, choroid together	uveitis (inflammation of uvea)
vacu	empty	e-vacu-ate (empty from)
vagin	sheath	vagin-itis (inflammation of vagina)
verd	green	verdi-gris (green of Greeks)
verm	worm	vermi-form (worm-shaped)
verruc	wart	verruci-form (wart-shaped)
vers, vert	to turn	versi-color (to turn color)
vesicul	blister	vesiculo-papular (vesicles and papules)
vir	a man	viri-potent (man able or power)
viv	alive	vivi-section (to cut live animals)
xeno	stranger	xeno-diagnosis (diagnosis using a stranger, an uninfected bug or animal)
xer	dry	xero-phthalmia (dry eyes)
zo	an animal	zoo-logy (study of animals)

APPENDIX B

Signs

A *sign* is an *objective* abnormality indicative of disease, discoverable by examination of the patient. By comparison, a *symptom* is *subjective* evidence of a disease as perceived by the patient and is related during the history.

1. Babinski's sign—extension of the great toe instead of normal flexion and abduction of the other toes in response to plantar stimulation; indicative of pyramidal tract involvement.
2. Bárány's sign—in evaluation of ear disease, water is used to irrigate the external canal. If cool water below the body temperature (65 degrees or lower) is used, nystagmus will be toward the opposite side; if warm water (above body temperature) is used to irrigate, nystagmus will be toward the irrigated side. No nystagmus occurs when the labyrinth is diseased.
3. Battle's sign—postauricular ecchymosis caused by fracture of the base of the skull.
4. Braxton Hicks contractions—irregular uterine contractions occurring after the third month of pregnancy.
5. Brudzinski's sign—(1) contralateral reflex in meningitis; on passive flexion of the leg on one side, a similar movement occurs in the opposite leg; (2) in meningitis, if the neck is passively flexed, the hips and knees flex spontaneously.
6. Chaddock's sign (or reflex)—when the external malleolar skin is irritated, the great toe extends upward (similar to Babinski's sign) in organic disease of the corticospinal tract.
7. Chadwick's sign—a bluish discoloration of the cervix and vagina caused by pregnancy.
8. Chvostek's sign—facial irritability in tetany. Unilateral spasm is produced by a tap over the facial nerve.
9. Clenched fist sign—the gesture of the patient with angina pectoris when he presses his clenched fist against his chest to indicate the constricting, pressing quality of pain. This is also termed Levine's sign.
10. Cullen's sign—periumbilical darkening of the skin as a result of intraperitoneal hemorrhage caused by conditions such as ruptured ectopic pregnancy or occurring in acute hemorrhagic pancreatitis.
11. de Musset's sign—rhythmic jerking movement of the head in aortic insufficiency.
12. Doll's eye sign—dissociation between the movements of the eyes and those of the head; the eyes are lowered as the head is raised, and the reverse.
13. Drawer sign—indicates laxity or disruption of an anterior or posterior cruciate ligament of the knee.

14. Ewart's sign—in large pericardial effusions, dullness, bronchial breathing, and bronchophony are present below the angle of the left scapula.
15. Eyelash sign—in apparent unconsciousness caused by functional disease such as hysteria, stroking the eyelashes will produce movement of the lids. No such reflex occurs in severe organic brain lesions such as stroke.
16. Grey Turner's sign—local discoloration (bruising) of the skin of the loins in acute hemorrhagic pancreatitis.
17. Groove sign—large, firm, fixed, tender lymph nodes in the groin above and below the inguinal ligament with a groove along the ligament; characteristic of lymphogranuloma venereum.
18. Hamman's sign—a crunching sound, synchronous with heartbeat heard in mediastinal emphysema and pneumopericardium.
19. Hill's sign—in aortic insufficiency, the exaggerated excess of femoral over brachial artery systolic pressure. In normal persons, the arterial systolic pressure in the leg is 10 to 20 mm Hg above that in the arm, whereas in those with aortic insufficiency, the difference may be 60 to 100 mm Hg.
20. Hoffmann's sign, or digital reflex—sudden nipping of the nail of the middle finger causes flexion of the terminal phalanx of the thumb. May be present or absent in healthy persons bilaterally. When sign is unilateral, it indicates pyramidal tract disease.
21. Homans' sign—pain at the back of the knee or calf when the foot is slowly and gently dorsiflexed (with the knee bent); it is indicative of thrombosis in the veins of the calf.
22. Joffroy's sign—absence of the forehead wrinkling when the eyeballs are rolled upward in Graves' disease.
23. Kehr's sign—violent pain in the left shoulder in some cases of rupture of the spleen.
24. Kernig's sign—when the patient lies on the back and the thigh is flexed to a right angle with the axis of the trunk, complete extension of the calf on the thigh is impossible because of back pain; it is a sign of meningitis.
25. Kestenbaum's sign—a decrease in the number of arterioles crossing optic disk margins; a sign of optic atrophy.
26. Kussmaul's sign—paradoxic increase in jugular venous distention during inspiration seen in patients with cardiac tamponade.
27. Lasègue's sign—when patient is supine with hip flexed, dorsiflexion of the ankle causes pain in the posterior thigh in sciatic nerve irritation.
28. Marcus Gunn's pupillary sign—a flashlight is shined into one pupil. After both pupils constrict, the flashlight is swung to the other pupil. If light fails to stimulate the same response in the other eye, both pupils dilate. Causes include cataract, optic nerve defects, and other conditions.
29. Möbius' sign—impairment of ocular convergence in Graves' disease.
30. Nikolsky's sign—sliding pressure of the thumb pressed against the skin separates the outer layer from the basal epidermis. Seen in pemphigus vulgaris and some other bullous diseases.
31. Osler's sign—circumscribed painful erythematous swellings, from the size of a pinhead to that of a pea, in the skin and subcutaneous tissues of the hands and feet, in endocarditis.
32. Pastia's sign—hemorrhagic transverse lines at the bend of the elbow, inguinal areas, or wrists in early scarlet fever. These persist and remain visible after desquamation.

33. Puddle sign—free abdominal (ascitic) fluid detected by having the patient assume a position on all fours. One flank is percussed by repeated light flicking of constant intensity. The bell of the stethoscope is placed over the most dependent portion of the abdomen and gradually moved toward the flank opposite the percussion. A sharp increase in the intensity of the sound picked up by the stethoscope indicates the level of fluid.
34. Romberg's sign—a patient standing with feet together is more unsteady with the eyes closed, indicating a loss of proprioceptive control. Seen in tabes dorsalis.
35. Rovsing's sign—pain in the right abdomen at McBurney's point induced in cases of appendicitis by pressure exerted over the left lower abdomen.
36. Stellwag's sign—infrequent and incomplete blinking in Graves' disease.
37. Trousseau's sign (phenomenon)—in latent tetany, the occurrence of carpal spasm elicited when the upper arm is compressed by a tourniquet or a blood pressure cuff.
38. Winterbottom's sign—swelling of the posterior cervical lymph nodes, characteristic of early stages of African sleeping sickness (trypanosomiasis).

APPENDIX C

Syndromes

A *syndrome* is a symptom complex associated with an illness; together they constitute the picture of the disease.

1. Acute brain syndrome—abnormalities of cerebral function (e.g., delirium, confusion, disorientation, restlessness) developing suddenly in a person who was previously psychologically normal.
2. Acute radiation syndrome—caused by exposure to large amounts of radiation marked by vomiting, beginning about 12 hours after exposure and followed 24 hours later by prostration, fever, and diarrhea. Later petechial and purpuric spots, extreme weakness, hypotension, tachycardia, profuse bloody diarrhea, and death may occur.
3. Adams-Stokes syndrome (disease)—characterized by heart block with slow or absent pulse, often accompanied by convulsions.
4. Afferent loop syndrome—gastrojejunal loop obstruction proximal to a gastrojejunostomy. Ingestion of food produces nausea, pain, and duodenal distention.
5. Amenorrhea-galactorrhea syndrome—nonphysiologic lactation resulting from endocrinologic causes or from a pituitary disorder.
6. Asherman's syndrome—synechiae (adhesions) within the endometrial cavity, often causing amenorrhea and infertility.
7. Banti's syndrome—chronic congestive splenomegaly with anemia as a sequel to portal hypertension (e.g., cirrhosis of the liver) or thrombosis of splenic veins.
8. Barlow syndrome—late apical systolic murmur, systolic click, or both, caused by massive protrusion of the posterior mitral valve leaflet into the left atrial cavity (floppy mitral valve syndrome).
9. Barrett's syndrome—chronic peptic ulcer of the lower esophagus, lined by columnar epithelium.
10. Bartter's syndrome—primary juxtaglomerular cell hyperplasia with secondary hyperaldosteronism, hypokalemic alkalosis, and elevated renin or angiotensin levels. The blood pressure is not elevated.
11. Behçet's syndrome—oral and genital ulcers, uveitis, and optic atrophy, with other findings suggesting vasculitis.
12. Brown-Séquard syndrome—damage to half of the spinal cord, causing paralysis and loss of discriminating joint sense on the side of the lesion, with loss of pain and temperature discrimination on the opposite side.
13. Budd-Chiari syndrome—the acute form is thrombosis of the hepatic vein with enlargement of the liver, development of massive ascites, and often dramatic

death. The chronic form is gradual liver enlargement, nausea, vomiting, edema, and finally death.

14. Carcinoid syndrome—a combination of symptoms produced by serotonin from carcinoid tumors. There are attacks of cyanotic flushing, diarrhea, bronchial spasm, edema, and ascites.
15. Carpal tunnel syndrome—pain and tingling, burning, and numbness in the hand in the distribution of the median nerve cause by compression of the median nerve in the carpal tunnel of the wrist.
16. Cerebellar syndrome—hereditary cerebellar ataxia.
17. Cervical syndrome—symptoms caused by pressure on nerves of the brachial plexus by a supernumerary rib that arises from the seventh cervical vertebra. Pain in the neck radiates into the shoulder, arm, or forearm.
18. Chédiak-Higashi syndrome—abnormalities of leukocytes with large inclusions.
19. Chinese restaurant syndrome—development of chest pain, feelings of facial pressure, and sensation of burning over portions of the body surface after dining on Chinese food to which monosodium glutamate was added to enhance flavor.
20. Churg-Strauss syndrome—allergic granulomatous angiitis, asthma, fever, and eosinophilia.
21. Conn's syndrome—primary hyperaldosteronism, characterized by muscular weakness, hypertension, persistent hypokalemia, and alkalosis.
22. Costochondral syndrome—pain in the chest with tenderness over one or more costochondral junctions.
23. Cronkhite-Canada syndrome—GI polyps with diffuse alopecia and nail dystrophy, sometimes with protein-losing enteropathy and malabsorption.
24. Cruveilhier-Baumgarten syndrome—cirrhosis of the liver, caput medusae, and venous hum and thrill.
25. Cushing's syndrome—excessive adrenocorticusum leading to fatness of the face, neck, and trunk, with accompanying buffalo hump, decalcification of bones, striae, diabetes, elevated blood pressure, and hypertrichosis.
26. Dandy-Walker syndrome—hydrocephalus in infants associated with obstruction of the foramina of Magendie and Luschka.
27. DiGeorge syndrome—congenital absence of the thymus and parathyroid glands without agammaglobulinemia but with frequent viral and fungal infections and with defects in development of the ears, nose, and mouth.
28. Down syndrome—mental retardation, skull abnormality, prominent epicanthal folds, and cardiac and hand abnormalities.
29. Dubin-Johnson syndrome—recurrence of mild jaundice caused by a defect in excretion of conjugated bilirubin.
30. Ehlers-Danlos syndrome—overelasticity and friability of the skin; hyperextensibility of the joints.
31. Eisenmenger's syndrome—pulmonary hypertension, ventricular septal defect, and cyanosis.
32. Fanconi's syndrome—type 1: refractory anemia, pancytopenia, hypoplasia of bone marrow, and congenital anomalies occurring in members of the same family. Type 2: renal disease with aminoaciduria, glycosuria, hyperphosphaturia, cystine deposition, and rickets.
33. Felty's syndrome—RA with splenomegaly, leukopenia, anemia, and thrombocytopenia.
34. Fetal alcohol syndrome—pattern of fetal malformation with growth deficiency and craniofacial anomalies with limb defects; found among infants of mothers who are alcoholics.

35. Fitz-Hugh–Curtis syndrome—gonococcal perihepatitis in women as a complication of gonorrhea.
36. Floppy valve syndrome—incompetence of the mitral valve resulting from myxomatous degeneration of the leaflets.
37. Froin's syndrome—xanthochromia of the CSF; a very high protein concentration without increased cells caused by a block in CSF flow from above.
38. Gardner's syndrome—inherited as a dominant trait, multiple tumors, including osteomas of the skull, epidermoid cysts, and fibromas, with colonic polyposis predisposing to carcinoma of the colon.
39. Gerstmann's syndrome—finger agnosia, agraphia, right-left disorientation, acalculia; caused by lesions between the occipital area and the angular gyrus.
40. Goodpasture's syndrome—Glomerulonephritis caused by antibasement-membrane antibodies associated with hemoptysis. Nephritis usually progresses to produce death from renal failure.
41. Guillain-Barré syndrome—infectious polyneuritis of unknown cause.
42. Hamman-Rich syndrome—interstitial fibrosis of the lung.
43. Horner's syndrome—ptosis, miosis, anhidrosis, and enophthalmos caused by paralysis of the cervical sympathetic nerves.
44. Hunt's syndrome (Ramsay Hunt)—herpes zoster infection of the seventh cranial nerve and geniculate ganglion showing zoster of the ear, often with facial nerve palsy.
45. Kartagener's syndrome—complete situs inversus associated with chronic sinusitis and bronchiectasis (autosomal recessive).
46. Kimmelstiel-Wilson syndrome—diabetic kidney disease, intercapillary glomerulosclerosis.
47. Klinefelter's syndrome—a chromosomal anomaly with a chromosome count of 47, small testes, and an increase in urinary gonadotropins.
48. Klippel-Feil syndrome—cervical vertebra fused, congenital short neck, abnormalities of the brainstem and cerebellum, low hairline, and limited neck motion.
49. Korsakoff's syndrome—confabulation to hide defective memory in chronic alcoholism.
50. Lambert-Eaton syndrome—progressive proximal muscle weakness in patients resulting from carcinoma.
51. Leriche's syndrome—occlusion of the distal aorta, with hip, thigh, and calf fatigue, along with impotence.
52. Lesch-Nyhan syndrome—deficiency of the enzyme hypoxanthine-guanine phosphoribosyltransferase in males, characterized by hyperuricemia and uric acid urolithiasis, choreoathetosis, mental retardation, spastic cerebral palsy, and self-mutilation of fingers and lips; X-linked recessive.
53. Löffler's syndrome—eosinophilia with transient infiltrates in the lungs.
54. Malabsorption syndrome—impaired absorption of a dietary substance such as fats, carbohydrates, proteins, iron, or vitamins that may lead to diarrhea, weakness, weight loss, or other specific manifestations.
55. Mallory-Weiss syndrome—laceration of the lower end of the esophagus caused by vomiting, which leads to bleeding.
56. Marfan syndrome—congenital disorder of connective tissue with abnormally long digits and extremities (arachnodactyly); subluxation of lens, and cardiovascular abnormalities.
57. Meigs' syndrome—fibroma of the ovary with ascites and hydrothorax.
58. Middle lobe syndrome—atelectasis with chronic pneumonitis of the middle lobe of the right lung.

59. Mikulicz's syndrome—salivary and lacrimal enlargement as seen in diseases such as sarcoidosis, tuberculosis, and leukemia.
60. Munchausen syndrome—fabrication by an itinerant malingerer of a clinically convincing simulation of disease.
61. Pancoast's syndrome—tumor in the region of the pulmonary apex resulting in neuritic pain of the arm, with muscle atrophy of the arm and Horner's syndrome on the same side.
62. Peutz-Jeghers syndrome—polyposis (actually hamartomas) of the small intestine and sometimes colon with melanin pigmentation of the buccal mucosa and the skin around the mouth and lips.
63. Pickwickian syndrome—obesity, hypoventilation, somnolence, and erythrocytosis.
64. Plummer-Vinson syndrome—dysphagia, atrophy of the papillae of the tongue, hypochromic anemia, and splenomegaly.
65. Postrubella syndrome—congenital defects resulting from maternal rubella during the first trimester of pregnancy; defects include microphthalmos, cataracts, deafness, mental retardation, patent ductus arteriosus, and pulmonary arterial stenosis.
66. Prader-Willi syndrome—congenital syndrome of unknown etiology characterized by short stature, mental retardation, polyphagia with marked obesity, and sexual infantilism.
67. Premenstrual syndrome—abnormal sensation of the breasts, abdominal pain, thirst, headache, nervous irritability, pelvic congestion, peripheral edema, and occasionally nausea and vomiting for 2 or 3 days before menstrual flow begins.
68. Reiter's syndrome—urethritis, iridocyclitis, arthritis, and skin lesions such as keratoderma blennorrhagicum and circinate balanitis.
69. Rendu-Osler-Weber syndrome—hereditary hemorrhagic telangiectasia.
70. Restless legs syndrome—twitching or restlessness that occurs in the legs after going to bed, frequently leading to insomnia, which may be relieved temporarily by walking about.
71. Reye's syndrome—loss of consciousness and seizures in children following an infection (often treated with aspirin); syndrome is sometimes fatal. Fatty changes are seen in the liver.
72. Riley-Day syndrome—familial dysautonomia.
73. Scalded skin syndrome—toxic epidermal necrolysis.
74. Sheehan's syndrome—postpartum pituitary necrosis with resultant findings caused by hormonal deficiency.
75. Shoulder-hand syndrome—pain in the shoulder with swelling and stiffness of the fingers sometimes occurring after myocardial infarction.
76. Sick sinus syndrome—chaotic atrial activity characterized by continual changes in P-wave configuration, with bradycardia alternating with recurring ectopic beats and runs of tachycardia.
77. Sjögren's syndrome—a symptom complex including keratoconjunctivitis sicca, dryness of mucous membranes, and telangiectasias or purpuric spots on the face; parotid enlargement.
78. Stein-Leventhal syndrome—polycystic ovary with secondary amenorrhea.
79. Stevens-Johnson syndrome—erythema and multiforme bullosum, often with large areas of skin sloughs, including mouth and anogenital membranes; headache, fever, and malaise.
80. Straight back syndrome—loss of the normal kyphosis of the thoracic spine,

producing a straight spine, an ejection murmur, and radiologic evidence of a widened cardiac silhouette.
81. Sudden infant death syndrome — abrupt and inexplicable death of an apparently healthy infant between the ages of 3 weeks and 5 months.
82. Superior vena cava syndrome — obstruction of the superior vena cava or its main tributaries by some condition (e.g., bronchogenic carcinoma, mediastinal neoplasm, or lymphoma), causing edema and engorgement of the vessels of the face, neck, and arms, a nonproductive cough, and dyspnea.
83. Takayasu's syndrome — pulseless disease primarily affecting blood vessels of the aortic arch.
84. Testicular feminization syndrome — a type of male pseudohermaphroditism characterized by complete female external genitalia, incompletely developed vagina often with a rudimentary uterus; female habitus at puberty but with scanty or absent axillary and pubic hair and amenorrhea.
85. Thorn's syndrome — salt-losing nephritis.
86. Tietze's syndrome — costal chondritis with swelling or tenderness of the end of the costal cartilage.
87. Toxic shock syndrome — a staphylococcal toxin–produced syndrome usually seen in menstruating women using superabsorbent tampons. It is characterized by fever, vomiting, diarrhea, and a scarlatiniform rash followed by desquamation. Decreased blood pressure and shock are seen.
88. Turner's syndrome — Phenotypic females with dwarfism, webbed neck, valgus of the elbows, and amenorrhea; sexual infantilism in genetic males with absent sex chromatin (XO).
89. Ulysses syndrome — the ill effects of extensive diagnostic investigations conducted because of a false-positive result in the course of routine laboratory screening.
90. Waterhouse-Friderichsen syndrome — fulminating meningococcal infections occurring mainly in children under 10 years of age, with vomiting, diarrhea, extensive purpura, cyanosis, circulatory collapse, and hemorrhage into the adrenal glands.
91. Wernicke's syndrome — a condition frequently encountered in chronic alcoholics largely caused by thiamine deficiency and characterized by disturbances in ocular motility, pupillary alterations, nystagmus, and ataxia with tremors.
92. Wilson's syndrome — hepatolenticular degeneration caused by abnormal copper metabolism.
93. Wolff-Parkinson-White syndrome — ECG pattern associated with paroxysmal tachycardia, a short PR interval, and an early QRS wave called the delta wave.
94. Yellow nail syndrome — nearly complete cessation of nail growth with thickening of the nails. There is an increase in the convexity, a loss of cuticles, and yellowing; may be associated with lymphedema and chronic bronchitis or bronchiectasis.
95. Zollinger-Ellison syndrome — a triad of severe peptic ulcers, gastric hyperacidity, and gastrin-secreting tumors of the pancreas.

APPENDIX D

Murmurs

A murmur is an auscultatory sound of cardiac or vascular origin, somewhat resembling the sound of forcible expiration with the mouth open. Murmurs may be benign or pathologic and be described in terms such as loud, harsh, functional, soft, or blowing.

1. Austin Flint murmur—a diastolic (presystolic) murmur similar to that of mitral stenosis, heard at the cardiac apex in some cases of aortic insufficiency. It is caused by the regurgitating stream from the aorta partially narrowing the mitral valve. The murmur differs from that of mitral stenosis in not being associated with an opening snap.
2. Cardiopulmonary murmur—an innocent extracardiac murmur related to movement of the heart, but disappearing when the breath is held.
3. Cooing murmur—musical murmur.
4. Diamond-shaped murmur—crescendo-decrescendo murmur; named for the diamond shape of the frequency intensity curve seen on the phonocardiogram. An example is the aortic stenosis murmur.
5. Early diastolic murmur—a murmur that begins with the second heart sound, such as the murmur of aortic insufficiency, early in diastole.
6. Ejection murmur—diamond-shaped systolic murmur ending before the second heart sound, produced by the ejection of blood into the aorta or pulmonary artery (e.g., aortic or pulmonic stenosis).
7. Extracardiac murmur—sounds typically heard over the precordium, originating from structures other than the heart. Examples include pericardial friction rubs and cardiopulmonary murmurs.
8. Graham Steell's murmur—early diastolic murmur of pulmonic insufficiency caused by pulmonary hypertension and mitral stenosis, best heard at Erb's point.
9. Hemic murmur—a cardiac or vascular murmur heard in anemic persons who have no valvular lesion. Also called a flow murmur.
10. Holosystolic murmur—pansystolic murmur.
11. Innocent murmur—a functional murmur without anatomic abnormality responsible for murmur.
12. Late systolic murmur—usually refers to a diamond-shaped murmur late in systole. May be accompanied by a mid or late systolic click if MVP is present.
13. Machinery murmur—the long "continuous" rumbling murmur of patent ductus arteriosus that is heard throughout systole and diastole. The sound resembles machine noise.

14. Middiastolic murmur—beginning after the AV valves have opened in diastole; is the murmur of mitral stenosis.
15. Musical murmur—having a musical quality.
16. Pansystolic murmur—holosystolic murmur occupies the entire systolic interval, from first to second sound.
17. Presystolic murmur—late diastolic murmur, heard at the end of ventricular diastole (during atrial contraction); usually occurs with narrowing of the AV valves.
18. Regurgitant murmur—caused by leakage (backward flow) of an incompetent cardiac valve.
19. Roger's murmur—loud pansystolic murmur maximal at the left sternal border, caused by a small VSD.
20. Still's murmur—an innocent musical murmur resembling a twanging string.

APPENDIX E

Role of Family History in Disease

General Questions to Ask

- Health status of parents, whether alive and well or deceased and, if so, the cause of death. Ask about specific diseases (see below).
- Health status of siblings, whether alive and well or deceased and, if so, the cause of death. Also, are living siblings afflicted with any chronic diseases.

Important Common Diseases to Ask About because of Increased Incidence in Families

- Diabetes mellitus
- Ischemic heart disease
- Hypercholesterolemia
- Hypertension
- Cancer (especially breast, colon)
- Sickle cell anemia
- Cystic fibrosis
- Chronic alcoholism
- Tuberculosis
- Milk intolerance caused by lactase deficiency

Some Relatively Frequent and Mendelian Disorders Affecting Adults

Major Manifestations in the Following System	Autosomal Dominant	Autosomal Recessive	X-Linked
Hematologic	• Hereditary hemorrhagic telangiectasia • Hereditary spherocytosis • von Willebrand's disease	• Sickle cell anemia • β-thalasemia • Job syndrome • Chédiak-Higashi syndrome	• Hemophilia A • Glucose-6-phosphate dehydrogenase deficiency • Chronic granulomatous disease of childhood
Gastrointestinal	• Acute intermittent porphyria	• Cystic fibrosis • Hemochromatosis • Wilson's disease	
Cardiovascular	• Familial hypercholesterolemia • Idiopathic hypertrophic subaortic stenosis		
Renal	• Adult polycystic kidney disease		
Neurologic	• Huntington's chorea	• Friedreich's ataxia	
Musculoskeletal	• Osteogenesis imperfecta • Myotonic dystrophy • Neurofibromatosis • Marfan syndrome	• Friedreich's ataxia	
Metabolic		• Phenylketonuria • Homocystinuria	

Index

A

a waves, 162, 163, 164
Abdomen, 199-261
 auscultation of, 227-229
 "boardlike," 236
 bruits over, causes of, 228
 and cardiovascular system abnormalities, 152-153
 of child, examination of, 491-492
 masses in, 233-234
 muscle rigidity of, 236
 pain in
  acute, 245-248, 257, 258-259
  character of, 200
  chronic, causes of, 248-259
  comparison of other types of pain with, 203-204
  factors precipitating and relieving, 203
  localizing, to intraabdominal sites, 235-236
  location of, 201-203
  other symptoms associated with, 204
  radiation of, 203
  severity of, patient assessment of, 203
  syndromes of, 245-259
 palpation of, 229-235
 percussion of, 224-227
 physical examination of, 218-237
 protuberant or distended, 219-221
 questions related to, 28
 tenderness of, 236-237
Abdominal aorta, palpation of, 166
Abdominal bruits, auscultation for, 228-229
Abdominal hernias, 223-224
Abdominal pain syndromes, 245-259
Abdominal reflexes, 408
Abdominal veins, dilated, causes of, 219
Abdominal wall pain, anterior, 256
Abducens nerve, testing of, 412
Abduction, 346

Abortion, 291
 causing pelvic pain, 288
Abrasions, corneal, 46
Abscess
 appendiceal, 233, 234
 causing exophthalmos, 46
 intracranial, causing nausea and vomiting, 207
 lung
  anaerobic, causing fecal breath odor, 95
  causing halitosis, 93
  causing hemoptysis, 76
  causing sputum production, 74
  causing night sweats, 92
 pelvic, rectal mass associated with, 234
 pericolic, abdominal masses with, 233
 perirectal, rectal mass associated with, 234
 peritonsillar, 66
  causing sore throat, 63
 retropharyngeal, 66
  causing croup syndrome, 115
 subphrenic
  causing chest pain, 79
  causing pleuritic chest pain, 91
 tubo-ovarian, rectal mass associated with, 235
Achalasia causing dysphagia, 209
Achilles reflex, 407
Acidosis; see Lactic acidosis; Metabolic acidosis
Acne vulgaris, 457
Acneiform rash, 465
Acoustic nerve, testing of, 412-413
Acquired immune deficiency syndrome
 causing candidal vaginitis, 296
 causing dilated chest veins, 96
 causing night sweats, 92
 oral thrush with, 462
 causing pneumonia, 91
 skin abnormalities in, 477, 478
 causing supraclavicular lymph nodes, 96

Acral-lentiginous melanomas, 471
Acrocyanosis, 148
Acromegaly
 and cardiovascular system abnormalities, 150
 causing exophthalmos, 46
 causing macroglossia, 65
Acromioclavicular joint arthritis, 359-360
Actinic keratosis, 471
Actinomycetes, sources of, 92
Actinomycosis causing sinus tracts, 104
Active range of motion, 352
Acuity, visual, testing, 55
"Acute abdomen"; see Abdominal pain
Adams-Stokes syndrome, 509
Adaptive behavior milestones, ages for attainment of, 481
Addicted patients, medical interview of, 18
Addison's disease, 63, 65
Additive arthralgia, 337
Adduction, 346
Adenoma, bronchial, causing hemoptysis, 77
Adenoviral pneumonia, 121
Adhesions, uterine, 285, 286
Adhesive capsulitis, 359
Adie's pupil, 48
Adnexa, abnormalities of, 313
Adrenal disorders and hypertension, 157
Adrenal insufficiency causing nausea and vomiting, 207
Adventitious sounds, causes of, 109
Advice giving, 20
Adynamic ileus causing protuberant abdomen, 220
Afferent loop syndrome, 509
Aganglionic megacolon causing constipation, 213
Aggressive behavior by patient, 14
Agoraphobia, 432, 433
Agranulocytosis causing oral ulcers, 62
AIDS; see Acquired immune deficiency syndrome

Airway, foreign body in, causing wheezing, 87
Airway disease
  obstructive, causing orthopnea, 80
  reactive, causing wheezing, 87
Airway obstruction, 90
  causing stridor, 88
Alcohol, use of, 390-391
  causing male impotence, 270
Alcohol withdrawal syndromes, 416
  tremors associated with, 395
Alcoholic cerebellar degeneration, 418
  causing intention tremor, 402
Alcoholic hepatitis, 251
  causing bruits, 229
  causing jaundice, 240
  causing liver enlargement, 231
Alcoholic liver disease, 238
  causing jaundice, 240-241
  causing liver enlargement, 231
Alcoholism, 390, 391
  causing atrophic testes, 274
  causing male infertility, 271
  causing parotid enlargement, 65
Alkaptonuria, brown sclerae in, 46
Allergic asthma, 112; see also Asthma
Allergic contact dermatitis, 459
Allergic reaction, anaphylactic, causing wheezing, 87
Allergic rhinitis
  causing nasal discharge, 60
  causing nasal polyps, 61
  causing rhinorrhea, 60
Allergy(ies), 90
  causing chemosis, 96
  causing cough, 73
  causing excessive lacrimation, 44
Alopecia, 449
  patchy, 462
Alopecia areata, 462
Aluminum-containing antacids causing chronic gastric retention and delayed gastric emptying, 207
Alzheimer's disease, 416
Amaurosis fugax, 39-40, 388
Amenorrhea, 282, 283-285
  with galactorrhea, 324
  as sign of pregnancy, 289
Amenorrhea-galactorrhea syndrome, 509
Aminoglycosides causing hearing loss, 57
Amitriptyline causing male impotence, 270
Amyl nitrite inhalation to enhance cardiac auscultation, 196-197
Amyloidosis
  causing liver enlargement, 231
  causing macroglossia, 65
  causing protuberant abdomen, 220
  causing splenomegaly, 232
Amyotrophic lateral sclerosis
  causing dysphagia, 209
  fasciculations caused by, 395
Anaerobic lung abscess causing fecal breath odor, 95

Anal fissure in child, 492
Analgesia, 396
Analgesic nephropathy causing abdominal pain, 247
Anaphylactic allergic reaction causing wheezing, 87
Anasarca, 147
  causing scrotal swelling, 269
Androgen excess causing hypertrichosis, 298
Androgen insensitivity syndrome causing amenorrhea, 284
Anemia
  arterial pulse volume in, 167
  causing dyspnea, 84
  eye signs associated with, 151
  causing fatigue, 143
  fatigue with, 345
  hemolytic
    chronic, and cardiovascular system abnormalities, 150
    yellow sclerae caused by, 46
  iron deficiency, tongue changes caused by, 65
  pernicious, 54, 65
  sickle cell, crisis in, causing abdominal pain, 247
Anesthesia, 398
Aneurysm
  aortic; see Aortic aneurysm
  dissecting, causing chest pain, 134
  causing eye pain, 43
  causing mydriasis, 48
  splenic artery, abdominal masses with, 233
  causing third nerve palsy, 50
Anger in patient, 14, 15
Angina
  atypical, causing chest pain, 127, 131
  and congestive heart failure, 132
  intestinal, causing bruits, 229
  pain from, location of, 202
  Prinzmetal's, 127, 132-133
  stable (typical), causing chest pain, 127, 130-131
  unstable, causing chest pain, 127, 131-132
  variant, 127, 132-133
  Vincent's, causing sore throat, 63
Angina decubitus, 131, 132
Angina equivalents, 131
Angina pectoris, heart sounds in, 179
Angiodysplasia
  of colon causing hematochezia, 215, 216
  causing maroon-colored stools, 217
Angioid streaks, 55
Angiokeratomas and cardiovascular system abnormalities, 152
Angiomas
  cherry, 472
  spider, 448
Anhidrosis in Horner's syndrome, 96
Anisocoria, 47

Ankle, 373-376
  palpation of, 375
  range of motion of, 355
Ankle clonus, 408
Ankylosing spondylitis, 367
  and cardiovascular system abnormalities, 150
  causing sacroiliac arthritis, 369
Annular lesions, 452
Anogenital warts, 272
Anorexia, 205
Anorexia nervosa, 205
  causing amenorrhea, 284
  causing chronic gastric retention and delayed gastric emptying, 207
Anorgasmia, 293
Answers, false, giving, 20
Antalgic gait, 370
Anterotemporal lobe lesions causing male impotence, 270
Antibiotics causing candidal vaginitis, 296
Anticholinergics, 207-209
  absent bowel sounds with, 227
  causing decreased salivation, 65
  causing hoarseness, 64
  causing protuberant abdomen, 220
Anticoagulation therapy causing hemoptysis, 78
Antidepressants
  causing galactorrhea, 324
  causing male impotence, 270
Antifreeze, ingestion of, causing dyspnea, 86
Antihypertensives causing male impotence, 270
Anuria, 266
Anxiety
  arterial pulse volume with, 167
  causing dyspnea, 139
  causing hyperventilation, 99
  patient demonstration of, 15
Anxiety disorders, generalized, 430-431
Aorta, 233-234
  abdominal, palpation of, 166
  bruits over, causes of, 228
  calcification of, causing bruits, 229
  coarctation of
    associated with Turner's syndrome, 150
    blood pressure measurements and, 157
  dilated, causing Oliver's sign, 104
  dissecting, associated with Marfan syndrome, 149
Aortic aneurysm, 229-234
  dissecting
    causing acute abdominal pain, 258
    causing chest pain, 128
    causing dysphagia, 209
    eye signs associated with, 151
    causing hoarseness, 64
    with Marfan syndrome, 149
    causing Oliver's sign, 104
    thoracic signs associated with, 152

Aortic bypass surgery causing male impotence, 270
Aortic insufficiency
  arterial pulse volume in, 167-168
  associated with Marfan syndrome, 149
Aortic regurgitation, 192
  arterial pulse volume in, 167, 168
  associated with ankylosing spondylitis, 150
  causing dyspnea, 137
  eye signs associated with, 151
  heart murmurs associated with, 184, 185
  heart sounds in, 178, 179
Aortic stenosis
  causing dyspnea, 137
  heart murmurs associated with, 184
  heart sounds in, 178, 179
  causing syncope, 145
  systolic murmurs associated with, 186, 187, 188
  thoracic signs associated with, 152
Aphasia, 388, 417
Aphthous ulcers, recurrent, 62, 63
Apical impulse, 170
Apnea, sleep, 100
  fatigue with, 345
Appearance
  assessment of, in psychiatric interview, 427
  general, questions related to, 26
Appendiceal abscess, 233, 234
Appendicitis, 247
  pain from, location of, 202
  causing testicular pain, 271
Arcuate scotomata, 44
Arcus, corneal, atherosclerosis associated with, 151
Arcus senilis, 47
  atherosclerosis associated with, 151
Areola, 322, 323
Argyll Robertson pupil, 48
  and cardiovascular system abnormalities, 151
Argyria, 90
Arrhythmias
  associated with myotonia dystrophica, 149
  giant *a* waves associated with, 164
  jugular venous waves in, 162
  sinus, 166, 167
  skin signs associated with, 152
  causing syncope, 145
Arterial occlusion, transient, to enhance cardiac auscultation, 196
Arterial pulse rate, 166
Arterial pulse rhythms, 166-167
Arterial pulse volume, 167-168
Arterial pulses, 164-168
Arteriosclerosis and blood pressure measurement, 156
Arteriovenous fistulas, pulmonary, extremity signs associated with, 153

Arteriovenous shunting causing clubbing of fingernails, 96
Arteritis
  Takayasu's, causing perforated nasal septum, 60
  temporal
    causing retinal artery occlusion, 41, 55
    headache associated with, 384
Arthralgia, 337
Arthritis, 377-381
  acromioclavicular joint, 359-360
  causing cervical spine abnormalities, 357
  degenerative, stiffness with, 344-345
  diseases causing, 339
  familial component in, 336
  gonococcal, in several joints, 341,
  knee involvement in, 373
  psoriatic, 335, 340, 366
  rheumatoid; *see* Rheumatoid arthritis
  sacroiliac, diseases causing, 369
  septic, causing sternoclavicular joint swelling, 104
  causing shoulder pain, 359
Arthropathy, pyrophosphate, 378-379
Ascites, 219, 220-221, 222
  rapid removal of, causing syncope, 146
Asherman's syndrome, 509
  causing amenorrhea, 285
Aspirated foreign body causing atelectasis, 105
Aspiration
  causing cough, 73
  of foreign body
    causing breathing difficulty in infant, 92
    causing croup syndrome, 114
    causing hemoptysis, 77
    causing pneumonia, 91, 92
Aspiration pneumonia, 117, 121; *see also* Pneumonia
Aspirin overdose
  causing dyspnea, 86
  causing hyperventilation, 99
Assurance, valid, 20
Astereognosis, 400
Asthenia, neurocirculatory, causing chest pain, 136
Asthma, 87, 90, 111, 112
  cardiac, 84, 87
  affecting chest expansion, 102
  and cough, 73
  causing dyspnea, 81
  causing prolonged exhalation, 97
  silent, 80
  triad, causing nasal polyps, 61
  causing wheezing, 80, 87
Ataxia
  cerebellar, 403
  Friedreich's, and cardiovascular system abnormalities, 149, 150
  sensory, 403
Ataxic breathing, 100

Atelectasis, 105, 111, 112
  causing decreased fremitus, 106
  examination techniques to determine, 110
Atherosclerosis
  coronary
    eye signs associated with, 151
    risk factors for, 129-130
  eye signs associated with, 151
  heart sounds in, 178, 179
  pulses associated with, 168-169
  retinal changes in, 158
Atherosclerotic heart disease, cigarette smoking causing, 92
Atherosclerotic peripheral vascular disease causing decreased or absent femoral pulses, 234
Atopic dermatitis, 453, 458-459
Atopy, 449, 458
Atrial contractions, premature, 164, 166, 167
Atrial fibrillation, 166-167
  jugular venous waves in, 163, 164
  paroxysmal, 142
Atrial myxoma
  eye signs associated with, 151
  causing syncope, 146
Atrial pulse tracing, 155
Atrial septal defect
  heart murmurs associated with, 184
  holosystolic murmurs associated with, 191
  jugular venous waves in, 163
  thoracic signs associated with, 152
Atrial tachycardia, paroxysmal, 142
Atrioventricular dissociation, jugular venous waves in, 164
Atrophic vaginitis, 286-287, 295, 297-298, 310
Atrophy, 446
  connective tissue, purpura associated with, 463
  optic, 52
Atropine causing mydriasis, 48
Atypical angina causing chest pain, 127, 131
Atypical pneumonia, 117, 121; *see also* Pneumonia
Auditory canal, external, examination of, 58, 59
Augenblick, 20
Auscultatory gap, 155-156
Auspitz's sign, 468
Austin Flint murmur, 192, 514
Automatic walking, 494
Autosomal dominant disorders, 517
Autosomal recessive disorders, 517
Avoidance behavior of clinician, 20
Axillae, palpation of, 330
Azoospermia, 269

B

Babinski's sign, 408-409, 506
Bacillus Calmette-Guerin immunization, 90, 91

Bacterial croup, 114; *see also* Croup
Bacterial endocarditis
   causing conjunctival petechiae, 45
   dermal manifestations of, 478
   petechiae in, 463
   causing retinal hemorrhages, 54
   causing Roth's spots, 54
   skin lesions associated with, 455, 456
Bacterial infections
   causing external otitis, 56
   causing hoarseness, 64
   causing nausea and vomiting, 207
   causing ocular discharge, 44
   of skin, 477
   causing splenomegaly, 232
   systemic, dermal manifestations of, 477, 478
Bacterial meningitis, 424
   causing hearing loss in child, 57
Bacterial pharyngitis causing sore throat, 63
Bacterial pneumonia, 121
Bacterial sepsis, dermal manifestations of, 478
Baker's cyst, 371
Balanitis, 272
   candidal, 462
   circinate, 334, 367
Ball-and-socket joint, 347
Ballottement
   to determine joint effusion, 372
   of patella, 349
Banti's syndrome, 509
Bárány's sign, 506
Barlow syndrome, 509
Barrel chest, 101, 103
Barrett's syndrome, 509
Bartholin's glands, 300, 301
Bartter's syndrome, 509
Basal cell carcinoma, 471
Battle's sign, 506
Beau's lines, 452, 454
Beclouded dementia, 422
Bed rest, prolonged, causing syncope, 146
Bedside manner, 6-8
Behavior
   general, assessment of, in psychiatric interview, 427
   of patients posing problems for physicians, 14
Behçet's syndrome, 509
   causing genital ulcers, 311
   causing oral ulcers, 62
   causing penile ulcer, 268, 272
   causing uveitis, 41
Bell's palsy causing failure of eyelids to close, 45
Benzodiazepines causing male impotence, 270
BGC; *see* Bacillus Calmette-Guerin, 90, 91
Biceps reflex, 404, 405
Bicipital groove, palpation of, 358
Bicipital tendinitis, 359, 360

Bifid pulse, 168
Bigeminal pulse, 167
Bileaflet heart valve, sounds associated with, 182
Biliary cirrhosis, Kayser-Fleischer rings in, 47
Biliary colic, 248, 249
Bimanual examination, 307-308
Binocular blindness, 42
Binocular diplopia, 42-43
Binocular loss of vision, 39
Biologic heart valve, sounds associated with, 182
Biot's breathing, 100
Bipolar depression, 428, 429
Bismuth poisoning, gingival signs of, 65
Bitemporal hemianopsia, 51
Bjork-Shiley heart valve, sounds associated with, 182
Blackheads, 457
Blackout; *see* Syncope
Bladder
   calculus of, causing dysuria, 263
   neoplasms of, causing hematuria, 266
   neurogenic, causing urinary incontinence, 265
Bleeding
   intraabdominal, causing pleuritic chest pain, 91
   menstrual, abnormal, 285
   postmenopausal, 286-287
   uterine, dysfunctional, 285
   vaginal, nonmenstrual, 286-287
Bleeding gums, 63
Blind patients, medical interview of, 17
Blindness
   binocular, 42
   cortical, 39, 42
   monocular, complete, 51
Blister(s)
   fever, 476
   of lip or mouth, 63
Blocked eustachian tube, 56
Blood dyscrasias
   causing bleeding gums, 63
   causing conjunctival petechiae, 45
Blood pressure, 153-157
   questions related to, 26
Blood volume, decreased, causing syncope, 146
Bloody fluid from breasts, 331
Blue sclerae, 46
   associated with osteogenesis imperfecta, 151
Blumer's shelf, 234
Blurred vision, 387
"Boardlike" abdomen, 236
Body position to enhance cardiac auscultation, 195-196
Boerhaave's syndrome causing free air in mediastinum, 111
Bone disease causing joint pain, 336
Bone pain, 336; *see also* Joint pain
Bone tumor, metastatic, and cough-induced rib fracture, 73

Borborygmi, 228
Bossing of skull, 488
Botulism causing dysphagia, 209
Bouchard's nodes, 365
Boutonniere deformity of finger, 349, 366
Bowel
   gangrenous, absent bowel sounds with, 227
   gas in, causing protuberant abdomen, 219, 220
   inflammatory disease of
     causing clubbing of fingernails, 96
     causing diarrhea, 211
     causing recurrent aphthous ulcers, 63
     causing sacroiliac arthritis, 369
   irritable, causing chronic abdominal pain, 253-254, 256
   strangulated, causing ecchymoses, 223
Bowel loops, 233-234
Bowel sounds, auscultation for, 227-228
Bowleg, 373
Brachioradialis reflex, 406
Bradycardia, 166
Bradypnea, 99, 100
Brain death, 410
   causing mydriasis, 48
Brain neoplasm causing quadrant hemianopsia, 52
Brain syndrome, acute, 509
Brain tumor
   causing chronic gastric retention and delayed gastric emptying, 206
   headache associated with, 384
   causing nausea and vomiting, 207
   causing nystagmus, 49
   causing papilledema, 54
Brainstem injury causing lack of pupillary reaction to light, 47
Brainstem reflexes, normal, 408
Braxton Hicks contractions, 290, 506
Breast(s), 316-332
   cancer of, 317, 318, 319, 331
     family history of, 325
     in men, 332
     risk factors for, 326
   cysts of, 331
   disease of, importance of past medical history in, 325
   enlarged, 322
     during pregnancy, 290
   fibrocystic disease of, 318, 319
   lumps in, 316-320
   lymphatic network draining, 319
   male, examination of, 331-332
   Paget disease of, 324, 328
   pain or tenderness of, 320, 322
     causes of, 79
     as sign of pregnancy, 290
   skin changes in, 327
Breath
   odor of, pulmonary diseases associated with, 93
   shortness of; *see* Dyspnea

Breath sounds, 108-109, 491
Breathing, 100
Bronchi, foreign body in, causing cough, 73
Bronchial adenoma causing hemoptysis, 77
Bronchial breath sounds, 108
Bronchiectasis, 111, 113, 117
  causing fecal breath odor, 95
  causing hemoptysis, 76, 78
  causing pneumonia, 91
  following pneumonia, 91
  causing sputum production, 74
Bronchiolitis, 113, 118
Bronchitis, 73-76, 90, 113, 117-118
  cigarette smoking causing, 92
Bronchoalveolar carcinoma causing sputum production, 74
Bronchogenic carcinoma, 114
  causing hemoptysis, 75, 77, 78
  causing hoarseness, 64
  causing Horner's syndrome, 48
Bronchophony, 110
Bronchopneumonia, 121
Bronchovesicular sounds, 108
Bronchus
  foreign body in, causing pneumonia, 91
  traction or pressure on, cough caused by, 73
Brown sclerae, 46
Brown-Séquard syndrome, 509
Brudzinski's sign, 423, 506
Bruits, 67
Brushfield's spots, 488
  and cardiovascular system abnormalities, 151
Buccal mucosa, physical examination of, 64-65
Budd-Chiari syndrome, 509-510
Buffalo hump, 101
Bulbar poliomyelitis
  causing chronic gastric retention and delayed gastric emptying, 206
  causing dysphagia, 209
Bulimia, 205
  causing amenorrhea, 284
  causing nausea and vomiting, 207
Bulla, 445
Bullous diseases, 473-475
Bullous myringitis, 58
  Mycoplasma pneumoniae infections causing, 56, 58
Bullous pemphigoid, 474-475
Bunion, 375, 376
Burning of eyes, 43, 44
Burns causing epiglottitis, 88
Burrow, 447
Bursitis, 349
  causing joint pain, 336, 337
  olecranon, 362
  causing shoulder pain, 359
  trochanteric, 370
Button hole deformity, 366

Bypass surgery causing male impotence, 270

C

c waves, 162, 163
Café-au-lait spots
  family history of, 444
  in hypertensive patient, 152
Calcific tendinitis, 359, 360
  causing arthritis, 339
Calcified aorta, signs of, 233
Calcium channel blockers causing dysphagia, 209
Calculus(i)
  bladder, causing dysuria, 263
  parotid duct, 65
  causing testicular pain, 271
Calluses of soles of feet, 375, 376
Campylobacter pylori colonization of stomach causing halitosis, 93
Cancer
  of breast; see Breast(s), cancer of
  chemotherapy for, causing candidal vaginitis, 296
  causing fatigue, 143
  laryngeal, smoking associated with, 92
  lip, pipe smoking associated with, 92
  lung; see Lung, cancer of
  muscle atrophy associated with, 395
  causing night sweats, 92
  causing nonmenstrual vaginal bleeding, 287
  of pancreas causing chronic abdominal pain, 252-253
  pancreatic, causing bruits, 229
  prostatic, 263
Candida infection causing balanitis, 272
Candidal balanitis, 462
Candidal vaginitis, 295, 296
Candidal vulvovaginitis, 462
Candidiasis, 462
  causing dysphagia, 209
  causing glossitis, 65
Cannabis causing male impotence, 270
Cannon a waves, 164
Capsulitis, 359
Carbon monoxide poisoning causing dyspnea, 85
Carcinoid syndrome, 510
Carcinoma
  basal cell, 471
  of breast, 318
  bronchoalveolar, causing sputum production, 74
  bronchogenic; see Bronchogenic carcinoma
  cecal, abdominal masses with, 233
  of cervix causing nonmenstrual vaginal bleeding, 286
  colonic, abdominal masses with, 233
  colorectal, causing hematochezia, 215-216
  endobronchial, causing pneumonia, 91
  esophageal, causing dysphagia, 209
  in situ, cervical, 312

Carcinoma—cont'd
  lung
    causing chest pain, 79
    causing dysphagia, 209
  oral, 62
  of pancreas causing jaundice, 243
  of penis, 268
  rectal mass associated with, 234
  squamous cell, 471
  of stomach, duodenum, or pancreas causing chronic gastric retention and delayed gastric emptying, 206
  causing supraclavicular lymph nodes, 96
  thyroid, causing thyroid enlargement, 67
  of tongue, 65
  of uterus causing nonmenstrual vaginal bleeding, 286
  vocal cord, causing hoarseness, 64
Cardiac asthma
  causing dyspnea, 84
  causing wheezing, 87
Cardiac cirrhosis, skin signs associated with, 152
Cardiac cycle, 159
Cardiac outflow tract obstruction causing syncope, 145-146
Cardiac pacemaker, jugular venous waves with, 163, 164
Cardinal positions of gaze, 49-50
Cardiomyopathy
  associated with Friedreich's ataxia, 149
  causing dyspnea, 138
  hypertrophic
    arterial pulse volume in, 168
    causing dyspnea, 141
    systolic murmurs associated with, 187, 188
  skin signs associated with, 152
Cardiopulmonary murmur, 514
Cardiovascular syphilis and cardiovascular system abnormalities, 151
Cardiovascular system, 126-197
Carditis, skin signs associated with, 152
Carey Coombs murmur, 194
Caries, dental, 65
  causing halitosis, 93
Carotid artery
  palpation of, 160, 164
  plaque in, causing retinal artery occlusion, 55
  stenosis of, 417
    causing amaurosis fugax, 39
  internal, 388
Carotid bruits, 67
Carotid sinus syncope, 146
Carpal tunnel syndrome, 364, 510
Carvallo sign, 195
Cataracts
  disorders associated with, 151
  causing loss of vision, 41

Cavernous sinus thrombosis
  causing exophthalmos, 46
  causing eye pain, 43
Cecum, carcinoma of, abdominal masses with, 233
Celiac axis compression causing bruits, 229
Cellulitis causing exophthalmos, 46
Central cyanosis, 89, 148
Central hearing loss, 56
Central retinal artery occlusion causing loss of vision, 41
Central scotomata, 44
Centrocecal scotomata, 44
Cerebellar ataxia, 403
Cerebellar degeneration, alcoholic, 418
  causing intention tremor, 402
Cerebellar disease, vertigo and, 57
Cerebellar dysfunction, signs of, 418
Cerebellar function and coordination, tests of, 400-404
Cerebellar infarction causing intention tremor, 402
Cerebellar syndrome, 510
Cerebellopontine angle tumors causing hearing loss, 57
Cerebral artery thrombosis causing homonymous hemianopsia, 52
Cerebral dysfunction causing Cheyne-Stokes respiration, 100
Cerebral embolism, 417
Cerebral thrombosis, middle, 417, 419
Cerebrospinal fluid rhinorrhea, 60
Cerebrovascular accident
  causing urinary incontinence, 265
  causing weakness, 388-389
Cerebrovascular disease
  causing anorexia, 205
  causing dysphagia, 209
Cerumen, excess, causing hearing loss, 57
Cervical carcinoma in situ, 312
Cervical disc disease causing chest pain, 129
Cervical fracture causing cervical spine abnormalities, 357
Cervical spine, 357
Cervical sympathetic nerves, 48
Cervical syndrome, 510
Cervix, 306
  abnormalities of, 311, 312
  neoplasms of, causing nonmenstrual vaginal bleeding, 286
Chaddock's reflex, 409
Chaddock's sign, 506
Chadwick's sign, 290, 506
Chalazion, 44, 45
Chancre, 466
  causing genital ulcers, 311
Chancroid
  causing genital ulcers, 311
  causing penile ulcer, 266, 272
Changing subject by clinician, 20
Chédiak-Higashi syndrome, 510
Chemicals causing oral ulcers, 62

Chemosis of conjunctivae, pulmonary causes of, 96
Chemotherapy
  causing candidal vaginitis, 296
  causing male infertility, 271
Cherry angiomas, 472
Chest, 96-97, 98, 99-111
  of child, examination of, 490-491
  deformities of, 102
  injuries to, history of, 90
  pain in, 79-80
    causes of, differentiating, 135
    gastrointestinal causes of, 135-136
    and heart disease, 126-136
    pleuritic, 79, 90, 91
    pulmonary causes of, 134-135
  questions related to, 27
  surgery on, causing free air in mediastinum, 111
Chest wall pain, causes of, 79
Cheyne-Stokes respiration, 100
Chickenpox, 451, 473
  petechiae in, 463
Chief complaint, 11
  format for recording, 31
Child(ren), 480-495
  medical interview of, 15-16
  vaginitis in, 296
Chinese restaurant syndrome, 510
Chlamydia trachomatis causing urethritis, 266
Chlamydia trachomatis pneumonia, 121
Chlamydial pneumonia, 121
Chlamydial vaginitis, 295, 297
Chloasma, 290
Cholangitis, sclerosing
  Kayser-Fleischer rings in, 47
  primary, causing jaundice, 244
Cholecystitis, 248
  and gallbladder symptoms, 232
  pain from, location of, 202
Choledocholithiasis
  causing chest pain, 136
  causing jaundice, 242
Cholelithiasis causing chronic abdominal pain, 249
olesteatoma causing hearing loss, 57
Chorea, gait with, 404
Chorioretinitis causing optic atrophy, 52
Choroidal tubercles, causes of, 96
Chromophobe tumor causing galactorrhea, 324
Churg-Strauss syndrome, 510
Chvostek's sign, 395, 506
Chylous ascites, 221
Cigar smoke, 92
Cigarette smoking causing pulmonary problems, 92
Ciliary ganglion lesion causing absent consensual response to light, 47
Cimetidine causing male impotence, 270
Circinate balanitis, 334, 367
Circinate lesions, 452
Cirrhosis
  cardiac, skin signs associated with, 152

Cirrhosis—cont'd
  causing epistaxis, 60
  causing gynecomastia, 331
  itching associated with, 449
  causing jaundice, 240
  of liver
    causing ascites, 220-221
    causing atrophic testes, 274
    causing jaundice, 243
    Kayser-Fleischer rings in, 47
    causing liver enlargement, 231
    causing splenomegaly, 232
Claudication, intermittent, pulses associated with, 169
Cleft palate, 489
Clenched fist sign, 506
Clicking of joints, 351
Clicks, systolic sounds and, 180-181
Climacteric, 285
Clinicians, responses of, and message conveyed to patient, 20
Clitoris, 300-301
Clonidine causing male impotence, 270
Clonus, ankle, 408
Closed drawer sign, 372
Clothing for physician, appropriate, 2
Clotting disorders causing conjunctival petechiae, 45
Club feet, 493
Clubbing
  of fingernails, causes of, 95-96
  of fingers and toes of child, 493
  of nails and cardiovascular system abnormalities, 153
Cluster headache, 384, 385
Coagulopathies causing epistaxis, 60
Coarctation of aorta
  blood pressure measurements and, 157
  causing decreased or absent femoral pulses, 234
  with Turner's syndrome, 150
Cocaine snorting causing nasal discharge, 60
Coccidioides immitis causing pneumonia, 121
Coccidioidomycosis, 121
  causing erythema nodosum, 96
  causing hemoptysis, 76
Codeine causing chronic gastric retention and delayed gastric emptying, 207
Cognitive function, assessment of, in psychiatric interview, 428
Cogwheel phenomenon, 395
Cold, common, 60, 90
Cold sore, 476
Colic
  biliary, 248, 249
  gallstone, causing chest pain, 136
  renal, 256
  pain from, location of, 202, 203
Colitis
  ischemic, causing hematochezia, 215, 217
  ulcerative; *see* Ulcerative colitis

Collagen diseases
    and Raynaud's phenomenon, 153
    causing Roth's spots, 54
    causing scleritis, 46
Collapsing pulse, 167
Collarette scale, 468
Colloid cyst causing thyroid enlargement, 67
Coloboma, 488
Colon
    angiodysplasia of, causing hematochezia, 215, 216
    carcinoma of, abdominal masses with, 233
    referred pain from, 203
Colonic polyps causing hematochezia, 215, 216
Color of skin, changes in, 448
Colorectal carcinoma causing hematochezia, 215-216
Coma, 414, 420-421
    deep, causing mydriasis, 48
    hyperglycemic, causing Kussmaul respirations, 99
    insulin, causing bradypnea, 99
Coma Scale, Glasgow, 415
Comatose patient, approach to, 420-421
Comedo, 447, 457
Common iliac artery, thrombosis of, causing decreased or absent femoral pulses, 234
Community-acquired pneumonia, 117, 122; see also Pneumonia
Complete abortion, 291
Complete heart block, jugular venous waves in, 163
Complete monocular blindness, 51
Compound nevi, 470
Compression, optic nerve, causing loss of vision, 41
Concepts, ability to handle, assessment of, 416
Conduction block associated with myotonia dystrophica, 149
Conductive hearing loss, 56
Condyloma acuminata, 272, 309
Condyloma lata, 309
Confluent lesions, 452
Confrontation testing, 50-51
Confusional states, acute, approach to patients with, 421-422
Congenital cyanotic heart disease, scoliosis associated with, 152
Congenital dislocation of hip, examination for, 493
Congenital heart disease
    causing dyspnea, 138
    extremity signs associated with, 153
    eye signs associated with, 151
Congenital heart lesions causing cyanosis, 149
Congenital syphilis, eye signs of, 46
Congestive cardiomyopathy causing dyspnea, 138

Congestive heart failure
    and angina, 132
    changes in retinal vessels caused by, 53
    causing chemosis, 96
    causing Cheyne-Stokes respiration, 100
    causing cough, 73
    causing cyanosis, 148
    causing dyspnea, 83
    causing nocturia, 264
    causing pedal edema, 147
    causing scrotal swelling, 269
Conjugate gaze, 49
Conjunctiva
    chemosis of, pulmonary causes of, 96
    diseases of, 45
    pale, in anemia, 151
    petechiae of, associated with bacterial endocarditis, 151
Conjunctivitis, 44, 45
Conn's syndrome, 510
Connective tissue atrophy, purpura associated with, 463
Connective tissue diseases, 459-461
    mixed, causing arthritis, 340
    causing uveitis, 41
Consciousness
    loss of, 385-387
    state of, assessment of, 415
Consensual pupillary response, 408
Consensual reaction to light, testing, 47
Consolidated lobar pneumonia, 121-122
Constipation, 211, 213
    as sign of pregnancy, 290
Constrictive pericarditis
    arterial pulse volume in, 168
    pericardial knock associated with, 181
Contact dermatitis, 453, 459
    causing external otitis, 56
Contact urticaria, 459
Continuous murmurs, 187, 194
Contraception, 291-292
Contraceptive device, intrauterine, 285, 286
Contraceptives, oral
    causing amenorrhea, 284
    and breast cancer, 325
    causing candidal vaginitis, 296
    use of, and hypertension, 157
Contractions
    atrial, premature, 164, 166, 167
    Braxton Hicks, 290, 506
    premature, 166, 167
    ventricular, premature, 163, 166, 167
Contractures, Dupuytren's, 365, 366
Convergence, testing, 48, 50
Convulsions, 387
Cooing murmur, 514
Cooper's ligament, 322
Cooperation, assessment of, 415
Coordination and cerebellar function, tests of, 400-404
COPD; see Obstructive pulmonary disease, chronic

Cor pulmonale, 114, 118
    associated with kyphoscoliosis, 149
    heart sounds in, 179
    causing jugular venous distention, 96
Cornea, 44, 46-47
Corneal arcus, atherosclerosis associated with, 151
Coronary artery disease, crease across earlobe associated with, 151
Coronary atherosclerosis
    eye signs associated with, 151
    risk factors for, 129-130
Coronary atherosclerotic heart disease, cigarette smoking causing, 92
Coronary insufficiency, 131
Coronary ostial stenosis, eye signs associated with, 151
Coronaviruses causing colds, 90
Corrigan's pulse, 167
Corrigan's water-hammer pulse and aortic regurgitation, 192
Corrosive esophagitis causing dysphagia, 209
Cortical blindness, 39, 42
Corticosteroids causing polyphagia, 205
Coryza, 90
Costochondral joint swelling, 104
Costochondral syndrome, 510
Costochondritis causing chest pain, 136
Cotton wool exudates, 54
Cough, 71-73
    productive, 74
Cough syncope, 73
Courvoisier's law, 232
Coxsackievirus, 473
Crackles, causes of, 109
Crackling of joints, 351
Cradle cap, 468
Cranial nerve palsies, 49-50
    causing mydriasis, 48
Cranial nerves, testing, 410-413
Craniotabes, 488
Cremasteric reflex, 408
Crepitations, causes of, 109
Crepitus, 350
Crescendo angina, 131
Crescendo murmur, 185
Crescendo-decrescendo murmur, 185
CREST syndrome, 460
Crohn's disease
    abdominal masses with, 233
    causing chronic gastric retention and delayed gastric emptying, 206
    causing genital ulcers, 311
    causing sacroiliac arthritis, 369
Cronkhite-Canada syndrome, 510
Crossed extension reflex, 494
Croup, 114-115, 119
Cruciate ligaments, examination of, 372, 373
Crusts, 446
Cruveilhier-Baumgarten syndrome, 510
Crying by patient, 14
Cryoglobulinemia causing retinal artery occlusion, 55

Cryptococcus neoformans causing pneumonia, 121
Cryptorchidism, 269, 275
 causing male infertility, 271
Cullen's sign, 506
Cushing's syndrome, 510
 causing breast striae, 328
 buffalo hump associated with, 101
 and cardiovascular system abnormalities, 150
 cataracts in, 151
 causing hypertrichosis, 298
 striae from, 219
Cutaneous nerves, 397
Cutaneous pain sensation, 396
Cyanosis, 88-90
 and cardiovascular system abnormalities, 153
 and heart disease, 148-149
Cyanotic heart disease
 causing clubbing of fingernails, 96
 congenital, scoliosis associated with, 152
Cyst(s), 445
 abdominal masses with, 233, 234
 Baker's, 371
 breast, 331
 colloid, causing thyroid enlargement, 67
 ovarian
  bleeding, causing pelvic pain, 288
  twisted, causing acute abdominal pain, 257
 pancreatic or gastric, aortic pulsation with, 233
 causing protuberant abdomen, 219
 renal, causing enlarged kidneys, 232
Cystic fibrosis, 115, 119
 causing dyspnea, 83
 causing male infertility, 271
 causing pneumonia, 91, 92
Cystitis, 263, 289
Cystocele, 298, 302
Cytotoxic drugs
 causing glossitis, 65
 causing oral ulcers, 62

D

DaCosta's syndrome causing chest pain, 129, 136
Dandy-Walker syndrome, 510
de Musset's sign, 506
Deaf patients, medical interview of, 17
Deafness, hearing loss and, 56-57
Death, brain, criteria for, 410
"Decompensated" hepatocellular disease, signs of, 238-239
Deep tendon reflexes, 404-407
Deformity, joint, 349
Degenerative arthritis, stiffness with, 344-345
Degenerative disease causing joint pain, 337

Delayed gastric emptying causing chronic abdominal pain, 250-252
Delirium
 approach to patient with, 421-422
 toxic, 416
Deltoid muscles, assessment of strength of, 393, 395-396
Delusional disorders, 437, 438
Delusions, 416
Demanding behavior of patient, 14
Dementia, 416, 437, 439, 440
 beclouded, 422
Demyelinating disease, 418
 causing chronic gastric retention and delayed gastric emptying, 206
 causing nystagmus, 49
 causing optic atrophy, 52
 causing optic neuropathy, 42
Denial, patient demonstration of, 15
Dental caries, 65
 causing halitosis, 93
Dental hygiene, poor, 92, 93
Dental malocclusion causing TMJ abnormalities, 356
Dentures causing oral ulcers, 62
Depression, 416, 428-429
 causing anorexia, 205
 patient demonstration of, 15
 with rheumatoid arthritis, 345
Depressive disorder, major, diagnostic criteria for, 429
DeQuervain's tenosynovitis, 362, 363
Dermal manifestations of systemic bacterial infections, 477, 478
Dermal nevi, 470
Dermatitis herpetiformis, 453, 474, 475
Dermatitis, 453, 458-459
 exfoliative, rash of, 465
 causing external otitis, 56
 seborrheic, 467, 468
Dermatoglyphics, 487
Dermatomyositis, 461
 causing arthritis, 340
 causing dysphagia, 209
Dermatophytes, 461
Dermatophytosis, 461-462
Dermis, 450
Diabetes causing mydriasis, 48
Diabetes insipidus causing polyuria, 264
Diabetes mellitus
 causing balanitis, 272
 causing candidal vaginitis, 296
 cataracts in, 151
 changes in vision associated with, 388
 causing chronic gastric retention and delayed gastric emptying, 207
 causing dysphagia, 209
 eye signs associated with, 151
 causing male impotence, 270
 causing nocturia, 264
 and periodontal disease, 65
 causing polyphagia, 205
 causing polyuria, 264

Diabetes mellitus—cont'd
 causing protuberant abdomen, 220
 pulses associated with, 168-169
 causing retinal exudates, 54
 causing retinal hemorrhages, 54
 skin ulcers in, 448
 causing third nerve palsy, 50
Diabetic ketoacidosis
 causing dyspnea, 85
 causing hyperpnea, 80
 causing Kussmaul respiration, 141
 causing nausea and vomiting, 207
Diabetic neuropathy causing syncope, 146
Diabetic proliferative retinopathy, 41
Diabetic retinopathy, 54
Diagnosis, 3
 errors in, causes of, 23-25
Diagnostic reasoning, 20-21
Diamond shaped murmur, 185, 514
Diaphragmatic excursion, 106
Diaphragmatic irritation causing chest pain, 79
Diaphragmatic paralysis causing orthopnea, 80
Diarrhea, 210-212
Diastasis recti, 219, 491
Diastolic dysfunction, 130
Diastolic murmurs, 184, 187, 191-194
 early, 514
Diathesis, hemorrhagic, causing hemoptysis, 78
Dietary factors causing diarrhea, 211
Diethylstilbestrol causing gynecomastia, 331-332
Differential diagnosis, 3
DiGeorge syndrome, 510
Digital reflex, 507
Digitalis causing gynecomastia, 332
Digitalis glycosides causing nausea and vomiting, 207
Dilated abdominal veins, causes of, 219
Dilation and curettage causing amenorrhea, 285
Dimpling of breasts, 322
Diphtheria
 causing dysphagia, 209
 causing pharyngeal membrane, 66
 causing sore throat, 63
Diplopia, 42-43, 50, 387
Direct hernia, 224
Disc, intervertebral, herniated, 368
Discharge
 nasal, 60
 from nipples, 324-325
 ocular, 44
 penile, 266, 268
 vaginal, 295-298
Discoid lesions, 452
Discoid lupus erythematosus, 460
Disconjugate gaze, 49
Discrete lesions, 452
Disease, 3

Dislocation of hip, congenital, examination for, 493
Dissecting aneurysm causing chest pain, 134
Dissecting aorta associated with Marfan syndrome, 149
Dissecting aortic aneurysm
 causing acute abdominal pain, 258
 causing chest pain, 128
Disseminated gonococcal disease, 334, 466
Distended abdomen, causes of, 219-221
Diuretics, 264
Diverticular disease
 causing diarrhea, 212
 causing hematochezia, 215, 216
Diverticulitis
 causing chronic abdominal pain, 252
 pain from, location of, 202
Diverticulum
 causing dysphagia, 209
 Meckel's, causing maroon-colored stools, 217
 Zenker's, causing halitosis, 93
Doll's eye sign, 506
Dorsal root ganglia, diseases of, causing male impotence, 270
Dorsalis pedis pulse, palpation of, 165
Dot-and-blot retinal hemorrhages, 54
Double questions, 20
Double vision, 42-43, 387
"Dowager's hump," 101, 367
Down syndrome, 486, 510
 and cardiovascular system abnormalities, 149, 150
 cataracts in, 151
 extremity signs associated with, 153
Doxapin causing male impotence, 270
Drawer sign, 506
Dress for physician, appropriate, 2
Drug eruptions, rash of, 465
Drug rash, 464, 465
Drug reactions, skin lesions associated with, 456
Drug-induced asthma, 112; *see also* Asthma
Drug-induced diarrhea, 212
Drug-induced fatigue, 143
Drug-induced respiratory depression causing bradypnea, 99
Drusen, 52
Dubin-Johnson syndrome, 510
Ductus arteriosus, patent, heart murmurs associated with, 194
Dullness as percussion sound, 107
Duodenal ulcer disease
 causing chronic gastric retention and delayed gastric emptying, 206
 causing hematemesis, 214
Duodenum
 carcinoma of, causing chronic gastric retention and delayed gastric emptying, 206

Duodenum—cont'd
 tumors of, causing pyloric outlet obstruction, 228
Dupuytren's contractures, 365, 366
Duroziez's murmur, 167
Duroziez's sign and aortic regurgitation, 192
Dust, inhalation of, causing cough, 73
Dysarthria, 388, 417
Dyscrasias, blood
 causing bleeding gums, 63
 causing conjunctival petechiae, 45
Dysdiadochokinesia, 402-403
Dysfunctional uterine bleeding, 285
Dysgeusia, 63
Dyshidrosis, skin lesions associated with, 456
Dysmenorrhea, 286
Dysmetria, testing, 401-402
Dyspareunia, 293
Dysphagia, 208-210
 thyroid enlargement causing, 67
Dysphonia, 388, 417
Dysplastic nevi, 470
Dyspnea, 80, 81-86
 differentiating causes of, 141
 and heart disease, 136-141
 nocturnal, paroxysmal, 80, 84, 139-140
 at rest, 139
Dysproteinemias
 changes in retinal vessels caused by, 53
 causing retinal artery occlusion, 55
 causing retinal vein occlusion, 55
 causing Roth's spots, 54
Dyssynergia, testing, 401-402
Dysuria
 in male, 263
 in urinary tract infection, 289

E

Ear, 56-59
 of child, examination of, 488-489
 pain in, 56
 questions related to, 27
Earlobe, disorders of, 58
Early diastolic murmur, 514
Eating disorders causing nausea and vomiting, 207
Eaton-Lambert syndrome, 345
Ecchymoses, 221, 223, 463
Eclampsia, 291
Ectopia lentis, Marfan syndrome associated with, 151
Ectopic pregnancy
 causing nonmenstrual vaginal bleeding, 286
 ruptured, causing acute abdominal pain, 257
Eczema, 458
Eczematoid lesions, 452
Eczematous diseases, 458-459

Edema
 breast, 328
 of conjunctivae, pulmonary causes of, 96
 and heart disease, 147-148
 laryngeal, causing wheezing, 87
 of neck of child, 490
 pedal, 147
 causing penile pain, 268
 pulmonary; *see* Pulmonary edema
Edinger-Westphal nucleus, lesion of, causing absent consensual response to light, 47
Effort dyspnea, 139
Effusion
 joint, 348-349
  ballottement to determine, 372
 pericardial
  associated with myxedema, 150
  pericardial friction rubs associated with, 182
 pleural; *see* Pleural effusion
Egophony, 110
Ehlers-Danlos syndrome, 510
 and cardiovascular system abnormalities, 149, 150
Eisenmenger's syndrome, 510
 causing cyanosis, 149
Ejection murmur, 514
Ejection sounds, 180
Elbow, 361-362
 range of motion of, 354
Elevation, leg, passive, to enhance cardiac auscultation, 196
Emboli
 pulmonary; *see* Pulmonary emboli
 retinal, and cardiovascular system abnormalities, 151
Embolism
 cerebral, 417
 causing homonymous hemianopsia, 52
 pulmonary; *see* Pulmonary embolism
Embolization of carotid artery causing amaurosis fugax, 39
Empathy, 8
Emphysema, 116, 119
 causing absent breath sounds, 109
 barrel chest in, 101
 affecting chest expansion, 102
 cigarette smoking causing, 92
 causing decreased fremitus, 106
 causing dyspnea, 81-82
 causing hyperresonance, 106
 mediastinal, causing chest pain, 135
 subcutaneous, 104
Empyema
 causing dullness to percussion, 107
 causing tracheal shift, 105
Encephalitis
 causing galactorrhea, 324
 causing nausea and vomiting, 207
 causing ptosis, 44
Encephalopathy, hepatic, 416

Endobronchial carcinoma causing pneumonia, 91
Endobronchial foreign body causing delayed chest movement, 102
Endocarditis
  causing arthralgia, 337
  bacterial; see Bacterial endocarditis
  and dental care, 152
  causing dyspnea, 137
  eye signs associated with, 151
  infective, extremity signs associated with, 153
  causing pulsatile liver, 231
Endocrine causes of male impotence, 270
Endocrine disease causing fatigue, 143
Endometriosis, 285, 286, 288
Endometrium, neoplasms of, causing nonmenstrual vaginal bleeding, 286
Enteritis
  infectious, 211, 215, 217
  regional; see Regional enteritis
Enuresis, 265
Eosinophilic gastroenteritis causing chronic gastric retention and delayed gastric emptying, 206
Epicondylitis, 362
Epidermal necrolysis, toxic, 465, 474
Epidermis, 450
Epididymis, 269, 271
Epigastric masses, 234
Epiglottitis, 88, 115, 119-120
  causing wheezing, 87
Epilepsy, 387
Epispadias, 272
Epistaxis, 60
  differentiation of, from hemoptysis, 75
Erection, sustained, causing penile pain, 268
Erosive gastritis causing hematemesis, 214
Erysipelas, 477
Erythema
  joint, 350
  toxic, rash of, 465
Erythema infectiosum, 451
Erythema marginatum, rheumatic fever associated with, 152
Erythema multiforme, 451, 453, 475
  causing oral ulcers, 62
  rash of, 465
  skin lesions associated with, 456
Erythema nodosum, causes of, 96
Esophageal carcinoma causing dysphagia, 209
Esophageal reflux causing chest pain, 135
Esophageal rings and web causing dysphagia, 209
Esophageal rupture, pain of, 80
Esophageal spasm
  causing chest pain, 129, 135
  causing dysphagia, 209
Esophageal stricture causing dysphagia, 209

Esophageal varices causing hematemesis, 214
Esophagitis
  corrosive, causing dysphagia, 209
  reflux
    causing chest pain, 129
    causing dysphagia, 209
Esophagus
  referred pain from, 201
  rupture of, causing free air in mediastinum, 111
Esotropia, 48
Essential hypertension, 157
Estrogens
  causing male impotence, 270
  causing male infertility, 271
  causing nonmenstrual vaginal bleeding, 287
Ethambutol causing optic neuropathy, 42
Ethanolism causing pancreatitis, 252
Ethylene glycol, ingestion of, causing dyspnea, 86
Eunuchism causing gynecomastia, 331
Eustachian tube, blocked, 56
Eversion, 346
Ewart's sign, 507
Examination, physical; see Physical examination
Exanthems, viral, causing serous otitis media, 56
Excoriation, 446
Exercise-induced amenorrhea, 284
Exercise-induced asthma, 112; see also Asthma
Exfoliation, diseases manifesting, 456
Exfoliative dermatitis, rash of, 465
Exhalation to enhance cardiac auscultation, 195
Exophthalmos, 46, 151
Exotropia, 48
Expiratory stridor, 489
Expressive aphasia, 417
Extension, 346
External auditory canal, examination of, 58, 59
External genitalia of female, examination of, 300-302
External otitis, causes of, 56
External rotation, 346
Extinction, sensory, 400
Extracardiac murmur, 514
Extraocular movements, 48-50
Extremities and cardiovascular system abnormalities, 153
Exudates, retinal, 54
Exudative pharyngitis causing halitosis, 93
Eye(s), 39-55
  and cardiovascular system abnormalities, 151
  of child, examination of, 488
  disorders of, vertigo and, 57
  questions related to, 26
Eye chart, Snellen, 55
Eyelash sign, 507

Eyelids, 44-45

F
Fabry's disease and cardiovascular system abnormalities, 150, 152
Face and cardiovascular system abnormalities, 150-151
Facial nerve, testing of, 412
Facial pain and chronic sinusitis, 60
Fainting; see Syncope
Faintness, etiology of, 386
Fallopian tubes, infections of, causing pelvic pain, 288-289
Fallot, tetralogy of; see Tetralogy of Fallot
False answers, giving, 20
Family history, 13
  format for recording, 31
  role of, in disease, 516
Fanconi's syndrome, 510
Fasciculations, 395
Fat necrosis causing dimpling of breast, 322
Fatigue, 143, 144, 345
Fatigue syndrome, chronic, 143, 345
Fatty liver
  causing jaundice, 240
  causing liver enlargement, 231
Fecal impaction causing urinary incontinence, 265
Fecal incontinence, 211, 212
Felty's syndrome, 510
Female, developmental markers in, 283
Female genitalia, 280-315
Femoral hernia, 223, 224, 277
Femoral pulses, decreased or absent, causes of, 234
Festinating gait, 404
Fetal alcohol syndrome, 510
Fever blister, 476
Fever, rheumatic; see Rheumatic fever
Fibrillation, atrial, 166-167
  jugular venous waves in, 163, 164
  paroxysmal, 142
Fibroadenomas of breast, 318, 319, 331
Fibrocystic breast disease, 318, 319
Fibroid tumors, 311-312
  uterine, causing menorrhagia, 285
Fibromuscular hyperplasia of renal arteries causing bruits, 229
Fibromyalgia, diagnosis of, criteria for, 351
Fibrosis
  cystic; see Cystic fibrosis
  pulmonary, 73, 91, 102
Fibrositis, 334
Fifth disease, 451
Finger-to-finger test, 401-402
Finger-to-nose test, 401-402
Fingernails, clubbing of, causes of, 95-96
Fingers, 364-366
  assessment of strength of, 393
  of child, clubbing of, 493
  deformities of, 349
First heart sound, 177

Fissure, 446
  anal, in child, 492
Fistulas, arteriovenous, pulmonary, extremity signs associated with, 153
Fitz-Hugh–Curtis syndrome, 511
Fixed drug eruptions, rash of, 465
Fixed split S_2, 178
Flail chest, 102
Flame-shaped retinal hemorrhages, 54
Flat foot, 375
Flatness as percussion sound, 107
Flexion, 346
Floppy valve syndrome, 511
Fluctuance of lesion, 451
Fluid removal causing syncope, 146
Fluid wave, eliciting, 226
Flush, hot, 285-286
Folic acid deficiency causing glossitis, 65
Fontanelles, assessment of, 487-488
Food poisoning causing nausea and vomiting, 207
Foot(feet), 373-376
  club, 493
  ulcers of, 375, 448
Foot drop, 403
Foreign body
  in airway causing wheezing, 87
  aspiration of
    causing atelectasis, 105
    causing breathing difficulty in infant, 92
    causing croup syndrome, 114
    causing hemoptysis, 77
  in bronchus causing pneumonia, 91
  in ear causing external otitis, 56
  endobronchial, causing delayed chest movement, 102
  causing excessive lacrimation, 44
  causing eye pain, 44
  causing oral ulcers, 62
  in trachea or bronchi causing cough, 73
Fourth heart sound, 179
Fracture
  cervical, causing cervical spine abnormalities, 357
  causing exophthalmos, 46
  rib; see Rib fracture
  skull, causing nasal discharge, 60
Freckles, 469
Free air in peritoneal cavity causing protuberant abdomen, 219, 220
Fremitus, tactile, 105-106
Frequency of urination, 289, 290
Friction rubs
  pericardial, 181-182
  peritoneal, 229
  pleural, causes of, 109-110
Friedreich's ataxia and cardiovascular system abnormalities, 149, 150
Froin's syndrome, 511
Frontal sinusitis, 60
Frozen shoulder, 359, 360
Functional dyspnea, 138
Funduscopic examination, 52-55

Fungal arthritis in single joint, 339
Fungal infections, 461-462
  causing external otitis, 56
  causing "hairy" tongue, 65
  of nails, 452, 454
  causing nausea and vomiting, 207
  causing splenomegaly, 232
Fungal pneumonia, 121
Funnel-chest deformity, 102, 103

G
Gait, 370, 403-404
Galactorrhea, causes of, 324
Gallbladder, 232, 233
  referred pain from, 201
Gallop, summation, 179
Gallop rhythm, 179
Gallstone colic causing chest pain, 136
Ganglia, 349, 362, 363
  ciliary, lesion of, causing absent consensual response to light, 47
  dorsal root, diseases of, causing male impotence, 270
Ganglionic blockers
  causing chronic gastric retention and delayed gastric emptying, 207
  causing protuberant abdomen, 220
Gangrenous bowel, absent bowel sounds with, 227
Gardner's syndrome, 511
Gardnerella vaginalis vaginitis, 296-297, 310
Gas(es)
  in bowel causing protuberant abdomen, 219, 220
  noxious, inhalation of, causing cough, 73
Gastritis, erosive, causing hematemesis, 214
Gastroenteritis
  eosinophilic, causing chronic gastric retention and delayed gastric emptying, 206
  increased bowel sounds with, 227
Gastroesophageal reflux, pain associated with, 200, 202
Gastroesophageal reflux disease causing wheezing, 87
Gastrointestinal disorders; see Abdomen
Gaucher's disease causing pingueculae, 47
Gaze, cardinal positions of, 49-50
Gaze palsy, 49
General appearance of patient, questions related to, 26
Generalized anxiety disorders, 430-431
Generalized lesions, 452
Genital ulcers, causes of, 311
Genitalia
  of child, examination of, 492
  female, 280-315
  male, 262-279
Genu recurvatum, 373, 374
Genu valgus, 373, 374
Genu varus, 373, 374
Geriatrics, medical interview in, 16-17

German measles, 465
Gerstmann's syndrome, 511
Gestalt, 20
Gestational trophoblastic neoplasia, 291
Giant *a* waves, 164
Gibbus, 101, 102, 367, 368
Gilbert syndrome causing jaundice, 244
Gingiva, physical examination of, 65
Gingivitis, 65
Gingivostomatitis
  caused by herpes simplex infections, 63
  herpetic, primary, 476
Gland(s); *see* specific gland
Glasgow Coma Scale, 415
Glaucoma causing loss of vision, 41
Globe, diseases of, 46
Globus hystericus causing dysphagia, 209
Glomerulonephritis, acute, causing hematuria, 266
Glomus tumor causing tinnitus, 57
Glossitis, 65
  causing hypogeusia, 63
Glossopharyngeal nerve, testing of, 413
Gloves, use of, 299
Golf elbow, 362
Gonadotropins, decreased secretion of, causing male infertility, 271
Goniometer, 352, 353
Gonococcal arthritis, 341, 378-379
Gonococcal disease, disseminated, 334, 466
Gonococcal urethritis causing penile pain, 266
Gonococcal vaginitis, 295, 297, 310
Gonococcemia, 466
  disseminated, causing sternoclavicular joint swelling, 104
  causing joint pain, 336
  skin lesions associated with, 456
Gonorrhea causing male infertility, 271
Goodell's sign, 290
Goodpasture's syndrome, 511
  causing hemoptysis, 77, 78-79
Gottron's papules, 461
Gout, 334, 343
  causing arthritis, 339, 341
  causing joint pain, 337
  tophi caused by, 58
Gouty arthritis, 343, 348, 378-379
Gouty podagra, 375, 376
Gouty tophi, 349
Grading of pulses, 168-169
Gradual loss of vision, causes of, 41-42
Graham Steell's murmur, 192, 193, 514
Gram-negative septicemia causing hyperventilation, 99
Grand mal seizures, 387
Granulomatosis, Wegener's
  causing hemoptysis, 77, 78-79
  causing oral ulcers, 62
  causing perforated nasal septum, 60
Grasp reflex, 410
Graves' disease, 46, 48, 67
Graves speculum, 303
Gravida, 281

Great vessels and heart, physical examination of, 157-197
Greek and Latin roots, 496-505
Grey Turner's sign, 223, 507
Groin of male, examination of, 276-277
Groove sign, 507
Grouped lesions, 452
Growth patterns, normal, 483-485
Guanethidine causing male impotence, 270
Guarding, involuntary, of abdomen, 236
Guillain-Barré syndrome, 511
Gums, 63-65
Gunshot wound causing hemoptysis, 77
Gynecologic causes of acute abdominal pain, 257
Gynecomastia, 331

H

h waves, 162
Haemophilus influenzae causing pneumonia, 121
Hair
  changes in, 449
  loss of, 462
  pubic, changes in, in female, 300
"Hairy" tongue, 65
Halitosis, pulmonary diseases associated with, 93
Hallucinations, assessment of, 416
Hallux valgus, 375
Haloperidol causing male impotence, 270
Hamman's sign, 111, 135, 507
Hamman-Rich syndrome, 511
Hand, 363, 364-366
  range of motion of, 354
Hand-foot-and-mouth disease, 473
  skin lesions associated with, 455
Handgrip, isometric, to enhance cardiac auscultation, 196
Hard retinal exudates, 54
Hay fever causing excessive lacrimation, 44
Head
  of child, examination of, 487-409
  and neck, 38-69
    examination of, checklist for, 68
  musculoskeletal examination of, 356
Headache, 383-385
  differential diagnosis of, considerations in, 22
  migraine, causing loss of vision, 40
Hearing
  changes in, 388
  testing, 59
Hearing loss, 56-57
Heart, 125-198
  anatomy of, 158
  auscultation of, 173, 175
  of child, examination of, 491
  congenital lesions of, causing cyanosis, 149
  congestive failure of; see Congestive heart failure

Heart—cont'd
  cyanotic chronic diseases of, causing clubbing of fingernails, 96
  examination of, techniques to improve, 173-175
  and great vessels, physical examination of, 157-197
  history taking related to, 126-149
  questions related to, 27-28
  surgery on, causing free air in mediastinum, 111
  valvular disease of, causing dyspnea, 140-141
Heart block
  complete, jugular venous waves in, 163
  eye signs associated with, 151
Heart disease
  congenital, 151, 153
  coronary atherosclerotic, cigarette smoking causing, 92
  cyanotic, congenital, scoliosis associated with, 152
  causing dyspnea, 83-84, 137-138
Heart failure
  congestive; see Congestive heart failure
  causing dyspnea, 139
  causing edema, 148
  eye signs associated with, 151
  causing fatigue, 143
  heart sounds in, 179
  hepatomegaly associated with, 152-153
  causing orthopnea, 80
  skin signs associated with, 152
Heart murmurs, 182-197
Heart sounds, 171-172, 174, 175-180
Heart valves, prosthetic, and blood pressure measurement, 156
Heaves, 170
Heberden's nodes, 334, 349, 365, 366
Heel spur, 375, 376
Heel-to-shin test, 402
Hematemesis, 213-214
  differentiation of, from hemoptysis, 75
Hematocele causing scrotal swelling, 269
Hematochezia, 210, 211, 214-218
Hematologic disorders causing oral ulcers, 62
Hematologic problems causing dyspnea, 84-85
Hematomas
  in abdominal wall causing abdominal wall pain, 256
  intracranial, causing nausea and vomiting, 207
Hematuria, 265-266
Hemianopsia, 51, 52
Hemic murmur, 514
Hemiparesis, 403, 404
Hemiplegia, 403
Hemochromatosis, and cardiovascular system abnormalities, 152
Hemoglobinuria, causes of, 265

Hemolytic anemia
  chronic, and cardiovascular system abnormalities, 150
  yellow sclerae caused by, 46
Hemolytic disorders causing splenomegaly, 232
Hemolytic uremic syndrome causing abdominal pain, 249
Hemophilia causing hemoptysis, 78
Hemophilus ducreyi causing penile ulcers, 266
Hemophilus influenzae
  causing consoldiated lobar pneumonia, 122
  causing epiglottitis, 88
Hemoptysis, 75-79
  and heart disease, 147
Hemorrhage
  retinal, 54
  splinter, 454
    under nails and cardiovascular system abnormalities, 153
  subarachnoid, causing papilledema, 54
  subconjunctival, 45
  vitreous, causing loss of vision, 41
Hemorrhagic diathesis causing hemoptysis, 78
Hemorrhagic measles, skin lesions associated with, 455
Hemorrhagic telangiectasia, hereditary
  causing epistaxis, 60
  mouth signs associated with, 151
Hemorrhagic varicella, skin lesions associated with, 455
Hemorrhoids causing hematochezia, 215
Hemostatic disorders causing retinal hemorrhages, 54
Hepatic encephalopathy, 416
Hepatitis
  alcoholic, 251
    causing bruits, 229
    causing jaundice, 240
    causing liver enlargement, 231
  causing jaundice, 241-242
  viral
    causing anorexia, 205
    causing dysgeusia, 63
    causing jaundice, 240
Hepatocellular disease, "decompensated," signs of, 238-239
Hepatojugular reflux, 161
Hepatoma causing bruits, 229
Hepatomegaly
  abdominal masses with, 233
  and cardiovascular system abnormalities, 152-153
Herald patch of pityriasis rosea, 468
Hereditary hemorrhagic telangiectasia
  causing epistaxis, 60
  mouth signs associated with, 151
Hereditary optic atrophy causing optic neuropathy, 42
Hernia(s)
  abdominal, 223-224

Hernia(s)—cont'd
  abdominal masses with, 233
  causing abdominal wall pain, 256
  femoral, 277
  inguinal, 276, 277
  umbilical, 491
Herniated nucleus pulposus, 368
Heroin causing male impotence, 270
Herpes genitalis causing penile ulcers, 266, 272
Herpes infections causing dysphagia, 209
Herpes simplex, 476
  causing genital ulcers, 311
  causing penile ulcers, 266
Herpes simplex infection causing oral ulcers, 62, 63
Herpes simplex vesicles, 475
Herpes simplex virus causing urethritis, 266
Herpes simplex virus vesicles, 451
Herpes zoster, 96, 473, 475
  causing abdominal pain, 249
  causing abdominal wall pain, 256
  causing chest pain, 129, 136
  causing external otitis, 56
Herpes zoster infection causing oral ulcers, 62
Herpetic gingivostomatitis, primary, 476
Herpetic infections causing sore throat, 63
Herpetic whitlow, 476
Herpetiform lesions of lip, 64
Hiccups, 88
Hidradenitis suppurativa, 457, 458
Hill's sign, 507
  and aortic regurgitation, 192
Hinge joint, 347
Hip, 368-370
  congenital dislocation of, examination for, 493
  extensor muscles of, assessment of strength of, 394
  range of motion of, 355
Hirschsprung's disease causing constipation, 213
Hirsutism, 449
  in women, 298
Histamine H_2-receptor antagonists causing male impotence, 270
Histiocytosis X causing oral ulcers, 62
Histoplasma capsulatum causing pneumonia, 121
Histoplasmosis
  causing erythema nodosum, 96
  causing hemoptysis, 76
  causing oral ulcers, 62
  causing uveitis, 41
History, 11-13
  format for recording, 31
  sexual, 269
Hives, 448-449, 472-473
Hoarseness, 64
Hodgkin's disease
  causing chylous ascites, 221
  causing splenomegaly, 232

Hoffmann's sign, 409, 507
Holosystolic murmurs, 184, 189-191, 514
Homans' sign, 507
Homonymous hemianopsia, 52
Honeymoon cystitis, 289
Hordeolum, 44, 45
Horner's syndrome, 48, 511
  eye signs of, 96
  causing ptosis, 44
Hospital-acquired pneumonia, 122
Hostile behavior by patient, 14
Hostile patients, medical interview of, 19-20
Hot flush, 285-286
Hum, venous, 191
Hunt's syndrome, 511
Hurler's syndrome and cardiovascular system abnormalities, 150
Hutchinson's triad, 46
Hydatidiform mole, 291
Hydrocele, 269
  transillumination of, 275
Hydrocephalus
  causing nausea and vomiting, 207
  normal pressure, causing urinary incontinence, 265
  causing papilledema, 54
Hydronephrosis causing enlarged kidneys, 232
Hymen, 301-301
  imperforate, 284, 286
Hypalgesia, 396
Hyperalgesia, 396
Hyperbilirubinemia, chronic idiopathic unconjugated, causing jaundice, 244
Hypercalcemia
  chronic, causing dysgeusia, 63
  causing polyuria, 264
Hypercholesterolemia, eye signs associated with, 151
Hyperemesis gravidarum, 290
Hyperesthesia, 398
Hyperglycemic coma causing Kussmaul respirations, 99
Hyperkinetic pulse, 167
Hypermenorrhea, 282
Hypernephroma
  causing enlarged kidneys, 232
  causing testicular displacement, 274
Hyperparathyroidism causing dysgeusia, 63
Hyperpathia, 398
Hyperpnea, 80, 99, 100, 139
Hyperprolactinemia causing male impotence, 270
Hyperresonance, 106
Hypertelorism, 488
Hypertension
  arterial pulse volume in, 167
  blood pressure measurements in patient with, 157
  changes in retinal vessels caused by, 53

Hypertension—cont'd
  complications of, 157
  with Cushing's syndrome, 150
  causing dyspnea, 138
  causing epistaxis, 60
  essential, 157
  eye signs associated with, 151
  heart sounds in, 178, 179
  intracranial, benign, causing papilledema, 54
  malignant, causing papilledema, 54
  portal
    dilated abdominal veins in, 219
    causing splenomegaly, 232
  pulmonary; *see* Pulmonary hypertension
  retinal changes in, 158
  causing retinal exudates, 54
  causing retinal hemorrhages, 54
  systemic, ocular changes caused by, 55
Hypertension headache, 384
Hyperthyroidism
  and cardiovascular system abnormalities, 150
  causing chemosis, 96
  eye signs associated with, 46, 151
  causing polyphagia, 205
  tremors associated with, 395
Hypertrichosis, 298
Hypertrophic cardiomyopathy
  arterial pulse volume in, 168
  causing dyspnea, 138, 141
  systolic murmurs associated with, 187, 188
Hypertrophic pyloric stenosis causing chronic gastric retention and delayed gastric emptying, 206
Hypertropia, 48
Hyperventilation, 99, 100
Hypesthesia, 398
Hypodermis, 450
Hypogammaglobulinemia causing pneumonia, 91
Hypogastric masses, 234
Hypogeusia, 63
Hypogonadism, hypogonadotropic, causing male infertility, 271
Hypogonadotropic hypogonadism causing male infertility, 271
Hypokalemia
  causing polyuria, 264
  causing weakness, 388
Hypomanic episodes, 420
Hypomenorrhea, 282
Hypospadias, 272, 273
Hypotelorism, 488
Hypotension, orthostatic, 156
Hypothalamic disorders causing male infertility, 271
Hypothyroidism
  absent bowel sounds with, 227
  characteristics of, 486
  causing chronic gastric retention and delayed gastric emptying, 207
  causing galactorrhea, 324

Hypothyroidism—cont'd
  causing hoarseness, 64
  causing protuberant abdomen, 220
Hypotropia, 48
Hypovolemia causing syncope, 146
Hypoxemic chronic obstructive pulmonary disease, changes in retinal vessels caused by, 53
Hysteria
  causing loss of vision, 39
  spurious muscle weakness caused by, 394

I

Ichthyosis, 472
Ichthyosis vulgaris, 472
Icterus, 221; *see also* Jaundice
  scleral, 46
Identifying data
  patient, format for recording, 31
  review of, before interview, 3-4
Idiopathic hypertrophic pyloric stenosis causing chronic gastric retention and delayed gastric emptying, 206
Idiopathic hypertrophic subaortic stenosis
  arterial pulse volume in, 168
  causing dyspnea, 141
Idiopathic secretory diarrhea, 212
Idiopathic thrombocytopenia causing hemoptysis, 78
Idiopathic ulcerative colitis causing hematochezia, 216
Idiopathic unconjugated hyperbilirubinemia, chronic, causing jaundice, 244
Idiophytid reactions, 461
  skin lesions associated with, 456
Idiosyncratic asthma, 112; *see also* Asthma
Ileus
  paralytic or adynamic, causing protuberant abdomen, 220
  referred pain from, 203
Iliac artery, common, thrombosis of, causing decreased or absent femoral pulses, 234
Illness, present, history of, 11-12
  format for recording, 31
Imipramine causing male impotence, 270
Immune deficiency syndrome; *see* Acquired immune deficiency syndrome
Immunization, bacillus Calmette-Guerin, 90, 91
Immunodeficiency causing pneumonia in child, 92
Impaction, fecal, causing urinary incontinence, 265
Imperforate hymen, 284, 286
Impetigo, 477
Impingement syndrome, 360
Impotence, male, 269, 270
Impulse, maximal, point of, 170, 171
Incarcerated hernia, 223

Incisional hernia, 223, 224
Incomplete abortion, 291
Incontinence
  fecal, 211, 212
  urinary, 265
Indirect hernia, 224
Induced abortion causing pelvic pain, 288
Induration of lesion, 451
Infant
  blood pressure measurement in, 155
  length of, measurement of, 486
Infarct, splenic, pain from, location of, 202
Infarction
  cerebellar, causing intention tremor, 402
  muscle, causing ecchymoses, 223
  myocardial; *see* Myocardial infarction
  pleural, causing pleural friction rub, 109
  pulmonary
    causing delayed chest movement, 102
    skin signs associated with, 152
  splenic, causing acute abdominal pain, 259
Infected teeth, ear pain caused by, 56
Infection(s)
  bacterial
    causing external otitis, 56
    causing ocular discharge, 44
    systemic, dermal manifestations of, 477, 478
  causing balanitis, 272
  chronic
    causing anorexia, 205
    causing fatigue, 143
  causing dysphagia, 209
  fungal, 461-462
    causing "hairy" tongue, 65
  causing glossitis, 65
  herpes simplex, causing oral ulcers, 62, 63
  herpes zoster, causing oral ulcers, 62
  causing hoarseness, 64
  maternal, causing hearing loss in child, 57
  of middle ear causing pain, 56
  Mycoplasma pneumoniae, causing bullous myringitis, 56, 58
  of nails, 452, 454
  causing nausea and vomiting, 207
  causing nonmenstrual vaginal bleeding, 286, 287
  oral, causing increased salivation, 65
  causing pelvic pain, 288-289
  respiratory; *see* Respiratory infection; Upper respiratory infections
  causing sore throat, 63
  causing splenomegaly, 232
  urinary tract, in female, 289
  Vincent's, 65
  viral
    causing dysgeusia, 63
    causing eye pain, 44

Infectious asthma, 112; *see also* Asthma
Infectious disease causing breathing difficulty in infant, 92
Infectious enteritis
  causing diarrhea, 211
  causing hematochezia, 215, 217
Infectious mononucleosis
  causing pharyngitis, 66
  causing sore throat, 63
  mouth signs associated with, 151
Infectious proctitis causing hematochezia, 215, 217
Infective endocarditis, extremity signs associated with, 153
Inferior vena cava, thrombosis of, causing scrotal swelling, 271
Infertility
  female, 293-294
  male, 269, 271
Infiltrative disorders causing splenomegaly, 232
Inflammation
  of buccal mucosa, 65
  cardinal signs of, 338
  of meatus causing dysuria, 263
  of mucous membranes causing cough, 73
Inflammatory bowel disease
  causing clubbing of fingernails, 96
  causing diarrhea, 211
  causing hematochezia, 215, 216
  causing recurrent aphthous ulcers, 63
  causing sacroiliac arthritis, 369
Inflammatory conditions causing increased salivation, 65
Inflammatory disease, pelvic; *see* Pelvic inflammatory disease
Influenza causing arthralgia, 337
Information, recording of, format for, 31-37
Ingestion
  of antifreeze causing dyspnea, 86
  of solvent causing breathing difficulty in infant, 92
Inguinal canals, examination of, 276-277
Inguinal hernia, 223-224, 276, 277
Inguinal pain and testicular mass, 272
Inhalation
  amyl nitrite, to enhance cardiac auscultation, 196-197
  of noxious gases causing cough, 73
  of smoke or noxious fumes causing hemoptysis, 77
Innocent murmurs, 191, 514
Insomnia, fatigue with, 345
Inspiration to enhance cardiac auscultation, 194-195
Inspiratory stridor, 489
Insulin coma causing bradypnea, 99
Intention tremor, 401-402
Intermittent claudication, pulses associated with, 169
Internal carotid artery stenosis, 388
Internal obstruction causing protuberant abdomen, 219, 220
Internal rotation, 346

Interphalangeal joint, 364-365
Interstitial keratitis, 46
Interstitial lung disease causing cough, 73
Intervertebral disc, herniated, 368
Interview, medical; see Medical interview
Intestinal angina causing bruits, 229
Intestinal obstruction, increased bowel sounds with, 227
Intestinal pseudo-obstruction
 causing chronic gastric retention and delayed gastric emptying, 206
 causing protuberant abdomen, 220
Intestine, mechanical obstruction of, 255
Intraabdominal bleeding causing pleuritic chest pain, 91
Intraabdominal tumors, striae from, 219
Intracranial abscess causing nausea and vomiting, 207
Intracranial hematoma causing nausea and vomiting, 207
Intracranial hypertension, benign, causing papilledema, 54
Intracranial lesion causing nausea and vomiting, 207
Intracranial pressure, increased, causing bradypnea, 99
Intraocular pressure, increased
 causing eye pain, 43
 causing loss of vision, 42
 causing mydriasis, 48
 causing papilledema, 54
Intrathoracic structures, pain in, causes of, 79
Intrathoracic tumor causing dysphagia, 209
Intrauterine contraceptive device, 285, 286
Intrauterine pregnancy causing nonmenstrual vaginal bleeding, 286
Inversion, 346
Involuntary guarding of abdomen, 236
Iridocyclitis causing eye pain, 44
Iridodonesis, Marfan syndrome associated with, 151
Iris
 lesions of, 452
 and pupils, diseases of, 47-48
Iritis
 and cardiovascular system abnormalities, 151
 causing eye pain, 44
 causing miosis, 48
Iron deficiency anemia, tongue changes caused by, 65
Iron preparations
 causing anorexia, 205
 causing nausea and vomiting, 207
Iron-containing medications causing melena, 218
Irreducible hernia, 223
Irrelevant questions, asking, 20
Irritable bowel syndrome, 204
 causing chronic abdominal pain, 253-254, 256

Irritable bowel syndrome—cont'd
 causing diarrhea, 212
Irritant dermatitis, 459
Irritation, meningeal, signs of, approach to patient with, 423
Ischemia, myocardial, causing syncope, 146
Ischemic attacks, transient, 418
 causing weakness, 388-389
Ischemic colitis causing hematochezia, 215, 217
Isometric handgrip to enhance cardiac auscultation, 196
Itching
 of eyes, 43, 44
 of skin, 448-449
 vaginal, 295-298

J

Janeway lesions and cardiovascular system abnormalities, 153
"Jar" tenderness of abdomen, 236-237
Jaundice, 221, 223, 237-244
 and cardiovascular system abnormalities, 152
 causing hematuria, 265
 yellow sclerae in, 46
Jaw, trauma to, causing TMJ abnormalities, 356
Jaw jerk, 408
Jendrassik's maneuver, 407
Jerk nystagmus, 49
Joffroy's sign, 507
Joint(s)
 acromioclavicular, arthritis of, 359-360
 auscultation of, 350-351
 deformity of, 349
 disease of, symptoms and signs of, 335
 effusion of, ballottement to determine, 372
 erythema and warmth of, 350
 examination of, 349
 inspection of, 347
 interphalangeal, 364-365
 metacarpophalangeal, 364-365
 pain in, 334, 335-343
 palpation of, 347-350
 septic
  causing arthritis, 339
  causing joint pain, 336, 337
  erythema and, 350
 stiffness in, 343-345
 swelling of, 348-349
 temporomandibular, 356, 357
 tenderness of, 350
 trauma to, causing joint pain, 336, 337
 types of, 347
Jones criteria for rheumatic fever, revised, 341-342
Jugular venous distention, causes of, 96
Jugular venous pressure, 160-162
Jugular venous pulse, 159-164
Jugular venous waves, 162-164
Junctional nevi, 470

Junctional rhythm, jugular venous waves in, 163
Juvenile rheumatoid arthritis, 334
 causing arthritis in several joints, 340

K

Kallmann's syndrome causing amenorrhea, 283
Kaposi's sarcoma, 472
Kartagener's syndrome, 511
 causing male infertility, 271
Kayser-Fleischer rings, 47
Kehr's sign, 507
Keloid, 219, 446
Keratitis, interstitial, 46
Keratoconjunctivitis sicca, 46
Keratoderma blenorrhagia, 334, 367
Keratosis, actinic, 471
Keratotic lesions, 452
Kernig's sign, 423, 507
Kestenbaum's sign, 507
Ketoacidosis, diabetic; see Diabetic ketoacidosis
Kidney
 bruits over, causes of, 228
 chronic disease of, 264
 colic of, 256
 pain from, location of, 202, 203
 cysts of, causing enlarged kidneys, 232
 disease of
  causing fatigue, 143
  and hypertension, 157
 enlarged, causes of, 232
 neoplasms of, causing hematuria, 266
 palpation of, 232-233
 papillary necrosis of, causing abdominal pain, 247
 polycystic disease of, causing enlarged kidneys, 232
 ptotic, 233
 tuberculosis of, causing hematuria, 266
Kidney failure
 acute, causes of, 267
 causing chemosis, 96
 chronic, causing anorexia, 205
 causing Kussmaul respirations, 100
 skin signs associated with, 152
Kimmelstiel-Wilson syndrome, 511
Klebsiella pneumoniae causing consolidated lobar pneumonia, 122
Klinefelter's syndrome, 511
 causing gynecomastia, 331
 causing male infertility, 271
 causing testicular failure, 275
Klippel-Feil syndrome, 511
Knee, 371-373, 374
 range of motion of, 355
Knife wound causing hemoptysis, 77
Knock, pericardial, 181
Knock-knee, 373, 374
Koebner's phenomenon, 468
Koilonychia, 454
Koplik's spots, 465
 on buccal mucosa, 65
Korotkoff sounds, 154, 155, 156

Korsakoff's syndrome, 511
Kussmaul respirations, 99, 100, 141
Kussmaul's sign, 161, 507
Kyphoscoliosis, 101-102, 346
  and cardiovascular system abnormalities, 149
Kyphosis, 101, 346, 366, 367, 368

L

Labia majora, 300, 301
Labia minora, 300, 301
Labyrinthine disorders, vertigo and, 57
Labyrinthine dysfunction, 388
Labyrinthitis
  acute, causing tinnitus, 57
  causing nausea and vomiting, 207
  causing nystagmus, 49
  toxic, vertigo and, 57
Lacrimal ducts, obstructed, causing excessive lacrimation, 44
Lacrimation, excessive, 44
Lactase deficiency causing chronic abdominal pain, 253
Lactic acidosis
  causing dyspnea, 86
  causing hyperpnea, 80
  causing Kussmaul respirations, 100
Lactose intolerance causing diarrhea, 212
Lambert-Eaton syndrome, 511
Language milestones, ages for attainment of, 481
Language problems, medical interview involving, 17
Laparoscopy causing protuberant abdomen, 220
Laryngitis
  causing cough, 73
  causing hoarseness, 64
Laryngotracheobronchitis, acute, history and physical findings in, 114
Larynx, 66
  cancer of, smoking associated with, 92
  edema of, causing wheezing, 87
Lasègue's sign, 369, 507
Late diastolic murmurs, 184
Late systolic ejection murmurs, 183, 184
Late systolic murmur, 514
Lateral sclerosis, amyotrophic
  causing dysphagia, 209
  fasciculations caused by, 395
Latin and Greek roots, 496-505
Laxative abuse causing diarrhea, 212
Lead poisoning, gingival signs of, 65
Leg, ulcers of, 448
Leg elevation, passive, to enhance cardiac auscultation, 196
Legionella pneumonia, 121
Legionella pneumophila
  causing consolidated lobar pneumonia, 122
  sources of, 92
Leiomyofibromas, 311-312
Lentigines, 469
  and cardiovascular system abnormalities, 152

Lentigo, 469
Leriche's syndrome, 511
  causing decreased or absent femoral pulses, 234
  causing male impotence, 270
  pulses associated with, 169
Lesch-Nyhan syndrome, 511
Leukemia
  causing bleeding gums, 63
  causing hemoptysis, 78
  myelogenous, chronic, causing liver enlargement, 231
  causing oral ulcers, 62
  causing pneumonia, 91
  causing retinal hemorrhages, 54
  causing Roth's spots, 54
  causing splenomegaly, 232
Leukoplakia of buccal mucosa and tongue, 65
Leukorhea during pregnancy, 290
Levine's sign, 130, 131
Libido, loss of, in male, 269
Lichen planus, 467, 469
Lichenification, 447, 458
Lid lag, 45
Lifts, 170
Ligament(s)
  Cooper's, 322
  cruciate, examination of, 372, 373
Light, reaction to, testing, 47
Light touch, assessment of, 398-399
Limb, upper, range of motion of, 353-354
Linear lesions, 452
Lip(s), 64-65
  cancer of, pipe smoking associated with, 92
Livedo reticularis, 451
Liver
  alcoholic disease of, 238, 240-241
  bruits over, causes of, 228
  chronic active disease of, causing jaundice, 241-242
  cirrhosis of
    causing ascites, 220-221
    causing atrophic testes, 274
    causing jaundice, 243
  disease of
    causing fatigue, 143
    causing liver enlargement, 231
    palpation indicating, 230-231
    parenchymal, causing anorexia, 205
    yellow sclerae in, 46
  enlarged
    and cardiovascular system abnormalities, 152-153
    causes of, 231
  fatty, causing jaundice, 240
  metastatic disease of, causing jaundice, 244
  palpation of, 229, 230-231
  percussion of, 225
  referred pain from, 203
Lobar pneumococcal pneumonia causing hemoptysis, 75

Lobar pneumonia
  consolidated, 121-122
  causing dullness to percussion, 107
Löffler's syndrome, 511
Lordosis, 102, 346, 367
Loud noise causing tinnitus, 57
Lower abdominal reflexes, 408
Lower extremities, assessment of strength of, 394
Lumbosacral strain, 367-368
Lump, breast, 316-320
Lung
  abscess of
    causing halitosis, 93
    causing hemoptysis, 76
    causing sputum production, 74
  anaerobic abscess of, causing fecal breath odor, 95
  cancer of, 114, 118
    causing dilated chest veins, 96
    causing hemoptysis, 77
    causing Horner's syndrome, 96
    smoking associated with, 92
  carcinoma of
    causing chest pain, 79
    causing dysphagia, 209
  of child, examination of, 491
  disease of, 71, 91, 93-95
    causing dyspnea, 139
    interstitial, causing cough, 73
    causing jugular venous distention, 96
  infarction of, causing delayed chest movement, 102
  lobes of, anatomy of, 98
  problems with, past history of, 90-92
  uncommon diseases of, with hereditary component, 94
Lupus erythematosus, 96
  and cardiovascular system abnormalities, 150
  discoid, 460
  causing retinal artery occlusion, 55
  causing scleritis, 46
  systemic, 334, 344, 380-381, 459-460
    causing arthritis, 340
    causing dysphagia, 209
    causing retinal hemorrhages, 54
    causing uveitis, 41
    skin lesions found in, 460
Lyme disease, 380-381
Lymph nodes, 66-67
  axillary, enlarged, 330
  enlargement of, associated with intrathoracic disease, 96
  supraclavicular, causes of, 96
Lymphangiectasia, intestinal, causing chylous ascites, 221
Lymphatic network draining breast, 319
Lymphatic obstruction causing edema, 148
Lymphogranuloma venereum causing penile ulcers, 268, 272
Lymphoma
  causing dysphagia, 209

Lymphoma—cont'd
  intraabdominal, causing chylous ascites, 221
  causing liver enlargement, 231
  rectal mass associated with, 234
  causing splenomegaly, 232
  causing supraclavicular lymph nodes, 96

M

Machinery murmur, 514
Macroglossia, 65
Macula
  degeneration of, 54
    causing loss of vision, 42
  disease of, causing Marcus Gunn response, 48
  funduscopic examination of, 54
Macules, 444, 464-466
  in child, 486
  diseases manifesting, 455
Maculopapular diseases, 464-466
Major depression, 428-429
Mal perforans ulcers of soles of feet, 375
Malabsorption causing polyphagia, 205
Malabsorption syndrome, 511
Malabsorptive disease causing diarrhea, 212
Male, breast of, examination of, 331-332
Male genitalia, 262-279
Malignancy causing genital ulcers, 311
Malignant breast tumors, 331
Malignant hypertension causing papilledema, 54
Malignant melanoma, 470-471
Mallory-Weiss syndrome, 511
Mallory-Weiss tear at cardioesophageal junction causing hematemesis, 214
Mammary souffle, 191
Mammography, 331
Manic episodes, 430
Marcus Gunn pupil, 47-48
Marcus Gunn's pupillary sign, 507
Marfan syndrome, 102, 149, 150, 151, 511
Marijuana smoke, effects of, 92
Maroon-colored stools, causes of, 217
Mass lesions causing eye pain, 43
Mastectomy, breast examination after, 331
Mastitis, plasma cell, causing dimpling of breast, 322
Maternal infection causing hearing loss in child, 57
Maxillary sinusitis, 60
Maximal impulse, point of, 170, 171
Measles, 463-465
  skin lesions associated with, 455
Meatus, inflammation of, causing dysuria, 263
Mechanical intestinal obstruction, 255
Meckel's diverticulum causing maroon-colored stools, 217

Mediastinal emphysema causing chest pain, 135
Mediastinal tumors, causing hoarseness, 64
Medical history, past, 12-13
  format for recording, 31
Medical interview
  components of, 11-13
  ending, 10
  in geriatrics, 16-17
  information from, format for recording, 31-37
  initiation of, 5-6
  language problems during, 17
  in pediatrics, 15-16
  and physical examination, 1-37
  during pregnancy, 16
  preparation for, 4-5
  review of identifying data before, 3-4
  in special situations, 13-20
  techniques for, 2-10
Mees' lines, 452, 454
Meeting with patient, preparing for, 2
Megacolon, aganglionic, causing constipation, 213
Meigs' syndrome, 511
Melanin spots
  on buccal mucosa, 65
  on lips, 64
Melena, 214-218
  malignant, 470-471
  causing optic nerve compression, 41
  rectal mass associated with, 234
Melioidosis, 121
Membrane(s)
  mucous
    inflammation of, causing cough, 73
    lesions involving, 454
  tympanic, examination of, 58, 59
Memory, assessment of, 416
Menarche, 282
Mendelian disorders, frequent, 517
Ménière's disease
  hearing changes associated with, 57, 388
  causing nystagmus, 49
  vertigo and, 57
Ménière's syndrome causing nausea and vomiting, 207
Menigitis, headache associated with, 384
Meningeal headache, 384
Meningeal irritation, signs of, approach to patient with, 423
Meningioma
  MRI of, 420
  causing optic nerve compression, 41
Meningismus, 384
Meningitis, 424
  bacterial, causing hearing loss in child, 57
  affecting breathing, 100
  causing cervical spine abnormalities, 357
  causing eye pain, 43
  causing nausea and vomiting, 207

Meningitis—cont'd
  causing papilledema, 54
Meningococcemia, 466
  petechiae in, 463
  skin lesions associated with, 455
Menopause, 282, 285-286
Menorrhagia, 282, 285
Menstrual bleeding, abnormal, 285
Menstruation, abnormalities of, 282-285
Mental status examination, 414, 415-420
Meperidine causing nausea and vomiting, 207
Mesenteric cysts, abdominal masses with, 233
Mesenteric thrombosis
  absent bowel sounds with, 227
  causing ecchymoses, 223
Mesenteric vascular occlusion, acute, causing acute abdominal pain, 259
Metabolic acidosis
  causing dyspnea, 86
  causing hyperpnea, 80
  causing Kussmaul respirations, 100
Metabolic diseases
  causing dyspnea, 85-86
  fatigue with, 345
Metacarpophalangeal joints, 364-365
Metamorphopsia, 44
Metastatic bone tumor and cough-induced rib fracture, 73
Metastatic liver disease causing jaundice, 244
Metatarsus varus, 493
Methadone causing male impotence, 270
Methemoglobinemia
  causing cyanosis, 148
  resembling cyanosis, 90
Methyl alcohol causing optic neuropathy, 42
Methyl alcohol intoxication causing scotomata, 44
Methyldopa
  causing galactorrhea, 324
  causing male impotence, 270
Metoclopramide causing male impotence, 270
Metronidazole
  causing anorexia, 205
  causing dysgeusia, 63
  causing glossitis, 65
  causing hematuria, 265
Metrorrhagia, 285
Mettelschmerz, 288
Microaneurysms, retinal, 54
Microtia, 58
Micturition syncope, 146
Midbrain lesions, 48, 50
Middiastolic murmurs, 184, 193-194, 515
Middle cerebral thrombosis, 417, 419
Middle ear disease, vertigo and, 57
Middle lobe syndrome, 511
Midsystolic ejection murmurs, 183

Migraine causing eye pain, 43
Migraine headache, 384
    causing loss of vision, 40
Migratory arthralgia, 337
Migratory joint pain, 334
Mikulicz's syndrome, 512
Milia, 447
Miliaria, 458
Miliaria crystallina, 458
Miliaria rubra, 458
Milk line and supernumerary nipples, 322-323
Mineral deficiencies, 63, 65
Miosis
    in Horner's syndrome, 96
    of pupils, 48
Miscarriage, 291
    causing pelvic pain, 288
Mitral regurgitation
    associated with Ehlers-Danlos syndrome, 149
    causing dyspnea, 137
    heart murmurs associated with, 184, 185
    heart sounds in, 179
    holosystolic murmurs associated with, 189-190
    systolic murmurs associated with, 187
Mitral stenosis
    causing dysphagia, 209
    causing dyspnea, 137
    flushed cheeks associated with, 151
    heart murmurs associated with, 184, 185
    causing hemoptysis, 78
    middiastolic murmurs associated with, 193
    opening snap of, 180, 181
    causing pulsatile liver, 231
Mitral valve disease, precordial pulsations associated with, 170
Mitral valve prolapse
    causing chest pain, 127, 133-134
    causing syncope, 145-146
    systolic clicks with, 181
    systolic murmurs associated with, 187, 188-189
    thoracic signs associated with, 152
Mitral valve stenosis causing hemoptysis, 147
Mixed connective-tissue disease causing arthritis, 340
Mixed sensory and motor neuropathy, common causes of, 419
Möbius' sign, 507
Mole(s), 469-470
    hydatidiform, 291
Molluscum contagiosum, 477
Mondor's disease of breast, 322, 328
Monilial infections causing sore throat, 63
Monoarticular arthralgia, 337
Monocular blindness, complete, 51
Monocular diplopia, 42
Monocular loss of vision, 39

Mononeuritis multiplex, 423
Mononucleosis, infectious
    causing pharyngitis, 66
    causing sore throat, 63
    mouth signs associated with, 151
Mood
    assessment of, 416
        in psychiatric interview, 427
    changes in, 390
Morning sickness, 290
Moro reflex, 494
Morphine causing chronic gastric retention and delayed gastric emptying, 207
Morton's neuroma, 375
Motility, ocular, and extraocular movements, 48-50
Motion, range of, 352-356
Motor functions, examination of, 391-396
Motor milestones, ages for attainment of, 481
Motor neuropathy, common causes of, 419
Mouth, 62-67
    and cardiovascular system abnormalities, 151-152
    of child, examination of, 489
    necrotic lesions of, causing halitosis, 93
    questions related to, 27
Mucosa, buccal, 64-65
Mucous membranes
    inflammation of, causing cough, 73
    lesions involving, 454
Mucus plugging
    causing absent breath sounds, 109
    causing atelectasis, 105
Müller's maneuver to enhance cardiac auscultation, 195
Multiforme lesions, 452
Multiple lumps in breast, 319-320
Multiple sclerosis, 418
    causing anorexia, 205
    changes in vision associated with, 388
    causing chronic gastric retention and delayed gastric emptying, 206
    causing dysphagia, 209
    causing intention tremor, 402
    causing nystagmus, 49
    causing optic atrophy, 52
    causing optic neuropathy, 42
    causing retrobulbar optic neuritis, 41
Mumps causing parotid enlargement, 65
Munchausen syndrome, 512
Murmurs, 514-515
    heart, 182-197
Murphy's sign, 232
Muscle(s)
    abdominal, rigidity of, 236
    extraocular, innervations and actions of, 49
    functions of, abnormal, assessment of, 392, 395-396
    infarction of, causing ecchymoses, 223

Muscle(s)—cont'd
    orbicularis oculi, paralysis of, causing failure of eyelids to close, 45
    overall function of, 356
    strength of, 351-352
        assessment of, 391-394
    tone of, assessment of, 392, 395
    weakness of, 351-352
Musculoskeletal disorders, terms applied to, 346
Musculoskeletal pain, 335-343
Musculoskeletal system, 333-381
    of child, examination of, 493
Musical murmur, 515
Musset's sign and aortic regurgitation, 192
Myasthenia gravis
    causing dysphagia, 209
    causing ptosis, 44
    causing weakness, 388
Mycobacterium tuberculosis, sources of, 92
Mycoplasma pneumonia, 121
Mycoplasma pneumoniae
    causing cough, 73
    infections of, causing bullous myringitis, 56, 58
    causing pneumonia, 122
Mydriasis, 48
Myelofibrosis, 231, 232
Myelogenous leukemia, chronic, causing liver enlargement, 231
Myocardial hypertrophy, heart sounds in, 179
Myocardial infarction
    causing chest pain, 127, 133
    heart sounds in, 177
    causing nausea and vomiting, 207
Myocardial ischemia, 129-133, 146
Myocarditis, heart sounds in, 177
Myochosis, 233
Myoglobinuria, causes of, 265
Myotonia dystrophica and cardiovascular system abnormalities, 149, 150
Myringitis, bullous, 58
    Mycoplasma pneumoniae infections causing, 56, 58
Myxedema
    and cardiovascular system abnormalities, 150
    causing dysphagia, 209
    causing nausea and vomiting, 207
Myxoma, atrial
    eye signs associated with, 151
    causing syncope, 146

N

Nails
    changes in, 449
    lesions associated with, 453-453
    pits in, 452, 454
    splinter hemorrhages under, and cardiovascular system abnormalities, 153
Narcotics causing miosis, 48

Nares, examination of, 60-61
Nasal discharge, 60, 90
Nasal hemianopsia, 52
Nasal polyps, 60-61
Nasal septum, examination of, 60-61
Nasal turbinates, examination of, 60-61
Nausea
  as sign of pregnancy, 289-290
  and vomiting, 205-208
Neck, 66-67
  of child, examination of, 68, 487-489, 490
  and head, 38-69
  physical examination of, 66-67
    giving clues to pulmonary disease, 96
  questions related to, 27
  range of motion of, 355
Necrolysis, epidermal, toxic, 465, 474
Necrosis, fat, causing dimpling of breast, 322
Necrotic lesions of mouth or throat causing halitosis, 93
Neisseria gonorrheae, 464, 466
Neisseria meningitidis, 463, 466
Neoplasia, trophoblastic, gestational, 291
Neoplasms
  bladder, causing hematuria, 266
  cervical, causing nonmenstrual vaginal bleeding, 286
  endometrial, causing nonmenstrual vaginal bleeding, 286
  causing hemoptysis, 77
  kidney, causing hematuria, 266
  causing protuberant abdomen, 219
  testicular, 275
Neoplastic disorders causing anorexia, 205
Nephropathy, analgesic, causing abdominal pain, 247
Nephrotic syndromes causing scrotal swelling, 269
Nerve(s)
  cranial, palsies of, 48, 49-50
  cutaneous, 397
  oculomotor, lesion of, causing absent consensual response to light, 47
  optic; see Optic nerve
  sympathetic, cervical, 48
Nervi erigentes, diseases of, causing male impotence, 270
Nervousness causing polyphagia, 205
Neuralgia, trigeminal, causing external otitis, 56
Neuritis
  optic, retrobulbar, causing loss of vision, 41
  retrobulbar, 388
  sciatic, 368
Neurocirculatory asthenia causing chest pain, 136
Neurodermatitis, 449
Neurofibromatosis, 444
  and cardiovascular system abnormalities, 152

Neurogenic bladder causing urinary incontinence, 265
Neurologic diseases
  causing dyspnea, 86
  causing fatigue, 143
  causing male impotence, 270
Neurologic examination, 382-425
  of child, examination of, 493
  essentials of, 391-420
  history taking associated with, 383-391
Neurologic impairment causing delayed chest movement, 102
Neurologic problems, common, recognition of, 417-420
Neuroma, Morton's, 375
Neuropathic joint disease causing joint pain, 337
Neuropathy(ies)
  diabetic, causing syncope, 146
  optic, causing loss of vision, 42
  peripheral, 389, 418-419
    approach to patient with, 423
    skin ulcers in, 448
Nevus(i), 469-470
Newborn, cyanosis in, 149
Niacin deficiency, 65
Night sweats, 92
Nikolsky's sign, 507
Nipples, 322-325, 330
Nocturia, 263, 264
Nocturnal dyspnea, paroxysmal, 80, 84, 139-140
Nodes
  Bouchard's, 365
  Heberden's, 334, 349, 365, 366
  Osler's, and cardiovascular system abnormalities, 153
Nodular melanoma, 471
Nodule, 445
  rheumatoid, 349
  subcutaneous, rheumatic fever associated with, 152
Nongonococcal urethritis causing penile pain, 266
Nonmenstrual vaginal bleeding, 286-287
Nonpalpable purpura, 463
Nonparalytic strabismus, 48
Nonproductive cough, 73
Nonsteroidal antiinflammatory drugs causing nausea and vomiting, 207
Nonsuppurative parotitis, 65
Nontoxic thyromegaly causing thyroid enlargement, 67
Nose, 60-62
  of child, examination of, 489
  questions related to, 26
Nose drops, chronic use of, causing nasal discharge, 60
Noxious fumes, inhalation of, causing hemoptysis, 77
Noxious gases, inhalation of, causing cough, 73

Nucleus, Edinger-Westphal, lesion of, causing absent consensual response to light, 47
Nucleus pulposus, herniated, 368
Numbness, causes of, 389
Nutrition, parenteral, total, causing anorexia, 205
Nystagmus, 48-49

O

Obesity
  and blood pressure measurement, 156-157
  heart sounds in, 172
  causing protuberant abdomen, 219
  striae in, 219
Objective vertigo, 57
Obsessive/compulsive disorder, 432, 433
Obstruction, intestinal, mechanical, 255
Obstructive airway disease causing orthopnea, 80
Obstructive pulmonary disease, chronic
  causing chemosis, 96
  causing cough, 73
  causing dilated chest veins, 96
  causing dyspnea, 80, 139
  heart sounds in, 172
  causing prolonged exhalation, 97
  causing wheezing, 87
Obturator hernia, 223, 224
Occlusion
  central retinal artery, causing loss of vision, 41
  mesenteric vascular, acute, causing acute abdominal pain, 259
Occupational asthma, 112; *see also* Asthma
Ocular discharge, 44
Ocular motility and extraocular movements, 48-50
Oculomotor nerve
  lesion of, causing absent consensual response to light, 47
  testing of, 411
Odynophagia, 208
Olecranon bursitis, 362
Olfactory nerve, testing of, 410
Oligomenorrhea, 282
Oligospermia, 269
Oliguria, 266
Oliver's sign, 104
Onycholysis, 452, 462
Onychomycosis, 462
Open drawer sign, 372
Open-ended questions, 8-9
Opening snap of mitral stenosis, 180, 181
Opiates
  causing chronic gastric retention and delayed gastric emptying, 207
  causing galactorrhea, 324
  causing nausea and vomiting, 207
Oppenheim's sign, 409
Optic atrophy, 52

Optic atrophy—cont'd
  hereditary, causing optic neuropathy, 42
Optic nerve
  compression of, by mass lesion causing loss of vision, 41
  degeneration of, causing lack of pupillary reaction to light, 47
  disease of, 44, 48
  lesions of, 51, 52
  testing of, 411
Optic nerve head, funduscopic examination of, 52, 53
Optic neuritis, retrobulbar, causing loss of vision, 41
Optic neuropathies causing loss of vision, 42
Optic tract lesion causing homonymous hemianopsia, 52
Oral contraceptives
  causing amenorrhea, 284
  and breast cancer, 325
  causing candidal vaginitis, 296
  and hypertension, 157
Oral infections causing increased salivation, 65
Oral thrush, 462
Orbicularis oculi muscles, paralysis of, causing failure of eyelids to close, 45
Orbicularis oculi reflex, 408
Orbital tumor causing exophthalmos, 46
Orchitis, 271, 274
Organic brain syndrome, patients with, medical interview of, 18
Organomegaly causing protuberant abdomen, 219
Orgasm, inhibitin of, 293
Orientation, assessment of, 415
Ornithosis, 121
Orthopnea, 80, 139
Orthostatic hypotension, 156
Osgood-Schlatter disease, 372
Osler's maneuver, 156
Osler's nodes and cardiovascular system abnormalities, 153
Osler's sign, 507
Osler-Weber-Rendu disease causing telangiectasia of lip, 64
Osteoarthritis, 334, 343, 348, 378-379
  fingers affected by, 349
  causing joint pain, 336
Osteogenesis imperfecta
  blue sclerae in, 46
  and cardiovascular system abnormalities, 150
  eye signs associated with, 151
Osteomyelitis causing joint pain, 336
Osteoporosis and cough-induced rib fracture, 73
Otitis, external, causes of, 56
Otitis media, 56
  acute, 489
  suppurative, chronic, causing hearing loss in child, 57

Otosclerosis causing hearing loss, 57
Ototoxic drugs causing hearing loss, 57
Ovarian failure, premature, causing amenorrhea, 285
Ovary
  cyst of
    abdominal masses with, 233, 234
    bleeding from, causing pelvic pain, 288
    twisted, causing acute abdominal pain, 257
  torsion of, causing pelvic pain, 288
Overtalkative behavior of patient, 14

P

P_2 shock, 170
Pacemaker, cardiac, jugular venous waves with, 163, 164
Paget disease of breast, 324, 328
Pain
  abdominal; see Abdomen, pain in
  abdominal wall, anterior, 256
  breast, 320, 322
  chest; see Chest pain
  ear, 56
  eye, 43-44
  facial, and chronic sinusitis, 60
  inguinal, and testicular mass, 272
  joint; see Joint pain
  musculoskeletal, 335-343
  pelvic, in female, 287-289, 314
  penile, 266, 268
  referred, 336
  severity of, patient assessment of, 203
  shoulder, 359
  testicular, 269, 271
  testing, 396
Palate, 64-65
  and cardiovascular system abnormalities, 151
  cleft, 489
Palmar grasp reflex, 494
Palmomental sign, 410
Palms, lesions involving, 454
Palpable purpura, 463
Palpation of chest, 104-106
Palpitations, 141-143
Palsy
  Bell's, causing failure of eyelids to close, 45
  cranial nerve, 448, 49-50
  gaze, 49
  pseudobulbar, causing dysphagia, 209
  third nerve, 50
Pancoast's syndrome, 512
Pancreas
  cancer of, 229, 252-253
  carcinoma of,
    causing chronic gastric retention and delayed gastric emptying, 206
    causing distension of gallbladder, 232
    causing jaundice, 243
  enlarged, 233
  referred pain from, 203

Pancreas—cont'd
  tumors of
    or cyst or pseudocyst of, aortic pulsation with, 233
    causing pyloric outlet obstruction, 228
Pancreatic exocrine insufficiency causing polyphagia, 205
Pancreatitis
  absent bowel sounds with, 227
  causing abdominal pain, 247
  acute, 250
  chronic, causing chronic abdominal pain, 252
  causing ecchymoses, 223
  causing pleuritic chest pain, 91
  causing pyloric outlet obstruction, 228
Panic disorders, 432
Pansystolic murmur, 189, 515
Papanicolaou smear, 306-308
Papillary necrosis, renal, causing abdominal pain, 247
Papilledema, 54
Papillitis, 54-55
Papules, 445, 464-466
  in child, 487
  diseases manifesting, 456
  Gottron's, 461
  satellite, 462
Papulosquamous disease, 464, 466-469
Papulosquamous lesions, 452
Para, 281
Paradoxic split S_2, 178
Paragonimus westermani, 121
Paralysis, 388-389
  of cervical sympathetic nerves causing miosis, 48
  diaphragmatic, causing orthopnea, 80
  of orbicularis oculi muscles causing failure of eyelids to close, 45
Paralytic ileus causing protuberant abdomen, 220
Paranoia in patient, 14
Paraphimosis, 273
Parasternal lift, 170
Parathyroid surgery causing hoarseness, 64
Paraurethral glands, 301
Paravertebral muscle prominence, 101
Parenchymal liver disease causing anorexia, 205
Parenteral nutrition, total, causing anorexia, 205
Paresthesia, causes of, 388, 389
Parkinson's disease, 418
Parkinsonism, 403
  causing anorexia, 205
  causing dysphagia, 209
  gait with, 404
  muscle tone in, 395
  tremors associated with, 395
Paronychia, 476
Parotid glands, physical examination of, 65

Parotid tumors causing parotid enlargement, 65
Parotitis, 65
Paroxysmal atrial fibrillation, 142
Paroxysmal atrial tachycardia, 142
Paroxysmal nocturnal dyspnea, 80, 84, 139-140
Passive leg elevation to enhance cardiac auscultation, 196
Passive range of motion, 352
Past medical history, 12-13
 format for recording, 31
Pastia's sign, 507
Patchy alopecia, 449, 462
Patella, ballottement of, 349
Patellar reflex, 406
Patent ductus arteriosus, heart murmurs associated with, 194
Patient(s)
 behavior of, posing problems for physicians, 14
 clinician responses and message conveyed to, 20
 general appearance of, questions related to, 26
 identifying data for, format for recording, 31
 preparing to meet, 2
 special, medical interview of, 15-20
Peau d'orange appearance of breast, 328
Pectoriloquy, whispered, 110
Pectus carinatum, 102, 103
Pectus excavatum, 102, 103
Pedal edema, 147
Pedersen speculum, 303
Pediatric patient, 480-495
 descriptive measurements of, 482
 growth patterns of, 483-485
 history taking related to, 480-481
 physical examination of, 482-494
Pediatrics, medical interview in, 15-16
Pelvic examination of woman, 309-314
 position for, 299
Pelvic floor relaxation, 302
Pelvic inflammatory disease
 causing acute abdominal pain, 257
 causing dysmenorrhea, 286
 causing menorrhagia, 285
 causing pelvic pain, 288-289
Pelvic masses, causes of, 313
Pelvic pain, 287-289, 314
Pelvic relaxation, 298
Pelvic veins, thrombosis of, causing scrotal swelling, 271
Pelvis, abscess of, rectal mass associated with, 234
Pemphigoid
 bullous, 474-475
 causing genital ulcers, 311
Pemphigus causing genital ulcers, 311
Pemphigus vulgaris, 474
Pendular nystagmus, 49
Penis, 272-273, 274
 carcinoma of, 268

Penis—cont'd
 diseases of, causing male impotence, 270
 pain, ulcers, and discharge associated with, 266, 268
 trauma to, causing male impotence, 270
Peptic ulcer, perforated, 255
Peptic ulcer disease
 causing chronic abdominal pain, 249
 causing hematemesis, 214
 causing maroon-colored stools, 217
 causing nausea and vomiting, 207
 pain associated with, 200
 with pyloric obstruction, 204
 causing pyloric outlet obstruction, 228
Perceptive hearing loss, 56
Percussion sounds, 107
Perforated nasal septum, 60
Perforated peptic ulcer, 255
Perforated viscera causing protuberant abdomen, 220
Periarticular swellings, 349
Pericardial disease, arterial pulse volume in, 168
Pericardial effusion
 arterial pulse volume in, 168
 associated with myxedema, 150
 pericardial friction rubs associated with, 182
Pericardial friction rubs, 181-182
Pericardial knock, 181
Pericarditis
 causing chest pain, 79, 128, 134
 constrictive
  arterial pulse volume in, 168
  pericardial knock associated with, 181
 eye signs associated with, 151
 pericardial friction rubs associated with, 182
 skin signs associated with, 152
Pericolic abscess, abdominal masses with, 233
Perimenopause, 285
Periodontal disease, 65
 causing bleeding gums, 63
Peripheral cyanosis, 89, 148
Peripheral neuropathy, 418-419
 approach to patient with, 423
 differential diagnosis of, 389
 skin ulcers in, 448
Peripheral vascular disease causing decreased or absent femoral pulses, 234
Perirectal abscess, rectal mass associated with, 234
Peristalsis, visible, 219
Peristaltic sounds, auscultation for, 227-228
Peritoneal cavity, free air in, causing protuberant abdomen, 219, 220
Peritoneal friction rubs, 229
Peritoneal irritation, abdominal tenderness associated with, 236-237

Peritonitis, absent bowel sounds with, 227
Peritonsillar abscess, 66
 causing sore throat, 63
Periungual telangiectasia, 448, 454
Pernicious anemia, 54, 65
Persistently split S_2, 178
Pertussis, cough caused by, 73
Pes cavus, 375, 376
Pes planus, 375, 376
Petechia, 28, 447, 263-264
 of conjunctiva, 45
  associated with bacterial endocarditis, 151
 from coughing, 73
 diseases manifesting, 455
 of soft palate, and cardiovascular system abnormalities, 151
Petit mal seizures, 387
Peutz-Jeghers syndrome, 512
 causing melanin spots on lips, 64
Peyronie's disease, 272, 273
 causing male impotence, 270
Phalen's test, 364
Pharyngeal lesions, ear pain caused by, 56
Pharyngitis
 bacterial, causing sore throat, 63
 exudative, causing halitosis, 93
 streptococcal, 66, 151
Pharynx, 66
 of child, examination of, 490
Phenothiazines causing male impotence, 270
Phenytoin
 affecting the mouth, 63, 65
 causing nystagmus, 49
Pheochromocytoma and von Recklinghausen's disease, 152
Phimosis, 268, 273
Phlegm, 74-75
Photophobia, 43, 44
Photosensitivity, rash of, 465
Physical examination
 as active process, 21, 28
 ending, 10
 information from, format for recording, 31-37
 medical interview and, 1-37
 of respiratory system, 92-111
 techniques for performing, 29-30
Physician(s)
 dress appropriate for, 2
 patient behavior posing problems for, 14
Physiologic dyspnea, 137
Pickwickian syndrome, 512
Pigeon-chest deformity, 102, 103
Pilonidal dimple, 492
Pingueculae, 47
Pinprick sensation, evaluation of, 396, 397
Pipe smoking, 92
Pits in nails, 452, 454

Pituitary disease causing amenorrhea, 284-285
Pituitary disorders causing male infertility, 271
Pituitary gonadotropic failure causing small testes, 274-275
Pituitary tumor causing bitemporal hemianopsia, 51
Pityriasis rosea, 451, 453, 467, 468-469
Pivot joint, 347
Plane joint, 347
Plantar tendinitis, 375
Plantar warts, 476
Plaque, 445
Plasma cell mastitis causing dimpling of breast, 322
Plateau shaped murmur, 185
Pleura, tumor of, causing pleural friction rub, 109
Pleural disease causing chest pain, 79
Pleural effusion, 115, 119
   causing absent breath sounds, 109
   causing cough, 73
   causing decreased fremitus, 106
   examination techniques to determine, 110
   causing flatness to percussion, 107
   causing pleural friction rub, 109-110
   causing tracheal shift, 105
Pleural fluid
   causing dullness to percussion, 107
   rapid removal of, causing syncope, 146
Pleural friction rub, causes of, 109-110
Pleural infarction causing pleural friction rub, 109
Pleural thickening causing decreased fremitus, 106
Pleurisy
   acute, causing chest pain, 128
   causing chest pain, 134
   causing delayed chest movement, 102
   friction rub in, 104
Pleuritic chest pain, 79
   history of, 90, 91
Pleuritic pain, location of, 202
Plummer-Vinson syndrome, 512
PMI; see Point of maximal impulse
Pneumatosis cystoides intestinalis causing protuberant abdomen, 220
Pneumaturia, 266
Pneumococcal pneumonia, 121
   lobar, causing hemoptysis, 75
Pneumocystis carinii pneumonia, 121
Pneumonia, 117, 120-122
   absent bowel sounds with, 227
   causing chest pain, 79
   causing Cheyne-Stokes respiration, 100
   consolidation in, examination techniques to determine, 110
   cough caused by, 73
   causing delayed chest movement, 102
   causing dyspnea, 82
   causing flatness to percussion, 107
   causing fremitus, 106

Pneumonia—cont'd
   causing hemoptysis, 76
   history of, 90, 91
   infant with, 92
   lobar, causing dullness to percussion, 107
   causing pleural friction rub, 109
   pneumococcal, lobar, causing hemoptysis, 75
   causing sputum production, 74
   zoster, 96
Pneumoperitoneum causing protuberant abdomen, 220
Pneumothorax, 105, 116, 119
   causing absent breath sounds, 109
   causing chest pain, 128, 135
   causing decreased fremitus, 106
   causing dyspnea, 83, 139
   examination techniques to determine, 110
   causing hyperresonance, 106
   tension, 105
Podagra, 334
   gouty, 375, 376
Point of maximal impulse, 170, 171
Poison ivy, 451, 475
Poisoning
   carbon monoxide, causing dyspnea, 85
   food, causing nausea and vomiting, 207
   lead or bismuth, gingival signs of, 65
Poliomyelitis
   bulbar
     causing chronic gastric retention and delayed gastric emptying, 206
     causing dysphagia, 209
   causing dysphagia, 209
Pollution-induced asthma, 112; see also Asthma
Polyarticular arthralgia, 337
Polychondritis, relapsing, auricular inflammation caused by, 58
Polycystic kidney disease causing enlarged kidneys, 232
Polycythemia rubra vera causing retinal vein occlusion, 55
Polydipsia, psychogenic, 264
Polymyalgia rheumatica, 334
Polymyositis, 461
   and cardiovascular system abnormalities, 150
Polyphagia, 205
Polyps
   colonic, causing hematochezia, 215, 216
   nasal, 60-61
   causing nonmenstrual vaginal bleeding, 287
   uterine, 285, 286
   vocal cord, causing hoarseness, 64
Polyuria, 264
Popliteal pulse, palpation of, 165-166
Porcine heart valve, sounds associated with, 182
Porphobilinogenuria, 265

Portal hypertension
   dilated abdominal veins in, 219
   causing splenomegaly, 232
Position sense, testing, 399
Positional vertigo, benign, 57
Positive Romberg sign, 404
Posterior tibial pulse, palpation of, 165
Postmenopausal bleeding, 286-287
Postpill amenorrhea, 284
Postrubella syndrome, 512
Posttussive syncope, 146
Pott's disease causing gibbus, 102
Practical skills, assessment of, 416
Prader-Willi syndrome, 486, 512
Precordial pulsations and shocks, 170
Precordium, 169-171
Prediverticular disease causing diarrhea, 212
Preeclampsia, 291
Pregnancy
   causing amenorrhea, 284
   causing anorexia, 205
   causing breast striae, 328
   causing candidal vaginitis, 296
   ectopic, ruptured, causing acute abdominal pain, 257
   high-risk, 290-291
   medical interview during, 16
   causing nausea and vomiting, 207
   normal, 289-290
   causing protuberant abdomen, 219
   tubal, ruptured, causing pelvic pain, 288
   causing vaginal bleeding, 286
Preinfarction angina, 131
Premature atrial contractions, 164, 166, 167
ture contractions, 166, 167
Premature ovarian failure causing amenorrhea, 285
Premature ventricular contractions, 163, 166, 167
Premenstrual syndrome, 286, 287, 512
Presbycusis causing hearing loss, 57
Presbyopia, 42
Present illness, history of, 11-12
   format for recording, 31
Pressure
   blood, questions related to, 26
   intraocular, increased, 42, 43
Presystolic murmurs, 184, 515
Priapism, 268, 270
Primitive reflexes, 410
Prinzmetal's angina, 127, 132-133
Proctitis, infectious, causing hematochezia, 215, 217
Productive cough, 74
Projectile vomiting, 208
Projection, patient demonstration of, 15
Prolapse, uterine, 298
Proliferative diabetic retinopathy, 41, 54
Pronation, 346
Propranolol causing male impotence, 270
Proptosis, 46

Prostate, 275-276
  cancer of, 263
Prostatectomy, complete, causing male impotence, 270
Prostatic hypertrophy, benign, 263, 264, 265
  causing abdominal pain, 247
  and changes in voiding pattern, 266
Prostatism, changes in voiding pattern and, 266
Prostatitis, 263, 276
Prosthetic heart valves and blood pressure measurement, 156
Prosthetic valve sounds, 182
Protein loss causing edema, 148
Protozoal infections causing nausea and vomiting, 207
Protuberant abdomen, causes of, 219-221
Proverbs, ability to handle, assessment of, 416
Pruritus, 448-449, 458, 472-473
Pruritus ani, 449
Pruritus vulvae, 449
Pseudobulbar palsy causing dysphagia, 209
Pseudocyesis, 220
Pseudocyst, pancreatic or gastric, aortic pulsation with, 233
Pseudogout, 378-379
  causing arthritis, 339, 341
Pseudopregnancy, 220
Pseudotumor cerebri causing papilledema, 54
Pseudoxanthoma elasticum
  angioid streaks in, 55
  and cardiovascular system abnormalities, 150
Psittacosis, 121
Psoriasis, 453, 467, 468
  and psoriatic arthritis, 335
Psoriatic arthritis, 335, 340, 366, 378-379
Psoriatic spondylitis causing sacroiliac arthritis, 369
Psychiatric disorders, common, 428-440
Psychiatric examination, 426-441
Psychiatric interview, 427-428
Psychiatric patients, medical interview of, 17
Psychogenic amenorrhea, 284
Psychogenic cough, 73
Psychogenic polydipsia, 264
Psychologic fatigue, 143
Psychotropic drugs causing male impotence, 270
Ptosis, 44-45
  and cardiovascular system abnormalities, 151
  unilateral, in Horner's syndrome, 96
Ptotic kidney, 233
Pubic hair, changes in, in female, 300
Puddle sign, 226-227, 508
Puffiness of face and cardiovascular system abnormalities, 150-151

Pulmonary arteriovenous fistulas, extremity signs associated with, 153
Pulmonary consolidation causing flatness to percussion, 107
Pulmonary disease, 71
  chronic obstructive, causing dyspnea, 81-83; *see also* Obstructive pulmonary disease, chronic
Pulmonary edema, 120
  causing dyspnea, 84, 140
  causing hemoptysis, 147
  causing sputum production, 74
Pulmonary emboli
  causing chest pain, 79
  causing cough, 73
  causing dyspnea, 82
  causing hemoptysis, 147
Pulmonary embolism, 116
  causing chest pain, 128, 134
  causing dyspnea, 139
  predisposing factors for, 134
Pulmonary fibrosis
  affecting chest expansion, 102
  cough caused by, 73
  after pneumonia, 91
Pulmonary hypertension, 120
  causing chest pain, 128, 135
  causing dyspnea, 138
  jugular venous waves in, 162, 163
  precordial pulsations associated with, 170
  primary, causing hemoptysis, 78
  and Raynaud's phenomenon, 153
Pulmonary infarctions, skin signs associated with, 152
Pulmonary oxygenation, inadequate, causing cyanosis, 148
Pulmonary stenosis, eye signs associated with, 151
Pulmonary thromboembolism causing hemoptysis, 77
Pulmonic regurgitation
  diastolic murmurs associated with, 192-193
  heart murmurs associated with, 184
Pulmonic stenosis
  heart murmurs associated with, 184
  heart sounds in, 179
  jugular venous waves in, 162, 163
  skin signs associated with, 152
  systolic murmurs associated with, 187, 188
Pulmonic valve shock, 170
Pulsatile liver, 231
Pulsatile tinnitus, 57
Pulsations, precordial, 170
Pulse
  arterial, 164-168
  Corrigan's water-hammer, and aortic regurgitation, 192
  femoral, decreased or absent, causes of, 234
  questions related to, 26
  venous, jugular, 159-164
Pulse deficit, 166

Pulse rate, arterial, 166
Pulse rhythms, arterial, 166-167
Pulse tracing, atrial, 155
Pulse volume, arterial, 167-168
Pulsus bigeminus, 167
Pulsus bisferiens, 168
Pulsus paradoxus, 168
Pulsus parvus et tardus, 188
Pupil(s), 47-48
Pupillary reaction to light, testing, 47
Pupillary response, 494
  consensual, 408
Purpura, 447, 463-464
  rash of, 465
  Schöenlein-Henoch, causing abdominal pain, 249
Purpura simplex, 463
Pustular diseases, 457
Pustule, 445
  in child, 487
Pyelonephritis
  causing abdominal pain, 247
  causing acute abdominal pain, 258
  causing nausea and vomiting, 207
  referred pain from, 203
  in urinary tract infection, 289
Pyloric obstruction, peptic ulcer disease with, 204
Pyloric outlet obstruction, 228
  disorders causing, 206
  increased bowel sounds with, 227
Pyloric stenosis, idiopathic hypertrophic, causing chronic gastric retention and delayed gastric emptying, 206
Pyramidal tract disease, abnormal reflexes associated with, 408-410
Pyrophosphate arthropathy, 378-379

Q

Q fever, 121
Quadrant hemianopsia, 52
Quadrantanopsia, 52
Questioning, techniques of, 8-10
Questions, 20
  answers to, assessment of, in psychiatric interview, 427
Quickening, 290
Quincke's pulse, 167-168
  and aortic regurgitation, 192

R

Radial artery, palpation of, 164-165
Radiation syndrome, acute, 509
Radiotherapy
  causing glossitis, 65
  causing oral ulcers, 62
Rales, causes of, 109
Ramsay Hunt syndrome, 511
Range of motion, 352-356
Rape, 294-295
Rapport in interview, establishing, 6-8
Rash(es), 447-448
  in child, 486
  drug, 465
"Raspberry" tongue, 65

Rat-bite fever, 463-464
Raynaud's disease
  and cardiovascular system abnormalities, 150
  causing dysphagia, 209
Raynaud's phenomenon, 460
  causing cyanosis, 148
  extremity signs associated with, 153
Reactive airway disease causing wheezing, 87
Rebound tenderness of abdomen, 236
Receptive aphasia, 417
Recording of information, format for, 31-37
Rectocele, 298, 302
Rectosigmoid operations causing male impotence, 270
Rectovaginal examination, 309
Rectum, 234-235, 278
Rectus abdominis nerve entrapment syndrome causing abdominal wall pain, 256
Rectus muscles, diastasis of, 491
Recurrent epistaxis, 60
Red reflex, 52
Reducible hernia, 223
Referred pain, 336
Reflexes, 404-410; *see also* specific reflex
  of child, 494
  digital, 507
  format for recording data for, 37
  red, 52
  vasomotor, impaired, causing syncope, 146
Reflux esophagitis
  causing chest pain, 129
  causing dysphagia, 209
Reflux
  esophageal, causing chest pain, 135
  gastroesophageal, pain associated with, 200, 202
  hepatojugular, 161
Regional enteritis, 254
  causing chronic gastric retention and delayed gastric emptying, 206
  causing hematochezia, 216
  causing pyloric outlet obstruction, 228
  causing recurrent aphthous ulcers, 63
Regression, patient demonstration of, 15
Regurgitant murmurs, 189, 515
Reiter's syndrome, 334, 367, 378-379, 512
  causing arthritis, 340-341
  causing balanitis, 272
  and cardiovascular system abnormalities, 151
  heel spurs in, 375
  iritis associated with, 151
  causing oral ulcers, 62
  causing sacroiliac arthritis, 369
  skin lesions associated with, 456
Renal artery stenosis causing bruits, 229
Renal colic, pain from, 202, 203
Renal failure
  chronic, causing retinal exudates, 54

Renal failure—cont'd
  causing epistaxis, 60
  causing hyperpnea, 80
Rendu-Osler-Weber syndrome, 512
  mouth signs associated with, 151
Reserpine causing male impotence, 270
Resonance, 106-107
Respiration
  Cheyne-Stokes, 100
  Kussmaul, 99, 100, 141
  questions related to, 26
Respiratory depression, drug-induced, causing bradypnea, 99
Respiratory disease, chronic, causing clubbing of fingernails, 96
Respiratory distress, 102
Respiratory expansion, 104
Respiratory infections, upper; *see* Upper respiratory infections
Respiratory rate, 97
Respiratory system, 70-124
Respiratory tract, upper, symptoms involving, 90
Responses of clinician and message conveyed to patient, 20
Restless legs syndrome, 512
Reticulated lesions, 452
Reticulated pattern on skin, 451
Retina
  changes in, in hypertension and atherosclerosis, comparison of, 158
  hemorrhages of, 54
  lesions of, causing complete monocular blindness, 51
Retinal artery(ies), 53
  central, occlusion of, causing loss of vision, 41
  occlusion of, 55
Retinal detachment, 40
Retinal emboli and cardiovascular system abnormalities, 151
Retinal exudates, 54
Retinal tear causing loss of vision, 40
Retinal veins, 53
  occlusion of, 55
  thrombosis of, causing retinal hemorrhages, 54
Retinitis pigmentosa and cardiovascular system abnormalities, 150
Retinoblastoma causing optic nerve compression, 41
Retinopathy, diabetic, 54
  proliferative, 41
Retraction, nipple, 323-324
Retrobulbar neuritis, 388
Retrobulbar optic neuritis, causing loss of vision, 41
Retropharyngeal abscess, 66
  causing croup syndrome, 115
Retrosternal chest pain, 79
Review of systems, 13
  format for recording, 31-32
Reye's syndrome, 512
Rhabdomyolysis causing ecchymoses, 223

Rheumatic fever, 334, 335, 378-379
  causing arthritis, 340
  erythema and, 350
  heart murmur associated with, 194
  causing joint pain, 336
  revised Jones criteria for, 341-342
  skin signs associated with, 152
Rheumatic valvular disease, eye signs associated with, 151
Rheumatoid arthritis, 334, 339, 378-379, 460
  and cardiovascular system abnormalities, 150
  depression with, 345
  diagnostic criteria for, 342
  fatigue with, 345
  finger deformities in, 349
  iritis associated with, 151
  causing joint pain, 336, 337
  juvenile, 334
  in multiple joints, 340
  causing scleritis, 46
  signs of, 348
  causing sternoclavicular joint swelling, 104
  symptoms of, 343
  causing TMJ abnormalities, 356
  causing uveitis, 41
Rheumatoid nodules, 349
Rhinitis
  allergic, 60, 61
  seasonal, causing excessive lacrimation, 44
  vasomotor, causing rhinorrhea, 60
Rhinophyma, 62, 457
Rhinorrhea, 60, 90
Rhinoviruses causing colds, 90
Rhonchus(i), causes of, 109
Rib fractures
  cough-induced, 73
  causing flail chest, 102
  causing hemoptysis, 77
Riboflavin deficiency causing glossitis, 65
Richter's hernia, 223, 224
Rickets, 102, 486
Riedel's lobe of liver, 230
Riedel's struma causing thyroid enlargement, 67
Rifampin causing hematuria, 265
Right-to-left shunts, extremity signs associated with, 153
Riley-Day syndrome, 512
Ringworm, 461
Rinne test of hearing, 59
Rocky Mountain spotted fever, 466
  skin lesions associated with, 455, 463, 464
Rodent ulcers, 471
Roger's murmur, 515
Romberg's sign, 508
  positive, 404
Root reflex, 494
Rosacea, 457
Rotation, external and internal, 346
Rotator cuff, 359, 360, 361
Roth's spots, 54

Roth's spots—cont'd
  associated with infective endocarditis, 151
Rovsing's sign, 508
Rubella, 464, 465
  causing arthralgia, 337
  infection of fetus, cataracts associated with, 151
Rubeola, 464, 465
Rumination, 208
Ruptured ectopic pregnancy causing acute abdominal pain, 257

S
S_1, 177
S_2, 177-178
S_3, 178-179
S_4, 179
S_4 shock, 170
Sacroiliac arthritis, diseases causing, 369
Sacroiliitis, 367
Saddle nose, 62
Salicylates causing bleeding gums, 63
Salivary glands, physical examination of, 65-66
Salivation, changes in, causes of, 65-66
Salt craving, 63
Sarcasm by patient, 14
Sarcoidosis, 334
  and cardiovascular system abnormalities, 150
  causing choroidal tubercles, 96
  causing erythema nodosum, 96
  iritis associated with, 151
  causing perforated nasal septum, 60
  causing splenomegaly, 232
  causing supraclavicular lymph nodes, 96
  causing uveitis, 41
Sarcoiliac joint, examination of, 366-367
Sarcoma, Kaposi's, 472
Satellite papules, 462
Scabies, itching associated with, 449
Scabs, 446
Scalded skin syndrome, 512
Scales, 446
  collarette, 468
  diseases manifesting, 456
Scalp, seborrhea of, 468
Scanning speech, 403
Scar(s), 446
  causing abdominal wall pain, 256
  corneal, 46
Scarlet fever
  color changes of tongue caused by, 65
  mouth signs associated with, 151
  skin lesions associated with, 456
Schamberg's disease, purpura associated with, 463
Schatzki ring causing dysphagia, 209
Schistosomiasis, itching associated with, 449
Schizophrenia, 416
Schizophrenic disorders, 435-437
Schöenlein-Henoch purpura causing abdominal pain, 249

Sciatic neuritis, 368
Sciatica, 368
  Lasègue's sign diagnosing, 369
Sclera, 46
  blue-colored, associated with osteogenesis imperfecta, 151
Scleritis, 46
  causing eye pain, 44
Scleroderma, 460-461
  causing arthritis, 340
  and cardiovascular system abnormalities, 150
  causing chronic gastric retention and delayed gastric emptying, 206
  causing dysphagia, 209
  causing protuberant abdomen, 220
Scleromalacia perforans, 46
Sclerosing cholangitis
  Kayser-Fleischer rings in, 47
  primary, causing jaundice, 244
Sclerosis
  lateral, amyotrophic
    causing dysphagia, 209
    fasciculations caused by, 395
  multiple; see Multiple sclerosis
  systemic, 460
    causing chronic gastric retention and delayed gastric emptying, 206
Scoliosis, 101, 346, 366, 367, 368
  and cardiovascular system abnormalities, 149
  and congenital cyanotic heart disease, 152
  and tetralogy of Fallot, 149
Scotomata, 43, 44
Scrotum, 274-275
  swelling of, 269, 271
Scybalous stools, 213
Seasonal rhinitis causing excessive lacrimation, 44
Seborrhea, 453
  scalp, 468
Seborrheic dermatitis, 467, 468
Second heart sound, 177-178
Second-wind phenomenon, 130
Seductive behavior of patient, 14
Seizures, 387
Seminiferous tubules, obstruction of, causing male infertility, 271
Sensation, testing, modalities of, 396
Sensorineural hearing loss, 56
Sensory ataxia, 403
Sensory examination, 396-400
Sensory extinction, 400
Sensory neuropathy, common causes of, 419
Sepsis
  bacterial
    dermal manifestations of, 478
    skin lesions associated with, 455, 456
  causing nausea and vomiting, 207
Septal defect
  atrial
    holosystolic murmurs associated with, 191

Septal defect—cont'd
  atrial—cont'd
    jugular venous waves in, 163
  ventricular
    causing dyspnea, 141
    holosystolic murmurs associated with, 190
Septal disease, extremity signs associated with, 153
Septic abortion, 291
Septic arthritis, 343, 348
  causing sternoclavicular joint swelling, 104
Septic joint
  causing arthritis, 339
  erythema and, 350
  causing joint pain, 336
Septicemia
  gram-negative, causing hyperventilation, 99
  mouth signs associated with, 151
Septum, nasal, examination of, 60-61
Serous otitis media, 56
Serpiginous lesions, 452
Sexual function, abnormalities in, in female, 292-294
Sexual history, 269
Sexual orientation, patients with differences in, medical interview of, 19
Sexual practices, 390-391
Sheehan's syndrome, 512
  causing amenorrhea, 284-285
  causing galactorrhea, 324
Shingles, pain of, 79; see also Herpes zoster
Shock(s)
  causing cyanosis, 148
  precordial, 170
Shortness of breath; see Dyspnea
Shoulder, 357-361
  range of motion of, 353
Shoulder-hand syndrome, 512
Shunting, arteriovenous, causing clubbing of fingernails, 96
Shunts, right-to-left, extremity signs associated with, 153
Sick sinus syndrome, 512
Sickle cell anemia crisis causing abdominal pain, 247
Sickle cell disease causing retinal vein occlusion, 55
SIDS; see Sudden infant death syndrome
Sight, complaints concerning, history of, 39-42
Signs, 3, 506-508; see also specific sign
Silence by patient, 14
Silent asthma, 80
"Silent" myocardial infarction, 133
Singultus, 88
Sinus(es), 61
  cavernous, thrombosis of, causing eye pain, 43
Sinus arrhythmia, 166, 167
Sinus tracts of chest, 104

Sinusitis
    acute, causing nasal discharge, 60
    chronic, 60, 61
    causing eye pain, 43
    causing halitosis, 93
    causing serous otitis media, 56
Sister Joseph nodule, 234
Sjögren's syndrome, 46, 65-66, 512
Skene's glands, 301
Skin, 442-479
    abnormalities of, in AIDS, 477, 478
    bacterial infections of, 477
    biology of, 450
    and cardiovascular system abnormalities, 152
    changes in, in breast, 327
    color of, changes in, 448
    diseases of, cardinal symptoms of, 447-449
    lesions of, 447-448
        in child, 486-487
        symptoms of, 443
    primary lesions of, descriptive terms for, 444-446
    secondary lesions of, descriptive terms for, 446-447
    ulcers of, 448
    viral infections of, 475-477
Skull fracture causing nasal discharge, 60
Sleep apnea, 100
    fatigue with, 345
Sleep pattern, changes in, 390
Small bowel, referred pain from, 201, 203
Smallpox, 455, 473
Smoke, inhalation of, 73, 77
Smoker's cough, 73
Smoking, 70
Snapping of joints, 351
Snellen eye chart, 55
Snout reflex, 410
Social history, 13
    format for recording, 31
Soft palate, petechiae of, and cardiovascular system abnormalities, 151
Soles, lesions involving, 454
Solvent, ingestion of, causing breathing difficulty in infant, 92
Somatization disorder, 434-435
Sore throat, 63
Souffle, mammary, 191
Spasm, esophageal
    causing chest pain, 129, 135
    causing dysphagia, 209
Spasmodic croup, acute, history and physical findings in, 114; see also Croup
Spasticity, 395
Speak, patients unable to, medical interview of, 17
Speculum examination, vaginal, 303-306
Speculums, vaginal, 303
Speech
    assessment of, in psychiatric interview, 427

Speech—cont'd
    changes in, 388
    problems with, assessment of, 417
    scanning, 403
    testing, 403
Sperm, defective or nonmotile, 269
Spermatic cord, 269
    torsion of, causing scrotal swelling, 271
Spermatocele, 269
Spermatogenesis, defective, causing male infertility, 271
Sphygmomanometer for blood pressure measurement, 154
Spider angiomas, 448
Spigelian hernia, 223, 224
Spinal cord
    diseases of, causing male impotence, 270
    injury to
        absent bowel sounds with, 227
        causing syncope, 146
Spine, 366-368
    cervical, 357
Spironolactone
    causing gynecomastia, 331-332
    causing male impotence, 270
Spleen
    bruits over, causes of, 228
    infarct of, pain from, location of, 202
    injury to, causing pleuritic chest pain, 91
    palpation of, 231-232
    percussion of, 225-226
    referred pain from, 203
    rupture or infarction of, causing acute abdominal pain, 258-259
Splenic artery, aneurysm of, abdominal masses with, 233
Splenomegaly, causes of, 232
Splinter hemorrhages, 454
    under nails and cardiovascular system abnormalities, 153
Splitting of S_2, 178, 181
Spondylitis
    ankylosing; see Ankylosing spondilitis
    psoriatic, causing sacroiliac arthritis, 369
Spontaneous abortion, 291
    causing pelvic pain, 288
Sprain, ankle, 375
Spur, heel, 375, 376
Sputum, 74-75
    blood-streaked; see Hemoptysis
Squamous cell carcinoma, 471
Stable (typical) angina causing chest pain, 127, 130-131
Staphylococcal scalded skin syndrome, 474
Starr-Edwards heart valve, sounds associated with, 182
Station, 403-404
Stein-Leventhal syndrome, 512
    causing hypertrichosis, 298
Stellwag's sign, 508

Stenosis
    aortic; see Aortic stenosis
    carotid artery, 417
    coronary ostial, eye signs associated with, 151
    heart sounds associated with, 172
    idiopathic hypertrophic subaortic
        arterial pulse volume in, 168
        causing dyspnea, 141
    internal carotid artery, 388
    mitral; see Mitral stenosis
    pulmonary, eye signs associated with, 151
    pulmonic; see Pulmonic stenosis
    tricuspid, jugular venous waves in, 162, 163
Stereognosis, 400
Sterility, 269
Sternoclavicular joint, swelling of, causes of, 104
Stethoscope
    for examination of heart and great vessels, 171-173
    use of, in auscultation of chest, 107-108
Stevens-Johnson syndrome, 475, 512
    causing oral ulcers, 62
"Stiff pipes," 156
Stiffness, joint, 343-345
Still's murmur, 515
Stokes-Adams attack, 143
Stokes-Adams syndrome, 145
Stomach
    Campylobacter pylori colonization of, causing halitosis, 93
    carcinoma of, causing chronic gastric retention and delayed gastric emptying, 206
    chronic retention of contents of, disorders causing, 206-207
    delayed emptying of
        causing chronic abdominal pain, 250-252
        disorders causing, 206-207
    referred pain from, 201
    tumors of
        cyst, or pseudocyst of, aortic pulsation with, 233
        causing pyloric outlet obstruction, 228
    ulcer disease of, causing hematemesis, 214
    varices of, causing hematemesis, 214
Stomatitis, 63
Stools, maroon-colored, causes of, 217
Strabismus, 488
    nonparalytic, 48
Straight back syndrome, 102, 367, 512-513
    and cardiovascular system abnormalities, 152
    systolic murmurs associated with, 191
Strain, lumbosacral, 367-368
Strangulated bowel causing ecchymoses, 223

"Strawberry" tongue, 65
Strength, muscle, 351-352, 391-394
Streptococcal pharyngitis, 66
    mouth signs associated with, 151
    causing sore throat, 63
Streptococcus pneumoniae, 121, 122
Stress causing amenorrhea, 284
Stretch marks on breasts, 328
Striae
    abdominal, 219
    breast, 328
    Wickham's, 469
Striae gravidarum, 290
Stricture, esophageal, causing dysphagia, 209
Stridor, 489
    and wheezing, 80, 87-88
Struma, Riedel's, causing thyroid enlargement, 67
Stye, 44, 45
Subarachnoid hemorrhage
    associated with headache, 384
    causing papilledema, 54
Subconjunctival hemorrhage, 45
Subcutaneous emphysema, 104
Subcutaneous nodules, rheumatic fever associated with, 152
Subjective vertigo, 57
Sublingual glands, physical examination of, 65
Subphrenic abscess, 79, 91
Succussion splash, auscultation for, 228
Suck reflex, 410
Sucking reflex, 494
Sudden infant death syndrome, 513
    sibling with, 92
Sudden loss of vision, causes of, 39-41
Suicidal ideas, 428
Sulfasalazine causing anorexia, 205
Sulfhemoglobinemia
    causing cyanosis, 148
    resembling cyanosis, 90
Summation gallop, 179
Superficial reflexes, 408, 410
Superior vena cava obstruction
    causing chemosis, 96
    jugular venous waves in, 163
Superior vena cava syndrome, 161, 513
Supernumerary nipples, milk line and, 322-323
Supination, 346
Suppurative otitis media, 56
    chronic, causing hearing loss in child, 57
Suppurative parotitis, 65
Supraclavicular lymph nodes, causes of, 96
Suprapatellar reflex, 407
Surgery
    chest or heart, causing free air in mediastinum, 111
    thyroid or parathyroid, causing hoarseness, 64
Sustained murmur, 185
Sutures, assessment of, 487-488

Swan neck deformity, 349, 366
Sweats, night, 92
Swelling
    joint, 348-349
    periarticular, 349
    scrotal, 269, 271
Swimmer's ear causing external otitis, 56
Swimmer's itch, 449
Sympathetic nerves, cervical, 48
Sympathomimetic drugs causing mydriasis, 48
Symptoms, 3
Syncope, 385-387
    carotid sinus, 146
    cough, 73
    and heart disease, 143-146
Syndromes, 3, 509-513; *see also* specific syndrome
Synovial thickening, 348
Syphilis, 466
    Argyll Robertson pupil caused by, 48
    and cardiovascular system abnormalities, 151
    congenital, eye signs of, 46
    eye signs associated with, 151
    causing genital ulcers, 311
    causing oral ulcers, 62
    causing penile ulcers, 266, 272
    causing perforated nasal septum, 60
    rash of, 464
    secondary, 467
        clues to, 453
        skin lesions associated with, 455
    causing supraclavicular lymph nodes, 96
Syringomyelia, 400
Systemic bacterial infections, dermal manifestations of, 477, 478
Systemic diseases, purpura associated with, 463
Systemic hypertension
    causing dyspnea, 138
    ocular changes caused by, 55
Systemic lupus erythematosus; *see* Lupus erythematosus, systemic
Systemic sclerosis, 460
    causing chronic gastric retention and delayed gastric emptying, 206
Systems, review of, 13
    format for recording, 31-32
Systolic dysfunction, 130
Systolic ejection murmurs, 183
Systolic ejection sounds, 180
Systolic heart murmurs, 186-191
Systolic murmur, late, 514
Systolic sounds and clicks, 180-181

T

Tabes dorsalis
    Argyll Robertson pupil caused by, 48
    causing male impotence, 270
    causing optic atrophy, 52
    causing syncope, 146
Tachycardia, 166
    atrial, paroxysmal, 142

Tachypnea, 99, 100
Tactile fremitus, 105-106
Takayasu's arteritis causing perforated nasal septum, 60
Takayasu's disease, pulses associated with, 169
Takayasu's syndrome, 513
Target lesions, 447
Taste, abnormal sensation of, 63
Tear(s)
    retinal, causing loss of vision, 40
    rotator cuff, 359, 360, 361
Teeth
    infected, ear pain caused by, 56
    physical examination of, 64-65
    questions related to, 27
Telangiectases, 447
    periungual, 454
Telangiectasia, 448
    on buccal mucosa, 65
    hemorrhagic, hereditary
        causing epistaxis, 60
        mouth signs associated with, 151
    of lip, 64
Telangiectatic lesions, 452
Temperature, questions related to, 26
Temperature sensation, testing, 400
Temporal arteritis
    headache associated with, 384
    causing central retinal artery occlusion, 41
    causing retinal artery occlusion, 55
Temporomandibular joint, 356, 357
    problems with, ear pain caused by, 56
Tenderness
    abdominal, 236-237
    breast, 320, 322
    joint, 350
Tendinitis, 336-337, 359, 360
    calcific, causing arthritis, 339
    plantar, 375
    trochanteric, 301
Tendon reflexes, deep, 404-407
Tennis elbow, 361
Tenosynovitis, 466
    DeQuervain's, 362, 363
    pain of, 336
Tension headache, 384
Tension pneumothorax, 105
Terry's nails, 452, 454
Tests (testing)
    of cerebellar function and coordination, 400-404
    finger-to-finger, 401-402
    finger-to-nose, 401-402
    of gait and station, 403-404
    heel-to-shin, 402
    of light touch sensation, 398-399
    for pain, 396
    Phalen's, 364
    of position sense, 399
    of reflexes, 404-410
    of speech, 403
    of temperature sensation, 400
    Trendelenburg, 370

Tests (testing)—cont'd
  of two-point discrimination, 400
  of vibration sense, 399, 400
Testes, 269, 274-275
Testicle
  mass in, inguinal pain and, 272
  pain in, 269, 271
  palpation of, 274, 275
Testicular failure of, causing male impotence, 270
Testicular feminization syndrome, 513
  causing amenorrhea, 284
Testosterone, 271
Tetanus causing dysphagia, 209
Tetany, 395
Tetralogy of Fallot
  causing cyanosis, 148, 149
  causing dyspnea, 138, 141
  jugular venous waves in, 162
  scoliosis associated with, 149
  causing syncope, 146
Thermography, breast, 331
Thiazide diuretics causing male impotence, 270
Thioridazine causing male impotence, 270
Third heart sound, 178-179
Third nerve palsies, 50
Thoracic kyphosis, 367, 368
Thoracic outlet syndrome causing chest pain, 129
Thorax and cardiovascular system abnormalities, 152
Thorn's syndrome, 513
Thought, content of, assessment of, in psychiatric interview, 428
Thought processes, assessment of, 416
Three-pillow orthopnea, 139
Thrills, 171
Throat
  and mouth, 62-67
  necrotic lesions of, causing halitosis, 93
Thrombocytopenia causing hemoptysis, 78
Thromboembolism, pulmonary, causing hemoptysis, 77
Thrombophlebitis, superficial, causing dimpling of breast, 322
Thrombosis
  cavernous sinus, 43, 46
  cerebral, middle, 417
  cerebral artery, causing homonymous hemianopsia, 52
  of common iliac artery causing decreased or absent femoral pulses, 234
  of inferior vena cava or pelvic veins causing scrotal swelling, 271
  mesenteric, absent bowel sounds with, 227
  retinal vein, causing retinal hemorrhages, 54
Thrush
  oral, 462

Thrush—cont'd
  of tongue, 489
Thumb, range of motion of, 354
Thyroid carcinoma causing thyroid enlargement, 67
Thyroid gland, 67
Thyroid surgery causing hoarseness, 64
Thyroiditis causing thyroid enlargement, 67
Thyromegaly, nontoxic, causing thyroid enlargement, 67
Thyrotoxicosis
  arterial pulse volume in, 167
  causing dysphagia, 209
Tibial pulse, posterior, palpation of, 165
Tics, 395
Tietze's syndrome, 79, 104, 513
  causing chest pain, 129, 136
Tinea, 461
  skin lesions associated with, 456
Tinea barbae, 461
Tinea capitis, 461-462
Tinea corporis, 451, 461
Tinea cruris, 461
Tinea pedis, 461
Tinea unguium, 461, 461
Tinea versicolor, 462
Tinel's sign, 364
Tinnitus, 57, 388
Titubation, 404
Toe walking, 493
Toes of child, clubbing of, 493
Tongue
  of child, examination of, 489
  physical examination of, 65
  ulcers and sores of, 62-63
Tonsillitis
  recurrent, causing sore throat, 63
  causing serous otitis media, 56
Tophi
  of auricle, 58
  gouty, 349
Torsion
  of ovary causing pelvic pain, 288
  of spermatic cord causing scrotal swelling, 271
Torticollis, 490
Total parenteral nutrition causing anorexia, 205
Totalis lesions, 452
Touch, light, assessment of, 398-399
Toxic delirium, 416
Toxic epidermal necrolysis, 465, 474
Toxic erythema, rash of, 465
Toxic shock syndrome, 456, 513
Trachea
  deviation of, 104-105
  foreign body in, causing cough, 73
  palpation of, 104
Tracheal breath sounds, 108
Tracheal deviation, thyroid enlargement causing, 67
Tracheal tug, 104
Tracheitis, 90, 117
  causing chest pain, 79

Tracheitis—cont'd
  causing cough, 73
Traction, response to, as reflex, 494
Traction diverticulum causing dysphagia, 209
Tranquilizers causing male impotence, 270
Transient arterial occlusion to enhance cardiac auscultation, 196
Transient epistaxis, 60
Transient ischemic attacks, 418
  causing weakness, 388-389
Translation, need for, during medical interview, 17
Traumatic arthritis, 343, 348
Traumatic rupture causing protuberant abdomen, 220
Tremors, 395-396
  intention, 401-402
Trench mouth, 65
Trendelenburg test, 370
Triad asthma causing nasal polyps, 61
Triceps muscle, assessment of strength of, 393
Triceps reflex, 404, 406
Trichomonal vaginitis, 295, 296, 310
Trichomonas infection causing balanitis, 272
Trichomonas vaginalis causing urethritis, 266
Tricuspid insufficiency
  jugular venous waves in, 162, 163, 164
  liver pulsations associated with, 153
Tricuspid regurgitation
  holosystolic murmurs associated with, 190-191
  causing pulsatile liver, 231
  systolic murmurs associated with, 187
Tricuspid stenosis
  heart murmurs associated with, 184
  jugular venous waves in, 162, 163
  middiastolic murmurs associated with, 193
Tricuspid valve, narrowing of, jugular venous waves in, 162
Tricyclic antidepressants causing protuberant abdomen, 220
Trigeminal nerve, testing of, 411
Trigeminal neuralgia causing external otitis, 56
Trigonitis in urinary tract infection, 289
Trochanteric bursitis, 370
Trochlear nerve, testing of, 411
Trophoblastic neoplasia, gestational, 291
Trousseau's phenomenon, 395
Trousseau's sign, 508
Tubal pregnancy, 286, 288
Tubercular arthritis in single joint, 339
Tuberculoma, MRI of, 420
Tuberculosis, 71, 121
  causing anorexia, 205
  causing chest pain, 79
  disseminated, causing choroidal tubercles, 96

Tuberculosis—cont'd
  causing erythema nodosum, 96
  causing hemoptysis, 76
  history of, 90, 91
  causing male infertility, 271
  causing night sweats, 92
  causing oral ulcers, 62
  causing perforated nasal septum, 60
  renal, causing hematuria, 266
  causing sputum production, 74
  causing supraclavicular lymph nodes, 96
  causing uveitis, 41
  vertebral, causing gibbus, 102
  vocal cord, causing hoarseness, 64
Tubo-ovarian abscess, rectal mass associated with, 235
Tumor(s), 469-472
  causing atelectasis, 105
  bone
    causing joint pain, 336
    metastatic, and cough-induced rib fracture, 73
  brain; see Brain tumor
  chromophobe, causing galactorrhea, 324
  causing delayed chest movement, 102
  causing dysphagia, 209
  glomus, causing tinnitus, 57
  intracranial, causing nausea and vomiting, 207
  intrathoracic, causing dysphagia, 209
  of liver causing liver enlargement, 231
  orbital, causing exophthalmos, 46
  pituitary, causing bitemporal hemianopsia, 51
  of pleura causing pleural friction rub, 109
  causing pyloric outlet obstruction, 228
  cerebellopontine angle, causing hearing loss, 57
  fibroid, 311-312
  gastric, aortic pulsation with, 233
  intraabdominal, striae from, 219
  mediastinal, causing hoarseness, 64
  pancreatic, aortic pulsation with, 233
  parotid, causing parotid enlargement, 65
Turbinates, nasal, examination of, 60-61
Turner's syndrome, 513
  causing amenorrhea, 283-284
  and cardiovascular system abnormalities, 149-150
  characteristics of, 486
Two-pillow orthopnea, 139
Two-point discrimination, testing, 400
Tympanic membrane, examination of, 58, 59
Tympany, 106-107
Typhus causing arthralgia, 337
Typical angina causing chest pain, 127, 130-131

U

Ulcer(ation), 446

Ulcer(ation)—cont'd
  aphthous, recurrent, 62, 63
  of buccal mucosa, 65
  corneal, 46
    causing eye pain, 44
  foot, 375
  genital, causes of, 311
  of lip, 64
  of nipples, 324
  oral, 62-63
  penile, 266, 268
  peptic; see Peptic ulcer
  rodent, 471
  skin, 448
  of tongue, 65
  vaginal, 286
Ulcerative colitis
  causing hematochezia, 216
  causing recurrent aphthous ulcers, 63
  causing sacroiliac arthritis, 369
  causing uveitis, 41
Ulnar deviation, 365, 366
Ultrasonography of breasts, 331
Ulysses syndrome, 513
Umbilical hernia, 223, 224, 491
Umbilicus, bruits over, causes of, 228
Unconjugated hyperbilirubinemia, chronic idiopathic, causing jaundice, 244
Unipolar depression, 428, 429
Unstable angina causing chest pain, 127, 131-132
Upper abdominal reflexes, 408
Upper limb, range of motion of, 353-354
Upper respiratory infections
  causing excessive lacrimation, 44
  causing hypogeusia, 63
  causing rhinorrhea, 60
  causing serous otitis media, 56
  causing sore throat, 63
  viral, vertigo and, 57
Upper respiratory tract symptoms, 90
Ureaplasma urealyticum causing urethritis, 266
Uremia
  causing Cheyne-Stokes respiration, 100
  frank, absent bowel sounds with, 227
Uremic syndrome, hemolytic, causing abdominal pain, 249
Urethra
  discharge from, in male, 266, 268
  female, 301, 302
  obstruction of, causing dysuria, 263
Urethritis
  causing dysuria, 263
  causing penile pain, 266
  in urinary tract infection, 289
Urethrocele, 298
Urgency, 263
Urinary frequency as sign of pregnancy, 290
Urinary incontinence, 265
Urinary tract infection in female, 289

Urination, frequency of, 263
Urticaria, 448-449, 472-473
  contact, 459
  rash of, 465
Uterus, 284-286, 311-313
  descent of, 302
  infections of, causing pelvic pain, 288-289
  lesions of, rectal mass associated with, 235
  positions of, 308
  prolapse of, 298
Uveitis causing loss of vision, 41

V

v waves, 162, 163, 164
Vagina
  abnormalities of, 310
    causing amenorrhea, 284
  bleeding from, nonmenstrual, 286-287
  discharge from, and itching, 295-298
  infections of, causing pelvic pain, 288-289
  speculum examination of, 303-306
  ulcers of, 286
Vaginal speculums, 303
Vaginismus, 293
Vaginitis
  atrophic, 286-287
  causes of, 310
  in childhood, 296
  and vaginal discharge, 295
Vagotomy causing chronic gastric retention and delayed gastric emptying, 206
Vagus nerve, testing of, 413
Valgus, 346
Valid assurance, 20
Valsalva's maneuver to enhance cardiac auscultation, 195
Valve sounds, prosthetic, 182
Valves, heart, prosthetic, and blood pressure measurement, 156
Valvular disease, rheumatic, eye signs associated with, 151
Valvular heart disease causing dyspnea, 140-141
Valvulitis, skin signs associated with, 152
Variant angina, 132-133
  causing chest pain, 127
Varicella, 455, 473
Varicella zoster, 473
Varicocele, 269, 271
Variola, 473
Varus, 346
Vas deferens, 269
  absence/atresia of, causing male infertility, 271
Vascular disease
  causing male impotence, 270
  peripheral, causing decreased or absent femoral pulses, 234
Vascular system, questions related to, 28

Vasculitis
    and cardiovascular system abnormalities, 150
    purpura associated with, 463
    rash of, 465
    causing retinal artery occlusion, 55
Vasomotor reflexes, impaired, causing syncope, 146
Vasomotor rhinitis causing rhinorrhea, 60
Vasovagal episodes, 144-145
Vasovagal syncope, 146
Veins
    abdominal, dilated, causes of, 219
    dilated, on chest, causes of, 96
    retinal, 53
        occlusion of, 55
Vena cava
    inferior, thrombosis of, causing scrotal swelling, 271
    superior, 161
        obstruction of
            causing chemosis, 96
            jugular venous waves in, 163
Vena cava syndrome
    facial puffiness associated with, 151
    superior, 161
Venereal warts, 476
Venoarterial shunting causing cyanosis, 148
Venous hum, 191
Venous pressure, jugular, 160-162
Venous pulse, jugular, 159-164
Venous waves, jugular, 162-164
Ventricular contractions, premature, 163, 166, 167
Ventricular dysfunction, heart sounds in, 179
Ventricular failure, left, causing hemoptysis, 77
Ventricular hypertrophy
    heaves and lifts associated with, 170
    jugular venous waves in, 162
Ventricular septal defect
    causing dyspnea, 141
    holosystolic murmurs associated with, 190
    thoracic signs associated with, 152
Vertebral column
    deformities of, 101
    disease of, causing chest pain, 129, 136
Vertebral tuberculosis causing gibbus, 102
Vertebral-basilar artery insufficiency, 418
Vertigo, 57-58, 388
Vesicles, 445
    diseases manifesting, 455
    herpes simplex virus, 451, 475
Vesicular breath sounds, 109
Vesicular diseases, 473
Vestibule, 300
Vibration sense, testing, 399, 400
Vincent's angina causing sore throat, 63
Vincent's infection, 65

Viral diseases causing joint pain, 336
Viral exanthems causing serous otitis media, 56
Viral hepatitis
    causing anorexia, 205
    causing dysgeusia, 63
    causing jaundice, 240
Viral illness causing chronic gastric retention and delayed gastric emptying, 207
Viral infections
    causing dysgeusia, 63
    causing eye pain, 44
    causing hoarseness, 64
    causing nausea and vomiting, 207
    of skin, 475-477
    causing splenomegaly, 232
Viral meningitis, differential diagnosis of, 424
Viral pneumonia, 121
Viral upper respiratory infection, vertigo and, 57
Viruses causing epiglottitis, 88
Viscera, perforated, causing protuberant abdomen, 220
Visible peristalsis, 219
Vision, changes in, 387-388
    history of, 39-42
Visual acuity, testing, 55
Visual fields, 50-52
Vital signs
    of pediatric patient, 482
    taking, 29
Vitamin B_{12} deficiency causing glossitis, 65
Vitamin C deficiency causing glossitis, 65
Vitamin deficiency(ies)
    causing dysgeusia, 63
    causing glossitis, 65
Vitiligo, 448
Vitreous hemorrhage causing loss of vision, 41
Vocal cords
    foreign body between, causing wheezing, 87
    lesions of, causing hoarseness, 64
Voiding pattern, changes in, and prostatism, 266
Vomiting
    nausea and, 205-208; see also Nausea and vomiting
    projectile, 208
    as sign of pregnancy, 289-290
von Recklinghausen's disease, 444
    and cardiovascular system abnormalities, 152
Vulva, abnormalities of, 309-310
Vulvovaginitis, 296
    candidal, 462

W

Waardenburg's syndrome, characteristics of, 486
Waddling gait, 370

Walking, automatic, 494
Walk-through angina, 130
Warmth, joint, 350
Warts, 272, 476
Water-hammer pulse, 167
    and aortic regurgitation, 192
Waterhouse-Friderichsen syndrome, 513
Weakness, 386
    muscle, 351-352
    musculoskeletal, 345
    neurologic, 388-389
Webbing of neck of child, 490
Weber's test of hearing, 59
Wegener's granulomatosis
    causing hemoptysis, 77, 78-79
    causing oral ulcers, 62
    causing perforated nasal septum, 60
Weight
    change in, as sign of pregnancy, 290
    loss of, causes of, 206
Weight-reduction amenorrhea, 284
Wernicke's syndrome, 513
Wernicke-Korsakoff syndrome, 416
    causing nystagmus, 49
Wheal, 445, 472
Wheeze, causes of, 109
Wheezing, 80, 87-88
Whispered pectoriloquy, 110
Whiteheads, 457
Whitlow, herpetic, 476
Whooping cough, 73
Why questions, 20
Wickham's striae, 469
Wilson's disease, Kayser-Fleischer rings in, 47
Wilson's syndrome, 513
Winterbottom's sign, 508
Wolff-Parkinson-White syndrome, 513
Wrist, 362-364
    assessment of strength of, 393
    range of motion of, 354

X

x descent, 162, 163
x' descent, 162, 163
Xanthelasma and cardiovascular system abnormalities, 151
Xerostomia in Sjögren's syndrome, 46
Xiphoid process, tender, 104
X-linked disorders, 517

Y

y descent, 162, 163
Yellow nail syndrome, 452, 454, 513
Yellow sclerae, 46

Z

Zenker's diverticulum, 93, 209
Zinc deficiency causing glossitis, 65
Zinc depletion causing dysgeusia, 63
Zollinger-Ellison syndrome, 513
Zoster, 473
    skin lesions associated with, 455
Zoster pneumonia, 96
Zosteriform lesions, 452